OXORN-FOOTE

Human Labor & Birth

FIFTH EDITION

Harry Oxorn, B.A., M.D., C.M., F.R.C.S.(C.)

Professor and Chairman
Department of Obstetrics and Gynecology
University of Ottawa
Obstetrician-Gynecologist-in-Chief
Ottawa Civic Hospital
Ottawa, Canada

Illustrations by Dorothy Irwin

Additional illustrations for the Fifth Edition by Valerie M. Oxorn

APPLETON-CENTURY-CROFTS/Norwalk, Connecticut

Copyright © 1986 by Appleton-Century-Crofts
A Publishing Division of Prentice-Hall, Inc.

86 87 88 89 / 10 9 8 7 6 5 4 3 2 1

Prentice-Hall of Australia, Pty. Ltd., Sydney
Prentice-Hall Canada, Inc.
Prentice-Hall Hispanoamericana, S.A., Mexico
Prentice-Hall of India Private Limited, New Delhi
Prentice-Hall International (UK) Limited, London
Prentice-Hall of Japan, Inc., Tokyo
Prentice-Hall of Southeast Asia (Pte.) Ltd., Singapore
Whitehall Books Ltd., Wellington, New Zealand
Editora Prentice-Hall do Brasil Ltda., Rio de Janeiro

Library of Congress Cataloging-in-Publication Data

Oxorn, Harry, 1920–
    Oxorn-Foote Human labor and birth.

    Rev. ed. of: Human labor and birth / Harry Oxorn.
4th ed. 1980.
    Includes bibliographies and index.
    1. Labor (Obstetrics) 2. Childbirth.
I. Foote, William R. (William Rodgers), 1908–
II. Title. III. Title: Human labor and birth.
[DNLM: 1. Delivery. 2. Labor. WQ 300 098h]
RG651.09 1986   618.4   85-18566
ISBN 0-8385-7665-6

Cover Design: M. Chandler Martylewski
Text Design: Jean M. Sabato-Morley

With contributions by

Mary D'Alton, M.B., B.Ch., F.R.C.S.(C.)
Assistant Professor of Obstetrics and Gynecology
University of Ottawa
Co-Director, High Risk Pregnancy Unit
Ottawa Civic Hospital
Ottawa, Canada

Denis K.L. Dudley, M.B., B.S., F.A.C.O.G., F.R.C.S.(C.)
Assistant Professor of Obstetrics and Gynecology
University of Ottawa
Director, High Risk Pregnancy Unit
Ottawa Civic Hospital
Ottawa, Canada

Peter Garner, M.B., F.R.C.P.(C.)
Assistant Professor of Obstetrics and Gynecology and Medicine
University of Ottawa
Attending Physician, Section of Maternal-Fetal Medicine
Ottawa Civic Hospital
Ottawa, Canada

Michael J. Hardie, M.B., F.R.C.P.(C.)
Assistant Professor of Obstetrics and Gynecology and Pediatrics
University of Ottawa
Chief, Division of Neonatology
Ottawa Civic Hospital
Ottawa, Canada

Henry F. Muggah, M.D., F.R.C.S.(C.)
Assistant Professor of Obstetrics and Gynecology
University of Ottawa
Director, Obstetrical and Gynecological Ultrasonographic Unit
Ottawa Civic Hospital
Ottawa, Canada

Donald C. Oxorn, M.D., C.M., F.R.C.P.(C.)
Lecturer in Anesthesiology
Dalhousie University
Attending Anesthesiologist
Halifax Infirmary
Halifax, Canada

Contents

Preface

A major change in the fifth edition is the introduction of new authors, physicians with special expertise in their fields. Six chapters are affected. Five are revisions of present material (Obstetric Analgesia and Anesthesia, Assessment of the Fetus in Utero, Ultrasonography and Radiography, Preterm Labor, and The Newborn Infant). The sixth (Medical Complications of Pregnancy: Intrapartum Management) was written de novo. In addition, two other new chapters deal with the Amniotic Fluid and the Puerperium. There are thirty new illustrations.

Special thanks are due to my secretary, Mrs. Sonia Lemkow, who typed, corrected errors, and retyped the manuscript again and again.

Pelvis: Bones, Joints, Ligaments

PELVIC BONES

The pelvis is the bony basin in which the trunk terminates and through which the body weight is transmitted to the lower extremities. In the female it is adapted for childbearing. The pelvis consists of four bones: the two innominates, the sacrum, and the coccyx. These are united by four joints.

Innominate Bones

The innominate bones are placed laterally and anteriorly. Each is formed by the fusion of three bones (ilium, ischium, pubis) around the acetabulum.

Ilium
The ilium is the upper bone: It has a body (which is fused with the ischial body) and an ala. Points of note concerning the ilium include:

1. The anterior superior iliac spine gives attachment to the inguinal ligament.
2. The posterior superior iliac spine marks the level of the second sacral vertebra. Its presence is indicated by a dimple in the overlying skin.
3. The iliac crest extends from the anterior superior iliac spine to the posterior superior iliac spine.

Ischium
The ischium consists of a body in which the superior and inferior rami merge.

1. The body forms part of the acetabulum.
2. The superior ramus is behind and below the body.
3. The inferior ramus fuses with the inferior ramus of the pubis.
4. The ischial spine separates the greater sciatic from the lesser sciatic notch. It is an important landmark. Part of the levator ani muscle is attached to it.
5. The ischial tuberosity is the lower part of the ischium and is the bone on which humans sit.

Pubis

The pubis consists of the body and two rami.

1. The body has a rough surface on its medial aspect. This is joined to the corresponding area on the opposite pubis to form the symphysis pubis. The levator ani muscles are attached to the pelvic aspect of the pubis.
2. The pubic crest is the superior border of the body.
3. The pubic tubercle, or spine, is the lateral end of the pubic crest. The inguinal ligament and conjoined tendon are attached here.
4. The superior ramus meets the body of the pubis at the pubic spine and the body of the ilium at the iliopectineal line. Here it forms a part of the acetabulum.
5. The inferior ramus merges with the inferior ramus of the ischium.

Landmarks can be identified:

1. The iliopectineal line extends from the pubic tubercle back to the sacroiliac joint. It forms the greater part of the boundary of the pelvic inlet.
2. The greater sacrosciatic notch is between the posterior inferior iliac spine above and the ischial spine below.
3. The lesser sacrosciatic notch is bounded by the ischial spine superiorly and the ischial tuberosity inferiorly.
4. The obturator foramen is delimited by the acetabulum, the ischial rami, and the pubic rami.

Sacrum

The sacrum is a triangular bone with the base above and the apex below. It consists of five vertebrae fused together; rarely, there are four or six. The sacrum lies between the innominate bones and is attached to them by the sacroiliac joints.

The upper surface of the first sacral vertebra articulates with the lower surface of the fifth lumbar vertebra. The anterior (pelvic) surface of the sacrum is concave, and the posterior surface convex.

The sacral promontory is the anterior superior edge of the first sacral vertebra. It protrudes slightly into the cavity of the pelvis, reducing the anteroposterior diameter of the inlet.

Coccyx

The coccyx (tail bone) is composed of four rudimentary vertebrae. The superior surface of the first coccygeal vertebra articulates with the lower surface of the fifth sacral vertebra to form the sacrococcygeal joint. Rarely, there is fusion between the sacrum and coccyx, with resultant limitation of movement.

The coccygeus muscle, the levator ani muscles, and the sphincter ani externus are attached to the coccyx from above downward.

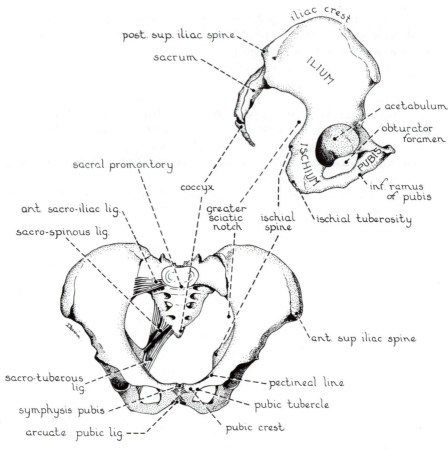

Figure 1. Bones and joints of the pelvis.

PELVIC JOINTS AND LIGAMENTS

The sacrum, coccyx, and two innominate bones are linked by four joints:
(1) the symphysis pubis, (2) the sacrococcygeal, and (3) the two sacroiliac synchondroses (Fig. 1).

Sacroiliac Joint

The sacroiliac joint lies between the articular surfaces of the sacrum
and the ilium. Through it the weight of the body is transmitted to the
pelvis and thence to the lower limbs. It is a synovial joint and permits a
small degree of movement. The capsule is weak, and stability is maintained especially by the muscles around it as well as by four primary
and two accessory ligaments.

Primary Ligaments

1. The anterior sacroiliac ligaments are short and transverse, running from the preauricular sulcus on the ilium to the anterior aspect of the ala of the sacrum.
2. The interosseus sacroiliac ligaments are short, strong transverse bands that extend from the rough part behind the auricular surface on the ilium to the adjoining area on the sacrum.
3. The short posterior sacroiliac ligaments are strong transverse bands that lie behind the interosseus ligaments.
4. The posterior sacroiliac ligaments are each attached to the posterosuperior spine on the ilium and to the tubercles on the third and fourth sacral vertebrae.

Accessory Ligaments

1. The sacrotuberous ligaments are attached on one side to the posterior superior iliac spine; posterior inferior iliac spine; tubercles on the third, fourth, and fifth sacral vertebrae; and lateral border of the coccyx. On the other side the sacrotuberous ligaments are attached to the pelvic aspect of the ischial tuberosity.
2. The sacrospinous ligament is triangular. The base is attached to the lateral parts of the fifth sacral and first coccygeal vertebrae, and the apex is attached to the ischial spine.

Sacrococcygeal Joint

The sacrococcygeal is a synovial hinge joint between the fifth sacral and the first coccygeal vertebrae. It allows both flexion and extension. Extension, by increasing the anteroposterior diameter of the outlet of the pelvis, plays an important role in parturition. Overextension during delivery may break the small cornua by which the coccyx is attached to the sacrum. This joint has a weak capsule, which is reinforced by anterior, posterior, and lateral sacrococcygeal ligaments.

Symphysis Pubis

The symphysis pubis is a cartilaginous joint with no capsule and no synovial membrane. Normally there is little movement. The posterior and superior ligaments are weak. The strong anterior ligaments are reinforced by the tendons of the rectus abdominis and the external oblique muscles. The strong inferior ligament in the pubic arch is known as the arcuate pubic ligament. It extends between the rami and leaves a small space in the subpubic angle.

MOBILITY OF PELVIS

During normal pregnancy, under the influence of progesterone and relaxin, there is increased flexibility of the sacroiliac joints and the symphysis pubis. Hyperemia and softening of the ligaments around the joints takes place also. The pubic bones may separate by 1 to 12 mm. Excessive mobility of the symphysis pubis leads to pain and difficulty in walking. It has been shown that, besides the local changes that may take place in the pelvic ligaments, a generalized change in the laxity of joints occurs in the association with pregnancy.

MALE AND FEMALE PELVIS

At birth there is no difference between the male and female pelvis. Sexual dimorphism does not take place until puberty. A female pelvis develops in offspring born with no gonads. Thus, ovaries and estrogen are not necessary for the formation of the female-type pelvis, but the presence of a testis that is producing androgen is essential for development of the male pelvis.

ADOLESCENCE

The pelvis of the adolescent girl is smaller than that of the mature woman. The pattern of growth of the pelvic basin is different from that of bodily stature. Among girls the growth in stature decelerates rapidly in the first year following menarche,and ceases within 1 or 2 years. The pelvic basin, on the other hand, grows more slowly and more steadily during late adolescence. At the same time it changes from an anthropoid to a gynecoid configuration. Thus, maturation of the reproductive system and attainment of adult size do not indicate that the growth and development of the pelvis are complete. The smaller pelvic capacity in adolescent girls may contribute to the higher incidence of fetopelvic disproportion and other dystocias in primigravidous girls below the age of 15.

BIBLIOGRAPHY

Aiman J: X-ray pelvimetry of the pregnant adolescent. Obstet Gynecol 48:281, 1976

Calguneri M, Bird HI, Wright V: Changes in joint laxity occurring during pregnancy. Ann Rheum Dis 41:126, 1982

Moerman ML: Growth of the birth canal in adolescent girls. Am J Obstet Gynecol 143:528, 1982

2

Floor of the Pelvis

The pelvic floor (Fig. 1) is a muscular diaphragm that separates the pelvic cavity above from the perineal space below. It is formed by the levator ani and coccygeus muscles and is covered completely by parietal fascia.

The urogenital hiatus is an anterior gap through which the urethra and vagina pass. The rectal hiatus is posterior, and the rectum and anal canal pass through it.

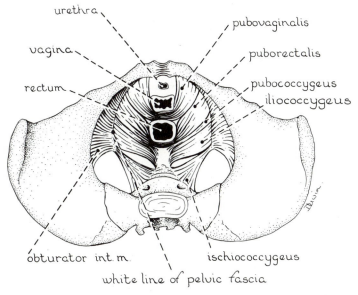

Figure 1. Pelvic floor.

PELVIC FLOOR FUNCTIONS

1. In humans it supports the pelvic viscera.
2. To build up effective intraabdominal pressure, the muscles of the diaphragm, abdominal wall, and pelvic floor must contract together.
3. The pelvic floor helps the anterior rotation of the presenting part and directs it downward and forward along the birth passage.

PELVIC FLOOR MUSCLES

1. Levators ani, each composed of two muscles:
   a. Pubococcygeus, which has three divisions: pubovaginalis, puborectalis, pubococcygeus proper
   b. Iliococcygeus
2. Coccygeus (ischiococcygeus)

Levator Ani Muscle

The levator ani muscle has a lateral origin and a central insertion, where it joins with the corresponding muscle from the other side. The direction of the muscle from origin to insertion is downward and medial. The origin of each levator ani is from the:

1. Posterior side of the pubis
2. Arcuate tendon of the pelvic fascia (the white line of the pelvic fascia)
3. Pelvic aspect of the ischial spine.

The insertion, from front to back, is into:

1. Vaginal walls
2. Central point of the perineum
3. Anal canal
4. Anococcygeal body
5. Lateral border of the coccyx

Pubococcygeus

The pubococcygeus is the most important, most dynamic, and most specialized part of the pelvic floor. It lies in the midline; is perforated by the urethra, vagina, and rectum; and is often damaged during delivery. It originates from the posterior side of the pubis and from the part of the white line of the pelvic fascia in front of the obturator canal. The muscle passes backward and medially in three sections: (1) pubovaginalis, (2) puborectalis and (3) pubococcygeus proper.

Pubovaginalis Muscle. The most medial section of the pubococcygeus, this muscle is shaped like a horseshoe, open anteriorly. The fibers make contact and blend with the muscles of the urethral wall, after which they form a loop around the vagina. They insert into the sides and back of the vagina and into the central point of the perineum.

The principal function of the pubovaginalis is to act as a sling for the vagina. Since the vagina helps to support the uterus and appendages, bladder and urethra, and rectum, this muscle is the main support of the female pelvic organs. Tearing or overstretching predisposes to prolapse, cystocele, and rectocele. The muscle also functions as the vaginal sphincter, and when it goes into spasm the condition is called *vaginismus*.

Puborectalis Muscle. The intermediate part of the pubococcygeus, this muscle forms a loop around the anal canal and rectum. The insertion is into the lateral and posterior walls of the anal canal between the sphincter ani internus and externus, with whose fibers the puborectalis joins. It inserts also in the anococcygeal body.

The puborectalis suspends the rectum, but since this organ does not support the other pelvic viscera, the puborectalis plays a small role in holding up the pelvic structures. The main work of this muscle is in controlling the descent of the feces, and in so doing it acts as an auxiliary sphincter for the anal canal. When the anococcygeal junction is pulled forward, the puborectalis increases the anorectal flexure and retards the descent of feces.

Pubococcygeus Proper. This muscle is composed of the most lateral fibers of the pubococcygeus muscle. It has a Y-shaped insertion into the lateral margins of the coccyx. When it contracts it pulls the coccyx forward, increasing the anorectal juncture. Thus, in combination with the external sphincter ani it helps control the passage of feces.

Iliococcygeus
The iliococcygeus muscles arise from the white line of the pelvic fascia behind the obturator canal. They join with the pubococcygeus muscle proper and insert into the lateral margins of the coccyx. These are less dynamic than the pubovaginalis and act more like a musculofascial layer.

Ischiococcygeus

The ischiococcygeus or coccygeus muscles originate from the ischial spines and insert into the lateral borders of the coccyx and the fifth sacral vertebra. These muscles supplement the levators ani and occupy most of the posterior portion of the pelvic floor.

PELVIC FLOOR DURING PARTURITION

When the presenting part has reached the proper level during the second stage of labor, the central point of the perineum becomes thin. The levator ani muscles and the anal sphincter relax, and the muscles of the pelvic floor are drawn over the advancing head. Tearing and overstretching these muscles weaken the pelvic floor and may cause extensive damage.

Perineum

3

The perineum is a diamond-shaped space that lies below the pelvic floor (Fig. 1). Its boundaries are as follows:

1. Superiorly: the pelvic floor, made up of the levator ani muscles and the coccygei
2. Laterally: the bones and ligaments that make up the pelvic outlet; from front to back, these are the subpubic angle, ischiopubic rami, ischial tuberosities, sacrotuberous ligaments, coccyx
3. Inferiorly: the skin and fascia

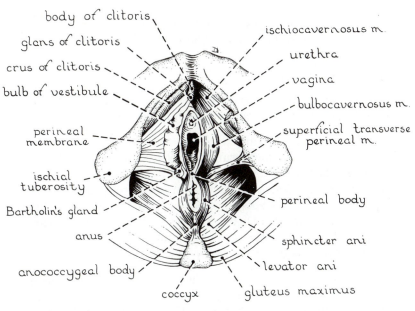

Figure 1. Perineum.

This area is divided into two triangles: anteriorly, the urogenital triangle; posteriorly, the anal triangle. These are separated by a transverse band composed of the transverse perineal muscles and the base of the urogenital diaphragm.

UROGENITAL TRIANGLE

The urogenital triangle is bounded:

1. In front: by the subpubic angle
2. At the sides: by the ischiopubic rami and the ischial tuberosities
3. Behind: by the transverse perineal muscles and the base of the urogenital diaphragm

The urogenital triangle contains:

1. Opening of the vagina
2. Terminal part of the urethra
3. Crura of the clitoris with the ischiocavernosus muscles
4. Vestibular bulbs (erectile tissue) covered by the bulbocavernosus muscles
5. Bartholin glands and their ducts
6. Urogenital diaphragm
7. Muscles that constitute the central point of the perineum (perineal body)
8. Perineal pouches, superficial and deep
9. Blood vessels, nerves, and lymphatics

Urogenital Diaphragm

The urogenital diaphragm (triangular ligament) lies in the anterior triangle of the perineum. It is composed of muscle tissue covered by fascia.

1. The two muscles are the deep transverse perineal and the sphincter of the membranous urethra.
2. The superior layer of fascia is thin and weak.
3. The inferior fascial layer is a strong fibrous membrane. It extends from a short distance beneath the arcuate pubic ligament to the ischial tuberosities. The fascial layers fuse superiorly and form the transverse perineal ligament. Inferiorly, they join in the central point of the perineum.

The deep dorsal vein of the clitoris lies in a small space between the apex of the urogenital diaphragm and the arcuate pubic ligament. Through the diaphragm pass the urethra, the vagina, blood vessels, lymphatics, and nerves.

Superficial Perineal Pouch

The superficial perineal pouch is a space that lies between the inferior layer of the urogenital diaphragm and Colles fascia.

Superficial Transverse Perineal Muscles
The superficial transverse perineal muscles are the superficial parts of the deep muscles and have the same origin and insertion. These are outside the urogenital diaphragm. Sometimes they are entirely lacking.

Ischiocavernosus Muscles
The ischiocavernosus muscles cover the clitoral crura. The origin of each is the inferior ramus of the pubis, and they insert at the lateral aspect of the crus. These muscles compress the crura, and by blocking the venous return cause the clitoris to become erect.

Bulbocavernosus Muscle
The bulbocavernosus muscle surrounds the vagina. With the external anal sphincter it makes a figure eight around the vagina and rectum. It is also called the bulbospongiosus. It originates from the central point of the perineum and inserts into the dorsal aspect of the clitoral body. The muscle passes around the orifice of the vagina and surrounds the bulb of the vestibule.

The bulbocavernosus muscle compresses the erectile tissue around the vaginal orifice (bulb of the vestibule) and helps in the clitoral erection by closing its dorsal vein. It acts as a weak vaginal sphincter. The real sphincter of the vagina is the pubovaginalis section of the levator ani.

Deep Perineal Pouch

The deep perineal pouch lies between the two fascial layers of the urogenital diaphragm.

Sphincter of the Membranous Urethra
The sphincter of the membranous urethra lies between the fascial layers of the urogenital diaphragm. It is also called the compressor of the urethra.

The voluntary fibers have their origin from the inferior rami of the ischium and pubis. They join with the deep transverse perineal muscles. Their action is to expel the last drops of urine.

The involuntary fibers surround the urethra and act as its sphincter.

Deep Transverse Perineal Muscles

The deep transverse perineal muscles lie between the layers of fascia of the urogenital diaphragm. They blend with the sphincter of the membranous urethra. The origin is the ischiopubic ramus on each side, and they insert at the central point of the perineum (perineal body).

ANAL TRIANGLE

The anal triangle is bounded:

1. Anteriorly: by the transverse perineal muscles and the base of the urogenital diaphragm
2. Laterally: by the ischial tuberosities and the sacrotuberous ligaments
3. Posteriorly: by the coccyx

The anal triangle contains the following:

1. Lower end of the anal canal and its sphincters
2. Anococcygeal body
3. Ischiorectal fossa
4. Blood vessels, lymphatics, and nerves

Sphincter Ani Externus

The sphincter ani externus has two parts.

1. The superficial portion surrounds the anal orifice. Its fibers are voluntary and act during defecation or in an emergency. The origin is the tip of the coccyx and the anococcygeal body. Insertion is in the central point of the perineum.
2. The deep part is an involuntary muscle that surrounds the lower part of the anal canal and acts as a sphincter for the anus. It blends with the levators ani and the internal anal sphincter. When inactive, the deep circular fibers are in a state of tonus, occluding the anal orifice.

Anococcygeal Body

The anococcygeal body is composed of muscle tissue (levators ani and external sphincter ani) and fibrous tissue. It is located between the tip of the coccyx and the anus.

PERINEAL BODY

The central point of the perineum or perineal body lies between the posterior angle of the vagina in front and the anus behind. In obstetrics it is referred to as the perineum. It is often torn at delivery. The following muscles meet to form this structure:

1. Sphincter ani externus
2. Two levator ani muscles
3. Superficial and deep transverse perineal muscles
4. Bulbocavernosus muscle

Uterus and Vagina

4

UTERUS

The normal uterus is a small muscular organ in the female pelvis. It is composed of three layers:

1. An outer, covering, serous peritoneal layer—the perimetrium
2. A thick middle layer made up of muscle fibers—the myometrium
3. An inner mucous layer of glands and supporting stroma—the endometrium—which is attached directly to the myometrium

The *myometrium* is made up of three layers of muscle:

1. An outer layer of mainly longitudinal fibers.
2. An inner layer whose fibers run, for the most part, in a circular direction.
3. A thick middle layer, whose fibers are arranged in an interlacing pattern and through which the blood vessels course. when these fibers contract and retract after the products of conception have been expelled, the blood vessels are kinked and constricted. In this way postpartum bleeding is controlled.

Uterine Shape

In the nonpregnant condition and at the time of implantation the uterus is pear-shaped. By the third month of gestation the uterus is globular. From the seventh month to term the contour is again pyriform.

Uterine Size

The uterus grows from the nonpregnant dimensions of about 7.5 × 5.0 × 2.5 cm to 28 × 24 × 21 cm. The weight rises from 30 to 60 g to 1000 g at the end of pregnancy. The uterus changes from a solid organ in the nullipara to a large sac, the capacity increasing from almost nil to 4000 ml.

Uterine Location

Normally the uterus is entirely in the pelvis. As it enlarges it gradually rises, and by the fourth month of gestation it extends into the abdominal region.

Uterine Divisions

1. The fundus (Fig. 1) is the part above the openings of the fallopian tubes.
2. The body (corpus) is the main part; it has thick walls, lies between the tubal openings and the isthmus, and is the main contractile portion. During labor the contractions force the baby downward, distend the lower segment of the uterus, and dilate the cervix.
3. The isthmus is a small constricted region of the uterus. It is about 5 to 7 mm in length and lies above the internal os of the cervix.
4. The cervix (Fig. 2) is composed of a canal with an internal os in its upper portion, separating the cervix from the uterine cavity, and an external os below, which closes off the cervix from the vagina. The cervix is about 2.5 cm in length. The lower part pierces the anterior wall of the vagina, and its tissue blends with that of the vagina.

Myometrium

Most of the uterine growth takes place in the myometrium of the body and fundus. During the first half of pregnancy the main factor in uterine growth is hyperplasia (formation of new muscle fibers). In the second half hypertrophy predominates (enlargement of existing myometrial cells). Individual myometrial fibers increase tenfold during pregnancy from a nonpregnant length of 50 to 100 μ to 500 to 800 μ during pregnancy. At term the estimated number of cells is 200 billion. The myometrial fibers are composed of four major proteins: myosin, actin, tropomysin, and troponin. The main stimulus to growth is provided by 17 β-estradiol, although some myometrial hypertrophy occurs in response to stretch.

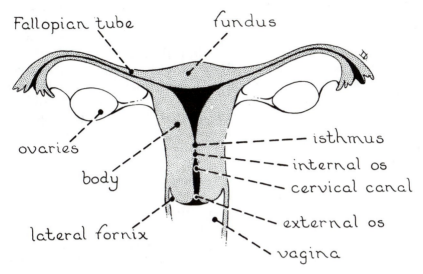

Figure 1. Uterus, cervix, vagina.

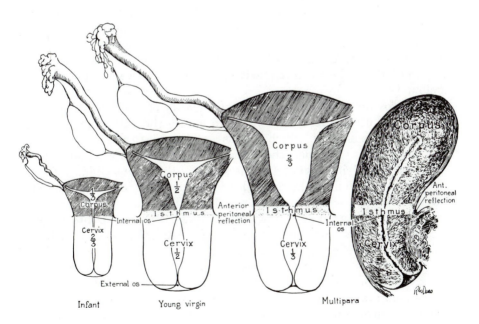

Figure 2. Normal uterus and cervix. (*From Pritchard, MacDonald and Gant. Williams Obstetrics, 17th ed., 1985. Courtesy of Appleton-Century-Crofts.*)

There is also an increase in the number and size of the blood vessels and lymphatics, as well as a marked overgrowth of connective tissue.

During early pregnancy the uterine walls are thicker than in the nonpregnant woman. As gestation continues the lumen becomes larger and the walls thinner. At the end of the fifth month they are 3 to 5 mm thick and remain so until term. Thus, during late pregnancy the uterus is a large muscular sac with thin, soft, easily compressible walls. This makes the corpus indentable and enables the fetus to be palpated. The walls of the uterus are so malleable that the uterus changes shape easily and markedly to accommodate to changes in fetal size and position.

Isthmus

The isthmus lies between the body of the uterus and the cervix. In the human its boundaries are not well defined, and it is important as a physiologic rather than as an anatomic entity. In the nonpregnant uterus it is 5 to 7 mm long. It differs from the corpus in that it is free of mucus-secreting glands. The upper limit of the isthmus corresponds to a constriction in the lumen of the uterus which marks the lower boundary of the body of the uterus (the anatomic internal os of Aschoff). The lower limit is the site of transition from the mucosa of the isthmus to the endocervical mucous membrane (histologic internal os).

While the isthmus is of small moment in the normal state, in pregnancy it plays an important role. As the uterus grows, the isthmus increases in length (Fig. 3) to about 25 mm and becomes soft and compressible. Hegar sign of early pregnancy depends upon palpation of the soft isthmus between the body of the uterus above and the cervix below.

The ovum implants, in the great majority of cases, in the upper part of the uterus. At about the third month the enlarging embryo grows into the isthmus, which unfolds and expands to make room for it. As this process continues, the isthmus is incorporated gradually into the general uterine cavity, and the shape of the uterus changes from pyriform to globular. The expanded isthmus forms part of the lower uterine segment of the uterus during labor. The histologic internal os becomes the internal os of pregnancy, while the anatomic internal os becomes the physiologic retraction ring of normal labor (and pathologic retraction ring of obstructed labor).

The unfolding of the isthmus continues until it has reached the firm cervix, where it stops. After the seventh month most of the enlargement takes place in the body and fundus, and the uterus becomes pear-shaped once more. At the onset of labor the lower uterine segment comprises about one-third of the whole uterus. While this area is not the passive part it was once thought to be, its contractions during normal labor are extremely weak when compared with those of the body.

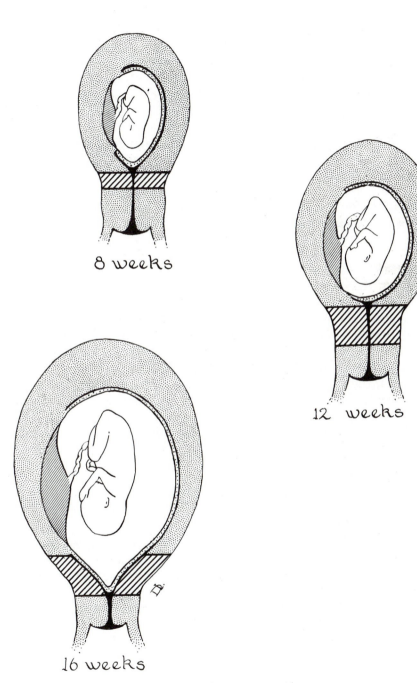

Figure 3. Isthmus of pregnant uterus.

Cervix

The cervix is composed mostly of connective tissue interspersed with muscle fibers. It feels hard and fibrous in the nonpregnant state. During pregnancy the cervix becomes progressively softer. This is caused by increased vascularity, general edema, and hyperplasia of the glands. The compound tubular glands become overactive and produce large quantities of mucus. The secretion accumulates in the cervical canal and thickens to form the so-called mucous plug. This inspissated mucus effectively seals off the canal from the vagina and prevents the ascent of bacteria and other substances into the uterine cavity. The plug is expelled early in labor.

At the end of gestation and during labor the internal os gradually disappears, and the cervical canal also becomes part of the lower uterine segment, leaving only the external os.

VAGINA

The vagina is a fibromuscular membranous tube surrounded by the vulva below, the uterus above, the bladder in front, and the rectum behind. Its direction is obliquely upward and backward. The cervix uteri enters the vagina through the anterior wall, and for this reason the anterior wall of the vagina (6 to 8 cm) is shorter than the posterior wall (7 to 10 cm). The protrusion of the cervix into the vagina divides the vaginal vault into four fornices: an anterior, a posterior, and two lateral fornices. The posterior fornix is much deeper than the others.

The wall of the vagina is made up of four layers:

1. The mucosa is the epithelial layer.
2. The submucosa is rich in blood vessels.
3. The muscularis is the third layer.
4. The outer connective tissue layer connects the vagina to the surrounding structures.

Even in the normal condition the vagina is capable of great distention, but in pregnancy this ability is increased many times. In the pregnant state there is greater vascularity, thickening and lengthening of the walls, and increased secretion, so that most women have varying quantities of vaginal discharge during the period of gestation.

5

Obstetric Pelvis

The pelvis is made up of the two innominate bones (which occupy the front and sides) and the sacrum and coccyx (which are behind). The bones articulate through four joints. The sacroiliac joint is the most important, linking the sacrum to the iliac part of the innominate bones. The symphysis of the pubis joins the two pubic bones. The sacrococcygeal joint attaches the sacrum to the coccyx.

The *false pelvis* lies above the true pelvis, superior to the linea terminalis. Its only obstetric function is to support the enlarged uterus during pregnancy. Its boundaries are:

1. Posteriorly: lumbar vertebrae
2. Laterally: iliac fossae
3. Anteriorly: anterior abdominal wall

The *true pelvis* (Fig. 1A) lies below the pelvic brim, or linea terminalis, and is the bony canal through which the baby must pass. It is divided into three parts: (1) the inlet, (2) the pelvic cavity, and (3) the pelvic outlet.

The *inlet* (pelvic brim) is bounded:

1. Anteriorly: by the pubic crest and spine
2. Laterally, by the iliopectineal lines on the innominate bones
3. Posteriorly, by the anterior borders of the ala and promontory of the sacrum

The *pelvic cavity* (Fig. 1B) is a curved canal.

1. The anterior wall is straight and shallow. The pubis is 5 cm long.
2. The posterior wall is deep and concave. The sacrum is 10 to 15 cm long.
3. The ischium and part of the body of the ilium are found laterally.

The *pelvic outlet* is diamond-shaped. It is bounded:

1. Anteriorly: by the arcuate pubic ligament and the pubic arch
2. Laterally: by the ischial tuberosity and the sacrotuberous ligament
3. Posteriorly: by the tip of the sacrum

The *pelvic inclination* (Fig. 1C) is assessed when the woman is in the upright position. The plane of the pelvic brim makes an angle of about 60° with the horizontal. The anterior superior iliac spine is in the same vertical plane as the pubic spine.

The *axis of the birth canal* (Fig. 1D) is the course taken by the presenting part as it passes through the pelvis. At first it moves downward and backward to the level of the ischial spines, which is the area of the bony attachment of the pelvic floor muscles. Here the direction changes and the presenting part proceeds downward and forward.

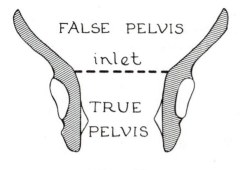

A. True pelvis.

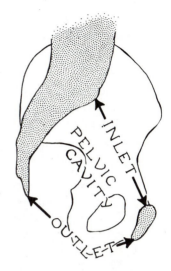

B. Pelvic cavity.

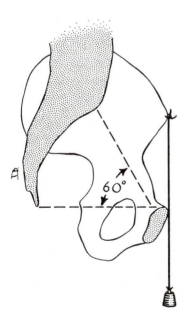

C. Pelvic inclination.

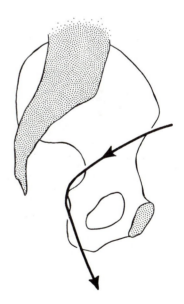

D. Axis of birth canal.

Figure 1. Pelvic cavity.

The *pelvic planes* (Fig. 2) are imaginary flat surfaces passing across the pelvis at different levels. They are used for the purposes of description. The important ones are as follows:

1. The plane of the inlet is also called the superior strait.
2. The pelvic cavity has many planes, two of which are the plane of greatest dimensions and the plane of least dimensions.
3. The plane of the outlet is also called the inferior strait.

The *diameters* are distances between given points. Important ones are the following:

1. Anteroposterior diameters.
2. Transverse diameters.
3. Left oblique: Oblique diameters are designated left or right according to their posterior terminal.
4. Right oblique.
5. Posterior sagittal diameter: This is the back part of the anteroposterior diameter, extending from the intersection of the transverse and anteroposterior diameters to the posterior limit of the latter.
6. Anterior sagittal diameter: This is the front part of the anteroposterior diameter, extending from the intersection of the transverse and anteroposterior diameter to the anterior limit of the latter.

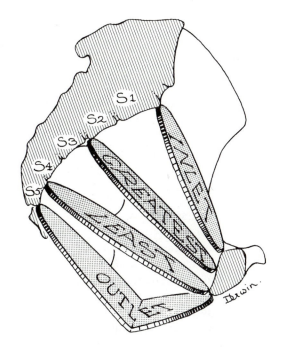

A. Sagittal section.

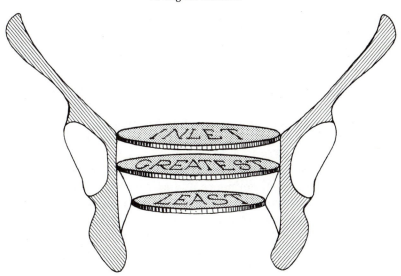

B. Coronal section.

Figure 2. Pelvic planes.

PELVIC INLET

Plane of Obstetric Inlet

The plane of the obstetric inlet is bounded:

1. Anteriorly: by the posterior superior margin of the pubic symphysis
2. Laterally: by the iliopectineal lines
3. Posteriorly: by the promontory and ala of the sacrum

Diameters of Inlet

The diameters of the inlet are as follows:
1. Anteroposterior diameters:
    a. The anatomic conjugate (Fig. 3) extends from the middle of the sacral promontory to the middle of the pubic crest (superior surface of the pubis). It measures 11.5 cm. It has no obstetric significance.
    b. The obstetric conjugate extends from the middle of the sacral promontory to the posterior superior margin of the pubic symphysis. This point on the pubis, which protrudes back into the cavity of the pelvis, is about 1 cm below the pubic crest. The obstetric conjugate is about 11.0 cm in length. This is the important anteroposterior diameter, since it is the one through which the fetus must pass.
    c. The diagonal conjugate extends from the subpubic angle to the middle of the sacral promontory. It is 12.5 cm in length. This diameter can be measured manually in the patient. It is of clinical significance because by subtracting 1.5 cm an approximate length of the obstetric conjugate can be obtained.
2. Transverse diameter is the widest distance between the iliopectineal lines and is 13.5 cm.
3. Left oblique diameter extends from the left sacroiliac joint to the right iliopectineal eminence and is about 12.5 cm.
4. Right oblique diameter extends from the right sacroiliac joint to the left iliopectineal eminence and is about 12.5 cm.
5. Posterior sagittal extends from the intersection of the anteroposterior and transverse diameters to the middle of the sacral promontory and is about 4.5 cm long.

PELVIC CAVITY

The pelvic cavity extends from the inlet to the outlet.

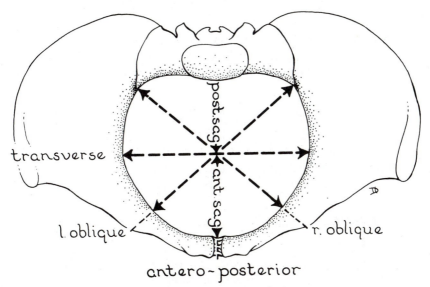

A. Anteroposterior view.

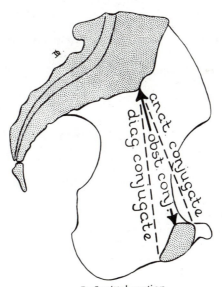

B. Sagittal section.

Figure 3. Pelvic inlet.

Plane of Greatest Dimensions

This is the roomiest part of the pelvis and is almost circular. Its obstetric significance is small. Its boundaries are:

1. Anteriorly: midpoint of the posterior surface of the pubis
2. Laterally: upper and middle thirds of the obturator foramina
3. Posteriorly: the junction of the second and third sacral vertebrae

The diameters of importance are:

1. The anteroposterior diameter extends from the midpoint of the posterior surface of the pubis to the junction of the second and third sacral vertebrae and measures 12.75 cm.
2. The transverse diameter is the widest distance between the lateral aspects of the plane and is 12.5 cm.

Plane of Least Dimensions

This is the most important plane of the pelvis (Fig. 4). It has the least room, and it is here that most instances of arrest of progress take place. This plane extends from the apex of the subpubic arch, through the ischial spines, to the sacrum, usually at or near the junction of the fourth and fifth sacral vertebrae. The boundaries are, from front to back:

1. Lower border of the pubic symphysis
2. White line on the fascia covering the obturator foramina
3. Ischial spines
4. Sacrospinous ligaments
5. Sacrum

The diameters of importance are:

1. Anteroposterior diameter, extending from the lower border of the pubic symphysis to the junction of the fourth and fifth sacral vertebrae and measuring 12.0 cm
2. Transverse diameter, lying between the ischial spines and measuring 10.5 cm
3. Posterior sagittal diameter, extending from the bispinous diameter to the junction of the fourth and fifth sacral vertebrae and measuring 4.5 to 5.0 cm

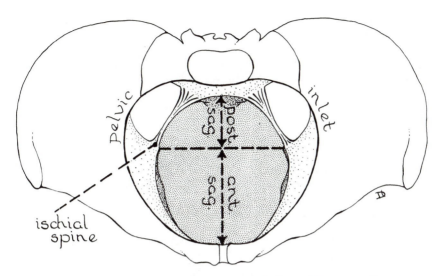

A. Anteroposterior view showing the anteroposterior and transverse diameters.

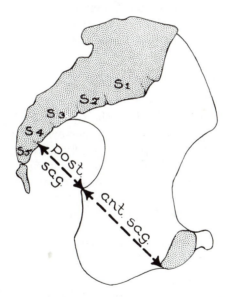

B. Sagittal section showing the anteroposterior diameter.

Figure 4. Pelvic cavity: the plane of least dimensions.

PELVIC OUTLET

The outlet is made up of two triangular planes, having as their common base and most inferior part the transverse diameter between the ischial tuberosities (Fig. 5).

Anterior Triangle

The anterior triangle has the following boundaries:

1. The base is the bituberous diameter (transverse diameter).
2. The apex is the subpubic angle.
3. The sides are the pubic rami and ischial tuberosities.

Posterior Triangle

The posterior triangle has the following boundaries:

1. The base is the bituberous diameter.
2. The obstetric apex is the sacrococcygeal joint.
3. The sides are the sacrotuberous ligaments.

Diameters of the Outlet

1. The anatomic anteroposterior diameter is from the inferior margin of the pubic symphysis to the tip of the coccyx. It measures about 9.5 cm. The obstetric anteroposterior diameter is from the inferior margin of the pubic symphysis to the sacrococcygeal joint. This measures 11.5 cm. Because of the mobility at the sacrococcygeal joint, the coccyx is pushed out of the way by the advancing presenting part, increasing the available space.
2. The transverse diameter is the distance between the inner surfaces of the ischial tuberosities and measures about 11.0 cm.
3. The posterior sagittal diameter extends from the middle of the transverse diameter to the sacrococcygeal junction and is 9.0 cm.
4. The anterior sagittal diameter extends from the middle of the transverse diameter to the subpubic angle and measures 6.0 cm.

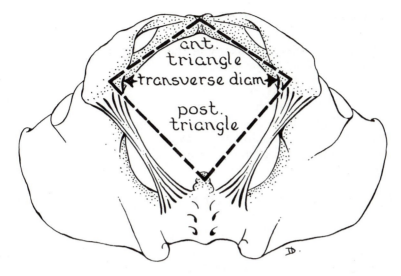

A. Inferior view.

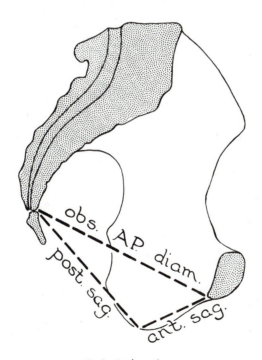

B. Sagittal section.

Figure 5. Pelvic outlet.

IMPORTANT MEASUREMENTS

In assessing the obstetric capacity of the pelvis the most important measurements are the following:

1. Obstetric conjugate of the inlet
2. Distance between the ischial spines
3. Subpubic angle and bituberous diameter
4. Posterior sagittal diameters of the three planes
5. Curve and length of the sacrum

CLASSIFICATION OF THE PELVIS

Variations in the female pelvis and in the planes of any single pelvis are so great that a rigid classification is not possible. A pelvis of the female type in one plane may be predominantly male in another. Many pelves are mixed in that the various planes do not conform to a single parent type.

For the purpose of classification the pelvis is named on the basis of the inlet, and mention is made of nonconforming characteristics. For example, a pelvis may be described as a female type with male features at the outlet.

We prefer the classification of Caldwell and Moloy (Table 1 and Figs. 6 through 8).

TABLE 1. CLASSIFICATION OF PELVIS (CALDWELL AND MOLOY)

	Gynecoid	Android	Anthropoid	Platypelloid
INLET				
Sex type	Normal female	Male	Ape-like	Flat female
Incidence	50%	20%	25%	5%
Shape	Round or transverse oval; transverse diameter is a little longer than the anteroposterior	Heart or wedge shaped	Long antero-posterior oval	Transverse oval
Anteroposterior diameter	Adequate	Adequate	Long	Short
Transverse diameter	Adequate	Adequate	Adequate but relatively short	Long
Posterior sagittal diameter	Adequate	Very short and inadequate	Very long	Very short
Anterior sagittal diameter	Adequate	Long	Long	Short

TABLE 1. (Cont.)

	Gynecoid	Android	Anthropoid	Platypelloid
Posterior segment	Broad, deep, roomy	Shallow; sacral promontory indents the inlet and reduces its capacity	Deep	Shallow
Anterior segment	Well rounded forepelvis	Narrow, sharply angulated forepelvis	Deep	Shallow

(continued)

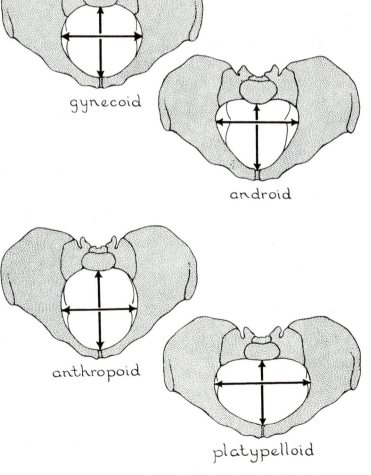

Figure 6. Pelvic inlet (Caldwell-Moloy classification).

TABLE 1. (Cont.)

	Gynecoid	Android	Anthropoid	Platypelloid
PELVIC CAVITY: MIDPELVIS				
Anteroposterior diameter	Adequate	Reduced	Long	Shortened
Transverse diameter	Adequate	Reduced	Adequate	Wide
Posterior sagittal diameter	Adequate	Reduced	Adequate	Shortened
Anterior sagittal diameter	Adequate	Reduced	Adequate	Short
Sacrum	Wide, deep curve; short; slopes backward; light bone	Flat; inclined forward; long; narrow; heavy	Inclined backward; narrow; long	Wide, deep curve; often sharply angulated with enlarged sacral fossa
Sidewalls	Parallel, straight	Convergent; funnel pelvis	Straight	Parallel
Ischial spines	Not prominent	Prominent	Variable	Variable
Sacrosciatic notch	Wide; short	Narrow; long; high arch	Wide	Short
Depth: iliopectineal eminence to tuberosities	Average	Long	Long	Short
Capacity	Adequate	Reduced in all diameters	Adequate	Reduced

(continued)

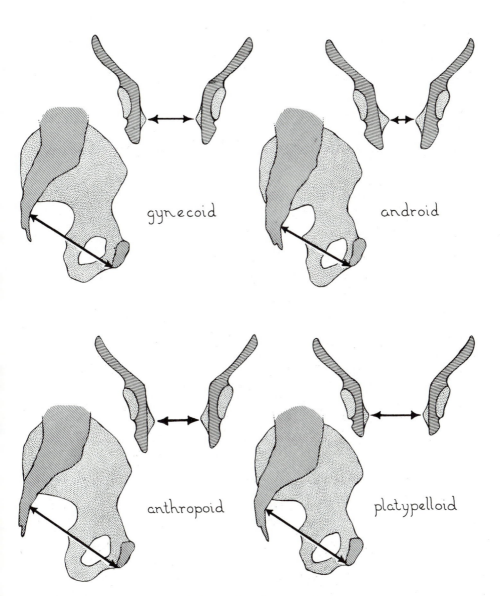

Figure 7. Midpelvis (Caldwell-Moloy classification).

TABLE 1. (Cont.)

	Gynecoid	Android	Anthropoid	Platypelloid
OUTLET				
Anteroposterior diameter	Long	Short	Long	Short
Transverse diameter (bituberous)	Adequate	Narrow	Adequate	Wide
Pubic arch	Wide and round; 90°	Narrow; deep; 70°	Normal or relatively narrow	Very wide
Inferior pubic rami	Short; concave inward	Straight; long	Long; relatively narrow	Straight; short
Capacity	Adequate	Reduced	Adequate	Inadequate
EFFECT ON LABOR				
Fetal head	Engages in transverse or oblique diameter in slight asynclitism; good flexion; OA is common	Engages in transverse or posterior diameter in asynclitism; extreme molding	Engages in anteroposterior or oblique; often occiput posterior	Engages in transverse diameter with marked asynclitism
Labor	Good uterine function; early and complete internal rotation; spontaneous delivery; wide pubic arch reduces perineal tears	Deep transverse arrest is common; arrest as OP with failure of rotation; delivery is often by difficult forceps application, rotation, and extraction; the narrow pubic arch may lead to major perineal tears	Delivery and labor usually easy; birth face to pubis is common	Delay at inlet
Prognosis	Good	Poor	Good	Poor; disproportion; delay at inlet; labor often terminated by cesarean section

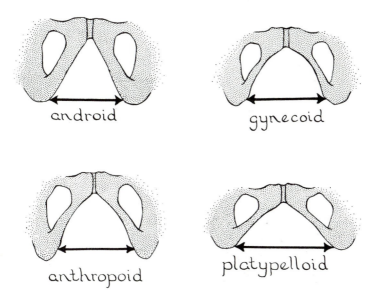

Figure 8. Pelvic outlet (Caldwell-Moloy classification).

6

The Passenger: Fetus

GENERAL CONSIDERATIONS

1. Resemblance to the adult human form may be perceptible at the end of 8 weeks and is obvious at the end of 12 weeks.
2. By the end of 12 weeks, and sometimes sooner, the sexual differences in the external genitalia may be recognized in abortuses.
3. Growth is greatest during the sixth and seventh months of intrauterine life.
4. Quickening (the perception by the pregnant woman of fetal movements in utero) occurs between the 16th and 20th weeks of pregnancy. The time of quickening is too variable to be of value in determining the expected date of confinement or when term has been reached. Active intestinal peristalsis is the most common phenomenon mistaken for quickening.
5. The fetal heart is audible by the 18th or 20th week.
6. The average length of the fetus at term is 50 cm.
7. Within wide variations the average male (7.5 pounds or 3400 g) is a little heavier at birth than the female (7.0 pounds or 3150 g).
8. In premature babies the circumference of the head is relatively large as compared with the shoulders. As the fetus matures the body grows faster than the head, so that at term the circumferences of the head and the shoulders are nearly the same.

FETAL OVOIDS

In its passage through the pelvis the fetus presents two oval parts, movable on each other at the neck. The oval of the head is longer in its anteroposterior diameter, while that of the shoulders and body is longer transversely. Thus, the two ovoids are perpendicular to each other.

FETAL HEAD

From the obstetric standpoint the fetal head (Fig. 1) is the most important part of the fetus. It is the largest, the least compressible, and the most frequently presenting part of the baby. Once the head has been born, rarely is there delay or difficulty with the remainder of the body.

Base of Skull

The bones of the base of the skull are large, ossified, firmly united, and not compressible. Their function is to protect the vital centers in the brain stem.

Vault of Skull: Cranium

The cranium is made up of several bones. Important ones are the occipital bone posteriorly, the two parietal bones on the sides, and the two temporal and the two frontal bones anteriorly. The bones of the cranial vault are laid down in membrane. At birth they are thin, poorly ossified, easily compressible, and joined only by membrane. This looseness of union of the bones (actually there are spaces between them) permits their overlapping under pressure. In this way the head can change its shape to fit the maternal pelvis, an important function known as *molding*. The top of the skull is wider posteriorly (biparietal diameter) than anteriorly (bitemporal diameter).

Sutures of Skull

Sutures are membrane-occupied spaces between the bones. They are useful in two ways (Fig. 1A):

1. Their presence makes molding possible.
2. By identifying the sutures on vaginal examination, the position of the baby's head can be diagnosed. The important sutures include the following.

Sagittal Suture
The sagittal suture lies between the parietal bones. It runs in an anteroposterior direction between the fontanelles and divides the head into left and right halves.

Lambdoidal Sutures
The lambdoidal sutures extend transversely from the posterior fontanelle and separate the occipital bone from the two parietals.

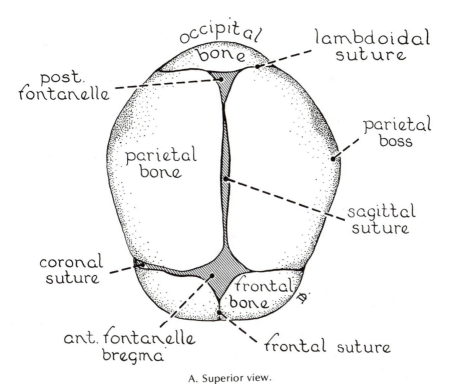

A. Superior view.

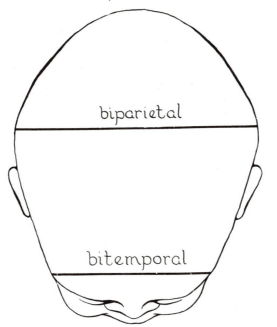

B. Transverse diameters.

Figure 1. Fetal skull.

Coronal Sutures
The coronal sutures extend transversely from the anterior fontanelle and lie between the parietal and frontal bones (Fig. 1).

Frontal Suture
The frontal suture is between the two frontal bones and is an anterior continuation of the sagittal suture. It extends from the glabella to the bregma.

Fontanelles

Where the sutures intersect are the membrane-filled spaces known as fontanelles. Two are important: the anterior and the posterior. These areas are useful clinically in two ways (Fig. 1A):

1. Their identification helps in diagnosing the position of the fetal head in the pelvis.
2. The large fontanelle is examined in assessing the condition of the child after birth. In dehydrated infants the fontanelle is depressed below the surface of the bony skull. When the intracranial pressure is elevated, the fontanelle is bulging, tense, and raised above the level of the skull.

Anterior Fontanelle
The anterior fontanelle (bregma) is at the junction of the sagittal, frontal, and coronal sutures. It is by far the larger of the two, measuring about 3 × 2 cm, and is diamond-shaped. It becomes ossified by 18 months of age. The anterior fontanelle facilitates molding. By remaining patent long after birth it plays a part in accommodating the remarkable growth of the brain.

Posterior Fontanelle
The posterior fontanelle (lambda) is located where the sagittal suture meets the two lambdoidals. The skull is not truly deficient at this point, and the area is a meeting point of the sutures rather than a true fontanelle. It is much smaller than the anterior one. The intersection of the sutures makes a Y with the sagittal suture as the base and the lambdoidals as the arms. This fontanelle closes at 6 to 8 weeks of age.

Landmarks of Skull

From posterior to anterior certain areas are identified (Fig. 2A).

1. Occiput: the area of the back of the head occupied by the occipital bone. It is behind and inferior to the posterior fontanelle and the lambdoidal sutures.

2. Posterior fontanelle.
3. Vertex: the area between the two fontanelles. It is the top of the skull and is bounded laterally by the parietal bosses.
4. Bregma or large anterior fontanelle.
5. Sinciput (or brow): the region bounded superiorly by the bregma and the coronal sutures, inferiorly by the glabella and the orbital ridges.

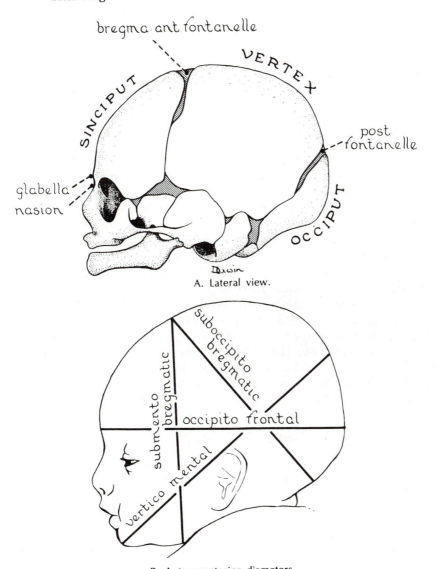

A. Lateral view.

B. Anteroposterior diameters.

Figure 2. Landmarks and diameters of fetal skull.

6. Glabella: the elevated area between the orbital ridges.
7. Nasion: the root of the nose.
8. Parietal bosses: two eminences, one on the side of each parietal bone. The distance between them is the widest transverse diameter of the fetal head.

Diameters of Fetal Skull

The diameters are distances between given points on the fetal skull (Fig. 2B). Their size varies, and the particular anteroposterior diameter that presents to the maternal pelvis depends on the degree of flexion or extension of the fetal head.

1. The biparietal diameter (Fig. 1B) is between the parietal bosses. It is the largest transverse diameter and measures 9.5 cm.
2. The bitemporal diameter lies between the lateral sides of the temporal bones. It is 8.0 cm in length and is the shortest transverse diameter of the skull.
3. The suboccipitobregmatic diameter extends from the undersurface of the occipital bone, where it meets the neck, to the center of the bregma. It is 9.5 cm long. It is the anteroposterior diameter that presents when the head is flexed well.
4. The occipitofrontal diameter presents in the military attitude, neither flexion nor extension. It extends from the external occipital protuberance to the glabella and is 11.0 cm long.
5. The verticomental diameter is involved in brow presentations (halfway extension of the head). It runs from the vertex to the chin, measures 13.5 cm, and is the longest anteroposterior diameter of the head.
6. The submentobregmatic is the diameter in face presentations (complete extension of the head). Reaching from the junction of the neck and lower jaw to the center of the bregma, it is 9.5 cm long.

Circumferences of Fetal Skull and Shoulders

1. In the occipitofrontal plane the circumference of the head is 34.5 cm.
2. In the suboccipitobregmatic plane it is 32 to 34 cm.
3. At term the bisacromial diameter of the shoulders is 33 to 34 cm.

Molding

Molding is the ability of the fetal head to change its shape and so adapt itself to the unyielding maternal pelvis (Fig. 3). This property is of the

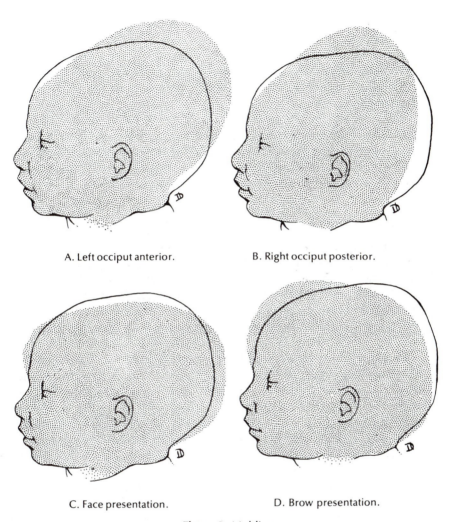

A. Left occiput anterior.   B. Right occiput posterior.

C. Face presentation.   D. Brow presentation.

Figure 3. Molding

greatest value in the progress of labor and descent of the head through the birth canal.

The fetal bones are joined loosely by membranes so that actual spaces exist between the edges of the bones. This permits the bones to alter their relationships to each other as pressure is exerted on the head by the bony pelvis; the bones can come closer to each other or move apart. The side-to-side relationships of the bones are changeable, and one bone is able to override the other. When such overlapping takes place, the frontal and occipital bones pass under the parietal bones. The posterior parietal bone is subjected to greater pressure by the sacral promontory; therefore it passes beneath the anterior parietal bone. A contributing factor to molding is the softness of the bones.

Compression in one direction is accompanied by expansion in another, and hence the actual volume of the skull is not reduced. Provided that molding is not excessive and that it takes place slowly, no damage is done to the brain.

Alteration of the shape of the head is produced by compression of the presenting diameter, with resultant bulging of the diameter that is at right angles. For example, in the occipitoanterior position the suboccipitobregmatic is the presenting diameter. The head therefore is elongated in the verticomental diameter, with bulging behind and above.

Caput Succedaneum

The caput succedaneum is a localized swelling of the scalp formed by the effusion of serum (Fig. 4). Pressure by the cervical ring causes obstruction of the venous return, so that the part of the scalp that lies within the cervix becomes edematous. The caput forms during labor and after the membranes have been ruptured. It is absent if the baby is dead, the contractions are poor, or the cervix is not applied closely to the head.

The location of the caput varies with the position of the head. In occipitoanterior (OA) positions the caput forms on the vertex, to the right of the sagittal suture in left (LOA), and to the left in right (ROA). As flexion becomes more pronounced during labor, the posterior part of the vertex becomes the presenting part and the caput is found in that region, a little to the right or left as before. Thus, when the position is LOA the caput is on the posterior part of the right parietal bone, and in ROA on the posterior part of the left parietal bone.

The size of the caput succedaneum is an indication of the amount of pressure that has been exerted against the head. A large one suggests strong pressure from above and resistance from below. A small caput is present when the contractions have been weak or the resistance feeble. The largest are found in contracted pelves after long, hard labor. In the presence of prolonged labor a large caput suggests disproportion or occipitoposterior position, while a small one indicates uterine inertia.

In performing rectal or vaginal examinations during labor one must take care to distinguish between the station of the caput and that of the skull. The enlarging caput may make the accoucheur believe that the head is descending, when in reality it means that advancement of the head is delayed or arrested. A growing caput is an indication for reassessing the situation.

The caput is present at birth, begins to disappar immediately afterward, and is usually gone after 24 to 36 hours.

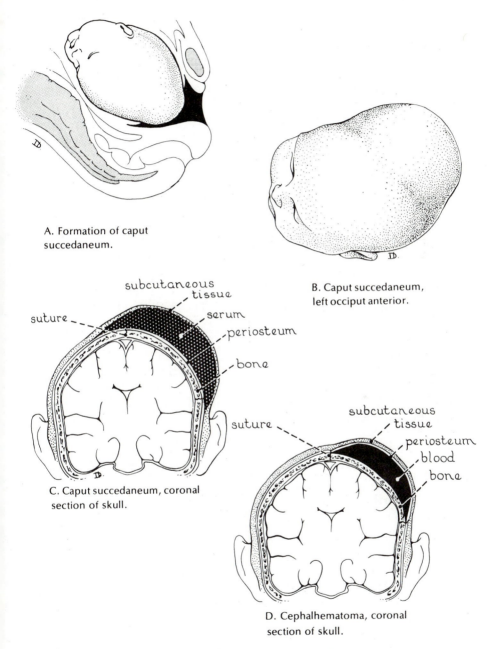

A. Formation of caput succedaneum.

B. Caput succedaneum, left occiput anterior.

C. Caput succedaneum, coronal section of skull.

D. Cephalhematoma, coronal section of skull.

Figure 4. Caput succedaneum (CS) and cephalhematoma.

Cephalhematoma

Cephalhematoma is a hemorrhage under the periosteum of one or more of the bones of the skull (Fig. 4D). It is situated on one or, rarely, both parietal bones and is similar in appearance to a caput succedaneum. A cephalhematoma is caused by trauma to the skull, including:

1. Prolonged pressure of the head against the cervix, perineum, or pubic bones
2. Damage from forceps blades
3. Difficult manual rotation of the head
4. Rapid compression and relaxation of the forces that act on the fetal head, as in precipitate births

This injury may occur also during normal spontaneous delivery.

Since the hemorrhage is under the periosteum, the swelling is limited to the affected bone and does not cross the suture lines; this is one way of distinguishing it from a caput succedaneum. The swelling appears within a few hours of birth, and since absorption is slow it takes 6 to 12 weeks to disappear. The blood clots early at the edges and remains fluid to the center. Rarely, ossification takes place in the clot and may cause a permanent deformity of the skull. The health of the child is not affected, and the brain is not damaged.

The prognosis is good. No local treatment is indicated. Vitamin K may be given to reduce further bleeding. The area should be protected from injury, but no attempt is made to evacuate the blood. Rarely, infection ensues with formation of an abscess that must be drained. The differential diagnosis of caput succedaneum and cephalhematoma includes these criteria:

Caput succedaneum	Cephalhematoma
Present at birth	May not appear for several hours
Soft, pits on pressure	Soft, does not pit
Diffuse swelling	Sharply circumscribed
Lies over and crosses the sutures	Limited to individual bones, does not cross suture lines
Movable on skull, seeks dependent portions	Fixed to original site
Is largest at birth and immediately begins to grow smaller, disappearing in a few hours	Appears after a few hours, grows larger for a time, and disappears only after weeks or months

Meningocele

A meningocele is a hernial protrusion of the meninges. It is a serious congenital deformity and must be distinguished from caput succedaneum and cephalhematoma. The meningocele always lies over a suture or a fontanelle and becomes tense when the baby cries.

Fetopelvic Relationships

7

DEFINITIONS

LIE   Relationship of the long axis of the fetus to the long axis of the mother.

PRESENTATION   The part of the fetus that lies over the inlet. The three main presentations are cephalic (head first), breech (pelvis first), and shoulder.

PRESENTING PART   The most dependent part of the fetus, lying nearest the cervix. During vaginal or rectal examination it is the area with which the finger makes contact first.

ATTITUDE   Relation of fetal parts to each other. The basic attitudes are flexion and extension. The fetal head is in flexion when the chin approaches the chest and in extension when the occiput nears the back. The typical fetal attitude in the uterus is flexion, with the head bent in front of the chest, the arms and legs folded in front of the body, and the back curved forward slightly.

DENOMINATOR   An arbitrarily chosen point on the presenting part of the fetus used in describing position. Each presentation has its own denominator.

POSITION   Relationship of the denominator to the front, back, or sides of the maternal pelvis.

LIE

The two lies are: (1) longitudinal, when the long axes of the fetus and mother are parallel; and (2) transverse, or oblique, when the long axis of the fetus is perpendicular or oblique to the long axis of the mother.

All terms of direction refer to the mother in the standing position. Upper means toward the maternal head, and lower toward the feet. Anterior, posterior, right, and left refer to the mother's front, back, right, and left, respectively.

Longitudinal Lies

Longitudinal lies are grouped into: (1) cephalic, when the head comes first; and (2) breech, when the buttocks or lower limbs lead the way (Table 1).

TABLE 1. FETOPELVIC RELATIONSHIPS ACCORDING TO FETAL POSITION

Presentation	Attitude	Presenting Part	Denominator
Longitudinal lie (99.5%)			
Cephalic (96 to 97%)	Flexion	Vertex (posterior part)	Occiput (O)
	Military	Vertex (median part)	Occiput (O)
	Partial extension	Brow	Forehead (frontum) (Fr)
	Complete extension	Face	Chin (mentum) (M)
Breech (3 to 4%)			
Complete	Flexed hips and knees	Buttocks	Sacrum (S)
Frank	Flexed hips, extended knees	Buttocks	Sacrum (S)
Footling: single, double	Extended hips and knees	Feet	Sacrum (S)
Kneeling: single, double	Extended hips; flexed knees	Knees	Sacrum (S)
Transverse or oblique lie (0.5%)			
Shoulder	Variable	Shoulder, arm, trunk	Scapula (Sc)

Cephalic Presentations

Cephalic presentations are classified into four main groups, according to the attitude of the fetal head:

1. Flexion is present when the baby's chin is near its chest (Fig. 1A). The posterior part of the vertex is the presenting part, and the occiput is the denominator.

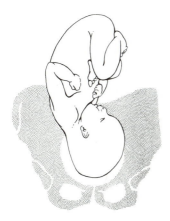

A. Flexion of head.

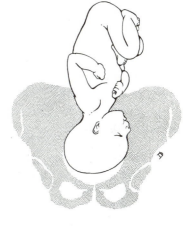

B. Military attitude.

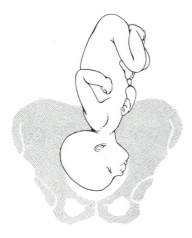

C. Brow presentation, partial extension.

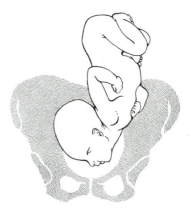

D. Face presentation, complete extension.

Figure 1. Attitude.

2. The position with neither flexion nor extension is called the military attitude or the median vertex presentation (Fig. 1B). The vertex (area between the two fontanelles) presents, and the occiput is the denominator.
3. In brow presentation (Fig. 1C) there is halfway extension. The frontum (forehead) leads the way and is also the denominator.
4. When extension is complete the presenting part is the face (Fig. 1D), and the denominator is the mentum (chin).

Breech Presentations

Breech or pelvic presentations are classified according to the attitudes at the hips and knees (Fig. 2).

1. The breech is complete when there is flexion at both hips and knees. The buttocks are the presenting part.
2. Flexion at the hips and extension at the knees change it to a frank breech. The lower limbs lie anterior to the baby's abdomen. The buttocks lead the way.
3. When there is extension both at the hips and at the knees we have a footling breech—single if one foot is presenting, and double if both feet are down.
4. Extension at the hips and flexion at the knees make it a kneeling breech, single or double. Here the knees present.

In all variations of breech presentation the sacrum is the denominator.

Transverse or Oblique Lie

Transverse or oblique lie (Fig. 3) exists when the long axis of the fetus is perpendicular or oblique to the long axis of the mother. Most often the shoulder is the presenting part, but it may be an arm or some part of the trunk, such as the back, abdomen, or side. The scapula is the denominator. The position is anterior or posterior depending on the situation of the scapulas, and right or left according to the location of the head.

POSITION

Position is the relationship of the denominator to the front, back, or sides of the mother's pelvis. The pelvic girdle has a circumference of 360°. The denominator can occupy any part of the circumference. In practice, eight points, 45° from each other, are demarcated, and the position of the fetus is described as the relationship between the denominator and one of these landmarks.

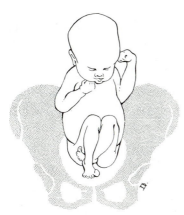

A. Complete breech.

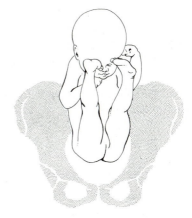

B. Frank breech.

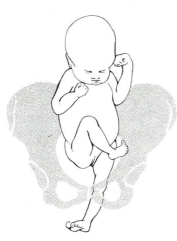

C. Footling breech.

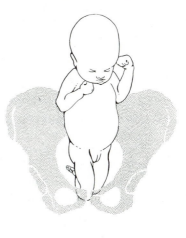

D. Kneeling breech.

Figure 2. Breech.

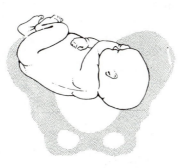

Figure 3. Transverse lie.

Three sets of terms are used to describe position: the *denominator;* *right* or *left,* depending upon which side of the maternal pelvis the denominator is in; and *anterior, posterior,* or *transverse,* according to whether the denominator is in the front, in the back, or at the side of the pelvis.

With the patient lying in the lithotomy position, the pubic symphysis is anterior and the sacrum posterior. Starting at the symphysis and moving in a clockwise direction, eight positions are described in succession, each 45° from the preceding one (Fig. 4A).

1. Denominator anterior (DA): The denominator is situated directly under the pubic symphysis.
2. Left denominator anterior (LDA): The denominator is in the anterior part of the pelvis, 45° to the left of the midline.
3. Left denominator transverse (LDT): The denominator is on the left side of the pelvis, 90° from the midline, at 3 o'clock.
4. Left denominator posterior (LDP): The denominator is now in the posterior segment of the pelvis and is 45° to the left of the midline.
5. Denominator posterior (DP): The denominator has rotated a total of 180 and is now in the posterior part of the pelvis, directly in the midline and directly above the sacrum.
6. Right denominator posterior (RDP): The denominator is in the posterior part of the pelvis, 45° to the right of the midline.
7. Right denominator transverse (RDT): The denominator is on the right side of the pelvis, 90° from the midline, at 9 o'clock.
8. Right denominator anterior (RDA): The denominator is in the anterior segment of the pelvis, 45° to the right of the midline.

Further rotation of 45° completes the circle of 360°, and the denominator is back under the symphysis pubis in the denominator anterior position.

This method of describing position is used for every presentation. Each presentation has its own denominator, but the basic descriptive terminology is the same.

Figure 4A demonstrates the various positions in which the vertex is the presenting part. The occiput (back of the head) is the denominator, and the eight positions (moving clockwise) are: OA—LOA—LOT—LOP—OP—ROP—ROT—ROA—OA.

In face presentations (Fig. 4B) the chin (mentum) is the denominator, and the sequence of positions is: MA—LMA—LMT—LMP—MP—RMP—RMT—RMA—MA.

A further example would be in breech presentations where the sacrum is the denominator (Fig. 4C). Here the eight positions are: SA—LSA—LST—LSP—SP—RSP—RST—RSA—SA.

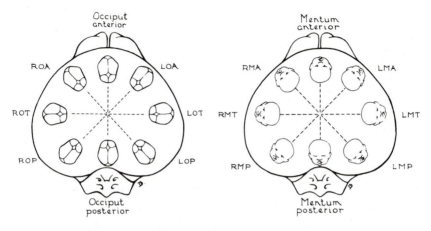

A. Occiput.   B. Face.

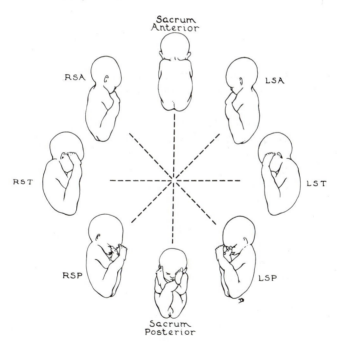

C. Breech.

Figure 4. Position.

CEPHALIC PROMINENCE

The cephalic prominence is produced by flexion or extension (Fig. 5). When the head is well flexed, the occiput is lower than the sinciput and the forehead is the cephalic prominence. When there is extension, the occiput is higher than the sinciput and the occiput or back of the head is the cephalic prominence. The cephalic prominence can be palpated through the abdomen by placing both hands on the sides of the lower part of the uterus and moving them gently toward the pelvis. When there is a cephalic prominence, the fingers abut against it on that side and on the other side meet little or no resistance. The location of the cephalic prominence aids in diagnosing attitude. When the cephalic prominence and the back are on opposite sides, the attitude is flexion. When the cephalic prominence and the back are on the same side, there is extension. When no cephalic prominence is palpable, there is neither flexion nor extension and the head is in the military attitude.

LIGHTENING

Lightening is the subjective sensation felt by the patient as the presenting part descends during the latter weeks of pregnancy. It is not synonymous with engagement, although both may take place at the same time. Lightening is caused by the tonus of the uterine and abdominal muscles and is part of the adaptation of the presenting part to the lower uterine segment and to the pelvis. In the latter weeks of pregnancy the cervix is taken up and the isthmus becomes part of the lower uterine segment. As this area expands, there is more room in the lower part of the uterus, and the fetus drops into it. Symptoms include:

1. Less dyspnea
2. Decreased epigastric pressure
3. A feeling that the child is lower
4. Increased pressure in the pelvis
5. Low backache
6. Urinary frequency
7. Constipation
8. Initial appearance or aggravation of already present hemorrhoids and varicose veins of the lower limbs
9. Edema of the legs and feet
10. More difficulty in walking

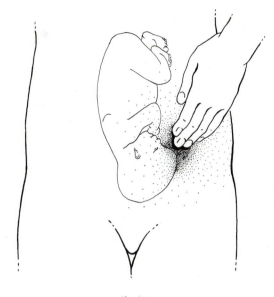

A. Flexion.

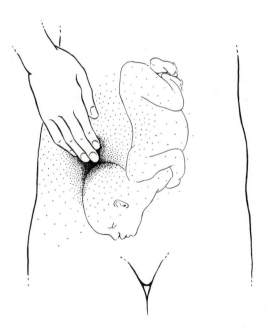

B. Extension.

Figure 5. Cephalic prominence.

GRAVIDITY AND PARITY

Gravidity

1. A *gravida* is a pregnant woman.
2. The word *gravida* refers to a pregnancy regardless of its duration.
3. A woman's *gravidity* relates to the total number of her pregnancies, regardless of their duration.
4. A *primigravida* is a woman pregnant for the first time.
5. A *secundagravida* is a woman pregnant for the second time.
6. A *multigravida* is a woman who has been pregnant several times.

Parity

1. The word *para* alludes to past pregnancies that have reached viability.
2. *Parity* refers to the number of past pregnancies that have gone to viability and have been delivered, regardless of the number of children involved. (For example, the birth of triplets increases the parity by only one.)
3. A *nullipara* is a woman who has never delivered a child that reached viability.
4. A *primipara* is a woman who has delivered one pregnancy in which the child has reached viability, without regard to the child's being alive or dead at the time of birth.
5. A *multipara* is a woman who has had two or more pregnancies that terminated at the stage when the children were viable.
6. A *parturient* is a woman in labor.

Gravida and Para

1. A woman pregnant for the first time is a primigravida and is described as gravida 1, para 0.
2. If she aborts before viability she remains gravida 1, para 0.
3. If she delivers a fetus that has reached viability she becomes a primipara, regardless of whether the child is alive or dead. She is now gravida 1, para 1.
4. During a second pregnancy she is gravida 2, para 1.
5. After she delivers the second child she is gravida 2, para 2.
6. A patient with two abortions and no viable children is gravida 2, para 0. When she becomes pregnant again she is gravida 3, para 0. When she delivers a viable child she is gravida 3, para 1.

7. Multiple births do not affect the parity by more than one. A woman who has viable triplets in her first pregnancy is gravida 1, para 1.

TPAL

A different way of describing the patient's obstetrical situation is as follows:

1. T: Term pregnancies
2. P: Preterm births
3. A: Abortions
4. L: Living children

Engagement, Synclitism, Asynclitism

8

ENGAGEMENT

By definition engagement (Fig. 1C) has taken place when the widest diameter of the presenting part has passed through the inlet. In cephalic presentations this diameter is the biparietal, between the parietal bosses. In breech presentation it is the intertrochanteric.

In most women, once the head is engaged the bony presenting part (not the caput succedaneum) is at or nearly at the level of the ischial spines. Radiologic studies have shown that this relationship is not constant and that in women with deep pelves the presenting part may be as much as a centimeter above the spines even though engagement has occurred.

The presence or absence of engagement is determined by abdominal, vaginal, or rectal examination. In primigravidas engagement usually takes place 2 to 3 weeks before term. In multiparas engagement may occur any time before or after the onset of labor. Engagement tells us that the pelvic inlet is adequate. It gives no information as to the midpelvis or the outlet. While failure of engagement in a primigravida is an indication for careful examination to rule out disproportion, abnormal presentation, or some condition blocking the birth canal, it is no cause for alarm. The occurrence of engagement in normal cases is influenced by the tonus of the uterine and abdominal muscles.

When the presenting part is entirely out of the pelvis and is freely movable above the inlet, it is said to be floating (Fig. 1A).

When the presenting part has passed through the plane of the inlet but engagement has not occurred, it is said to be dipping (Fig. 1B).

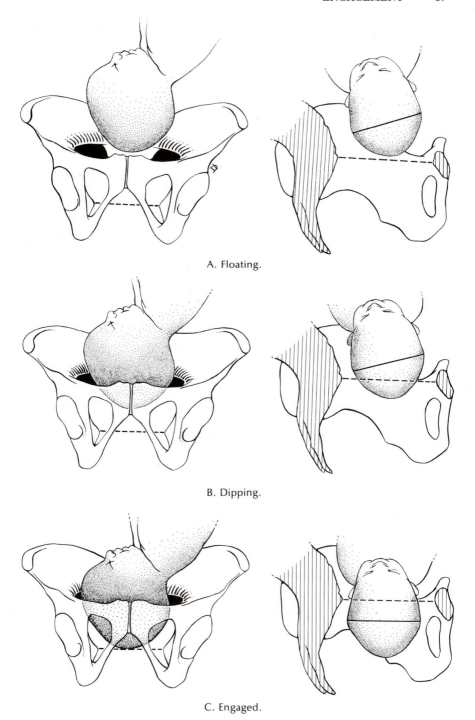

A. Floating.

B. Dipping.

C. Engaged.

Figure 1. Process of engagement.

STATION

Station is the relationship of the presenting part to an imaginary line drawn between the ischial spines (Fig. 2). The location of the buttocks in breech presentations or the bony skull (not the caput succedaneum) in cephalic presentations at the level of the spines indicates that the station is zero. Above the spines the station is minus one, minus two, and so forth, depending on how many centimeters above the spines the presenting part is. At spines minus five it is at the inlet. Below the spines it is plus one, plus two, and so forth. There are various relationships between station and the progress of labor.

1. In nulliparas entering labor with the fetal head well below the spines, further descent is often delayed until the cervix is fully dilated.
2. In nulliparas beginning labor with the head deep in the pelvis, descent beyond the spines often takes place during the first stage of labor.
3. An unengaged head in a nullipara at the onset of labor may indicate disproportion and warrants investigation. This condition is not rare, however, and in many cases descent and vaginal delivery take place.
4. The incidence of disproportion is more common when the head is high at the onset of labor.
5. Patients who start labor with high fetal heads usually have lesser degrees of cervical dilatation. There is a tendency for lower stations to be associated with cervices that are more effaced and dilated, both at the onset of labor and at the beginning of the active phase.
6. Other factors being equal, the higher the station the longer the labor.
7. Dysfunctional labor is more frequent when the station is high.
8. The high head that descends rapidly is usually not associated with abnormal labor.

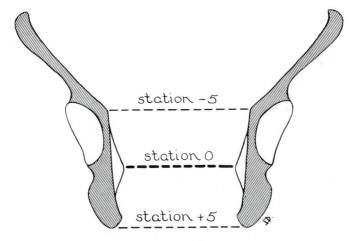

A. Anteroposterior view.

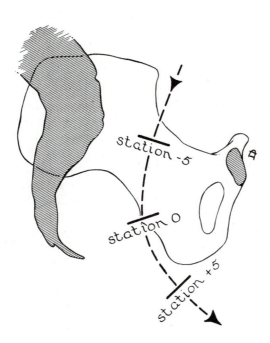

B. Lateral view.

Figure 2. Station of the presenting part.

SYNCLITISM AND ASYNCLITISM

Engagement in Synclitism

In cephalic presentations engagement has occurred when the biparietal diameter has passed through the inlet of the pelvis. The fetal head engages most frequently with its sagittal suture (the anteroposterior diameter) in the transverse diameter of the pelvis. Left occiput transverse is the most common position at engagement.

When the biparietal diameter of the fetal head is parallel to the planes of the pelvis, the head is in *synclitism*. The sagittal suture is midway between the front and the back of the pelvis. When this relationship does not obtain, the head is in *asynclitism*.

Engagement in synclitism takes place when the uterus is perpendicular to the inlet and the pelvis is roomy (Fig. 3). The head enters the pelvis with the plane of the biparietal diameter parallel to the plane of the inlet, the sagittal suture lies midway between the pubic symphysis and the sacral promontory, and the parietal bosses enter the pelvis at the same time.

Posterior Asynclitism (Litzmann Obliquity)

In most women the abdominal wall maintains the pregnant uterus in an upright position and prevents it from lying perpendicular to the plane of the pelvic inlet. As the head approaches the pelvis, the posterior parietal bone is lower than the anterior parietal bone, the sagittal suture is closer to the symphysis pubis than to the promontory of the sacrum, and the biparietal diameter of the head is in an oblique relationship to the plane of the inlet. This is posterior asynclitism (Fig. 4). It is the usual mechanism in normal women and is more common than engagement in synclitism or anterior asynclitism.

As the head enters the pelvis, the posterior parietal bone leads the way, and the posterior parietal boss (eminence) descends past the sacral promontory. At this point the anterior parietal boss is still above the pubic symphysis and has not entered the pelvis. Uterine contractions force the head downward and into a movement of lateral flexion. The posterior parietal bone pivots against the promontory, the sagittal suture moves posteriorly toward the sacrum, and the anterior parietal boss descends past the symphysis and into the pelvis. This brings the sagittal suture midway between the front and back of the pelvis, and the head is now in synclitism.

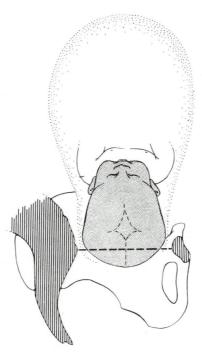

Figure 3. Synclitism at the inlet.

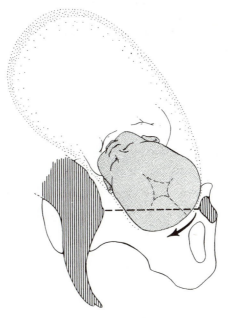

Figure 4. Posterior asynclitism.

Anterior Asynclitism (Nägele Obliquity)

When the woman's abdominal muscles are lax and the abdomen is pendulous so that the uterus and baby fall forward, or when the pelvis is abnormal and prevents the more common posterior asynclitism, the head enters the pelvis by anterior asynclitism (Fig. 5). In this mechanism the anterior parietal bone descends first, the anterior parietal boss passes by the pubic symphysis into the pelvis, and the sagittal suture lies closer to the sacral promontory than to the pubic symphysis. When the anterior parietal bone becomes relatively fixed behind the symphysis, a movement of lateral flexion takes place so that the sagittal suture moves anteriorly toward the symphysis and the posterior parietal boss squeezes by the sacral promontory and into the pelvis. The mechanism of engagement in anterior asynclitism is the reverse of that with posterior asynclitism.

There is a mechanical advantage to the head's entering the pelvis in asynclitism. When the two parietal bosses enter the pelvic inlet at the same time (synclitism), the presenting diameter is the biparietal of 9.5 cm. In asynclitism the bosses come into the pelvis one at a time, and the diameter is the subsuperparietal of 8.75 cm. Thus, engagement in asynclitism enables a larger head to pass through the inlet than would be possible if the head entered with its biparietal diameter parallel to the plane of the inlet (Fig. 6).

Whenever there is a small pelvis or a large head, asynclitism plays an important part in enabling engagement to take place. Marked and persistent asynclitism, however, is abnormal. When asynclitism is maintained until the head is deep in the pelvis, it may prevent normal internal rotation.

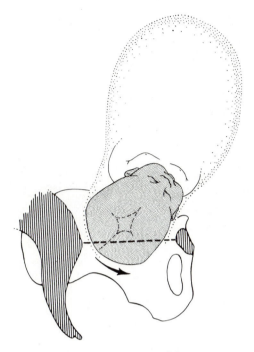

Figure 5. Anterior asynclitism.

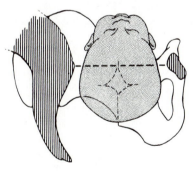

Figure 6. Synclitism in the pelvis.

Examination of the Patient

9

ABDOMINAL INSPECTION AND PALPATION

The position of the baby in utero is determined by inspecting and palpating the mother's abdomen, with these questions in mind:

1. Is the lie longitudinal, transverse, or oblique?
2. What presents at or in the pelvic inlet?
3. Where is the back?
4. Where are the small parts?
5. What is in the uterine fundus?
6. On which side is the cephalic prominence?
7. Has engagement taken place?
8. How high in the abdomen is the uterine fundus?
9. How big is the baby?

The patient lies on her back with the abdomen uncovered (Fig. 1). In order to help relax the abdominal wall muscles the shoulders are raised a little and the knees are drawn up slightly. If the patient is in labor the examination is carried out between contractions.

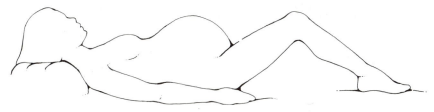

Figure 1. Position of patient for abdominal palpation.

First Maneuver: What Is the Presenting Part?

The examiner stands at the patient's side and grasps the lower uterine segment between the thumb and fingers of one hand to feel the presenting part (Fig. 2A). The other hand may be placed on the fundus to steady the uterus. This maneuver should be performed first. Since the head is the part of the fetus that can be identified with the most certainty, and since it is at or in the pelvis in 90 percent of cases, the logical thing to do first is to look for the head in its most frequent location. Once it has been established that the head is at the inlet, two important facts are known: (1) that the lie is longitudinal, and (2) that the presentation is cephalic.

An attempt is made to move the head from side to side to see whether it is outside the pelvis and free (floating) or in the pelvis and fixed (engaged). In contrast to the breech, the head is harder, smoother, more globular, and easier to move. A groove representing the neck may be felt between the head and the shoulders. The head can be moved laterally without an accompanying movement of the body. When the head is in the fundus and when there is sufficient amniotic fluid, the head can be ballotted. When a floating rubber ball is forced under water, it returns to the surface as soon as it is released; so the fetal head can be pushed posteriorly in the amniotic fluid, but as soon as the pressure on it is relaxed it rises back and abuts against the examining fingers.

Second Maneuver: Where Is the Back?

The examiner stands at the patient's side facing her head. The hands are placed on the sides of the abdomen, using one hand to steady the uterus while the other palpates the fetus (Fig. 2B). The location of the back and of the small parts is determined.

The side on which the back is located feels firmer and smoother and forms a gradual convex arch. Resistance to the palpating fingers (as pressure is exerted toward the umbilicus) is even in all regions.

On the other side the resistance to pressure is uneven, the fingers sinking deeper in some areas than they do in others. The discovery of moving limbs is diagnostic.

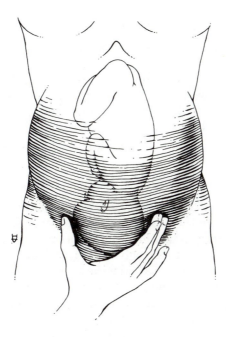

A. First maneuver: What is the presenting part?

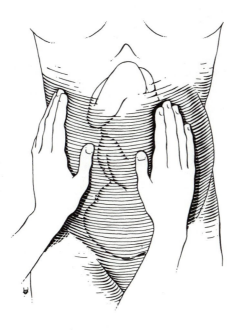

B. Second maneuver: Where is the back?

Figure 2. Abdominal palpation.

Third Maneuver: What Is in the Fundus?

The hands are moved up the sides of the uterus and the fundus is palpated (Fig. 2C). In most cases the breech is here. It is a less definite structure than the head and is not identified as easily. The breech is softer, more irregular, less globular, and not as mobile as the head. It is continuous with the back, there being no intervening groove. When the breech is moved laterally the body moves as well. Finding moving small parts in the vicinity of the breech strengthens the diagnosis.

Fourth Maneuver: Where Is the Cephalic Prominence?

The examiner turns and faces the patient's feet. Gently the fingers are moved down the sides of the uterus toward the pubis (Fig. 2D). The cephalic prominence is felt on the side where there is greater resistance to the descent of the fingers into the pelvis. In attitudes of flexion the forehead is the cephalic prominence. It is on the opposite side from the back. In extension attitudes the occiput is the cephalic prominence and is on the same side as the back. In addition it is noted whether the head is free and floating or fixed and engaged.

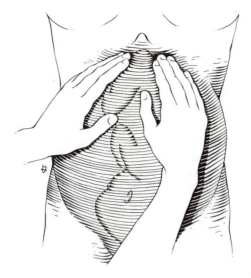

C. Third maneuver: What is in the fundus?

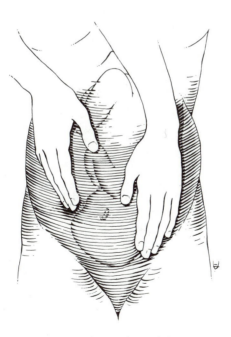

D. Fourth maneuver: Where is the cephalic prominence?

Figure 2. (cont.) Abdominal palpation.

Relationship of Head to Pelvis

1. The floating head lies entirely above the symphysis pubis, so that the examining fingers can be placed between the head and the pubis. The head is freely movable from side to side.
2. When the head is engaged, the biparietal diameter has passed the inlet and only a small part of the head may be palpable above the symphysis. The head is fixed and cannot be moved laterally. Sometimes it is so low in the pelvis that it can barely be felt through the abdomen.
3. The head may be midway between the previous two locations. Part of it is felt easily above the symphysis. It is not freely movable but is not fixed; nor is it engaged. The head is described as lying in the brim of the pelvis, or dipping. (See Chapter 8 under *Engagement* and Figures 1A, 1B, and 1C.)

AUSCULTATION OF FETAL HEART

The fetal heart should be auscultated every 15 minutes during the first stage of labor, and every 3 to 5 minutes in the second stage. It is heard best by using a fetoscope (Fig. 3). Information gained by listening to the fetal heart falls into two main groups. It tells us something about (1) the general health of the baby in utero, and (2) the presentation and position of the fetus.

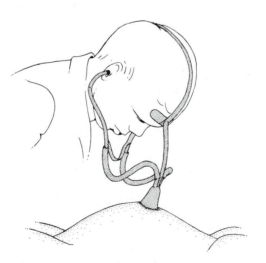

Figure 3. Auscultation of the fetal heart beat.

General Health of the Fetus

The general health of the fetus can be estimated by observing the rate and rhythm of its heart.

1. The presence of the fetal heart sound indicates that the baby is alive.
2. The normal heart rate is 120 to 160 beats/minute. The fetal heart becomes slower at the height of a uterine contraction and speeds up after the contraction has worn off. A fetal heart rate of less than 100 or more than 160/minute with the uterus at rest suggests fetal distress. A slow rate has a greater significance than a rapid one.
3. The rhythm is regular and of a "tic toc" quality. Irregularity is a sign of fetal embarrassment.
4. The loudness of the fetal heart, contrary to popular belief, is not a sign of fetal vigor. It depends upon the following:
   a. The relationship between the fetal back and the mother's abdomen. When the baby's back is near the anterior abdominal wall, the fetal heart is strong and near. This is so in anterior positions. In posterior positions, on the other hand, the fetal heart gives the impression of being far away.
   b. In obese women with thick abdominal walls the fetal heart is not heard clearly.
   c. An excessive amount of amniotic fluid muffles the fetal heart tones.
5. Other sounds may be heard:
   a. The funic souffle, which is synchronous with the fetal heart, is caused by the blood rushing through the umbilical arteries.
   b. The uterine (maternal) souffle pulses at the same speed as the maternal pulse and results from the blood passing through the large blood vessels of the uterus.
6. Failure to hear the fetal heart may result from one of the following:
   a. Too early in the pregnancy. The fetal heart is heard only rarely before the 18th week.
   b. Fetal death. Inability to hear the baby's heart in a patient in whom it has been audible previously is a suggestion of fetal death. Usually fetal activity has ceased.
   c. Maternal obesity.
   d. Polyhydramnios (an excessive amount of amniotic fluid).
   e. A loud maternal souffle that obscures the fetal heart tones, making it difficult or impossible to identify them.

    f. Posterior position of the occiput, where the fetal back is away from the anterior abdominal wall.

    g. At the height of a strong uterine contraction.

    h. Defective stethoscope.

    i. An excessive amount of noise in the room.

    j. Error by observer. In some instances one listener is unable to hear the fetal heart tones, while another can hear them clearly.

7. Ultrasound. When the fetal heart is not heard using the fetal stethoscope, ultrasonic equipment should be employed. By the Doppler technique the beating of the fetal heart can be detected reliably after 8 weeks. By the use of real-time imaging fetal movement can be seen as early as 6 to 7 weeks.

Presentation and Position

In most cases there is a constant relationship between the location of the baby's heart and the fetal position in the uterus. In attitudes of flexion the fetal heart sound is transmitted through the scapula and the back of the shoulder. It is therefore heard loudest in that area of the mother's abdomen to which the fetal back is closest. In attitudes of extension the fetal heart beat is transmitted through the anterior chest wall of the baby.

In cephalic presentations the fetal heart beat is loudest below the umbilicus; in anterior positions it is clearest in one or the other lower quadrant of the mother's abdomen. The relationship of the fetal back and the fetal heart to the midline of the maternal abdomen is similar. As the one comes nearer to or moves away from the midline, so does the other. In posterior positions the fetal heart is loudest in the maternal flank on the side to which the back is related. In breech presentation the point of maximum intensity of the baby's heart sound is above the umbilicus.

The position of the fetal heart changes with descent and rotation. As the baby descends, so does the fetal heart. The anterior rotation of an occipitoposterior position can be followed by listening to the fetal heart as it moves gradually from the maternal flank toward the midline of the abdomen.

The location of the fetal heart (Fig. 4) may be used to check, but should not be relied upon to make, the diagnosis of presentation and position. Occasionally the point of maximum intensity of the fetal heart beat is not in the expected location for a given position. For example, it is not unusual in breech presentations for the fetal heart to be heard loudest below the umbilicus, instead of above it. The diagnosis made by

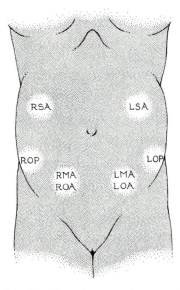

Figure 4. Location of the fetal heart beat in relation to the various positions.

careful abdominal palpation is the more reliable finding. Locating the fetal heart sound in an unexpected place is an indication for reexamination by palpation of the position of the infant. If the findings on palpation are confirmed, the locale of the fetal heart tones should be disregarded.

The Role of Continuous Electronic Fetal Heart Monitoring

The achievements of electronic monitoring of the fetal heart rate have been impressive. Unfortunately, excessive reliance has been placed on the machinery and clinical judgment denigrated. Good clinical evaluation encompassing all factors and data must be the final arbiter in selecting the optimal management for the particular patient.

It has been shown that for almost all normal cases, and even for some high-risk pregnancies, intermittent human auscultation of the fetal heart rate is almost as effective as continuous monitoring. To achieve this degree of excellence it is necessary that an almost one-to-one relationship exist between the patient and the nurse, that the auscultator be experienced, and that the fetal heart be evaluated rigidly every 15 minutes in the first stage and every 5 minutes in the second stage of labor. Auscultation of the fetal heart every 1 to 2 hours, not infrequently seen on a busy obstetrical service, is inadequate.

Indications for Electronic Fetal Heart Monitoring

1. Clinically detected abnormalities of the FHR
2. Meconium in the amniotic fluid
3. Stimulation of labor by oxytocin
4. Preterm labor
5. Slow progress in labor
6. Patients at high risk for uteroplacental insufficiency including those with:
   a. Previous stillbirth
   b. Hypertension and preeclampsia
   c. Intrauterine growth retardation
   d. Postterm pregnancy
   e. Abnormal presentation
   f. Rh affected infant
   g. Diabetes
   h. Premature rupture of the membranes
   i. Multiple gestation

RECTAL EXAMINATION

Because some obstetricians believe that there is danger of infection during vaginal examinations, the course of labor in normally progressing cases is followed by rectal examinations. During pregnancy and especially during labor the muscles of the pelvic floor soften and are more easily dilated, so that rectal examination is easier to perform. However, rectal examination is painful and should be done only as often as is necessary for the safe conduct of labor.

Rectal examination during labor has several drawbacks:

1. It is less accurate than vaginal examination and must not be relied on in problem cases.
2. The condition and dilatation of the cervix is often difficult to determine, especially when a bag of waters is present.
3. The caput succedaneum may be mistaken for the skull, resulting in erroneous diagnoses of station.
4. It is unreliable in breech presentation.
5. During examination the posterior wall of the vagina is pushed against the cervix, bringing the vaginal bacteria into direct contact with the cervix.
6. Rectal examination is painful and aggravates hemorrhoids.

VAGINAL EXAMINATION

Several recent studies demonstrated that there is no greater danger of infection with vaginal than with rectal examination. Points in favor of the vaginal examination in the management of labor are as follows:

1. Vaginal examination is more accurate than rectal examination in determining the condition and dilatation of the cervix, station and position of the presenting part, and relationship of the fetus to the pelvis.
2. Vaginal examination takes less time, requires less manipulation, and gives more information than the rectal approach.
3. Cultures taken during the puerperium from women whose vaginas were sterile on admittance to hospital showed no higher incidence of positive results in those who had vaginal examinations during labor than those who had only rectal evaluations.
4. Clinical studies have shown that maternal morbidity is no higher following vaginal than following rectal examinations.
5. Vaginal examination causes less pain.
6. Vaginaphobia leads to the dangerous attitude of always waiting a little longer before doing a necessary vaginal examination during labor.
7. Prolapse of the umbilical cord can be diagnosed early, as can compound presentations.
8. It is important to remember that a clean or sterile glove is different from the contaminated finger of Semmelweis's time, when doctors went from infected surgical cases to the maternity ward without using aseptic precautions.

The examination must be done gently, carefully, thoroughly, and under aseptic conditions. Sterile gloves should be used. We prefer the lithotomy or dorsal position, finding the examination and orientation easier. It is the best position for determining proportion between the presenting part and the pelvis.

Palpation of Cervix

1. Is the cervix soft or hard?
2. Is it thin and effaced or thick and long?
3. Is it easily dilated or is it resistant?
4. Is it closed or open? If it is open, estimate the length of the diameter of the cervical ring.

Presentation

1. What is the presentation—breech, cephalic, shoulder?
2. Is there a caput succedaneum, and is it small or extensive?
3. What is that station? What is the relationship of the presenting part (not the caput succedaneum) to a line between the ischial spines? If it is above the spines it is -1, -2 or -3 cm. If it is below the spines it is $+1$, $+2$, or $+3$ cm.

Position

1. If it is a breech, where is the sacrum? Are the legs flexed or extended?
2. With a cephalic presentation, identify the sagittal suture (Fig. 5A). What is its direction? Is it in the anteroposterior, oblique, or transverse diameter of the pelvis?
3. Is the sagittal suture midway between the pubis and the sacrum (synclitism); is it near the sacral promontory (anterior asynclitism); or is it near the pubic symphysis (posterior asynclitism)?
4. Is the bregma right or left, anterior or posterior? (It is diamond-shaped and is the meeting point of four sutures) (Fig. 5A.)
5. Where is the posterior fontanelle (Fig. 5B)? (It is Y-shaped and has three sutures.)
6. Is the head in flexion (occiput lower than sinciput) or is there extension (sinciput lower than occiput)?
7. In cases where there is difficulty in identifying the sutures, palpation of an ear (Fig. 5D) helps establish the direction of the sagittal suture and thus the anteroposterior diameter of the long axis of the head. The tragus points to the face.

Membranes

Feeling the bag of waters is evidence that the membranes are intact. The drainage of fluid, passage of meconium, and grasping of fetal hair in a clamp indicate that the membranes have ruptured.

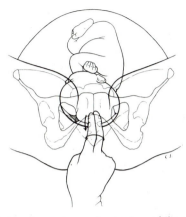

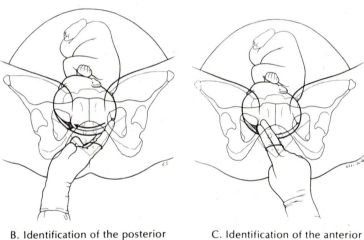

A. Determining the station and palpation of the sagittal suture.

B. Identification of the posterior fontanelle.

C. Identification of the anterior fontanelle.

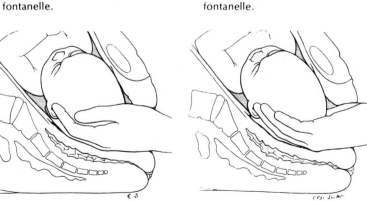

D. Palpation of the posterior ear.

Figure 5. Diagnosis of station and position. (*From Douglas and Stromme. Operative Obstetrics, 4th ed., 1982. Courtesy of Appleton-Century-Crofts.*)

General Assessment of Pelvis

1. Can the sacral promontory be reached? The diagonal conjugate can be measured clinically. It extends from the inferior margin of the pubic symphysis to the middle of the sacral promontory, and its average length is 12.5 cm. During the vaginal examination the promontory is palpated. When the distal end of the finger reaches the middle of the promontory, the point where the proximal part of the finger makes contact with the subpubic angle is marked (Figs. 6A, B, and C). The fingers are withdrawn from the vagina, and the distance between these two points is measured. By deducting 1.5 cm from the diagonal conjugate (Fig. 6C), the approximate length of the obstetric conjugate can be obtained. In many women the promontory cannot be reached, and this is accepted as evidence that the anteroposterior diameter of the inlet is adequate. If the promontory can be felt, the obstetric conjugate may be short.
2. Is the pelvic brim symmetrical?
3. Are the ischial spines prominent and posterior?
4. Is the sacrum long and straight or short and concave?
5. Are the side walls parallel or convergent?
6. Is the sacrosciatic notch wide or narrow?
7. Is there any bony or soft tissue encroachment into the cavity of the pelvis?
8. How wide is the subpubic angle? The distance between the ischial tuberosities (average 10.5 cm) can be measured roughly by placing a fist between them (Fig. 6D). If this can be done the transverse diameter of the outlet is considered adequate.
9. Are the soft tissues and the perineum relaxed and elastic or hard and rigid?

Fetopelvic Relationship

1. How does the presenting part fit the pelvis?
2. If engagement has not taken place, can the presenting part be pushed into the pelvis by fundal and suprapubic pressure?
3. Does the presenting part ride over the pubic symphysis?

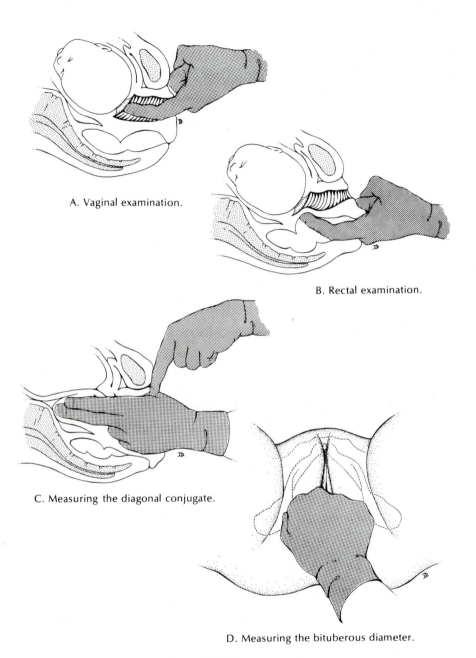

A. Vaginal examination.

B. Rectal examination.

C. Measuring the diagonal conjugate.

D. Measuring the bituberous diameter.

Figure 6. Pelvic assessment.

X-RAY EXAMINATION

In some problem cases radiologic pelvimetry can provide valuable information about the following:

1. Shape and type of pelvis
2. Internal measurements of pelvis
3. Presentation, position, and station of fetus
4. Relationship of fetus to pelvis
5. Estimate of fetal size

10

Anterior Positions of the Occiput and the Normal Mechanism of Labor

LEFT OCCIPUT ANTERIOR: LOA

LOA is a common longitudinal cephalic presentation (Fig. 1). The attitude is flexion, the presenting part is the posterior part of the vertex and the posterior fontanelle, and the denominator is the occiput (O).

Diagnosis of Position: LOA

Abdominal Examination

1. The lie is longitudinal. The long axis of the fetus is parallel to the long axis of the mother.
2. The head is at or in the pelvis.
3. The back is on the left and anterior and is palpated easily except in obese women.
4. The small parts are on the right and are not felt clearly.
5. The breech is in the fundus of the uterus.
6. The cephalic prominence (in this case the forehead) is on the right. When the attitude is flexion, the cephalic prominence and the back are on opposite sides. The reverse is true in attitudes of extension.

Fetal Heart

The fetal heart is heard loudest in the left lower quadrant of the mother's abdomen. In attitudes of flexion the fetal heart rate is transmitted through the baby's back. The point of maximum intensity varies with the degree of rotation. As the child's back approaches the midline of the maternal abdomen, so does the point where the fetal heart is heard most strongly. Therefore in a left anterior position it is heard below the umbilicus and somewhere to the left of the midline, depending on the exact situation of the back.

Vaginal Examination

1. The station of the head is noted—whether it is above, at, or below the ischial spines.
2. If the cervix is dilated, the suture lines and the fontanelles of the baby's head can be felt. In the LOA position the sagittal suture is in the right oblique diameter of the pelvis.
3. The small posterior fontanelle is anterior and to the mother's left.
4. The bregma is posterior and to the right.
5. Since the head is probably flexed, the occiput is a littler lower than the brow.

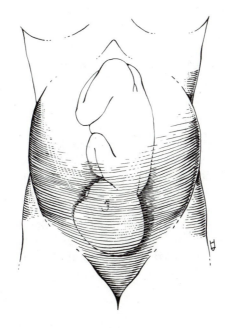

A. Abdominal view.

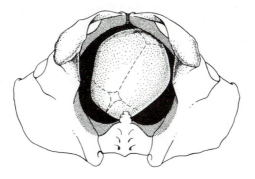

B. Vaginal view.

Figure 1. Left occiput anterior.

Normal Mechanism of Labor: LOA

The mechanism of labor as we know it today was described first by William Smellie during the eighteenth century. It is the way the baby adapts itself to and passes through the maternal pelvis. There are six movements, with considerable overlapping. The following description is for left anterior positions of the occiput.

Descent

Descent, which includes engagement in the right oblique diameter of the pelvis, continues throughout normal labor as the baby passes through the birth canal. The other movements are superimposed on it. In primigravidas considerable descent should have taken place before the onset of labor (Figs. 2A and B) in the process of engagement, provided there is no disproportion and the lower uterine segment is well formed. In multiparas engagement may not take place until good labor has set in. Descent is brought about by the downward pressure of the uterine contractions, aided in the second stage by the bearing-down efforts of the patient, and to a minimal extent by gravity.

Flexion

Partial flexion exists before the onset of labor, since this is the natural attitude of the fetus in utero. Resistance to descent leads to increased flexion. The occiput descends in advance of the sinciput, the posterior fontanelle is lower than the bregma, and the baby's chin approaches its chest (Figs. 3A and B). This usually takes place at the inlet, but it may not be complete until the presenting part reaches the pelvic floor. The effect of flexion is to change the presenting diameter from the occipitofrontal of 11.0 cm to the smaller and rounder suboccipitobregmatic of 9.5 cm. Since the fit between fetal head and maternal pelvis may be snug, the reduction of 1.5 cm in the presenting diameter is important.

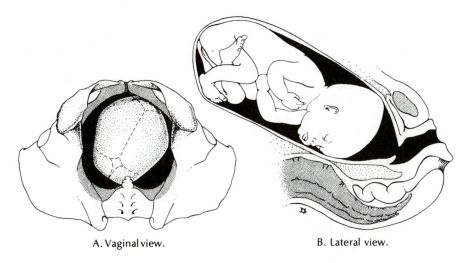

A. Vaginal view.   B. Lateral view.

Figure 2. Mechanism of labor: LOA. Onset of labor.

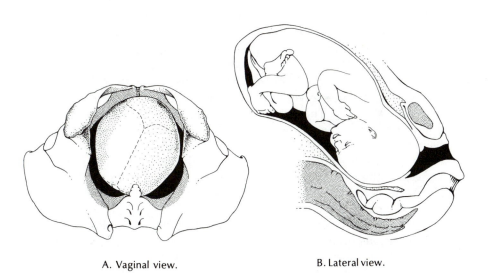

A. Vaginal view.   B. Lateral view.

Figure 3. Descent and flexion of the head.

Internal Rotation

In the majority of pelves the inlet is a transverse oval. The anteroposterior diameter of the midpelvis is a little longer than the transverse diameter. The outlet is an anteroposterior oval, as is the fetal head. The long axis of the fetal head must fit into the long axis of the maternal pelvis. Hence the head, which entered the pelvis in the transverse or oblique diameter, must rotate internally to the anteroposterior diameter in order to be born. This is the purpose of internal rotation (Fig. 4).

The occiput now leads the way to the midpelvis, where it makes contact with the pelvic floor (the levator ani muscles and fascia). Here the occiput rotates 45° to the right (toward the midline). The sagittal suture turns from the right oblique diameter to the anteroposterior diameter of the pelvis: LOA to OA. The occiput comes to lie near the pubic symphysis and the sinciput near the sacrum.

The head rotates from the right oblique diameter to the anteroposterior diameter of the pelvis. The shoulders, however, remain in the left oblique diameter. Thus the normal relationship of the long axis of the head to the long axis of the shoulders is changed, and the neck undergoes a twist of 45°. This situation is maintained as long as the head is in the pelvis.

We do not know accurately why the fetal head, which entered the pelvis in the transverse or oblique diameter, rotates so that the occiput turns anteriorly in the great majority of cases and posteriorly in so few. One explanation is based on pelvic architecture. Both the bones and the soft tissues play a part. The ischial spines extend into the pelvic cavity. The sidewalls of the pelvis anterior to the spines curve forward, downward, and medially. The pelvic floor, made up of the levator ani muscles and fascia, slopes downward, forward, and medially. The part of the head that reaches the pelvic floor and ischial spines first is rotated anteriorly by these structures. In most cases the head is well flexed when it reaches the pelvic floor, and the occiput is lower than the sinciput. Hence the occiput strikes the pelvic floor first and is rotated anteriorly under the pubic symphysis.

This does not explain why some well flexed heads in the LOT and ROT positions (proved by x-ray) do not rotate posteriorly. Nor do the theories based upon pelvic architecture explain the situation in which, in the same patient, the head rotates anteriorly during one labor and posteriorly in another. In truth we do not know the exact reasons internal rotation takes place in the way it does. In most labors internal rotation is complete when the head reaches the pelvic floor, or soon after. Early internal rotation is frequent in multiparas and in patients having efficient uterine contractions. Internal rotation takes place mainly during the second stage of labor.

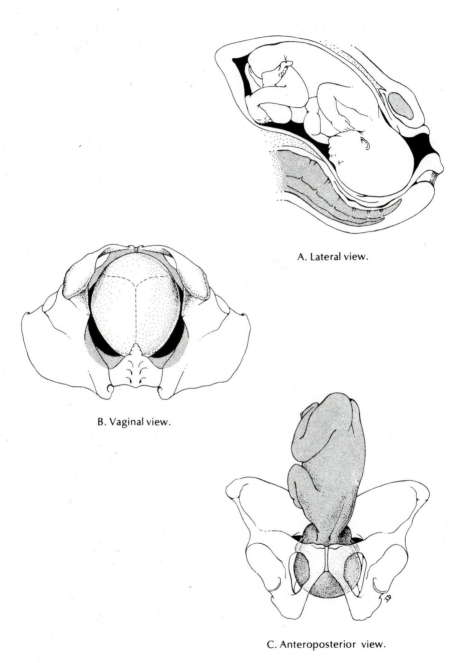

A. Lateral view.

B. Vaginal view.

C. Anteroposterior view.

Figure 4. Internal rotation: LOA to OA.

Extension

Extension (Fig. 5) is basically the result of two forces: (1) uterine contractions exerting downward pressure and (2) the pelvic floor offering resistance. It must be pointed out that the anterior wall of the pelvis (the pubis) is only 4 to 5 cm long, while the posterior wall (the sacrum) is 10 to 15 cm. Hence the sinciput has a greater distance to travel than the occiput. As the flexed head continues its descent there is bulging of the perineum followed by crowning. The occiput passes through the outlet slowly, and the nape of the neck pivots in the subpubic angle. Then by a rapid process of extension the sinciput sweeps along the sacrum, and the bregma, forehead, nose, mouth, and chin are born in succession over the perineum.

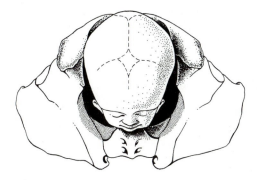

A. Vaginal view.

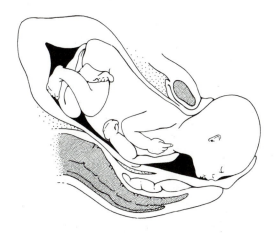

B. Lateral view.

Figure 5. Extension of the head: birth.

Restitution

When the head reaches the pelvic floor the shoulders enter the pelvis (Fig. 6). Since the shoulders remain in the oblique diameter while the head rotates anteriorly, the neck becomes twisted. Once the head is born and is free of the pelvis, the neck untwists and the head restitutes back 45° (OA to LOA) to resume the normal relationship with the shoulders and its original position in the pelvis.

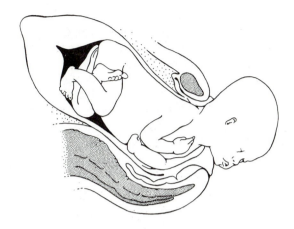

A. Lateral view.

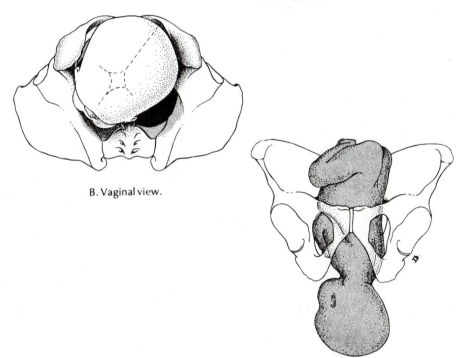

B. Vaginal view.

C. Anteroposterior view.

Figure 6. Restitution: OA to LOA.

External Rotation

External rotation of the head is really the outward manifestation of internal rotation of the shoulders. As the shoulders reach the pelvic floor the lower anterior shoulder is rotated forward under the symphysis, and the bisacromial diameter turns from the left oblique to the anteroposterior diameter of the pelvis. In this way the long diameter of the shoulders can fit the long diameter of the outlet. The head, which had already restituted 45° to resume its normal relationship to the shoulders, now rotates another 45° to maintain it: LOA to LOT (Fig. 7).

A summary of the mechanism of labor to this point is seen in Figure 8.

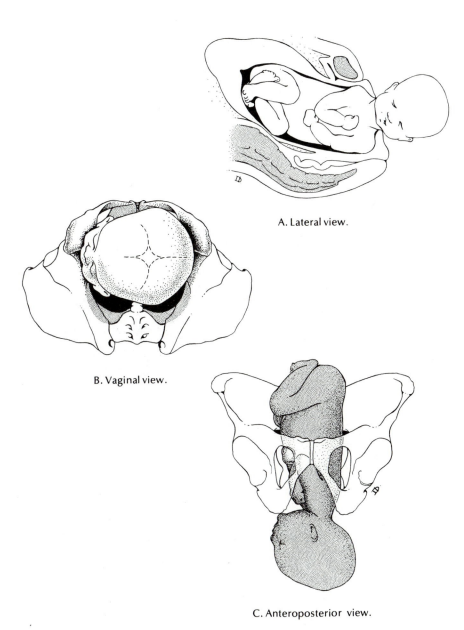

A. Lateral view.

B. Vaginal view.

C. Anteroposterior view.

Figure 7. External rotation: LOA to LOT.

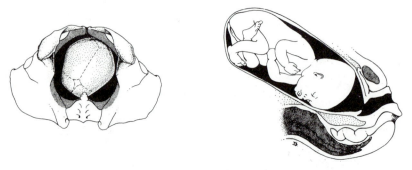

A. Onset of labor.

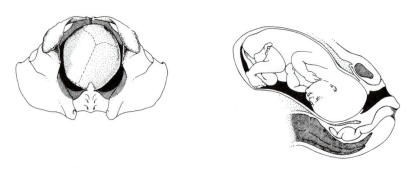

B. Descent and flexion.

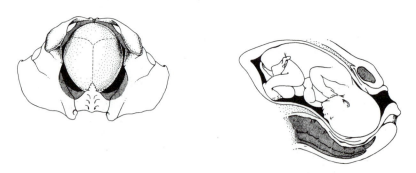

C. Internal rotation: LOA to OA.

Figure 8. Summary of mechanism of labor: LOA.

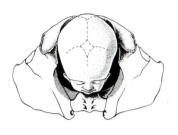 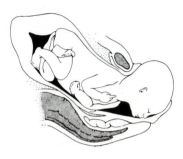

D. Extension.

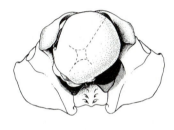 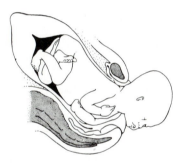

E. Restitution: OA to LOA.

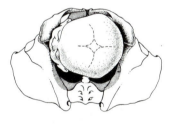 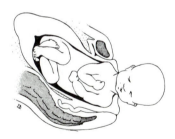

F. External rotation: LOA to LOT.

Figure 8. (cont.) Summary of mechanism of labor: LOA.

Mechanism of Shoulders

When the head appears at the outlet, the shoulders enter the inlet. They engage in the oblique diameter opposite that of the head. For example, in LOA, when the head engages in the right oblique diameter of the inlet the shoulders engage in the left oblique.

The uterine contractions and the bearing-down efforts of the mother force the baby downward. The anterior shoulder reaches the pelvic floor first and rotates anteriorly under the symphysis. Anterior rotation of the shoulders takes place in a direction opposite to that of anterior rotation of the head. The anterior shoulder is born under the pubic symphysis and pivots there (Fig. 9A). Then the posterior shoulder slides over the perineum by a movement of lateral flexion (Fig. 9B).

Birth of Trunk and Extremities

Once the shoulders have been born the rest of the child is delivered by the mother's forcing down, with no special mechanism, and with no difficulty.

Molding

In LOA the presenting suboccipitobregmatic diameter is diminished, and the head is elongated in the verticomental diameter (Fig. 10).

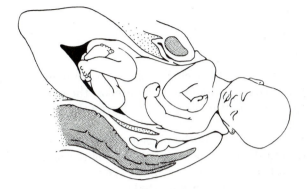

A. Birth of anterior shoulder.

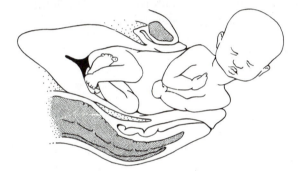

B. Birth of posterior shoulder.

Figure 9. Birth of the shoulders.

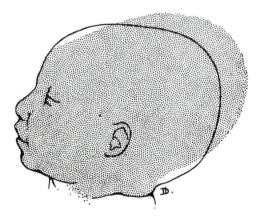

Figure 10. Molding: LOA.

BIRTH OF PLACENTA

Separation of Placenta

Within a few minutes of delivery of the child the uterine contractions begin again. Because the fetus is no longer in the uterus, the extent of the retraction of the upper segment is larger than during the first and second stages. This retraction decreases greatly the area where the placenta is attached (Fig. 11A). The size of the placenta itself, however, is not reducible. The resultant disparity between the size of the placenta and its area of attachment leads to a cleavage in the spongy layer of the decidua, and in this way the placenta is separated from the wall of the uterus (Fig. 11B). During the process of separation blood accumulates between the placenta and uterus. When the detachment is complete the blood is released and gushes from the vagina.

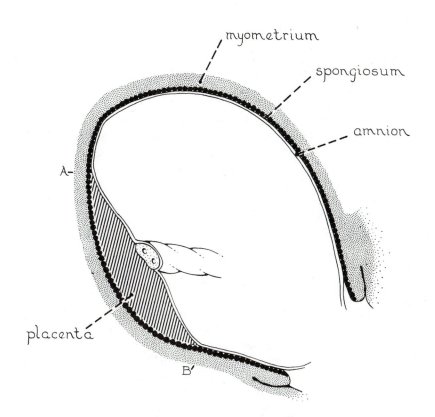

A. Placenta attached to uterine wall.

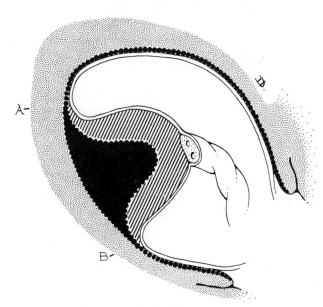

B. Placenta separated from uterine wall.

Figure 11. Birth of the placenta.

Expulsion of Placenta

Soon after the placenta has separated it is expelled into the vagina by the uterine contractions. From here it is delivered by the bearing-down efforts of the patient. Two methods of expulsion have been described. In the Duncan method the lower edge of the placenta comes out first, with the maternal and fetal surfaces appearing together, and the rest of the organ slides down. In the Schultze method the placenta comes out like an inverted umbrella, the shiny fetal side appearing first, and the membranes trailing after. Although the Schultze mechanism suggests fundal implantation, while the Duncan method intimates that the placenta was attached to the wall of the uterus, the exact birth mechanism of the placenta is of little practical significance.

Control of Hemorrhage

The blood vessels that pass through the myometrium are tortuous and angular. The muscle fibers are arranged in an interlacing network through which the blood vessels pass. After the placenta has separated, retraction leads to a permanent shortening of the uterine muscle fibers. This compresses, kinks, twists, and closes the arterioles and venules in the manner of living ligatures. The blood supply to the placental site is effectively shut off, and bleeding is controlled. If the uterus is atonic and fails to retract properly after separation of the placenta, the vessels are not closed off, and postpartum hemorrhage may take place.

CLINICAL COURSE OF LABOR: LOA

Almost always an LOA turns 45° to bring the occiput under the pubic arch, from where spontaneous delivery takes place. Occasionally, because of minor degrees of disproportion, a rigid perineum, or generalized fatigue, the patient may not be able to complete the second stage.

Arrests may take place in two positions:

1. It can occur after rotation to occiput anterior (OA) is complete, so that the sagittal suture is in the anteroposterior diameter.
2. Rotation may fail, the fetal head remaining in the original LOA position, with the sagittal suture in the right oblique diameter of the pelvis.

Management of arrested occipitoanterior positions consists of the following steps:

1. If rotation to OA has occurred, the forceps are applied to the sides of the baby's head, which is then extracted. (See Chapter 25 for details of technique.)

2. If rotation has failed, the forceps are applied to the sides of the baby's head. First the head is rotated with the forceps from LOA to OA and then it is extracted. (See Chapter 25 for details of technique.)

RIGHT OCCIPUT ANTERIOR: ROA

ROA is less common than LOA. The physical findings and the mechanism of labor are similar but opposite to LOA. The difference lies in the fact that in ROA the occiput and back of the fetus are on the mother's right side, while the small parts are on the left.

11

Clinical Course of Normal Labor

DEFINITIONS

LABOR   A function of the female by which the products of conception (fetus, amniotic fluid, placenta, and membranes) are separated and expelled from the uterus through the vagina into the outside world.

PRETERM LABOR   The onset of regular uterine contractions accompanied by cervical effacement and/or dilatation and fetal descent in a gravid woman whose period of gestation is less than 37 completed weeks (less than 259 days) from the first day of the last menstrual period.

EUTOCIA   Normal labor. Labor is considered normal when the child presents by the vertex of the head, when there are no complications, and when the labor is completed by the natural efforts of the mother. It should take no longer than 24 hours.

DYSTOCIA   Abnormal labor.

EXPECTED DATE OF CONFINEMENT   On an average this is 280 days from the first day of the last menstrual period or 267 days from conception. It is calculated by going back 3 months from the first day of the last menses and adding 7 days.

ONSET OF LABOR

Causes of Onset of Labor

Hippocrates' concept that the fetus determines the time of its birth has been proven correct in some animals. In humans, however, it appears that the placenta and fetal membranes play the major role in the initiation of labor, while the fetus may modulate the timing of labor. While the exact cause of and mechanism for the provoking of labor are not known, evidence is mounting in support of a hormonal basis.

In the sheep it is clear that maturation of the fetal hypothalamo-hypophyseal-adrenal axis during late pregnancy is responsible for initiating labor by inducing changes in the pattern of placental steroid genesis and, ultimately, by increasing the production of intrauterine prostaglandin. Birth can be induced by infusing ACTH or glucocorticoids to the fetal lamb in utero before term has been reached. These preterm fetuses are viable, and are able to expand their lungs, indicating that the fetal glucocorticoids play a role in pulmonary maturation as well as in parturition. In sheep, as in humans, the nature of the stimulus that leads to increased pituitary-adrenal activity in late pregnancy is not known.

At the present time there is no evidence that the human fetus plays the same pivotal role in determining the time it is born as does the sheep. The belief that anencephaly and adrenal hypoplasia predispose to prolongation of pregnancy has been challenged. In both humans and monkeys the administration of glucocorticoids does not bring on labor, nor is there evidence to show that fetal cortisol sets off parturition in humans.

Estrogen. Although there is some evidence that estrogen may be involved in human parturition, its main source and its mode of action has not been established.

Progesterone. In some animals progesterone plays a part in maintaining uterine quiescence. In primates the role of progesterone is unclear. The concentrations of progesterone in the maternal plasma do not seem to decrease before the spontaneous onset of labor. There is, to the contrary, some evidence that the levels of free progesterone may rise as parturition approaches.

Oxytocin. The sensitivity of the uterus to oxytocin increases in late pregnancy, as does the pulsatile release of oxytocin as labor progresses. However, the role of oxytocin in the initiation of human parturition is unclear. Fetal production of oxytocin has been demonstrated, but the pathways by which the peptide reaches the myometrium have not been established.

Prostaglandin. Three lines of evidence support the part played by prostaglandin in human parturition: (1) There is an increase in the production of prostaglandin at term. (2) Myometrial contractility and preterm labor can be suppressed by the use of inhibitors of the synthesis of prostaglandin. (3) Exogenous prostaglandins stimulate the primate uterus to contract. Whether the primary effect of prostaglandin at term is exerted by increased biosynthesis, by increased myometrial sensitivity, or both, is not yet known.

Phenomena Preliminary to the Onset of Labor

1. Lightening occurs 2 to 3 weeks before term and is the subjective sensation felt by the mother as the baby settles into the lower uterine segment.
2. Engagement takes place 2 to 3 weeks before term in primigravidas.
3. Vaginal secretions increase in amount.
4. Loss of weight is caused by the excretion of body water.
5. The mucous plug is discharged from the cervix.
6. Bloody show is noted.
7. The cervix becomes soft and effaced.
8. Persistent backache is present.
9. False labor pains occur with variable frequency.

TRUE AND FALSE LABOR

Signs of True Labor

1. Uterine contractions occur at regular intervals. Coming every 20 or 30 minutes at the beginning, the contractions get closer together. As labor proceeds the contractions increase in duration and severity.
2. The uterine systoles are painful.
3. Hardening of the uterus is palpable.
4. Pain is felt both in the back and in the front of the abdomen.
5. True labor is effective in dilating the cervix.
6. The presenting part descends.
7. The head is fixed between pains.
8. Bulging of the membranes is a frequent result.

False Labor Pains

False labor pains are inefficient contractions of the uterus or painful spasms of the intestines, bladder, and abdominal wall muscles. They appear a few days to a month before term. They are sometimes brought on by a digestive upset or a strong laxative. Usually they start on their own. They are irregular and short, and are felt more in the front than in the back.

There may be either no accompanying uterine contraction at all, or one that lasts only a few seconds. The uterus does not become stony hard and can be indented with the finger. These contractions are inefficient in pushing down the presenting part and do not bring about progressive effacement and dilatation of the cervix.

False labor pains can have the harmful effect of tiring the patient, so that when true labor does begin she is in poor condition, both mentally and physically. The treatment is directed to the cause if there is one, or the physician can prescribe an efficient sedative that stops the false labor pains but does not interfere with true labor.

True Labor	False Labor
Pains at regular intervals	Irregular
Intervals gradually shorten	No change
Duration and severity increase	No change
Pain starts in back and moves to front	Pain mainly in front
Walking increases the intensity	No change
Association between the degree of uterine hardening and intensity of pain	No relationship
Bloody show often present	No show
Cervix effaced and dilated	No change in cervix
Descent of presenting part	No descent
Head is fixed between pains	Head remains free
Sedation does not stop true labor	Efficient sedative stops false labor pains

The strength of the uterine contractions can be estimated clinically by using the following criteria (Table 1):

TABLE 1: STRENGTH OF UTERINE CONTRACTIONS

	Frequency	Duration	Indentibility of Uterus
Good	q 2–3 min	45–60 sec	None
Fair	q 4–5 min	30–45 sec	Slight
Poor	q 6+ min	<30 sec	Easy

STAGES OF LABOR

First Stage. From the onset of true labor to complete dilatation of the cervix. It lasts 6 to 18 hours in a primigravida, and 2 to 10 hours in a multipara.

Second Stage. From complete dilatation of the cervix to the birth of the baby. It takes 30 minutes to 3 hours in a primigravida, and 5 to 30 minutes in the multipara. The median duration is slightly under 20 minutes in multiparas, and just under 50 minutes for primigravidas.

Third Stage. From the birth of the baby to delivery of the placenta. It takes 5 to 30 minutes.

Fourth Stage. From the birth of the placenta until the postpartum condition of the patient has become stabilized.

First Stage of Labor

The first stage of labor lasts from the onset of true labor to full dilatation of the cervix. The contractions are intermittent and painful, and the uterine hardening is felt easily by a hand on the abdomen. The pains become more frequent and more severe as labor proceeds. As a rule they begin in the back and pass to the front of the abdomen and the upper thighs.

Effacement and Dilatation of the Cervix

During most of pregnancy the cervix uteri is about 2.5 cm in length and closed. Toward the end of the period of gestation progressive changes occur in the cervix, including softening, effacement (shortening), dilatation, and movement from a posterior to an anterior position in the vagina. The internal os starts to disappear as the cervical canal becomes part of the lower segment of the uterus. The extent to which these changes have taken place correlates with the proximity of the onset of labor and with the success of attempts to induce labor.

Ideally, the cervix should be ripe at the onset of labor. A ripe cervix is (1) soft, (2) less than 1.3 cm in length, (3) admits a finger easily, and (4) is dilatable. The presence of a ripe cervix is one indication that the uterus is ready to begin labor. During labor the cervix shortens further and the external os dilates. When the cervix has opened enough (average 10 cm) to permit passage of the fetal head it is described as being fully dilated (Fig. 1).

Ripening of the cervix is a gradual process that merges into labor. The rigid collagen bundles rearrange themselves in a more flexible pattern so that the fibers are able to slide over each other more freely. During pregnancy this process takes place gradually, resulting in softening, shortening, and partial dilatation of the cervix. These changes may begin as early as the 24th to 28th week of pregnancy. The mechanisms that control cervical ripening are not well understood, but they are linked with those that control parturition. Factors that play a part include the Braxton-Hicks contractions (usually painless) of the uterus pulling on the cervix, and hormones such as estrogen, progesterone, relaxin, oxytocin, and prostaglandin.

The changes in the cervix during pregnancy can be correlated to the time of onset of labor. Women whose cervices ripen early are likely to begin labor before 40 weeks. When the cervix remains unripe until late in pregnancy, prolongation of the gestation past 40 weeks is common.

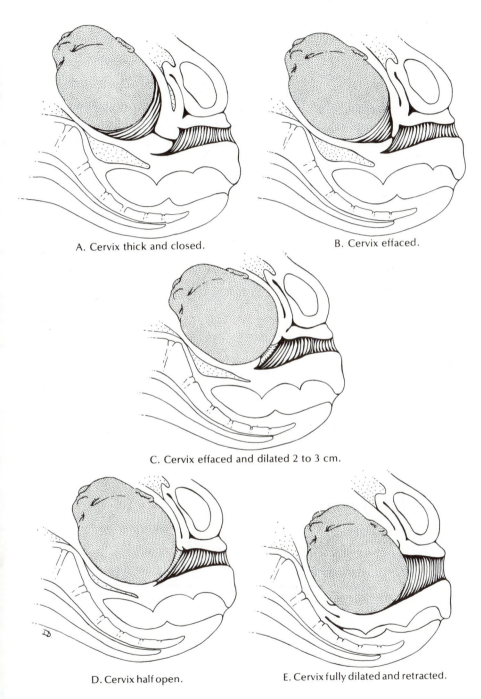

A. Cervix thick and closed.

B. Cervix effaced.

C. Cervix effaced and dilated 2 to 3 cm.

D. Cervix half open.

E. Cervix fully dilated and retracted.

Figure 1. Dilatation of the cervix.

Phases of the First Stage of Labor

The Latent Phase. There is a variable but substantial period after labor begins when little appears to be happening (Fig. 2). However, the contractions are becoming coordinated, stronger, polarized, and more efficient. At the same time the cervix is becoming softer, pliable, and more elastic. The average latent phase lasts 8.6 hours in nulliparas, and 5.3 hours in multiparas (Table 2). The normal latent phase does not exceed 20 hours in the former and 14 hours in the latter. Patients who enter labor with a ripe cervix have a shorter latent phase than those whose cervix is unripe.

The Active Phase. The dilatation of the cervix has reached 3 to 4 cm. Although there may be no great change in the uterine contractions, the cervix has undergone important alterations that make it more responsive, and dilatation proceeds rapidly. The average length of the active phase is 5.8 hours in nulliparas and 2.5 hours in multiparas, with the limits of normal being 12 and 6 hours (Table 2).

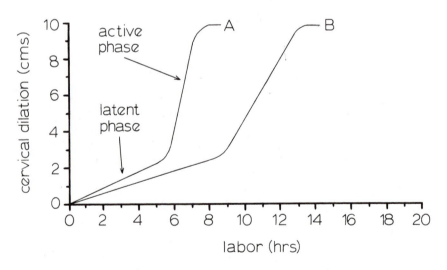

Figure 2. First stage of labor: Friedman curve.

TABLE 2. LENGTHS OF THE PHASES OF LABOR

	Primigravidas		Multiparas	
	Average	**Upper Normal**	**Average**	**Upper Normal**
Latent phase	8.6 hrs	20 hrs	5.3 hrs	14 hrs
Active phase	5.8 hrs	12 hrs	2.5 hrs	6 hrs
First stage of labor	13.3 hrs	28.5 hrs	7.5 hrs	20 hrs
Second stage labor	57 min	2.5 hrs	18 min	50 min
Rate of cervical dilatation during active phase	Under 1.2 cm/hr is abnormal		Under 1.5 cm/hr is abnormal	

Descent of the Presenting Part. During the latent and early active phase of cervical dilatation fetal descent may be minimal. Once the phase of rapid cervical dilatation has begun, steady fetal descent usually begins. The greatest degree of descent takes place when the cervix nears full dilatation and in the second stage of labor. Once descent begins it should be progressive. Descent of less than 1 cm per hour in nulliparas and 2 cm per hour in multiparas is abnormal and investigation is indicated.

Bag of Waters: Membranes

The fetus lies in a sac with an inner layer of amnion and an outer covering of chorion. The sac is filled with the amniotic fluid. As labor proceeds and the internal os becomes effaced and opens, the membranes separate from the lower uterine segment. The lower pole of the membranes bulges a little with each contraction and may adopt various shapes:

1. The protruding part may have the shape of a watch glass (Fig. 3A) containing a small amount of amniotic fluid. This is called the forewaters.
2. In other cases the membranes point into the cervix like a cone (Fig. 3B).
3. Still again, the bag may hang into the vagina (Fig. 3C).
4. In some cases the membranes are applied so tightly to the fetal head that no bag forms (Fig. 3D).

Frequently the membranes rupture near the end of the second stage, but this event can take place at any time during or before labor. When the membranes rupture, the fluid may come away with a gush or may dribble away. On occasion it is difficult to know whether the membranes are ruptured or intact. Methods of determining whether the bag of waters has ruptured include:

1. Observation of the escape of fluid from the vagina spontaneously or as a result of manual pressure on the uterus.
2. Putting a speculum in the vagina and seeing whether fluid is coming from the cervix. The amount may be increased by pressure on the fundus of the uterus.
3. The passage of meconium.
4. Use of Nitrazine paper to determine the pH of the vaginal fluid. The vagina, normally acidic, becomes neutral or alkaline when contaminated with alkaline amniotic fluid. Hence an alkaline pH in the vagina suggests that the membranes are ruptured.
5. Use of special staining of vaginal fluid, followed by microscopic search for components of amniotic fluid, including lanugo hairs, fetal squamous cells, and fat. Quinaldine blue stains fetal cells only faintly, while vaginal squamous cells become dark.
6. The arborization test depends on the property of dried amniotic fluid to form crystals in an arborization pattern. A few drops of vaginal fluid are aspirated from the vagina by a bulb syringe and are placed on a clean, dry glass slide. After waiting 5 to 7 minutes for drying to take place, the slide is examined under the low power microscope for identification of the arborization pattern.

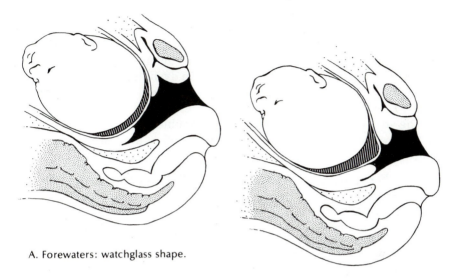

A. Forewaters: watchglass shape.

B. Forewaters: cone into the cervix.

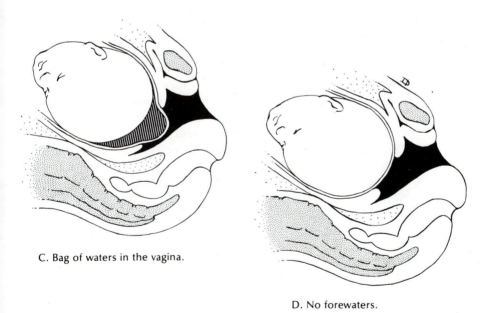

C. Bag of waters in the vagina.

D. No forewaters.

Figure 3. The membranes.

A bag of waters that hangs into the vagina is of little or no help in dilating the cervix; it may impede labor by filling the vagina and preventing descent of the fetal head. The intact bag of amniotic fluid does little to help labor progress. In normal cases after the membranes have ruptured (spontaneously or artificially) the uterine contractions are more efficient and labor progresses faster. In dysfunctional labor, however, or in the presence of an unripe cervix (one that is thick, hard, and closed), amniotomy is ineffectual in shortening labor and may complicate the situation by introducing an irreversible factor.

Several conditions should be present before amniotomy is performed:

1. Labor is in progress, as indicated by observed change in the cervix.
2. The cervix is at least 3 cm dilated.
3. The head is fixed in the pelvis and applied to the cervix.

Management: First Stage of Labor

1. As long as the patient is healthy, the presentation normal, the presenting part engaged, and the fetus in good condition, the parturient may walk about or may be in bed, as she wishes. There is evidence to suggest that uterine action is more efficient, the duration of labor shorter, the need for analgesia less, and the necessity of augmenting labor by oxytocin less in women who are ambulatory during labor as compared with those who remain in bed.
2. The patient's condition and progress is checked periodically. The pulse, temperature, and blood pressure are measured every 4 hours or more often if necessary.
3. The fetal heart is auscultated every 15 minutes if normal and more frequently if irregular or slow.
4. The progress of labor is followed by abdominal, rectal, or vaginal examination to note the position of the baby, station of the presenting part, and dilatation of the cervix. These examinations should be done only often enough to ensure safe conduct of labor.
5. Enema: It is a routine in many hospitals to give the patient an enema when she is admitted to the labor ward. The purpose is to stimulate uterine contractions, to clean the rectum, and to prevent fecal contamination of the infant and the genital tract. Recent studies have shown that giving an enema made no difference in the incidence of fecal contamination. Many women

object to having an enema. It is, probably, necessary to administer an enema only to those women who have a full rectum or who have not had a bowel movement in the last 24 hours.

6. Overdistention of the bladder is obviated by urging the patient to pass urine every few hours. Occasionally catheterization may be necessary, mainly for the patient's comfort. The distensible part of the bladder is largely abdominal during the active phase of labor, and it is rare for a full bladder to interfere with progress in a normal case. Since catheterization does not improve the progress of labor and does increase the risk of infection, it should be carried out only when absolutely necessary.

7. Adequate amounts of fluid and nourishment are essential. In most normal labors sugared drinks or clear soups can be taken by mouth. Since solid foods remain in the stomach during labor, tend to be vomited, and increase the danger of aspiration, they should not be given. If the patient is unable to take enough orally, an intravenous infusion of crystalloid solution is given.

8. The patient must rest and maintain her self-restraint. This is important, for lost control is difficult to regain. The attendants can help the patient by continual reassurance, frequent encouragement, and judicious sedation. Such relaxation helps the patient rest, assists her in keeping control, and accelerates the progress of labor. When the pains are severe an analgesic preparation may be given. Since there is a limit to the amount of drugs that can be administered without harming the baby or interfering with labor, these must be given in logical dosage and sequence. (It has been said that the best sedative for a woman in labor is to see her doctor at the side of the bed.)

9. During the first stage the patient is impressed continually with the importance of relaxing with the contractions. Bearing down must be avoided, as it does nothing to improve progress. Bearing down comes into its own use when the cervix is fully dilated and not before. During the first stage it has only bad effects:
   a. It delays cervical dilatation.
   b. It tires the patient needlessly.
   c. It forces down the uterus and stretches the supporting ligaments, predisposing to later prolapse.

10. Measures to improve the character and the efficiency of the contractions include:
   a. Hot soapsuds enema.
   b. Artificial rupture of the membranes.
   c. Oxytocin.

d. Ambulation: Walking about during labor stimulates the cervix and reflexly intensifies the uterine contractions. It has been shown that in ambulant patients the duration is shorter, the need for analgesia is less, and the incidence of abnormalities of the fetal heart lower than in recumbent women.

11. Artificial rupture of membranes: Amniotomy for the purpose of inducing labor has been practiced for centuries, but its use to augment established labor is more recent. Many physicians perform amniotomy as soon as patients are admitted to hospital in well-established labor. Without this interference the membranes remain intact until the second stage of labor in some two-thirds of patients.

  a. Advantages of amniotomy:

    i. It enables the condition of the amniotic fluid to be observed, especially the presence or absence of meconium.

    ii. Where continuous FHR monitoring is indicated the electrode can be placed directly on the fetal scalp, providing a better tracing than is obtained by an electrode on the mother's abdomen.

    iii. A recording catheter can be placed inside the uterus and can measure intrauterine pressure directly and accurately.

    iv. It may shorten the duration of labor. It is believed that the better application of the fetal head to the cervix improves the pattern of dilatation and, also, that direct pressure on the cervix leads to improved uterine contractions by reflex action. Recent evidence suggests that anmiotomy and stimulation of the lower genital tract leads to increased production of prostaglandins, and that these improve uterine contractions.

  b. Disadvantages of amniotomy. There is some feeling that early amniotomy may be harmful to the fetus:

    i. The increased pressure differentials around the fetal head may lead to deformities of the skull.

    ii. The reduction in the amount of amniotic fluid may increase compression of the umbilical cord.

  c. While early amniotomy may accelerate cervical dilatation, it may also result in reduced placental blood flow. The benefit of a shorter labor may be outweighed by potentially harmful effects on the fetus, such as reduction in the pH of the blood. Some workers have noted changes in the FHR patterns following amniotomy.

Most obstetricians feel that in properly selected cases the advantages of amniotomy outweigh the disadvantages.

12. While an intravenous infusion is useful in normal labor, it is mandatory in the difficult cases for the following reasons:

a. Fluids and nourishment can be given without provoking emesis. The woman who cannot take adequate fluids by mouth or who is nauseated or vomiting can be maintained in a state of good hydration.

b. Analgesics in small amounts can be administered for rapid effect.

c. When uterine action is inefficient pitocin added to the solution improves labor.

d. When there is excessive bleeding in the third or fourth stages, oxytocic agents can be given quickly.

e. Blood and plasma expanders may be infused without delay.

f. Once hypotension has occurred the veins often collapse and it is difficult to insert a needle. Having an infusion already underway obviates this problem.

g. Recent evidence has suggested that infusions of glucose-containing solutions given to the mother may be harmful to the fetus. Glucose crosses the placenta easily, while insulin does not. The fetal pancreas can respond to a load of glucose by increasing the output of insulin. The sequence of events appears to be: Maternal hyperglycemia $\longrightarrow$ fetal hyperglycemia $\longrightarrow$ fetal hyperinsulinemia $\longrightarrow$ fetal hypoglycemia. Because glucose offers, in most cases, no benefit to the mother that solutions without glucose do not, and because both hyper- and hypoglycemia may be bad for the fetus and the newborn infant, glucose should not be infused to the prepartum or intrapartum patient unless there are indications to do so. If an infusion of glucose is necessary, the rate of the infusion before delivery should not exceed 20 g per hour, and the maternal level of glucose should not be above 120 mg per dl at the time of delivery. Infants whose mothers have been given an excessive amount of glucose must be monitored for hypoglycemia in the first two hours of life.

Passage of Meconium in Cephalic Presentations

The passage per vaginam of meconium or meconium-stained amniotic fluid when the fetal presentation is cephalic may be a sign of fetal distress. It is believed to result from relaxation of the rectal sphincter and increased peristalsis as a consequence of fetal hypoxia. However, the passage of meconium may represent nothing more than fetal maturity. In most cases no cause is found.

The incidence of meconium staining is around 5 percent. The occurrence of stillbirth, when this is the only sign, is low, but the number of newborns requiring resuscitation is higher than the overall incidence.

When meconium is passed the fetal heart must be observed closely. Should there be a significant alteration in the rate and rhythm of the fetal heart, immediate delivery may be needed to save the child. Operative delivery is not indicated on the basis of meconium staining alone, however.

In breech presentations the passage of meconium is caused by pressure of the uterine contractions on the fetal intestines and is not accepted as a sign of anoxia or fetal distress.

Second Stage of Labor

The second stage of labor lasts from the end of the first stage, when the cervix has reached full dilatation, to the birth of the baby. As the patient passes through the end of the first stage and into the second stage, the contractions become more frequent and are accompanied by some of the worst pain of the whole labor. Once the second stage is achieved the discomfort is less.

There are clinical indications that the second stage has started:

1. There is an increase in bloody show.
2. The patient wants to bear down with each contraction.
3. She feels pressure on the rectum accompanied by the desire to defecate.
4. Nausea and retching occur frequently as the cervix reaches full dilatation.

These signs are not infallible, and the condition of the cervix and station of the presenting part must be confirmed by rectal or vaginal examination.

Position for Delivery

The adaptability of the human female has led to a wide variation of the delivery positions used by various cultures. There is no single correct position; each has its good and bad features.

During the second and third stages of labor the expulsive powers include (1) involuntary uterine contractions, (2) voluntary efforts of the abdominal, thoracic, and diaphragmatic muscles, and (3) action of the levator ani muscles.

Positions for giving birth may be grouped:

Upright or Vertical. Included are the standing, sitting, squatting, and upright-kneeling positions. Most delivery positions illustrated in historic texts show the parturient in an upright posture with abducted thighs, indicating that women preferred to be delivered with their trunks vertical. This is evidence that the adoption of a squatting position increases both the transverse and the anteroposterior diameters of the outlet of the pelvis. Studies have shown that the woman can create 30 percent more intraabdominal pressure in the vertical than in the horizontal position. Benefits of the vertical position include a reduction in the length of labor, a lower incidence of instrumental birth, a decreased need for anesthesia, and a lower incidence of fetal hypoxia.

Horizontal or Semihorizontal. In this group are the lateral, prone, semirecumbent, knee-elbow, and dorsal positions. These were developed by obstetricians with the aim of achieving ease and efficiency in dealing with complications and administering drugs to relieve pain. However, they may not be best for normal deliveries.

Advantages and Disadvantages of Various Positions

Squatting Position. This position is recorded in the earliest pictures of birth scenes. It has the advantage of enlarging the pelvic outlet. A woman can increase the efficiency of the forces of labor by pulling her knees upward, and this is easier to do when squatting. The disadvantages are that in the squatting position it is difficult for the accoucheur to control the birth and to manage complications, and it may be impossible to administer sedatives and analgesics during labor.

Lateral Position.   This is shown in Fig 4A. Advantages include:

1. Ease, convenience, and comfort for the woman
2. Relaxation of pelvic muscles, which facilitates descent of the fetal head
3. Ease in controlling the head as it advances over the perineum, with fewer lacerations occurring
4. Natural drainage of secretions or vomitus from the pharynx
5. Absence of pressure by the pregnant uterus on the inferior vena cava, thus precluding the supine hypotensive syndrome

This is not, however, a good position in which to handle complicated forceps deliveries. Lacerations of the vagina and cervix are awkward to repair. Complications of the third stage are difficult to manage.

Dorsal (Supine) Position. The woman lies on her back with the knees flexed (Fig. 4B). The dorsal position is advantageous for those multiparas who do not need an episiotomy, as they can be delivered without having to put their legs in stirrups. Episiotomy and forceps operations are not performed easily. The dorsal position is potentially harmful to the fetus during labor and delivery. Should the supine hypotensive syndrome occur, fetal hypoxia and bradycardia may result. A firm wedge placed under the patient's right side will, by producing a 15° left tilt, reduce the incidence of hypotension.

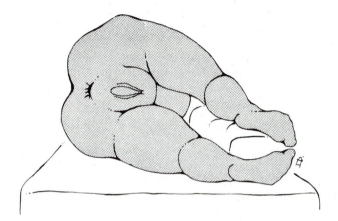

A. Left lateral position.

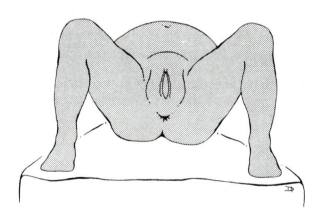

B. Dorsal position.

Figure 4. Positions for delivery.

Lithotomy Position. Here the woman lies on her back, her legs in stirrups, and her buttocks close to the lower edge of the table (Fig. 4C).
Advantages include:

1. Asepsis is more complete.
2. The fetal heart can be auscultated without change of position.
3. Anesthesia can be provided efficiently—general, conduction, and local.
4. The perineum can be protected and lacerations prevented.
5. This is a good position for the use of forceps, for the repair of episiotomy and lacerations, and for conduction of the third stage of labor.

Disadvantages include:

1. Risk of the supine hypotensive syndrome.
2. The use of stirrups or leg supports may lead to sacroiliac or lumbosacral strain, thrombosis in the veins of the lower limbs, and damage to the nerves, especially the peroneal, as a result of prolonged pressure.
3. There is danger of aspiration of vomitus.

Semisitting Position. An adjustable backrest can be used on a standard delivery table during the second and third stages of labor. Women are most comfortable with their backs raised at an angle of between 30° and 45° from the horizontal, which places them in a modified sitting posture (Fig. 4D). The efficiency of the expulsive forces are increased by directing them toward the pelvis and by making use of the forces of gravity. For the obstetrician this position is compatible with modern methods of obstetric care.

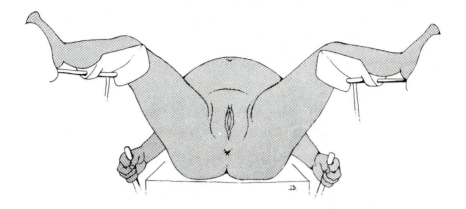

C. Lithotomy position.

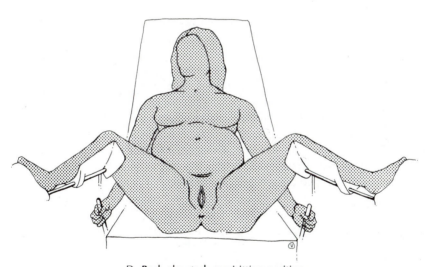

D. Back elevated: semisitting position.

Figure 4. (cont.) Positions for delivery.

Supine Hypotensive Syndrome

The clinical picture is one of hypotension when, in the late stages of pregnancy, the woman lies on her back; there is rapid recovery when she turns on her side. Other symptoms include nausea, shortness of breath, faintness, pallor, tachycardia, and increased femoral venous pressure.

When the pregnant, near-term woman lies on her back, the flaccid uterus bulges over the vertebral column and compresses the inferior vena cava. This leads to an increased volume of blood in the lower limbs, but a decreased return to the heart, lowered pressure in the right atrium, diminished cardiac output, and hypotension. Reduced perfusion of the uterus and placenta leads to fetal hypoxia and changes in the fetal heart rate. During a uterine contraction the uterus sits on the spine and does not press on the large blood vessels. Complete relief of symptoms occurs when the baby has been delivered.

Bearing Down by the Patient

During the first stage, labor progresses faster and the patient feels less pain if she breathes slowly and deeply during each uterine contraction and avoids bearing down. The more effective the relaxation, the more rapid the cervical dilatation. In the second stage, on the other hand, the patient has to work hard. She must force down with each contraction and rest between them. The more effectively she bears down, the shorter the second stage. During the early part of the second stage the abdominal muscles, which are responsible for the bearing-down efforts, are under the patient's complete control. Later she sometimes finds it impossible to stop bearing down even if she wants to. This action is more efficient if the patient braces herself against a solid object. On delivery tables hand bars are provided. When the contraction comes on the patient takes one or two deep breaths and then holds her breath to fix the diaphragm. She then pulls on the hand bars, and at the same time bears down as hard and for as long a period as she can. This is shown in Fig. 4C. With each contraction the pressure on the perineum and rectum stimulates the patient to move toward the head of the table and out of the best position. Shoulder braces prevent this.

Descent, Crowning, and Spontaneous Birth of the Head

With each contraction the head advances and then recedes as the uterus relaxes. Each time a little ground is gained. The introitus becomes an anteroposterior slit, .then an oval, and finally a circular opening (Figs. 5A-C). The pressure of the head thins out the perineum. Feces may be forced out of the rectum. As the anus opens, the anterior wall of the rectum bulges through. With descent the occiput comes to lie under the pubic symphysis. The head continues to advance and recede with the contractions, until a strong one forces the largest diameter of the head through the vulva (crowning), as seen in Figure 5D. Once this has occurred there is no going back, and by a process of extension (Fig. 5E) the head is born, as the bregma, forehead, nose, mouth, and chin appear over the perineum (Fig. 5F). At the stage where the head is passing through the introitus, the patient has the sensation of being torn apart. Laceration of the vulva sometimes occurs.

The head then falls back toward the anus. Once it is out of the vagina it restitutes (Fig. 5G) as the neck untwists. After a few moments, external rotation takes place (Fig. 5H) as the shoulders move from the oblique to the anteroposterior diameter of the pelvis.

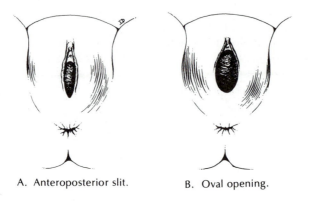

A. Anteroposterior slit.   B. Oval opening.

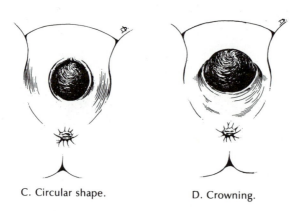

C. Circular shape.   D. Crowning.

Figure 5. Dilatation of the introitus and birth of the head.

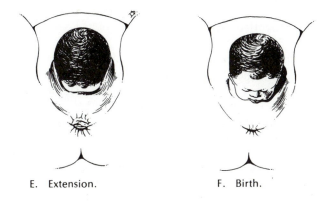

E. Extension.   F. Birth.

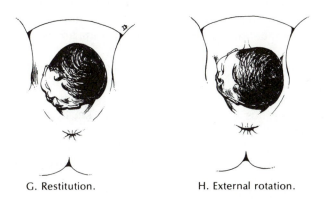

G. Restitution.   H. External rotation.

Figure 5. (cont.) Dilatation of the introitus and birth of the head.

Assisted Delivery of Head

Many women can deliver their babies spontaneously in bed without assistance. There are advantages, however, of having an accoucheur in attendance and of having the patient on a delivery table. (1) Should an unexpected complication arise, immediate action can be carried out. (2) The obstetrician is able to assist the patient so that the incidence of large and uncontrolled lacerations is reduced.

Controlled Birth of Head. Procedures designed to promote leisurely egress of the fetal head should be performed. Slow, gradual birth of the head reduces the incidence of lacerations. The attendant must guard against a sudden bursting out of the head, as this leads to large and jagged lacerations, which in the extreme may extend through the anal sphincter and into the rectum.

1. Management of bearing-down efforts: Correct management of the bearing-down efforts of the parturient is important. The two forces responsible for birth of the child are uterine contractions and bearing-down forces. The uterine contractions are involuntary, but the bearing-down forces can be controlled. During the first part of the second stage the patient must bear down during the uterine contractions to expedite progress. However, during the actual delivery too rapid emergence of the fetal head can be slowed by the patient's panting rapidly through the open mouth during the contraction. When the patient breathes in and out rapidly, the diaphragm moves, making it impossible for effective intraabdominal pressure to be built up, and so the power to bear down is lost.

2. Manual pressure: In most cases the speed of delivery can be reduced by gentle manual pressure against the baby's head. Occasionally the propulsive force is so great that it is impossible,or even dangerous, to try slowing the birth. The head should never be held back forcibly.

3. Ritgen maneuver: The objective of this maneuver is to encourage extension of the fetal head and thus expedite its birth. This procedure is performed ideally between uterine contractions. During this interval the head can be delivered slowly, gradually, and under the obstetrician's complete control. Further, the soft tissues are more relaxed and tissue damage is less. The maneuver cannot be carried out before the occiput has come under the symphysis. It is done when the suboccipitofrontal diameter is ready to be born.

    The operator's hand, covered with a towel or a pad, is placed so that the fingers are behind the maternal anus (Fig. 6A). Extension of the fetal head is furthered by pressing against the baby's face, preferably the chin, through the rectum. The bregma, forehead, and face are born in that order. The other hand is placed against the baby's head to control the speed of its delivery. Sometimes fundal pressure is needed to deliver the head, or if the patient is awake she can bear down gently.

4. Hooking out the chin: Occasionally the chin gets stuck against the perineum. It is extracted by inserting the fingers into the vagina, over the cheek and under the chin, which is then brought out over the perineum (Fig. 6B).

5. Episiotomy: When large lacerations seem inevitable it is better to make an incision into the perineum (episiotomy). In this way the direction and size of the cut can be controlled, and tears into the rectum can be obviated.

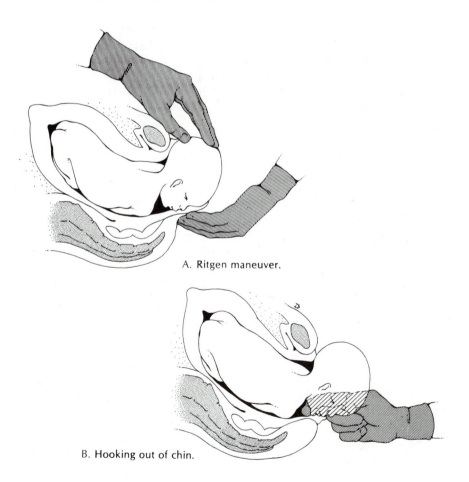

A. Ritgen maneuver.

B. Hooking out of chin.

Figure 6. Birth of head.

Following Delivery of Head

1. The head should be supported as it restitutes and rotates externally.
2. The face should be wiped gently and mucus aspirated from the mouth and throat by a small, soft, rubber bulb syringe.
3. The region of the neck is explored for coils of umbilical cord. If the cord is around the neck loosely it can be slipped over the head. If it is coiled around the neck tightly, it must be clamped doubly, cut between the clamps, and then unwound.
4. Meconium aspiration syndrome must be prevented. When thick meconium has been passed there is a danger that the fetus will aspirate it during the first deep postnatal breath. Therefore, in cases where meconium is present the following steps should be taken:
   a. As soon as the head is born, and before the baby breathes, the nostrils, nasopharynx, mouth, and hypopharynx are suctioned thoroughly.
   b. After the delivery is complete the laryngoscope is employed to see whether there is meconium at or below the level of the vocal cords.
   c. If there is, all the meconium should be suctioned out before any resuscitative measures, such as positive pressure breathing, are performed.

Birth of Body

Shoulders. By the time the shoulders are ready for delivery, restitution has occurred and external rotation is taking place. During a uterine contraction the patient is asked to bear down. If the patient is anesthetized or unable to force down, pressure is exerted by an attendant on the fundus of the uterus. At the same time the head of the baby is grasped with the hands on the parietal bones or with one hand over the face and the other on the occiput (Fig. 7A); the head is then depressed toward the rectum. This enables the anterior shoulder to emerge under the symphysis pubis. (Fig. 7B). When this has been achieved the head is raised so that the posterior shoulder can be born over the perineum (Fig. 7C). It must be emphasized that the operator merely lowers and lifts the baby's head to facilitate birth of the shoulders. He does not exert great traction, as this carries with it the danger of damaging the nerve plexus in the neck. The force that actually pushes out the shoulder is provided by the bearing-down efforts of the mother if she is awake, or by pressure on the fundus by an assistant if the mother is asleep.

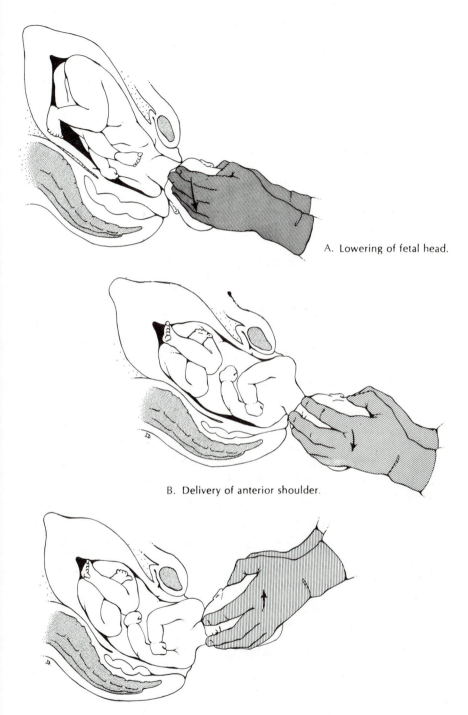

A. Lowering of fetal head.

B. Delivery of anterior shoulder.

C. Delivery of posterior shoulder.

Figure 7. Delivery of the shoulders.

Trunk and Lower Limbs. Once the head and shoulders have been delivered, the rest of the body slips out easily, usually with a gush of aminiotic fluid.

Third Stage of Labor

Birth of Placenta
Delivery of the placenta occurs in two stages: (1) separation of the placenta from the wall of the uterus and into the lower uterine segment and/or the vagina, and (2) actual expulsion of the placenta out of the birth canal.

Separation of Placenta. Placental separation takes place, as a rule, within 5 minutes of the end of the second stage. Signs suggesting that detachment has taken place include:

1. Gush of blood from the vagina
2. Lengthening of the umbilical cord outside the vulva
3. Rising of the uterine fundus in the abdomen as the placenta passes from the uterus into the vagina
4. Uterus becoming firm and globular

Expulsion of Placenta. When these signs have appeared the placenta is ready for expression. If the patient is awake, she is asked to bear down while gentle traction is made on the umbilical cord. If the patient is asleep or unable to bear down, pressure is made on the uterine fundus and the placenta expressed. A popular and effective method of delivering the placenta is by the Brandt-Andrews maneuver. This procedure involves exerting gentle traction on the cord by one hand, while the uterus is lifted gently out of the pelvis by suprapubic pressure on the uterus with the other. It is wise to avoid rough manipulations of the uterus before placental separation has taken place. Such actions do not hasten delivery of the placenta and may lead to excessive bleeding (Fig. 8).

The actual birth of the placenta takes place in one of two ways: (1) Duncan method (dirty Duncan), when the rough maternal edge comes first; or (2) Schultze mechanism (shiny Schultze), when the placenta comes out like an inverted umbrella with the glistening fetal membranes leading the way.

Delivery of the Membranes. In most cases, as the placenta is born, the membranes peel off from the endometrium and are delivered spontaneously. Occasionally this does not take place, and the membranes are removed by gentle traction with forceps (Fig. 9). Retention of bits of membrane does not seem to lead to any untoward effects.

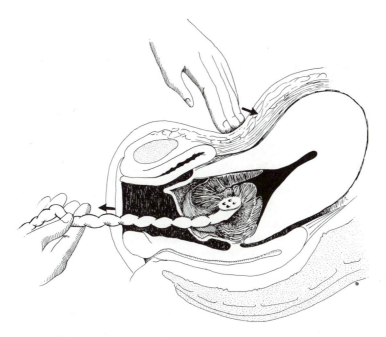

Figure 8. Brandt-Andrews maneuver: Delivery of placenta.

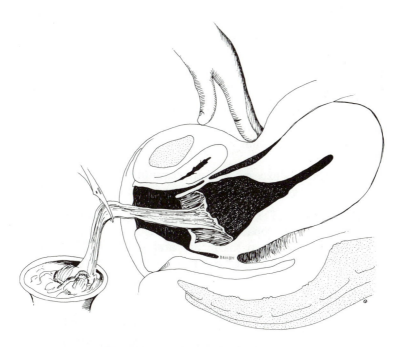

Figure 9. Delivery of the membranes.

Examination of Delivered Placenta. Examination of the delivered placenta is performed to see that no parts are missing—i.e., left in the uterus. Torn blood vessels along the edge suggest that an accessory lobe may have remained in the uterus. Some obstetricians feel that examination of the placenta does not ensure that fragments have not been left behind, and they explore the uterine cavity manually after each delivery.

Delayed Separation and Delivery of Placenta. Delayed separation and delivery of the placenta may occur in several situations:

1. Placenta separated but trapped in the uterus by the cervix
2. Placenta separated incompletely
3. Placenta not separated at all
4. Placenta acreta, where the decidua is deficient and the chorionic villi have grown into the myometrium

Manual Removal of Placenta. At one time invasion of the postpartum uterus was believed to be so dangerous a procedure that a placenta that did not deliver spontaneously was left in situ even for days. Today we feel that prolonged retention of the afterbirth increases the danger of infection and hemorrhage. Current practice is to remove the placenta manually if it does not deliver within 30 minutes of the birth of the baby, provided bleeding is not excessive. If hemorrhage is profuse, the placenta must be removed immediately. The average blood loss during the third stage is 200 to 250 ml.

Manual Exploration of Uterus
Manual exploration of the uterus is mandatory:

1. When examination of the placenta is inconclusive or there is suspicion that something has been left in the uterus
2. After a traumatic delivery to rule out lacerations of the uterus and cervix
3. When there is excessive postpartum bleeding
4. When a congenital anomaly of the uterus is suspected

A frequent cause of excessive bleeding is the attempt to deliver the placenta before it has separated. Kneading or massaging the uterus roughly when it is not ready to contract and retract may lead to partial separation of the placenta, and postpartum hemorrhage.

Oxytocics
Oxytocics are drugs that stimulate the uterus to contract. Posterior pituitary extract causes clonic rhythmic contractions. The ergot alkaloids provoke a tonic type of contraction. The purpose of using these substances is to hasten placental delivery and so reduce uterine blood loss.

It is doubtful that the amount of blood lost during the delivery and the immediate postpartum period has any relationship to the rapidity of placental separation. In most cases detachment of the placenta from the wall of the uterus takes place within 5 minutes of the birth of the baby. After delivery of the placenta the uterine contractions decrease in strength and frequency; the normal puerperal uterus does not remain in a tonically contracted state, yet no excessive blood loss occurs. This suggests that the routine use of ecbolic drugs is unnecessary in normal deliveries and should be reserved for women who have conditions that increase the risk of postpartum hemorrhage, including: (1) overdistended uterus (multiple pregnancy, polyhydramnios), (2) high parity, (3) history of previous postpartum hemorrhage, (4) prolonged labor, especially when associated with ineffective uterine contractions, (5) deep general anesthesia, (6) difficult operative delivery, (7) induction or augmentation of labor by oxytocin.

Pitocin and Syntocinon. Pitocin was originally the trade name for posterior pituitary extract that had been purified by removing the vasopressor substances almost completely. Today both Pitocin and Syntocinon are trade names for synthetic oxytocin. These substances may be given in several ways:

1. After birth of the baby, 10 units intramuscularly
2. After delivery of the placenta, 10 units intramuscularly
3. As an intravenous infusion using 5 to 10 units of oxytocin per liter of 5 percent glucose in water, given either before or after placental separation.

Ergometrine. Ergometrine is given most commonly after the end of the third stage, either intramuscularly in the amount of 0.5 mg, or intravenously in a dose of 0.125 or 0.25 mg. A popular method of using ergometrine is to give·0.125 mg intravenously when the anterior shoulder has emerged from the symphysis pubis and the rest of the baby can be delivered at will. The birth of the rest of the baby is delayed 10 to 15 seconds. This gives the ergometrine time to reach the uterus and stimulate it to contract. The baby's buttocks are still in the uterine cervix and hold it open, so that the placenta is expelled from the uterus literally on the baby's heels. The aim of this technique is to speed expulsion of the placenta and reduce bleeding. Before employing this method the presence of twins must be ruled out. A rare complication is spasm of the cervix trapping the placenta. In such a case one must wait for the spasm to wear off.

Repair of Lacerations

The cervix, vagina, and perineum must be examined carefully, lacerations repaired, and bleeding controlled.

Fourth Stage of Labor

The patient is kept in the delivery suite for 1 hour postpartum under close observation. She is checked for bleeding, the blood pressure is measured, and the pulse is counted. The third stage and the hour after delivery are more dangerous to the mother than any other time.

Before the doctor leaves the patient he must do the following:

1. Feel the uterus through the abdomen to be sure it is firm and not filling with blood.
2. Look at the introitus to see that there is no hemorrhage.
3. See that the mother's vital signs are normal and that she is in good condition.
4. Examine the baby to be certain that it is breathing well and that the color and tone are normal.

ASEPSIS AND ANTISEPSIS

Anatomic Factors

The birth passage is divided into three parts:

1. The vulva and vaginal orifice, which are loaded with bacteria of all kinds.
2. The vagina, which contains some vaginal bacteria with their acidic secretion, a few fungi, and a number of leukocytes.
3. The uterine cavity, which is separated from the vagina by the mucous plug. There are no organisms here.

Natural Safeguards

1. During the first and second stages there is an increase in the vaginal secretion, which cleans the passage.
2. When the membranes rupture, the amniotic fluid flushes out the vagina.
3. As the baby passes through the vagina it distends the walls. Usually the birth of the baby is accompanied by another discharge of amniotic fluid, which helps wash out the vagina.
4. As the membranes and placenta pass through the vagina they also exert a cleaning, mop-like action.

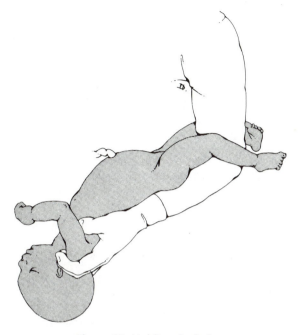

Figure 10. Holding the baby.

IMMEDIATE CARE OF NEWBORN BABY

The following measures are designed to assist the infant in accomplishing the adaptations to extrauterine life.

Clearing the Airway

As soon as the head is born, and before the baby takes its first breath, the nasopharynx and the oropharynx must be suctioned to prevent aspiration of mucus and debris into the trachea when breathing begins. This procedure is especially important when meconium is present. If there is thick meconium, the larynx should be examined by means of a laryngoscope and the trachea aspirated under direct vision.

Once the infant is born it should be held head down for a few moments to promote drainage of mucus. The best way of holding the baby is to place it with the back on the attendant's forearm; one leg is tucked between the doctor's arm and his side to prevent the infant from rolling off; the neck is between the third and fourth fingers; the shoulders rest on the palmar surfaces of the fingers; and the baby's head is below the operator's hand (Fig. 10). The advantages of this method are:

1. The infant is held securely and cannot slip between the fingers.
2. The head is maintained in slight extension, straightening the trachea and helping drainage.
3. The baby is held in a fixed position so that the trachea can be milked down, the mucus aspirated from the mouth and throat, and any other needed procedure carried out with the infant's swinging like a pendulum, as it does when held by the ankles.
4. The baby is then placed on the mother's abdomen and, if necessary, further suctioning is carried out.

The infant is transferred to a warmed bassinet that has been placed in a 20° head down position to facilitate the drainage of liquid material from the oropharynx by gravity.

Initiation of Respiration

As it passes through the vaginal canal, the baby's chest is compressed by the pelvic floor, and much of the fluid in the lungs is expressed. The remaining fluid is removed from the lungs after birth via the capillaries and lymphatics. When the vaginal squeeze does not take place, such as in premature infants and those born by cesarean section, more fluid remains in the lungs, and may be an embarrassment to the fetus. Once the baby is born the rebound of the chest wall acts to fill the lungs with air. Spontaneous respiration commences, in most cases, within 1 minute after birth. By 2 to 10 minutes the respiratory center in the brain, stimulated by the mixed acidosis, hypoxia, and hypercarbia that develops during the delivery, initiates rhythmic breathing at a rate of about 40 breaths per minute. The first inspiration is usually followed by a cry. In the healthy newborn infant the best way of stimulating respiration is by gentle slapping of the soles of the feet. More drastic measures may be harmful.

Umbilical Cord

The umbilical cord is tied doubly with tapes or with special mechanical ties. The cord is then cut. The timing of the clamping will affect the volume of blood transfused from the placenta into the fetal circulation. Early clamping reduces the neonatal blood volume and the red blood cell mass. Iron stores are thereby reduced and the potential for anemia increased. Late clamping, on the other hand, by increasing the transferred volume of red blood cells, may predispose to hyperviscosity and jaundice. Many physicians prefer to delay tying the cord until it stops pulsating. If this is done the infant must be held lower than the level of the placenta (at the introitus) or the blood will not reach him.

Thermoregulation

Born into the cool environment of the delivery room, the infant suffers an enormous loss of heat. This occurs primarily by evaporation because the skin is wet with amniotic fluid. Once the skin is dry the loss of heat is mainly by a process of radiation. Hypothermia is dangerous because it may lead to hypoxia, hypoglycemia, metabolic acidosis, and kernicterus. To prevent this, excessive loss of heat must be prevented. The infant should be dried and placed under a radiant heater. This is especially important for immature or depressed babies. For the normal, vigorous infant wrapping in a warm blanket is often sufficient.

When the newborn baby becomes cold he attempts to compensate by increasing the production of thyroid hormone and catecholamines. This leads to an increase in the consumption of oxygen and of glycolysis, and the breakdown of thermogenic brown fat. Norepinephrine is a pulmonary vasoconstrictor, and may interfere with the normal perinatal increase in pulmonary blood flow. Free fatty acids, formed by the breakdown of triglycerides, bind to albumen, and may compete with bilirubin for binding sites; this can be significant if the infant becomes jaundiced.

Apgar Score

Assessment by Apgar scoring is carried out at 1 minute and at 5 minutes after birth (Table 3). If the infant is still depressed at 5 minutes the scoring is repeated every 5 minutes until his condition is satisfactory. A score of 7 to 10 is considered normal, a score of 3 to 6 indicates mild to moderate depression, and a score of 0 to 2 severe depression. The management of the individual infant can conveniently be based on the Apgar Score.

Apgar scoring is simple to perform and its usefulness has been confirmed for over 30 years. It is not, however, a reliable index of asphyxia, which may be assessed better from the acid-base state of the infant at birth. This is evaluated from arterial and venous blood samples taken from a clamped section of umbilical cord.

TABLE 3. APGAR SCORING OF NEWBORNS

Sign	0 Points	1 Point	2 Points
Heart rate	Absent	Under 100	Over 100
Respiratory effort	Absent	Slow, irregular	Good, crying
Muscle tone	Limp	Flexion of extremities	Active motion
Reflex irritability: response to catheter in nostril	No response	Grimace	Cough or sneeze
Color	Blue-white	Body pink, extremities blue	Completely pink

Physical Examination

Prior to discharge from the case room a complete physical examination is carried out. This includes the use of a suction catheter to confirm patency of the nasal choanae. The catheter may be advanced through the esophagus into the stomach, thereby excluding esophageal atresia. The gastric fluid is aspirated and the volume measured. Excessive fluid in the stomach (greater than 15 ml) suggests the possibility of a small bowel obstruction.

Care of the Eyes

Before the baby is transferred to the nursery the eyes must be treated to prevent the development of ophthalmia neonatorum. The traditional agent has been a 1% solution of silver nitrate. Occasionally this causes chemical conjunctivitis. Acceptable alternatives include tetracycline and erythromycin ointments. These antibiotics have the advantage of being active against Chlamydia, which are, today, a commoner cause of eye infections than the gonococcus.

Vitamin K

Hemorrhagic disease of the newborn is a condition which results from a deficiency of vitamin K-dependent clotting factors. This can be prevented by the intramuscular injection after birth of 1 mg of water soluble vitamin K.

Family Interaction

Over the past 10 years a great deal of interest has been directed towards the developing relationship between the infant and the mother in the initial hours of life. It has been suggested that there is a "maternal-sensitive period" beginning immediately after birth, and that more contact at this time increases the attachment of mother to baby. There is evidence that, in this way, maternal behavior towards her baby is influenced and remains closer not only over a period of hours and days, but for months and even years.

The attachment of the father to the baby has not been studied as intensively as that of the mother, but it seems clear that the presence of the father at the delivery and after birth does affect his feelings and behavior towards his child.

It is, therefore, important that mother, father, and even other members of the family should be encouraged to spend some time with their baby in a relaxed and quiet atmosphere. Mother can nurse the infant at this time.

Asphyxia Neonatorum

(See Chapter 51.)

BIBLIOGRAPHY

Atwood, RJ: Parturitional posture and related birth behaviour. Acta Obstet Gynecol Scand (Suppl) 57, 1976

Challis JRG, Mitchell BF: Hormonal control of preterm and term parturition. Seminars Perinatal 5:192, 1981

Drover JW, Casper RF: Initiation of parturition in humans. Can Med Assoc J 128:387, 1983

Kenepp NB, Kumar S, Shelley WC, et al: Fetal and neonatal hazards of maternal hydration with 5% dextrose before cesarean section. Lancet 1:1150, 22 May 1982

Kerr-Wilson RHJ, Groesbeck PP, Orr JW: The effect of a full bladder on labor. Obstet Gynecol 62:319, 1983

Marx GF, Bassell GM: Hazards of the supine position in pregnancy. Clin Obstet Gynaecol 9: 255, 1982

Mendiola J, Grylack LJ, Scanlon JW: Effects of intrapartum maternal glucose infusion on the normal fetus and newborn. Anesth Analg 6:32, 1982

Ostheimer GW: Resuscitation of the newborn infant. Clin Perinatol 9:177, 1982

Peltonen T: Placental transfusion: Advantage and disadvantage. Eur J Pediat 137:141, 1981

Russell JGB: The rationale of primitive delivery positions. Brit J Obstet Gynaecol 89:712, 1982

Shepherd JH, Knuppel RA: The role of prostaglandins in ripening the cervix and inducing labor. Clin Perinatol 8:49, 1981

Stewart P, Kennedy JH, Calder AA: Spontaneous labour: When should the membranes be ruptured? Brit J Obstet Gynaecol 89:39, 1982

12

Transverse Positions of the Occiput

LEFT OCCIPUT TRANSVERSE: LOT

Engagement is more frequent in the transverse diameter of the inlet than in the oblique, and left occiput transverse (LOT) is the most common position at the onset of labor (Fig. 1).

Diagnosis of Position: LOT

Abdominal Examination

1. The lie is longitudinal.
2. The head is at or in the pelvis.
3. The back is on the left and toward the mother's flank.
4. The small parts are on the right and sometimes can be felt clearly.
5. The breech is in the fundus of the uterus.
6. The cephalic prominence (forehead) is on the right.

Fetal Heart
The fetal heart is heard loudest in the left lower quadrant of the mother's abdomen.

Vaginal Examination

1. The sagittal suture is in the transverse diameter of the pelvis. If the head is in synclitism (Fig. 1B), the sagittal suture is midway between the symphysis pubis and the promontory of the sacrum. If there is anterior asynclitism (Fig. 1D) the sagittal suture is nearer the sacral promontory, while with posterior asynclitism (Fig. 1C) it is closer to the pubic symphysis.
2. The small posterior fontanelle is toward the mother's left, at 3 o'clock.
3. The bregma is on the right, at 9 o'clock.
4. If there is flexion the occiput is lower than the brow. If flexion is poor the occiput and brow are almost at the same level in the pelvis.

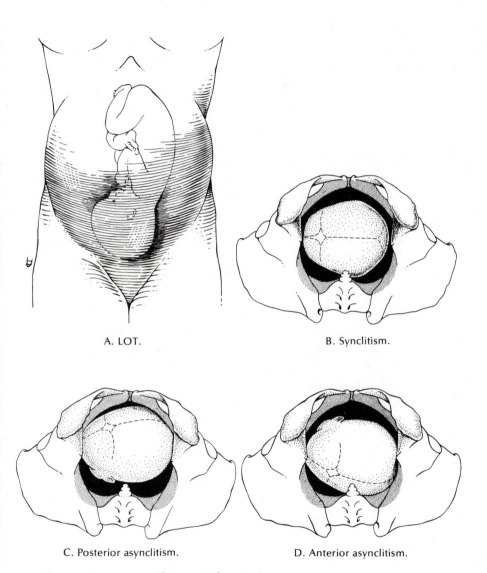

A. LOT.   B. Synclitism.

C. Posterior asynclitism.   D. Anterior asynclitism.

Figure 1. Left occiput transverse.

Mechanism of Labor: LOT

Descent
Descent includes engagement, which may have taken place before labor (Figs. 2A and B). Descent continues throughout labor.

Flexion
Resistance to descent causes the head to flex (Fig. 2B) so that the chin approaches the chest. This reduces the presenting diameter by 1.5 cm. The occipitofrontal diameter of 11.0 cm is replaced by the suboccipito-bregmatic diameter of 9.5 cm.

Internal Rotation
The head enters the pelvis with the sagittal suture in the transverse diameter of the inlet and the occiput at 3 o'clock. The occiput then rotates 90° to arrive under the pubic symphysis. The sinciput comes to lie anterior to the sacrum. The sequence is LOT to LOA to OA (Figs. 2A and B). The shoulders lag behind 45° so that when the sagittal suture of the head is in the anteroposterior diameter of the pelvis the shoulders are in the left oblique. Thus the neck is twisted.

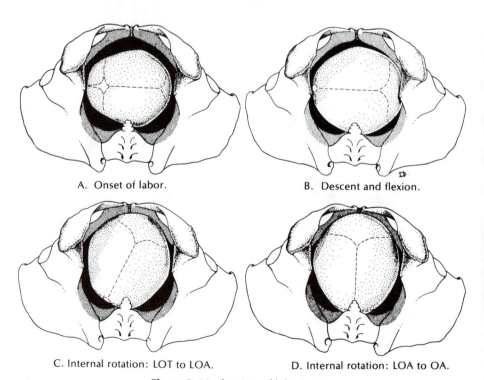

A. Onset of labor.   B. Descent and flexion.

C. Internal rotation: LOT to LOA.   D. Internal rotation: LOA to OA.

Figure 2. Mechanism of labor: LOT.

Extension
Birth is by extension (Figs. 2E and F). The nape of the neck pivots under the pubis, while the vertex, bregma, forehead, face, and chin are born over the perineum.

Restitution
When the head has made its exit, the neck untwists and the head turns back 45° to the left, resuming the normal relationship with the shoulders—OA to LOA (Fig. 2G).

External Rotation
The shoulders now rotate 45° to the left to bring their bisacromial diameter into the anteroposterior diameter of the pelvis. The head follows the shoulder and rotates externally another 45° to the left—LOA to LOT (Fig. 2H).

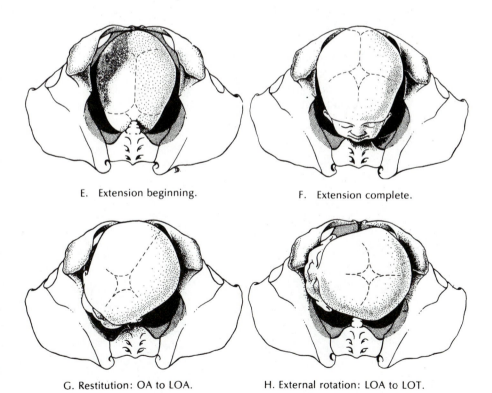

E. Extension beginning.   F. Extension complete.

G. Restitution: OA to LOA.   H. External rotation: LOA to LOT.

Figure 2. (cont.) Mechanism of labor: LOT.

Birth of Shoulders, Trunk, and Placenta

Birth of the shoulders, trunk, and placenta is the same as described in Chapter 10, "Anterior Positions of the Occiput and the Normal Mechanism of Labor." A summary of the mechanism of labor (LOT) is presented in Figure 3.

CLINICAL COURSE OF LABOR: LOT

Most fetuses that begin labor in the LOT position rotate the head 90° (LOT to LOA to OA) to bring the occiput under the pubic symphysis, from which position spontaneous delivery takes place.

Arrest of Progress

Arrest of progress can occur in any of these situations:

1. Anterior rotation of 90° to the OA position, but spontaneous delivery does not take place.
2. Anterior rotation of 45°, with cessation of progress in the LOA position.
3. No rotation. The head is arrested with the sagittal suture in the transverse diameter of the pelvis. This is known as transverse arrest.
4. In the rare case posterior rotation takes place, LOT to LOP. The mechanism of labor then becomes that of occipitoposterior positions.

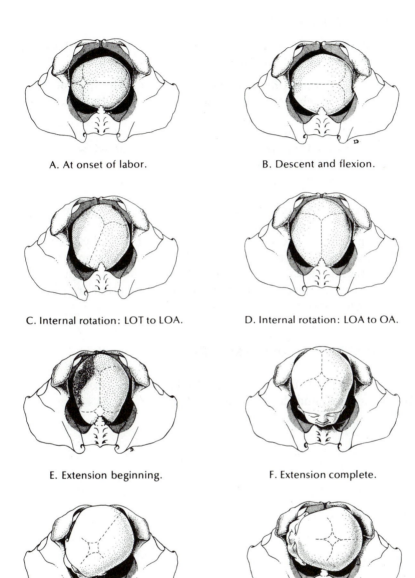

A. At onset of labor.

B. Descent and flexion.

C. Internal rotation: LOT to LOA.

D. Internal rotation: LOA to OA.

E. Extension beginning.

F. Extension complete.

G. Restitution: OA to LOA.

H. External rotation: LOA to LOT.

Figure 3. Summary of the mechanism of labor: LOT.

Management of Arrested Cases

Providing the prerequisites for operative vaginal delivery are present, the following treatment is carried out:

1. Arrest in OA position: Forceps are applied to the sides of the fetal head, which is then extracted (see Chapter 25 for technical details).
2. Arrest as LOA: Forceps are applied to the fetal head, which is then rotated 45° to the OA position and extracted (see Chapter 25 for technical details).
3. Transverse arrest: LOT: Two operative techniques are available.
   a. Manual rotation, 90°, LOT to LOA to OA, followed by forceps extraction (see Chapter 26 for technique).
   b. Application of the forceps to the sides of the baby's head, rotation by the forceps of 90°, LOT to LOA to OA, and then extraction by the forceps (see Chapter 26 for technique).
4. Arrest as an occiput posterior is treated like other occiput posterior deliveries (see Chapters 13 and 27).

RIGHT OCCIPUT TRANSVERSE: ROT

ROT is similar to LOT. The difference is that the back and occiput are on the mother's right, and the limbs are on her left.

13

Posterior Positions of the Occiput

GENERAL CONSIDERATIONS

Definition

The occiput and the small posterior fontanelle are in the rear segment of the maternal pelvis, and the brow and bregma are in the anterior segment.

Incidence

The incidence of this position is 15 to 30 percent. The exact incidence of posterior positions is difficult to ascertain, since most of them rotate anteriorly and are considered erroneously as being originally occipito-anterior. The posterior positions that rotate anteriorly with no difficulty are often not diagnosed, and only the persistent posteriors are recognized regularly. Right occiput posterior (ROP) is five times as common as left occiput posterior (LOP).

Etiology

The etiology of posterior positions of the occiput is the same as the etiology of other abnormal positions. Cephalopelvic disproportion is a frequent and serious complicating factor which must be considered at all times. The shape of the pelvic inlet influences the position of the occiput. Where the forepelvis is narrow there is a tendency for the back of the head with its long biparietal diameter to be pushed to the rear, so that the front of the head with its short bitemporal diameter can be accommodated by the small forepelvis. Hence posterior positions of the occiput are found often in android and anthropoid pelves.

RIGHT OCCIPUT POSTERIOR: ROP

Diagnosis of Position: ROP

Abdominal Examination

1. The lie is vertical. The long axis of the fetus is parallel to the long axis of the mother (Fig. 1).
2. The head is at or in the pelvis.
3. The fetal back is in the right maternal flank. In most cases it cannot be outlined clearly.
4. The small parts are easily felt anteriorly on the left side. The maternal abdomen has been described as being alive with little hands and feet.
5. The breech is in the fundus of the uterus.
6. The cephalic prominence is on the left. It is not felt as easily as in anterior positions, because flexion is less marked.

Fetal Heart

Fetal heart tones are transmitted through the scapula and hence are heard in the right maternal flank, on the same side as the baby's back. Frequently the fetal heart sounds are indistinct. They can be transmitted through the baby's chest and in some cases are loudest in the left anterior lower quadrant of the abdomen. The location of the fetal heart sounds is not a reliable sign in determining how the baby is placed; hence a carefully made diagnosis of posterior position should not be changed because of the situation of the fetal heart. As the back rotates anteriorly, the fetal heart tones approach the midline of the abdomen.

Vaginal Examination

1. The sagittal suture is in the right oblique diameter of the pelvis.
2. The small posterior fontanelle is in the right posterior segment of the pelvis.
3. The bregma is anterior and to the left of the symphysis pubis.
4. Since flexion is imperfect, the fontanelles may be close to the same level in the pelvis.
5. Where there is difficulty in diagnosis, the pinna (auricle) of the ear is found pointing to the occiput.

X-ray Examination

Occasionally x-ray is helpful when diagnosis is in doubt.

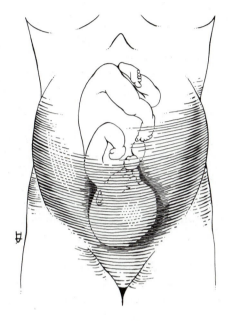

A. Abdominal view.

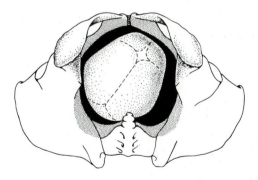

B. Vaginal view.

Figure 1. Right occiput posterior.

Mechanism of Labor: ROP

Rotation of varying degree and direction can take place:

1. Anterior rotation
   a. Long arc rotation of 135°, ROP to ROT to ROA to OA. This occurs in 90 percent of occipitoposterior positions. The baby is born as an occipitoanterior.
   b. Rotation of 90°, ROP to ROT to ROA.
   c. Rotation of 45°, ROP to ROT. The result is deep transverse arrest.
2. No rotation. The position remains ROP.
3. Posterior rotation of 45°, ROP to OP, with the occiput turning into the hollow of the sacrum.

Spontaneous delivery can take place after:

1. Anterior rotation to OA with normal birth
2. Posterior rotation to OP with face to pubis delivery

Arrest can occur:

1. High in the pelvis, with failure to engage. These are often problems of disproportion.
2. In the midpelvis, with complete or partial failure of rotation.
   a. Deep transverse arrest, ROT
   b. Arrest with the sagittal suture in the right oblique diameter of the pelvis, ROP
   c. Arrest with the occiput in the hollow of the sacrum, OP
3. Arrest at the outlet.

Long Arc Rotation: 135° to the Anterior

Descent. The head enters the inlet with the sagittal suture in the right oblique diameter (Fig. 2A), and unless obstruction is encountered descent continues throughout labor. Engagement may be delayed, and the entire labor may take longer than in normal anterior positions.

Flexion. Flexion (Fig. 2B) is imperfect and often is not complete until the head reaches the pelvic floor. The partial flexion and the resulting larger diameter of the presenting part contribute to the labor's being longer and harder for both mother and child.

Internal Rotation. The occiput rotates 135° anteriorly under the symphysis pubis—ROP to ROT to ROA to OA (Figs. 2C-E).

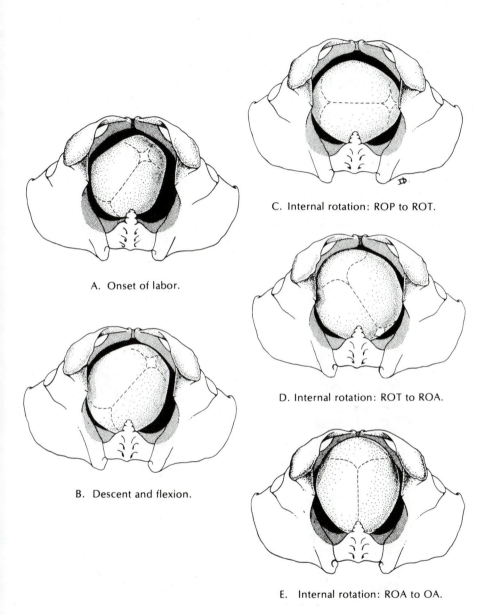

A. Onset of labor.

B. Descent and flexion.

C. Internal rotation: ROP to ROT.

D. Internal rotation: ROT to ROA.

E. Internal rotation: ROA to OA.

Figure 2. ROP: long arc rotation.

Extension. The nape of the neck pivots in the subpubic angle, and the head is born by extension (Figs. 2F and G). The bregma, forehead, nose, mouth, and chin pass over the perineum in order.

Restitution. Restitution (OA to ROA) takes place to the right (Fig. 2H). The extent of restitution depends on how far the shoulders have followed the head during internal rotation. In most cases the shoulders turn with the head, lagging behind only 45°, and restitution is the usual 45°. Occasionally the shoulders may lag behind more or may swing back. The head then restitutes 90° or even 135°.

External Rotation. The anterior shoulder strikes the pelvic floor and rotates 45° toward the pubic symphysis so that the bisacromial diameter of the shoulders is in the anteroposterior diameter of the outlet. The head follows the shoulders, and the occiput rotates 45° to the right transverse position—ROA to ROT (Fig. 2I).

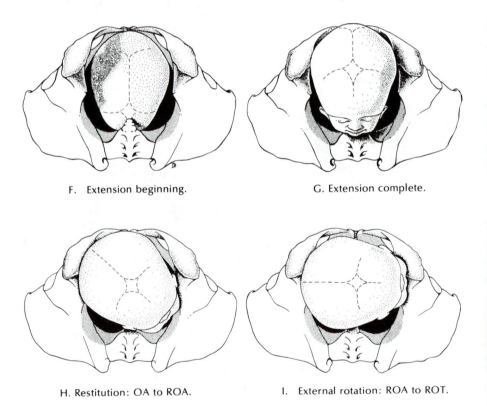

F. Extension beginning.   G. Extension complete.

H. Restitution: OA to ROA.   I. External rotation: ROA to ROT.

Figure 2. (cont.) ROP: long arc rotation.

Short Arc Rotation: 45° to the Posterior

Descent. The head enters the inlet with the sagittal suture in the right oblique (Fig. 3A). Descent continues throughout labor.

Flexion. Flexion (Fig. 3B) is imperfect, resulting in a longer presenting diameter.

Internal Rotation. The occiput turns posteriorly 45° (ROP to OP) into the hollow of the sacrum (Fig. 3C). The sagittal suture is in the antero-posterior diameter of the pelvis. The bregma is behind the pubis.

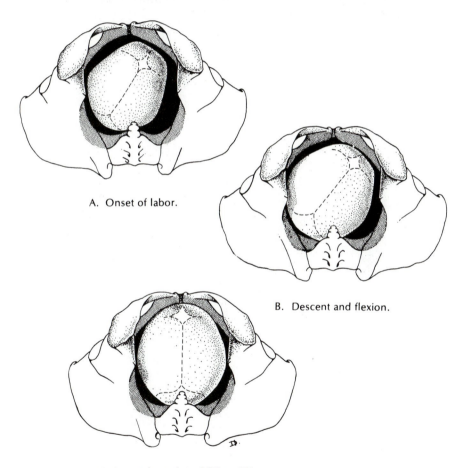

A. Onset of labor.

B. Descent and flexion.

C. Internal rotation: ROP to OP.

Figure 3. ROP: short arc rotation.

Birth of Head. Birth of the head is by a combination of flexion and extension (Fig. 3D-G).

There are two mechanisms of flexion:

1. Where there is good flexion the area anterior to the bregma pivots under the symphysis pubis. The presenting diameter is the suboccipitofrontal of 10.5 cm. The bregma, vertex, small fontanelle, and occiput are born by further flexion.
2. Where flexion is incomplete the root of the nose pivots under the symphysis. The presenting diameter is the larger occipitofrontal of 11.5 cm. This bigger diameter is more traumatic than the smaller one. By flexion, the forehead, bregma, vertex, and occiput are born over the perineum.

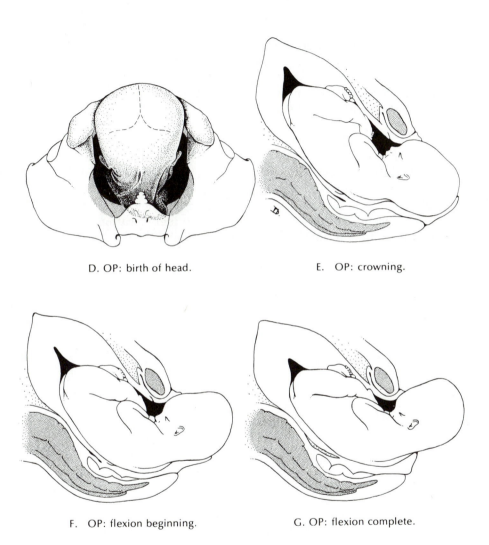

D. OP: birth of head.

E. OP: crowning.

F. OP: flexion beginning.

G. OP: flexion complete.

Figure 3. (cont.) ROP: short arc rotation.

Once the top and back of the head have been born by flexion, the occiput falls back toward the anus, and the nose, mouth, and chin are born under the symphysis pubis by extension (Figs. 3H and I).

Restitution of the occiput is 45° to the right oblique (OP to ROP) to resume the normal relationship of the head to the shoulders (Fig. 3J).

The anterior shoulder strikes the pelvic floor and rotates 45° toward the symphysis pubis, to bring the bisacromial diameter of the shoulders into the anteroposterior diameter of the pelvis (external rotation). The head follows, and the occiput rotates 45° to the right transverse position—ROP to ROT (Fig. 3K).

Molding

In persistent occipitoposterior positions the head is shortened in the occipitofrontal and lengthened in the suboccipitobregmatic and mentobregmatic diameters. The head rises steeply in front and in back. The caput succedaneum is located over the bregma. Molding (Fig. 4) and extensive edema of the scalp make accurate identification of the sutures and fontanelles difficult, thereby obscuring the diagnosis.

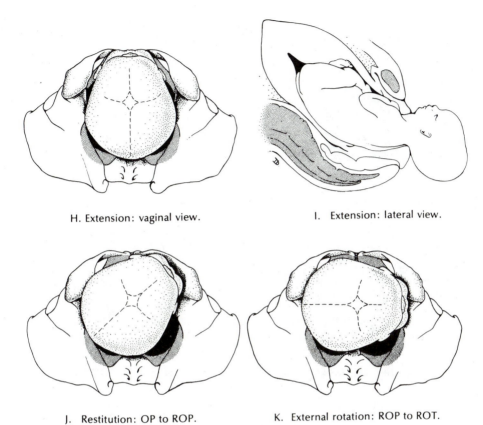

H. Extension: vaginal view.

I. Extension: lateral view.

J. Restitution: OP to ROP.

K. External rotation: ROP to ROT.

Figure 3. (cont.) ROP: short arc rotation.

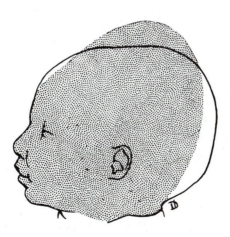

Figure 4. Molding: ROP.

Summaries

Summaries of both long arc and short arc rotations may be reviewed in Figures 5 and 6, respectively.

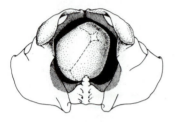

A. ROP: onset of labor.

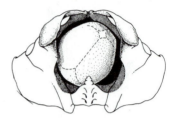

B. Descent and flexion.

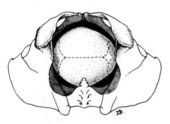

C. Internal rotation: ROP to ROT.

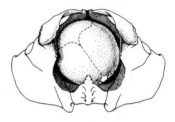

D. Internal rotation: ROT to ROA.

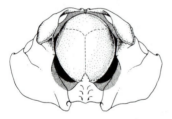

E. Internal rotation: ROA to OA.

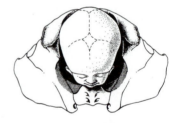

F. Extension.

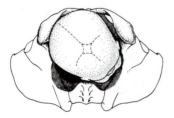

G. Restitution: OA to ROA.

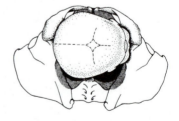

H. External rotation: ROA to ROT.

Figure 5. Summary of long arc rotation: ROP to OA.

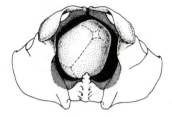

A. ROP: onset of labor.

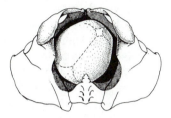

B. Descent and flexion.

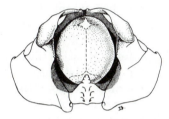

C. Internal rotation: ROP to OP.

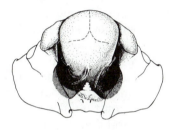

D. Birth by flexion.

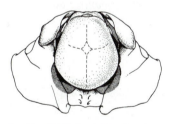

E. Head falls back in extension.

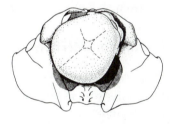

F. Restitution: OP to ROP.

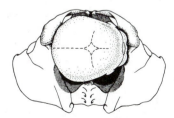

G. External rotation: ROP to ROT.

Figure 6. Summary of short arc rotation: ROP to OP.

Management of the Progressing Case

1. Expectant observation is the best policy. Given sufficient time, most posterior positions of the occiput rotate anteriorly, and the baby is delivered spontaneously or by low forceps. Thus as long as the fetus and mother are in good condition and labor is progressing, there is no justification for interference. The safe and wise rule is to leave occipitoposterior positions to nature, supplying only supportive measures until there is a definite indication for intervention.
2. While it is believed that anterior rotation is helped by the mother's lying on the same side as the fetal limbs, most women remain in the position of greatest comfort.
3. Because the labor may be long and difficult for mother and child, care must be exercised to ensure adequate intake of fluids and nourishment. More judicious use of analgesia and sedation is required than in normal occipitoanterior positions.
4. When the head is delivered in the posterior position (face to pubis) the large back part of the head (biparietal diameter of 9.5 cm) causes greater stretching and more lacerations of the perineum than does the narrow anterior part of the head (bitemporal diameter of 8.0 cm). For this reason a large episiotomy is indicated. Frequently there is arrest at the perineum, and low forceps is the management of choice to save mother and child from the effects of a prolonged period of bearing down.

Indications for Interference

Maternal Distress
Maternal distress is fatigue or exhaustion and is accompanied by the following signs:

1. Pulse above 100 beats/minute
2. Temperature above 100°F
3. Dehydration, dry tongue, dry skin, concentrated urine
4. Loss of emotional stability

Fetal Distress
Fetal distress is shown by:

1. Irregular fetal heart rate
2. Fetal heart rate below 100 or over 160 beats/minute between uterinecontractions
3. Passage of meconium in a vertex presentation

Lack of Progress

The cessation of descent and/or rotation indicates that labor is arrested and that interference is mandatory. Reasons for failure of descent and rotation include:

1. Cephalopelvic disproportion
2. Android midpelvis
3. Ineffective uterine contractions
4. Deflexion of the head
5. Uterine contraction ring preventing the shoulders from rotating anteriorly
6. Multiparity, pendulous abdomen, poor abdominal and uterine tone
7. A weak pelvic floor, failing to guide the occiput anteriorly

While the basic strategy of nonintervention is, up to a point, a wise one, it is not safe to wait too long; fine judgment is needed to decide the point at which further delay is undesirable or even harmful. Where the standard signs of fetal or maternal distress are present, the decision to interfere is based on clear-cut grounds. However, when the contractions are long, strong, and too frequent, the risk of intracranial damage is present and operative therapy must be instituted sooner, even though the fetal heart sounds are normal and no meconium has been passed.

Methods of Operative Vaginal Delivery in Arrested Occipitoposterior Position

Vaginal delivery by forceps is the procedure of choice, but only if the following prerequisites have been fulfilled:

1. The fetal head must be engaged—i.e., the biparietal diameter has passed through the pelvic inlet, and the bony presenting part has reached the level of the ischial spines.
2. There must be no cephalopelvic disproportion.
3. The cervix must be fully dilated.
4. The membranes have to be ruptured.
5. Accurate diagnosis of position and station is essential.

Under these conditions, arrest of progress in the second stage of labor (cervix is fully dilated) of 2 hours in a primigravida and 1 hour in a multipara is an indication for reevaluation of the situation and consideration of operative delivery. The following choices are available:

1. No fetal or maternal distress
   a. Labor is permitted to continue. If the uterine contractions are weak an infusion of oxytocin is established.

    b. The fetal head is low in the pelvis: delivery is effected by forceps. (See Chapter 27 for the techniques.)

    c. The fetal head is high in the pelvis and disproportion is suspected: cesarean section is performed.

2. Fetal distress
Immediate delivery is carried out, either by forceps or by cesarean section.

With forceps the fetal head can be delivered in the posterior position or it can be rotated to the anterior position before being extracted. The various maneuvers are described in Chapter 27. If an attempt at delivery with forceps fails, cesarean section is performed.

Management When Conditions for Immediate Vaginal Delivery Are Not Present

Fetopelvic Disproportion
If there has been no progress in the face of efficient uterine contractions and a diagnosis of fetopelvic disproportion has been made, cesarean section should be performed.

Intact Membranes
Intact membranes do not always help labor and often even seem to retard it. Therefore, before the progress of labor can be considered halted, the membranes should be ruptured artificially and the patient given a further trial of labor. With these measures the patient frequently makes good progress in rotation and descent, and spontaneous delivery takes place.

Ineffective Uterine Contractions
Ineffective uterine contractions result in slow advance or none at all. There are two main groups of cases: (1) myometrial fatigue resulting from long labor and (2) inefficient uterine action, a condition frequently associated with posterior positions of the occiput, as well as with other malpresentations.

Two types of therapy are available: (1) the uterus can be rested or (2) it can be stimulated. Since in most cases the patient is weary, she should be helped to rest. Ten milligrams of morphine sulfate or 100 mg of Demerol gives the patient an hour or two of sleep, and an infusion of a liter (or more if needed) of crystalloid solution improves her state of hydration. In many instances good labor starts soon after the patient awakens.

If effective labor does not begin, the uterus may be stimulated. The best method of doing this is to add 5 units of oxytocin to a liter of crystalloid solution and to give this as an intravenous infusion. The drip is started slowly, at a rate of about 10 drops/minute, and the effect on the contractions and the fetal heart is observed. The subsequent speed is governed by the effect. The aim is to achieve good uterine contractions every 2 to 3 minutes, lasting 45 to 60 seconds (see Chapter 39).

Undilated Cervix

The causes and management of failure of the cervix to dilate fully or to progress beyond 4 to 5 cm fall into several groups (see Chapter 38).

1. When the basic etiology is cephalopelvic disproportion, treatment by cesarean section is best for mother and child.
2. Artificial rupture of the bag of waters, by bringing the presenting part into closer apposition with the cervix, brings about more rapid dilatation in many instances.
3. When inefficient uterine action does not open the cervix, treatment is instituted to correct the defective contractions.
4. When some intrinsic disease of the cervix prevents it from dilating, cesarean section must be performed.

Malpresentations

14

GENERAL ETIOLOGIC FACTORS

Accidental Factors

This classification is used when there is no discovered cause for the malpresentation.

Maternal and Uterine Factors

1. Contracted pelvis. This is the most important factor.
2. Pendulous maternal abdomen. If the uterus and fetus are allowed to fall forward, there may be difficulty in engagement.
3. Neoplasms. Uterine fibromyomas or ovarian cysts can block the entry to the pelvis.
4. Uterine anomalies. In a bicornuate uterus the nonpregnant horn may obstruct labor in the pregnant one.
5. Abnormalities of placental size or location. Conditions such as placenta previa are associated with unfavorable positions of the fetus.
6. High parity

Fetal Factors

1. Large baby
2. Errors in fetal polarity, such as breech presentation and transverse lie
3. Abnormal internal rotation. The occiput rotates posteriorly or fails to rotate at all.

4. Fetal attitude: extension in place of normal flexion
5. Multiple pregnancy
6. Fetal anomalies, including hydrocephaly and anencephaly
7. Polyhydramnios. An excessive amount of amniotic fluid allows the baby freedom of activity, and it may assume abnormal positions.
8. Prematurity

Placenta and Membranes

1. Placenta previa
2. Cornual implantation
3. Premature rupture of membranes

EFFECTS OF MALPRESENTATIONS

Effects on Labor

The less symmetrical adaptation of the presenting part to the cervix and to the pelvis plays a part in reducing the efficiency of labor.

1. The incidence of fetopelvic disproportion is higher.
2. Inefficient uterine action is common. The contractions tend to be weak and irregular.
3. Prolonged labor is seen frequently.
4. Pathologic retraction rings can develop, and rupture of the lower uterine segment may be the end result.
5. The cervix often dilates slowly and incompletely.
6. The presenting part stays high.
7. Premature rupture of the membranes occurs often.
8. The need for operative delivery is increased.

Effects on the Mother

1. Because greater uterine and intraabdominal muscular effort is required, and because labor is often prolonged with attendant lack of rest and inadequate nourishment, maternal exhaustion is common.
2. There is more stretching of the perineum and soft parts, and there are more lacerations.
3. Bleeding is more profuse, originating from:
   a. Tears of the uterus, cervix, and vagina

   b. The placental site, maternal exhaustion leading to uterine atony
4. There is a greater incidence of infection. This is caused by:
   a. Early rupture of the membranes
   b. Excessive blood loss
   c. Tissue damage
   d. Frequent rectal and vaginal examinations
5. The patient's discomfort seems out of proportion to the strength of the uterine contractions. She complains bitterly of pain before the uterus is felt to harden, and continues to feel the pain after the uterus has relaxed.
6. Paresis of the bowel and bladder add to the patient's suffering.

Effects on the Fetus

1. The fetus fits the pelvis less perfectly, making its passage through the pelvis more difficult and leading to excessive molding.
2. The long labor is harder on the baby, with a greater incidence of anoxia, brain damage, asphyxia, and intrauterine death.
3. There is a higher incidence of operative delivery, increasing the danger of trauma to the baby.
4. Prolapse of the umbilical cord is more common than in normal positions.

Face Presentation

15

GENERAL CONSIDERATIONS

Definition

The lie is longitudinal, the presentation is cephalic, the presenting part is the face, the attitude is one of complete extension, the chin (mentum, M) is the denominator and leading pole, and the presenting diameter is the submentobregmatic of 9.5 cm. In face presentations the part be-tweeen the glabella and chin presents; in brow presentations it is the part between the glabella and bregma. However, positions intermediate to these are seen.

Incidence

The incidence is less than 1 percent (1 in 250) and is higher in multiparas than primigravidas. Primary face presentations are present before the onset of labor and are rare. Most face presentations are secondary, extension taking place during labor generally at the pelvic inlet. About 70 percent of face presentations are anterior or transverse, while 30 percent are posterior.

Etiology

Anything that delays engagement in flexion can contribute to the etiology of attitudes of extension. There is an association between attitudes of extension and cephalopelvic disproportion, and since this is a serious combination the presence of a small pelvis or a large head must be ruled out with certainty. Rare causes of extension include thyroid neoplasms, which act by pushing the head back; multiple coils of cord around the

183

neck, which prevent flexion; and spasm or shortening of the extensor muscles of the neck. Anencephalic fetuses frequently present by the face. In many cases no cause can be found.

ANTERIOR FACE PRESENTATIONS

The following descriptions apply to the left mentum anterior (LMA) presentation. The mechanism for the right mentum anterior (RMA) presentation is similar to that for LMA except that the chin, small parts, and fetal heart are on the right side, while the back and cephalic prominence are on the left.

Diagnosis of Position: LMA

Abdominal Examination

1. The long axes of the fetus and mother are parallel (Fig. 1A).
2. The head is at the pelvis. Early in labor the head is not engaged.
3. The back is on the right side of the mother's abdomen, but since it is posterior, it is often felt indistinctly. The small parts are on the left and anterior. Extension of the spine causes the chest to be thrown out and the back to be hollowed.
4. The breech is in the fundus.
5. The cephalic prominence (the occiput) is on the right. An important diagnostic sign of extension attitudes is that the back and the cephalic prominence are on the same side. When flexion is present, the cephalic prominence and the back are on opposite sides.
6. It must be kept in mind that in anterior face presentations the baby's back and occiput are posterior. When the chin is posterior, on the other hand, the back and occiput are anterior.

Fetal Heart
The fetal heart tones are transmitted through the anterior chest wall of the fetus and are heard loudest in the left lower quadrant of the maternal abdomen, on the same side as the small parts.

Vaginal Examination

1. The clue to diagnosis is a negative finding—i.e., absence of the round, even, hard vertex. In place of the dome of the skull with its identifying suture lines and fontanelles, there is a softer and irregular presenting part. One suspects face or breech. Identifi-

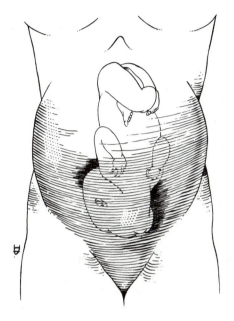

A. Abdominal view.

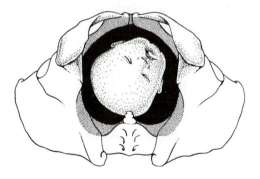

B. Vaginal view.

Figure 1. Left mentum anterior.

cation of the various parts of the face clinches the diagnosis. After prolonged labor marked edema may confuse the picture.

2. The long axis of the face is in the right oblique diameter of the pelvis (Fig. 1B).
3. The chin is in the left anterior quadrant of the maternal pelvis.
4. The forehead is in the right posterior quadrant of the pelvis.
5. Vaginal examination must be performed gently to avoid injury to the eyes.

X-ray Examination
Occasionally radiologic examination is necessary in nonprogressing labors to diagnose the position and to estimate pelvic capacity.

Late Diagnosis
Because most face presentations make good progress, the diagnosis may not be made until the face has reached the floor of the pelvis or until advance has ceased.

Mechanism of Labor: LMA

Extension
For some reason the head does not flex. Instead, it extends (Fig. 2), so that in place of an LOP or ROP there is an RMA or an LMA. The baby enters the pelvis chin first. The presenting diameter in face presentations (submentobregmatic) and in well-flexed head presentations (suboccipitobregmatic) is 9.5 cm in each case. This is one of the reasons why most anterior face presentations come to spontaneous delivery.

Descent
With the chin as the leading part, engagement takes place in the right oblique diameter of the pelvis. Descent is slower than in flexed attitudes. The face is low in the pelvis before the biparietal diameter has passed the brim. When the forward leading edge of the presenting face is felt at the level of the ischial spines, the tracheobregmatic diameter is still above the inlet.

Internal Rotation
With descent and molding, the chin reaches the pelvic floor, where it is directed downward, forward, and medially. As it rotates 45° anteriorly toward the symphysis (LMA to MA), the long axis of the face comes into the anteroposterior diameter of the pelvis (Figs. 2C and D). With further descent the chin escapes under the symphysis. The shoulders have remained in the oblique diameter, so the neck is twisted 45°. An essen-

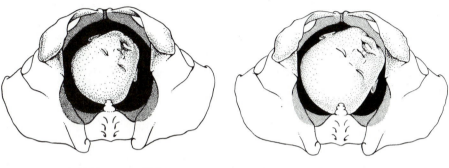

A. LMA: onset of labor.   B. Extension and descent.

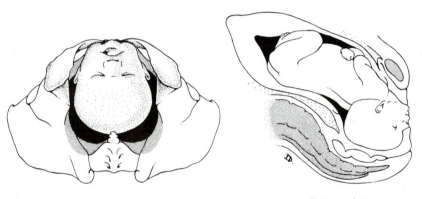

C. Vaginal view.   D. Lateral view.

C and D.   Internal rotation: LMA to MA.

Figure 2. Mechanism of labor.

tial feature of internal rotation is that the chin must rotate anteriorly and under the symphysis, or spontaneous delivery is impossible. Anterior rotation does not take place until the face is well applied to the pelvic floor and may be delayed until late in labor. The attendant must not give up hope too soon.

Flexion

The head is born by flexion (Figs. 2E-G). The submental region at the neck impinges under the symphysis pubis. With the head pivoting around this point, the mouth, nose, orbits, forehead, vertex, and occiput are born over the perineum by flexion. The head then falls back (Figs. 2H and I).

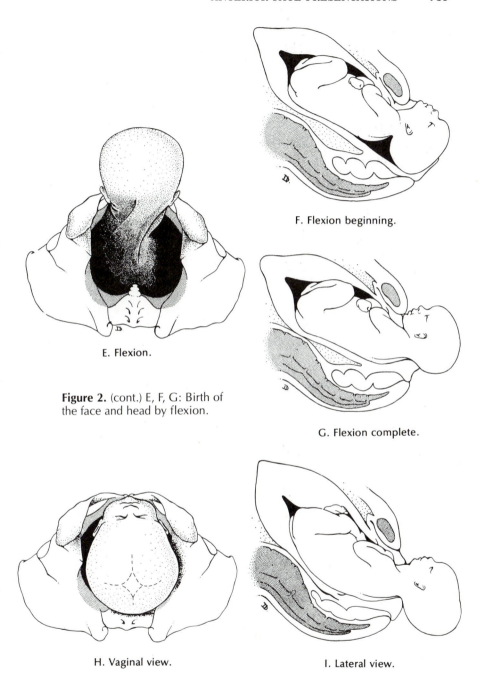

F. Flexion beginning.

E. Flexion.

Figure 2. (cont.) E, F, G: Birth of the face and head by flexion.

G. Flexion complete.

H. Vaginal view.

I. Lateral view.

Figure 2. (cont.) H, I: Head falls back in extension.

Restitution
As the head is released from the vagina, the neck untwists and the chin turns 45° back toward the original side (Fig. 2J).

External Rotation
The anterior shoulder reaches the pelvic floor and rotates toward the symphysis to bring the bisacromial diameter from the oblique to the anteroposterior diameter of the outlet. The chin rotates back another 45° to maintain the head in its correct relationship to the shoulders (Fig. 2K).

Molding
Molding (Fig. 3) leads to an elongation of the head in its anteroposterior diameter and flattening from above downward. The forehead and occiput protrude. The extension of the head on the trunk disappears after a few days.

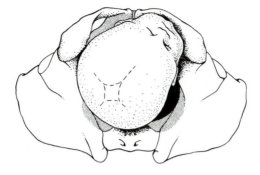

J. Restitution: MA to LMA.

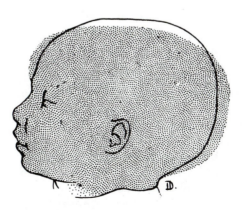

K. External rotation: LMA to LMT.

Figure 2. (cont.) Restitution and external rotation.

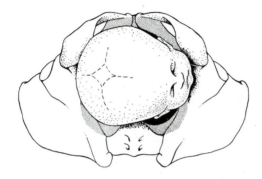

Figure 3. Molding: face presentation.

Prognosis: Anterior Face Presentations

Labor

Because thc face is a poor dilator, and because attitudes of extension are less favorable, labor takes longer than in normal occipitoanterior positions. The labor is conducted with this in mind. Delay takes place at the inlet, but once the face presentation and the labor are well established steady progress is the rule. Over 90 percent of anterior face presentations deliver per vaginam without complications. Figure 4 summarizes the mechanism of labor with the LMA presentation.

Mother

The mother has more work to do, suffers more pain, and receives greater lacerations than in normal positions.

Fetus

The baby does well in most cases, but the prognosis is less favorable than in normal presentations. The outlook for the child can be improved by early diagnosis, carefully conducted first and second stages of labor, and the restriction of operative vaginal deliveries to easily performed procedures. Cesarean section is preferable to complicated, difficult, and traumatic vaginal operations.

The membranes rupture early in labor, and the face takes the brunt of the punishment so that it becomes badly swollen and misshapen. Its appearance is a great worry to the parents. The edema disappears gradually, and the infant takes on a more normal appearance. Edema of the larynx may result from prolonged pressure of the hyoid region of the neck against the pubic bone. For the first 24 hours the baby must be watched carefully to detect any difficulty in breathing.

Management of Anterior Face Presentations

1. *Disproportion*: Disproportion is managed by cesarean section.
2. *Normal pelvis*: In a normal pelvis anterior face presentations are left alone for these reasons:
   a. Most deliver spontaneously or with the aid of low forceps.
   b. Should conversion (flexion) be successful, the anterior face presentation is replaced by an occipitoposterior one (LMA to ROP or RMA to LOP). This does not improve the situation and may make it worse.
   c. If conversion is partially successful, the face is changed to a brow presentation. In this case a face presentation, which usually delivers spontaneously, is replaced by a brow, which cannot.

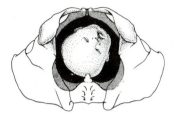

A. LMA: onset of labor.

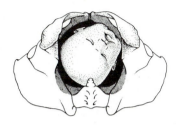

B. Extension and descent.

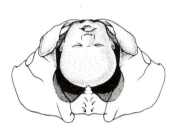

C. Internal rotation: LMA to MA.

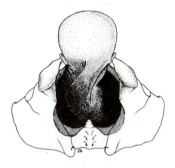

D. Flexion.

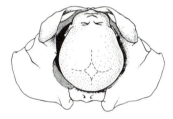

E. Extension.

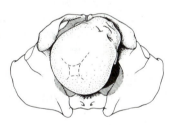

F. Restitution: MA to LMA.

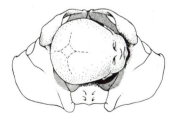

G. External rotation: LMA to LMT.

Figure 4. Summary of mechanism of labor: LMA.

3. *Arrest*
   a. Low in the pelvis, well below the ischial spines: Extraction with low forceps
   b. High in the pelvis: Cesarean section

TRANSVERSE FACE PRESENTATIONS

The long axis of the face is in the transverse diameter of the pelvis, with the chin on one side and the forehead on the other (Fig. 5).

The following descriptions apply to the left mentum transverse (LMT) presentation. The mechanism of labor for the right mentum transverse (RMT) presentation is the same as that for LMT except that the chin, small parts, and fetal heart are on the right, while the back and cephalic prominence are on the left.

Diagnosis of Position: LMT

Abdominal Examination

1. The long axis of the fetus is parallel to that of the mother.
2. The head is at the pelvis.
3. The back is on the right, toward the maternal flank. The small parts are on the left side.
4. The breech is in the fundus.
5. The cephalic prominence (the occiput) is on the right, the same side as the back.

Fetal Heart
The fetal heart is heard loudest in the left lower quadrant of the mother's abdomen.

Vaginal Examination

1. The long axis of the face is in the transverse diameter of the pelvis.
2. The chin is to the left, at 3 o'clock.
3. The forehead is to the right, at 9 o'clock.

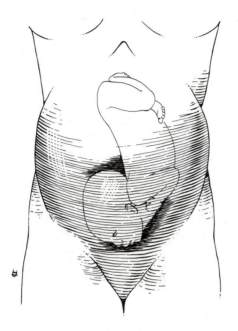

A. Abdominal view.

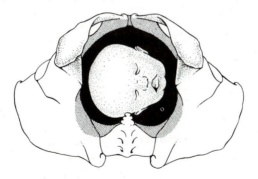

B. Vaginal view.

Figure 5. Left mentum transverse.

Mechanism of Labor: LMT

A summary of the mechanism of labor for the LMT presentation is given in Figure 6.

Extension
Extension to LMT occurs instead of flexion to ROT.

Descent
Engagement takes place in the transverse diameter of the pelvis. Descent is slow.

Internal Rotation
The chin rotates 90° anteriorly to the midline (LMT to LMA to MA). The chin comes under the symphysis.

Flexion
The submental region of the neck impinges in the subpubic angle. Birth is by flexion, after which the head falls backward.

Restitution
As the neck untwists, the head turns back 45°.

External Rotation
The shoulders turn from the oblique into the anteroposterior diameter of the pelvis, and the head rotates back another 45°.

Clinical Course of Labor and Management: LMT

1. Anterior rotation takes place in the majority of cases, LMT to LMA to MA. The treatment is the same as LMA. Delivery is spontaneous or assisted by low forceps.
2. Arrest as LMT low in the pelvis.
   a. Rotation to LMA manually or by forceps, followed by extraction of the head by forceps.
   b. If rotation is difficult or fails, cesarean section is performed.
3. Arrest as LMT high in the pelvis is treated by cesarean section.

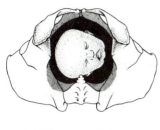

A. LMT: onset of labor.

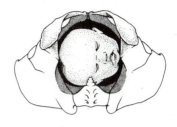

B. Descent.

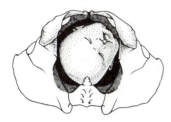

C. Internal rotation: LMT to LMA.

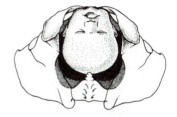

D. Internal rotation: LMA to MA.

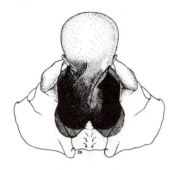

E. Birth by flexion.

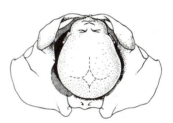

F. Extension.

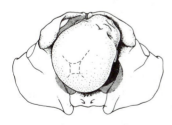

G. Restitution: MA to LMA.

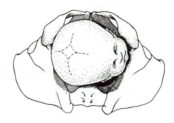

H. External rotation: LMA to LMT.

Figure 6. Mechanism of labor: LMT.

POSTERIOR FACE PRESENTATIONS

Some 30 percent of face presentations are posterior. Most of these rotate anteriorly. The flexed counterpart of the posterior face is the anterior occiput; thus LMP flexes to ROA and RMP to LOA. Persistent posterior face presentations become arrested, as they cannot deliver spontaneously. The descriptions here are for the left mentum posterior (LMP) presentation.

Diagnosis of Position: LMP

Abdominal Examination

1. The long axis of the fetus is parallel to the long axis of the mother (Fig. 7A).
2. The head is at the pelvis.
3. The back is anterior and to the right. The small parts are on the left and posterior.
4. The breech is in the fundus of the uterus.
5. The cephalic prominence (occiput) is to the right and anterior. It is on the same side as the back.

Fetal Heart
The fetal heart tones, transmitted through the anterior shoulder, are heard loudest in the left lower quadrant of the mother's abdomen.

Vaginal Examination

1. The long diameter of the face is in the left oblique diameter of the pelvis.
2. The chin is in the left posterior quadrant of the pelvis (Fig. 7B).
3. The forehead is in the right anterior quadrant.

Mechanism of Labor: LMP

There are two basic mechanisms:
1. Long arc rotation, with the chin rotating 135° to the anterior. About two-thirds of posterior face presentations do this and deliver spontaneously or with the aid of low forceps.
2. Short arc rotation of 45° to the posterior, with the chin ending up in the hollow of the sacrum. These cases become arrested as persistent posterior face presentations.

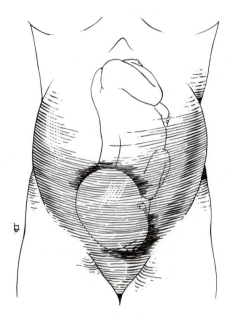

A. Abdominal view.

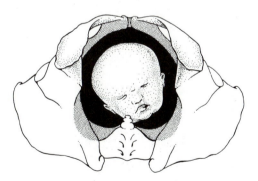

B. Vaginal view.

Figure 7. Left mentum posterior.

Long Arc Rotation: 135° to the Anterior

Extension
Extension to LMP (Fig. 8) occurs instead of flexion to ROA.

Descent
Descent is slow. The presenting part remains high while the essential molding takes place. Without extreme molding the vertex cannot pass under the anterior part of the pelvic inlet.

Internal Rotation
The slow descent continues; the marked molding enables the chin to reach the pelvic floor, where it rotates 135° to the anterior and comes to lie under the symphysis. Since the original position was LMP, the sequence is LMP to LMT to LMA to MA in rotations of 45° between each step.

Flexion
The submental area pivots under the symphysis, and the head is born by flexion. The head then falls backward.

Restitution
The chin rotates back 45° as the neck untwists.

External Rotation
With the rotation of the shoulders from the oblique into the anteroposterior diameter of the pelvis, the chin turns back another 45°.

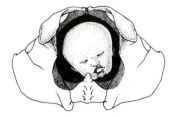

A. LMP: descent.

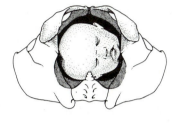

B. Internal rotation: LMP to LMT.

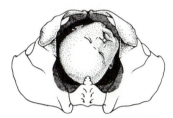

C. Internal rotation: LMT to LMA.

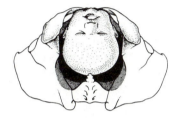

D. Internal rotation: LMA to MA.

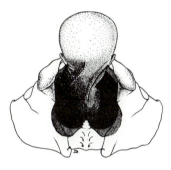

E. Birth by flexion.

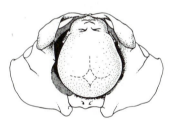

F. Head falls back in extension.

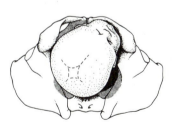

G. Restitution: MA to LMA.

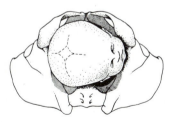

H. External rotation: LMA to LMT.

Figure 8. LMP: long arc rotation.

Short Arc Rotation: 45° to the Posterior

Extension
Extension to LMP takes place (Fig. 9).

Descent
Descent occurs with the help of extreme molding.

Internal Rotation
The chin rotates 45° posteriorly into the hollow of the sacrum (LMP to MP). Impaction follows and the progress of labor comes to a halt. Flexion cannot take place and further advancement is not possible, except in the rare situation where the baby is so small that the shoulders and head can enter the pelvis together.

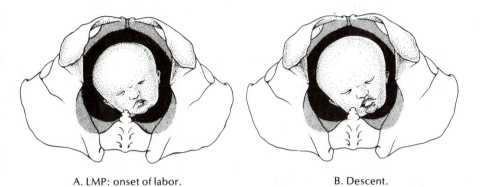

A. LMP: onset of labor.   B. Descent.

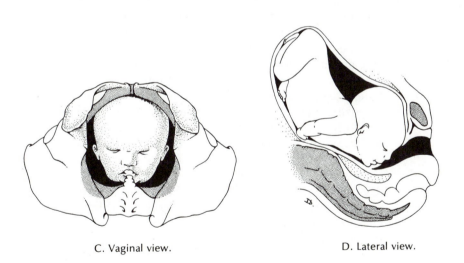

C. Vaginal view.   D. Lateral view.

C and D. Internal rotation: LMP to MP.

Figure 9. LMP: short arc rotation.

Prognosis: Posterior Face Presentations

The prolonged labor and difficult rotation are traumatic to both baby and mother. When the chin rotates posteriorly the prognosis is poor unless the situation is corrected. Maternal morbidity is directly proportional to the degree of difficulty of the birth. High forceps or version and extraction carry with them the most morbid postpartum courses.

Management of Posterior Face Presentations

1. *Disproportion:* Disproportion is managed by cesarean section.
2. *Trial of labor:* Since two-thirds of posterior faces rotate anteriorly and deliver spontaneously, and since internal rotation may not be completed until later in labor when the face is distending the pelvic floor, plenty of time should be allowed for the rotation to be accomplished. Interference must not be premature.
3. *Persistent posterior face:* Since face presentations that have remained posterior cannot be delivered spontaneously, operative interference is necessary.
    a. Cesarean section is the modern treatment of choice, giving the best results for both mother and child.
    b. Flexion (conversion) from mentoposterior to occipitoanterior may be considered if cesarean section cannot be performed. One method of accomplishing this is by the *Thorn maneuver* (Fig. 10). The cervix must be fully dilated. With the vaginal hand the operator flexes the fetal head. With his other hand he pushes on the breech to flex the body. At the same time an assistant presses against the baby's thorax or abdomen to try and jack-knife the infant's body. This procedure is performed under anesthesia, and must be done soon after the membranes rupture. If the amniotic fluid has drained away, the dry uterine cavity and snug fit of the uterus around the baby make it difficult or impossible to carry out this treatment. Once flexion has been accomplished, the head is pushed into the pelvis and held in place.
    c. Rotation to mentum anterior can sometimes be achieved by the use of forceps, but the operation is difficult and may be traumatic.

BIBLIOGRAPHY

Benedetti TJ, Lowensohn RI, Truscott AM: Face presentation at term. Obstet Gynecol 55:199, 1980

Duff P: Diagnosis and management of face presentation. Obstet Gynecol 57:105, 1981

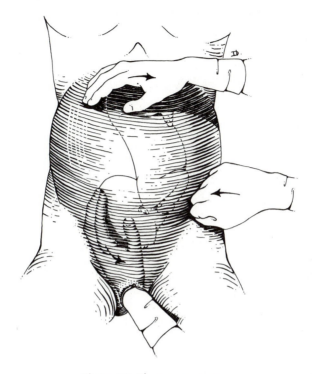

Figure 10. Thorn maneuver.

16

Brow Presentation

GENERAL CONSIDERATIONS

Definition

Brow presentation is an attitude of partial (halfway) extension, in contrast to face presentation in which extension is complete. The presenting part is the area between the orbital ridges and the bregma. The denominator is the forehead (frontum: Fr). The presenting diameter is the verticomental, which, at 13.5 cm, is the longest anteroposterior diameter of the fetal head.

Incidence

The incidence is under 1 percent, ranging from 1:3000 to 1:1000. Primary brow presentations—those that occur before labor has started—are rare. The majority are secondary—i.e., they occur after the onset of labor. Often the position is transitory, and the head either flexes to an occiput presentation or extends completely and becomes a face presentation.

Etiology

The causes are similar to those of face presentation and include anything that interferes with engagement in flexion.

1. Cephalopelvic disproportion is of great significance.
2. Some fetal conditions prevent flexion.
   a. Tumors of the neck, e.g., thyroid
   b. Coils of umbilical cord around the neck
   c. Fetal anomalies

3. Increased fetal mobility.
   a. Polyhydramnios
   b. Small or premature baby
4. Premature rupture of membranes when the head is not engaged. It is trapped in an attitude of extension.
5. Uterine abnormalities.
   a. Neoplasm of lower segment
   b. Bicornuate uterus
6. Abnormal placental implantation: placenta previa.
7. Iatrogenic: external version.
8. Idiopathic: nearly 30 percent are unexplained.

LEFT FRONTUM ANTERIOR: LFrA

Diagnosis of Position: LFrA

Abdominal Examination

1. The lie is longitudinal (Fig. 1A).
2. The head is at the pelvis but is not engaged.
3. The back is on the mother's right and posterior; it may be difficult to palpate. The small parts are on the left and anterior.
4. The breech is in the fundus of the uterus.
5. The cephalic prominence (occiput) and the back are on the same side (the right).

Fetal Heart
Fetal heart sounds are heard best in the left lower quadrant of the maternal abdomen.

Vaginal Examination

1. The anteroposterior diameter of the head is in the right oblique diameter of the pelvis (Fig. 1B).
2. The brow, the area between the nasion and the bregma, presents and is felt in the left anterior quadrant of the pelvis.
3. The vertex is in the right posterior quadrant.
4. The bregma (anterior fontanelle) is palpated easily.
5. The frontal suture is felt, but the sagittal suture is usually out of reach.
6. Identification of the supraorbital ridges is a key to diagnosis.

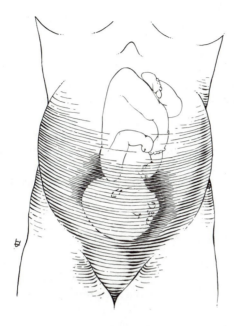

A. Abdominal view.

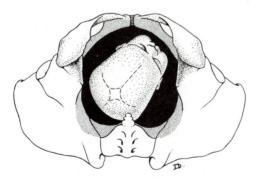

B. Vaginal view.

Figure 1. Left frontum anterior.

X-ray Examination
When labor has been prolonged and the landmarks on the fetal head are obscured by edema and molding, x-ray pelvimetry is helpful in making the diagnosis and assessing the pelvis.

Late and Failed Diagnosis
The difference, on vaginal examination, between the hard, smooth dome of the skull and the soft irregular face is great enough to diagnose the abnormal position or at least to suspect it. On the other hand, the feel of the vertex and that of the forehead may be similar, and molding and edema add to the difficulty of differentiation. Hence anything short of a most careful abdominal and vaginal examination with a high index of suspicion fails to identify the malposition. A good rule is that whenever there is failure of progress, one should examine the patient thoroughly, keeping brow presentation in mind.

Mechanism of Labor: LFrA

Presenting diameter is the verticomental, measuring 13.5 cm. It is the longest anteroposterior diameter of the head. When engagement takes place it is accompanied by extensive molding, and when progress occurs it is slow.

Spontaneous delivery is rare, and can take place only when there is the combination of a large pelvis, strong uterine contractions, and a small baby. In these cases the following mechanism of labor occurs (Fig. 2):

Extension
The head extends and the verticomental diameter presents, with the forehead leading the way.

Descent
Descent is slow and late. Usually the head does not settle into the pelvis until the membranes have ruptured and the cervix has reached full dilatation.

Internal Rotation
The forehead rotates anteriorly 45° so that the face comes to lie behind the pubic symphysis (LFrA to FrA). A considerable amount of internal rotation may take place between the ischial spines and the tuberosities.

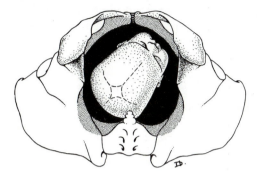

A. LFrA: Onset of labor.

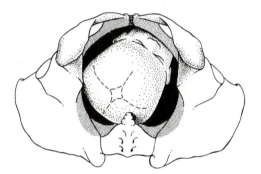

B. Descent.

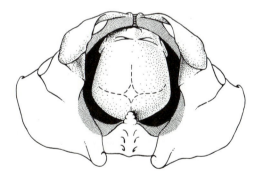

C. Internal rotation: LFrA to FrA.

Figure 2. Labor: LFrA. Descent, internal rotation.

Flexion

The face impinges under the pubis, and as the head pivots round this point the bregma, vertex, and occiput are born over the perineum (Figs. 3A-C).

Extension

The head then falls back in extension (Figs. 4A and B), and the nose, mouth, and chin slip under the symphysis.

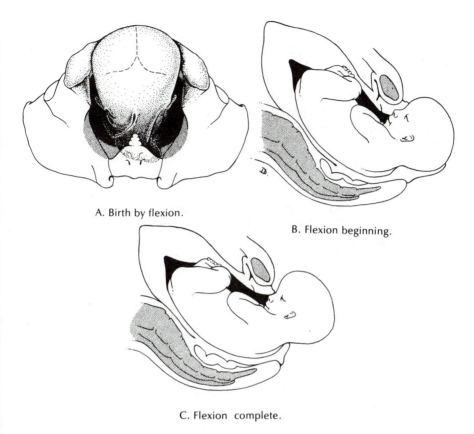

A. Birth by flexion.

B. Flexion beginning.

C. Flexion complete.

Figure 3. Birth of brow and head by flexion.

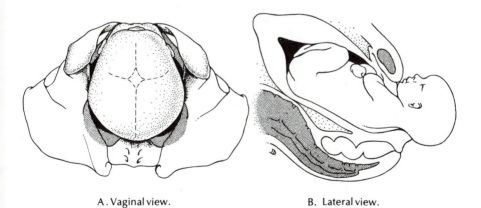

A. Vaginal view.

B. Lateral view.

Figure 4. Head falls back in extension.

Restitution
The neck untwists, and the head turns 45° back to the original side (Fig. 5A).

External Rotation
As the shoulder rotates anteriorly from the oblique to the anteroposterior diameter of the pelvis, the head turns back another 45° (Fig. 5B).

Molding
Molding is extreme (Fig. 6). The verticomental diameter is compressed. The occipitofrontal diameter is elongated markedly, so that the forehead bulges greatly. The face is flattened, and the distance from the chin to the top of the head is long. This is exaggerated by the large caput succedaneum that forms on the forehead.

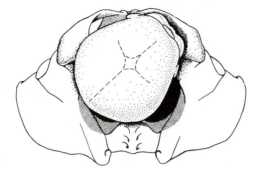

A. Restitution: FrA to LFrA.

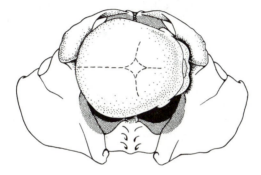

B. External rotation: LFrA to LFrT.

Figure 5. Restitution, external rotation.

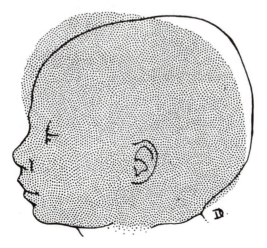

Figure 6. Molding: brow presentation.

PROGNOSIS: BROW PRESENTATIONS

Labor

In most cases brow presentations do not deliver spontaneously. If the malposition is detected early in labor and if appropriate therapeutic measures are undertaken, the fetal and maternal results are good. Failure to recognize the problem leads to prolonged and traumatic labor.

Mother

Passage of a brow through the pelvis is slower, harder, and more traumatic to the mother than any other presentation. Perineal laceration is inevitable and may extend high into the vaginal fornices or into the rectum because of the large diameter offered to the outlet.

Fetus

Fetal mortality is high. The excessive molding may cause irreparable damage to the brain. Mistakes in diagnosis and treatment are the main causes of the poor fetal prognosis.

MANAGEMENT OF BROW PRESENTATIONS

X-ray pelvimetry helps in making the diagnosis and in assessing the pelvis.

1. *Trial of labor:* Since brow presentation may be transitory, a trial of labor is permissible in the hope that flexion to an occiput presentation or complete extension to a face presentation will take place.
2. *Persistent brow presentation:* Since brow presentations cannot deliver spontaneously, operative interference is necessary.
   a. Cesarean section is the treatment of choice, giving the best results for both mother and child.
   b. Flexion of the head may be attempted, especially in multiparas. This procedure is carried out when the cervix is dilated and soon after the membranes have ruptured. If success is not immediate, the procedure must be abandoned in favor of cesarean section without delay.

17

Median Vertex Presentation: Military Attitude

DEFINITION

There is neither flexion nor extension; the occiput and the brow are at the same level in the pelvis. The presenting part is the vertex. The denominator is the occiput. The presenting diameter is the occipitofrontal, which at 11.0 cm is longer than the more favorable suboccipitobregmatic of 9.5 cm. Hence progress is slower and arrest a little more frequent. In many cases the military attitude is transitory, and the head flexes as it descends. Occasionally extension to a brow or face presentation takes place.

DIAGNOSIS OF POSITION: MEDIAN VERTEX PRESENTATION

Abdominal Examination

1. The long axes of fetus and mother are parallel (Fig. 1A).
2. The head is at or in the pelvic inlet.
3. The back is in one flank, the small parts on the opposite side.
4. The breech is in the fundus.
5. Since there is neither flexion nor extension there is no marked cephalic prominence on one side or the other.

Fetal Heart
The fetal heart tones are heard loudest in the lower quadrant of the mother's abdomen, on the same side as the fetal back.

Vaginal Examination

1. The sagittal suture is felt in the transverse diameter of the pelvis, as LOT or ROT (Fig. 1B).
2. The two fontanelles are equally easy to palpate and identify. They are at the same level in the pelvis.

X-ray Examination
Occasionally radiologic examination is needed to diagnose the position and to assess the pelvis.

MECHANISM OF LABOR: MEDIAN VERTEX PRESENTATION

Engagement takes place most often in the transverse diameter of the inlet. The head descends slowly, with the occiput and the brow at the same level (there is neither flexion nor extension) and with the sagittal suture in the transverse diameter of the pelvis, until the median vertex reaches the pelvic floor. Now several terminations are possible:

1. Most often the head flexes, the occiput rotates to the anterior, and delivery takes place as an occipitoanterior position.
2. The head may become arrested in the transverse diameter of the pelvis. Operative assistance is necessary for deep transverse arrest.
3. The head may rotate posteriorly with or without flexion. The occiput turns into the hollow of the sacrum and the forehead to the pubis. The mechanism is that of persistent occipitoposterior positions. Delivery may be spontaneous or by operative methods.

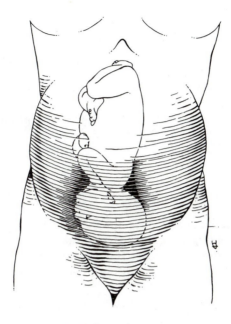

A. Abdominal view.

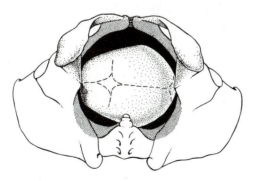

B. Vaginal view.

Figure 1. Median vertex presentation: LOT.

4. In rare instances delivery can occur with the sagittal suture in the transverse diameter.
5. Occasionally the head extends, and the mechanism becomes a face or brow presentation.

PROGNOSIS: MEDIAN VERTEX PRESENTATION

While labor is a little longer and harder than normal on mother and child, the prognosis is reasonably good. Many cases flex and proceed to normal delivery.

MANAGEMENT OF MEDIAN VERTEX PRESENTATION

1. Since flexion occurs so frequently, there should be no interference as long as progress is being made.
2. When flexion takes place the management is that of occipitoanterior (see Chapter 10) or occipitoposterior (see Chapter 13) positions.
3. Cases in which the head extends are treated as face (see Chapter 15) or brow (see Chapter 16) presentations.
4. When arrest occurs in the military attitude, and the head is low in the pelvis, vaginal delivery may be attempted by flexing the head manually, rotating the occiput to the anterior, and extracting the head by forceps (see Chapter 26).
5. Where there is disproportion, when the head is high in the pelvis, or where an attempt at vaginal delivery fails, cesarean section should be performed.

Breech Presentation

18

GENERAL CONSIDERATIONS

Definition

Breech presentation is a longitudinal lie with a variation in polarity. The fetal pelvis is the leading pole. The denominator is the sacrum. A right sacrum anterior (RSA) is a breech presentation where the fetal sacrum is in the right anterior quadrant of the mother's pelvis, and the bitrochanteric diameter of the fetus is in the right oblique diameter of the pelvis (Fig. 1).

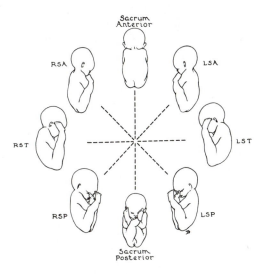

Figure 1. Positions of breech presentation.

Incidence

Breech presentation at delivery occurs in 3 to 4 percent of pregnancies. However, prior to 28 weeks the incidence is about 25 percent. As term is approached the incidence decreases. In most cases the fetus converts to the cephalic presentation by 34 weeks of gestation. Some 15 percent of babies presenting by the breech when labor has begun are preterm, three times the overall rate of preterm labor.

Etiology

As term approaches, the uterine cavity, in most cases, accommodates the fetus best in a longitudinal lie with a cephalic presentation. In many cases of breech presentation no reason for the malpresentation can be found and, by exclusion, the cause is ascribed to chance. Some women deliver all their children as breeches, suggesting that the pelvis is so shaped that the breech fits better than the head.

Breech presentation is more common at the end of the second trimester than near term; hence fetal prematurity is associated frequently with this presentation.

Maternal

Factors that influence the occurrence of breech presentation include: (1) the uterine relaxation associated with high parity; (2) polyhydramnios, in which the excessive amount of amniotic fluid makes it easier for the fetus to change position; (3) oligohydramnios, where, because of the small amount of fluid, the fetus is trapped in the position assumed in the second trimester; (4) uterine anomalies; (5) neoplasms, such as leiomyomata of the myometrium; (6) while contracted pelvis is an uncommon cause of breech presentation, anything that interferes with the entry of the fetal head into the pelvis may play a part in the etiology of breech presentation.

Placental

Placental site: There is some evidence that implantation of the placenta in either cornual-fundal region tends to promote breech presentation. There is a positive association of breech with placenta previa.

Fetal

Fetal factors that influence the occurrence of breech presentation include: (1) multiple pregnancy, (2) hydrocephaly, (3) anencephaly, (4) any fetal anomaly, (5) intrauterine fetal death.

Notes and Comments

1. The patient feels fetal movements in the lower abdomen and may complain of painful kicking against the rectum.

2. Engagement before the onset of labor is uncommon. The patient rarely experiences lightening.

3. The uneven fit of breech to pelvis predisposes to early rupture of the membranes, with the danger of umbilical cord prolapse. The incidence of the latter, which is 4 to 5 percent, is higher with footling breeches. It is wise, therefore, when the bag of waters breaks to make a sterile vaginal examination to determine the exact state of the cervix and to make certain that the cord has not prolapsed.

4. In theory the breech is a poor dilator in comparison with the well flexed head, and labor, descent, and cervical dilatation are believed to take longer. While this is true in some cases, the mean duration of labor of 9.2 hours in primigravidas and 6.1 hours in multiparas suggests that in the majority of cases labor is not prolonged.

5. In frank breeches the baby's lower limbs, which are flexed at the hips and extended at the knees, lie anterior to and against the baby's abdomen. This has the effect of a splint and by decreasing the maneuverability of the baby may result in delay or arrest of progress.

6. On the one hand, the frank breech has the disadvantage of a large and less maneuverable presenting part and may have difficulty passing through the pelvis. On the other hand, it dilates the soft parts to the greatest degree and makes the most room for the head. The small footling breach slips through the pelvis easily but makes less provision for the aftercoming head.

7. One of the dangers to the fetus in breech presentation is that the largest and least compressible diameter comes last.

8. There is an added risk in premature infants because the head is relatively larger in proportion to the rest of the body than in full-term babies. Thus while the small body slips through with no difficulty, it does not dilate the soft parts sufficiently to allow the head to pass easily.

9. Since the posterior segment of the pelvis is roomier than the anterior segment, the posterior parts of the baby are usually born first.

10. Because of the rapid passage of the head through the pelvis there is no time for molding to take place. The fetal head is round and symmetrical.

11. The baby which lay in utero as a frank breech lies with its hips flexed and the feet near its face for some time after birth.
12. The external genitalia are edematous.
13. The passage of meconium in a breech presentation does not have the same significance of fetal distress as in vertex presentation. The meconium is squeezed out of the intestine by the uterine contractions pressing the lower part of the baby's body against the pelvis.

CLASSIFICATION

There are four types of breech presentation:

1. *Complete*: Flexion at thighs and knees (Fig 2A).
2. *Frank*: Flexion at thighs; extension at knees. This is the most common variety and includes almost two-thirds of breech presentations (Fig. 2B).
3. *Footling*: Single or double, with extension at thighs and knees. The foot is the presenting part (Fig. 2C).
4. *Kneeling*: Single or double, with extension at thighs, flexion at knees. The knee is the presenting part (Fig. 2D).

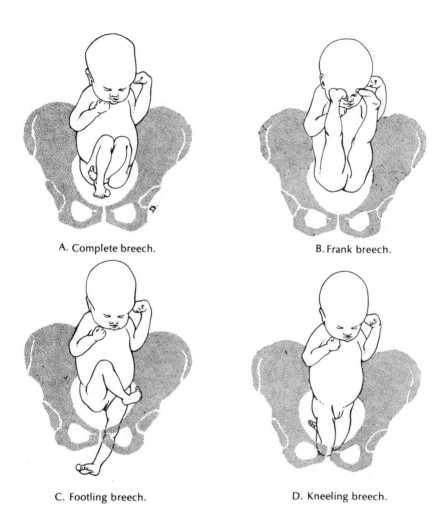

A. Complete breech.

B. Frank breech.

C. Footling breech.

D. Kneeling breech.

Figure 2. Attitudes of breech presentation.

RIGHT SACRUM ANTERIOR: RSA

Diagnosis of Position

Abdominal Examination

1. The lie is longitudinal (Fig. 3A).
2. A soft, irregular mass lies over the pelvis and does not feel like the head. One suspects breech. In a frank breech the muscles of the thighs are drawn taut over the underlying bones, giving an impression of hardness not unlike the head and leading to diagnostic errors.
3. The back is on the right near the midline. The small parts are on the left, away from the midline, and posterior.
4. The head is felt in the fundus of the uterus. If the head is under the liver or the ribs, it may be difficult to palpate. The head is harder and more globular than the breech, and sometimes it can be balloted. Whenever a ballotable mass is felt in the fundus, breech presentation should be suspected.
5. There is no cephalic prominence, and the breech is not ballotable.

Fetal Heart

The fetal heart tones are heard loudest at or above the umbilicus and on the same side as the back. In RSA the fetal heart is heard best in the right upper quadrant of the maternal abdomen. Sometimes the fetal heart is heard below the umbilicus; hence the diagnosis made by palpation should not be changed because of the location of the fetal heart.

Vaginal Examination

1. The presenting part is high.
2. The smooth, regular, hard head with its suture lines and fontanelles is absent. This negative finding suggests a malpresentation.
3. The presenting part is soft and irregular. The anal orifice and the ischial tuberosities are in a straight line (Fig. 3B). The breech may be confused with a face.
4. Sometimes in frank breeches the sacrum is pulled down and is felt by the examining finger. It may be mistaken for the head because of its bony hardness.
5. The sacrum is in the right anterior quadrant of the pelvis, and the bitrochanteric diameter is in the right oblique.
6. Sometimes a foot is felt and must be distinguished from a hand.

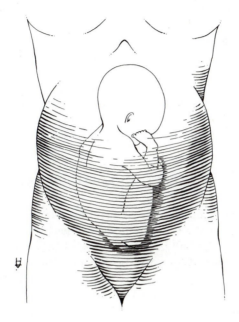

A. Abdominal view.

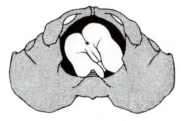

B. Vaginal view.

Figure 3. Right sacrum anterior.

Ultrasonography

This is an important tool in the management of breech presentation, especially in the following areas: (1) confirmation of the clinical diagnosis; (2) diagnosis of hyperextension of the fetal head; (3) evaluation of the size of the fetal head; (4) estimation of fetal weight; (5) diagnosis of major congenital anomalies, such as hydrocephaly, anencephaly, spina bifida.

X-ray

Radiography is no longer indicated in the diagnosis of breech presentation or fetal anomalies unless ultrasonography is unavailable. However, it is useful in assessing pelvic structure and capacity.

MECHANISMS OF LABOR: BREECH PRESENTATIONS

Cephalic and breech presentations are like triangles. When the head presents, the base of the triangle leads the way: The largest and most unyielding part of the baby comes first, and the parts that follow are progressively smaller. When the breech presents, on the other hand, the apex of the triangle comes first and the succeeding parts are progressively bigger, with the relatively large head being last. In cases of cephalopelvic disproportion, by the time it is realized that the head is too big for this pelvis, the rest of the baby has been born and vaginal delivery must be carried on, with sad results for the baby.

In breech presentations there are three mechanisms of labor: (1) the buttocks and lower limbs, (2) the shoulders and arms, and (3) the head.

Mechanism of Labor: RSA

Buttocks and Lower Limbs

Descent.   Engagement has been achieved when the bitrochanteric diameter has passed through the inlet of the pelvis. In RSA the sacrum is in the right anterior quadrant of the maternal pelvis, and the bitrochanteric diameter is in the right oblique diameter of the pelvis (Figs. 4A and B). Since the breech is a less efficient dilator than the head, descent is slow and the breech may remain high until labor has been in progress for some time. In many instances the breech does not come down until the cervix is fully dilated and the membranes are ruptured.

Flexion. In order to facilitate passage of the breech through the pelvis, lateral flexion takes place at the waist. The anterior hip becomes the leading part. Where the breech is frank, the baby's legs act as a splint along the body and, by reducing lateral flexion and maneuverability, may prevent descent into the pelvis.

Internal Rotation of Breech. The anterior hip meets the resistance of the pelvic floor and rotates forward, downward, and toward the midline (Figs. 5A and B). The bitrochanteric diameter rotates 45° from the right oblique diameter of the pelvis to the anteroposterior. The sacrum turns away from the midline, from the right anterior quadrant to the right transverse (RSA to RST).

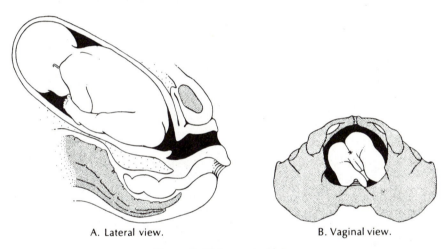

A. Lateral view.   B. Vaginal view.

Figure 4. RSA: onset of labor.

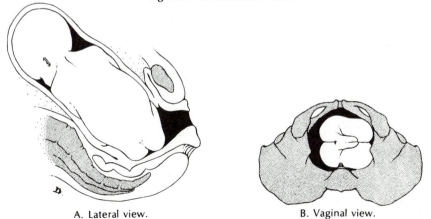

A. Lateral view.   B. Vaginal view.

Figure 5. Descent and internal rotation of buttocks.

Birth of Buttocks by Lateral Flexion. The anterior hip impinges under the pubic symphysis, lateral flexion occurs, and the posterior hip rises and is born over the perineum. The buttocks then fall toward the anus and the anterior hip slips out under the symphysis (Fig 6).

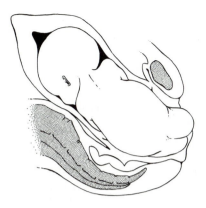

A. Breech crowning.

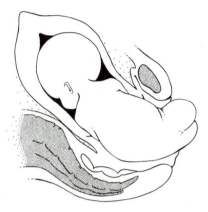

B. Birth of posterior buttock.

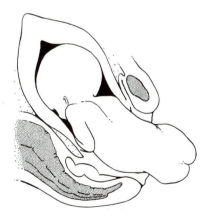

C. Birth of anterior buttock.

Figure 6. Birth of the buttocks.

Shoulders and Arms

Engagement. Engagement of the shoulders takes place in the right oblique diameter of the pelvis, as the sacrum rotates RST to RSA (Fig. 7A).

Internal Rotation of Shoulders. The anterior shoulder rotates under the symphysis, and the bisacromial diameter turns 45° from the right oblique to the anteroposterior diameter of the outlet. The sacrum goes along, RSA to RST (Fig.7B).

Birth of Shoulders by Lateral Flexion. The anterior shoulder impinges under the symphysis and the posterior shoulder and arm are born over the perineum as the baby's body is lifted upward (Fig. 7C). The baby is then lowered and the anterior shoulder and arms pass out under the symphysis.

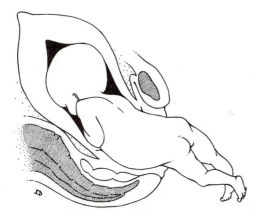

A. Feet born, shoulders engaging.

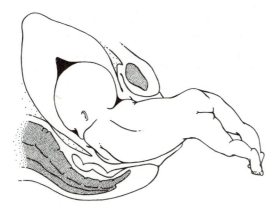

B. Descent and internal rotation of shoulders.

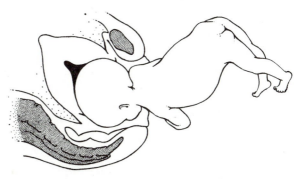

C. Posterior shoulder born: head has entered the pelvis.

Figure 7. Birth of the shoulders.

Head

Descent and Engagement. When the shoulders are at the outlet, the head is entering the pelvis (Fig. 8A). It enters the pelvis with the sagittal suture in the left oblique diameter. The occiput is in the right anterior quadrant of the pelvis.

Flexion. Flexion of the head takes place just as in any other presentation. It is important that flexion is maintained.

Internal Rotation. The head strikes the pelvic floor and rotates internally so that it comes to the outlet with the sagittal suture in the anteroposterior diameter, the brow in the hollow of the sacrum, and the occiput under the symphysis (Fig 8B). The sacrum rotates toward the pubis, so that the back is anterior.

Birth of Head by Flexion. The diameters are the same as in occipitoanterior positions but in reverse order. The nape of the neck pivots under the symphysis and the chin, mouth, nose, forehead, bregma, and occiput are born over the perineum by a movement of flexion (Fig 8C).

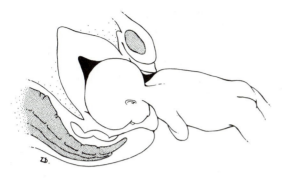

A. Anterior shoulder born; descent of head.

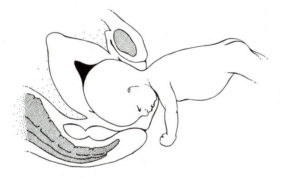

B. Internal rotation and beginning flexion of the head.

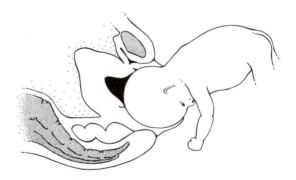

C. Flexion of the head complete.

Figure 8. Birth of the head.

Mechanism of Labor: Sacrum Directly Anterior

Descent. Engagement takes place with the bitrochanteric diameter in the transverse diameter of the inlet. The sacrum is directly anterior, behind the symphysis pubis (SA).

Flexion. Flexion is the same as in RSA.

Internal Rotation. The bitrochanteric diameter rotates 90° from the transverse diameter of the pelvis to the anteroposterior. The sacrum turns away from the midline to the transverse (SA to RST).
    The rest of the mechanism of labor is the same as in RSA.

Mechanism of Labor: Sacrum Posterior

In the rare case, the sacrum and head rotate posteriorly so that the occiput is in the hollow of the sacrum and the face is behind the pubis. If the head is flexed (Fig. 9A), delivery occurs with the occiput posterior. The nasion pivots in the subpubic angle, and the nape of the neck, occiput, and vertex roll over the perineum. The face then emerges from behind the pubis. This method of delivery is helped by lifting up the child's body.
    If the head is extended (Fig. 9B), the chin impinges behind the pubis and the submental area of the neck pivots in the subpubic angle. For delivery to take place the infant's body must be raised by the accoucheur so that the occiput, vertex, and forehead can pass over the perineum, in that order.
    Delivery of the head from this position can be difficult. The best management of this complication lies in its prevention. Once the breech has been born, any tendency for the sacrum to rotate posteriorly must be restrained by the attendant and the breech encouraged to turn with the sacrum anteriorly toward the symphysis pubis.

Mechanism of Labor in Footling and Kneeling Breech

The mechanism of labor is the same as has been described in RSA with the difference being that in complete and frank breech presentations the buttocks form the leading part. In footling presentations it is one or both feet, and in kneeling breeches it is the knees.

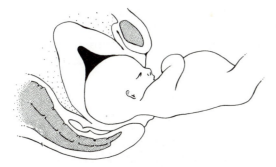

A. Head flexed.

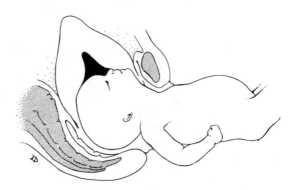

B. Head extended.

Figure 9. Arrest of head: sacrum posterior.

PROGNOSIS: BREECH PRESENTATIONS

Mother

When spontaneous delivery takes place the maternal prognosis is good. Genital tract lacerations and hemorrhage may be caused by excessively rapid and forceful delivery of the baby through a pelvis that is too small or in which the soft parts have not been dilated sufficiently.

Fetus

The fetal mortality associated with vaginal delivery of full-term breech presentations is three times that of cephalic presentations. The worst prognosis is in premature breeches. The perinatal mortality is highest in double footling presentations and lowest when the breech is frank. Factors influencing the perinatal mortality include (1) prematurity, (2) congenital abnormalities, (3) prolapse of the umbilical cord, (4) fetal asphyxia from other causes, and (5) fetal injury.

Prolapse of the umbilical cord is more common than in cephalic presentation, especially when the presentation is footling and when the mother is multiparous. Frank breech has the lowest incidence.

The danger of injury is as great in multiparas as in primigravidas. In difficult deliveries the risk of damage to the baby is 20 percent; in easy births it is 3.5 percent. The fetal outcome is worse when the diagnosis is not made before the onset of labor.

Intracranial hemorrhage, more common with breech than with cephalic presentations, is a major cause of fetal mortality. Sometimes the unmolded head has to pass rapidly and with difficulty through a borderline pelvis.

Significant long-term major abnormalities of the central nervous system are increased in breeches born per vaginam. These include (1) cerebral palsy, (2) epilepsy, (3) mental retardation, and (4) hemiplegia.

Time of Death. About 15 percent of fetal deaths occur during labor. The remainder are divided more or less equally between fetal death in utero before the onset of labor, congenital anomalies incompatible with life, and neonatal death.

Causes of Death or Damage to the Baby

1. Prematurity is the major etiologic factor in the perinatal morbidity and mortality of infants presenting by the breech. The

risk of death during labor is much higher for premature fetuses in breech than cephalic presentation.

2. Congenital malformation. The incidence of anomalies among fetuses presenting by the breech is twice that seen in cephalic presentations, 6.3 versus 2.4 percent. Known fetal disorders associated with breech presentation include congenital dislocation of the hip, hydrocephaly, anencephaly, and meningomyelocele, as well as some less common anomalies.

3. Asphyxia.
   a. Prolonged compression of the umbilical cord between the pelvis and the aftercoming head.
   b. Actual prolapse of the cord.
   c. Aspiration of amniotic fluid and vaginal contents caused by active breathing before the head has been born.
   d. Prolonged and hard labor.

4. Injury to brain and skull.
   a. The aftercoming head passes through the pelvis rapidly. Instead of gradual molding taking place over several hours, there is rapid and sometimes excessive compression and decompression occurring within a few minutes. The ligaments of the brain are subjected to sudden and marked stretching, with the risk of laceration and intracranial hemorrhage. Injury to the brain may follow delivery through an incompletely dilated cervix or through a pelvis whose adequacy has been estimated incorrectly.
   b. Minute hemorrhages.
   c. Fractures of the skull.
   d. Minimal brain dysfunction.One study has reported that the frequency of learning and motor defects is higher in infants delivered vaginally as breech presentations than in infants delivered as cephalic presentations.These include difficulties in reading and writing, and disturbances in hearing, sight, and speech.It is not known whether the basic etiologic factor is anoxia or trauma. Unfortunately this study has not matched a number of important variables, and a cause-and-effect relationship has not been proved. A study in the Netherlands of the neurologic status of children born by vaginal delivery, involving 256 cases and matched controls, found that significant differences between the study and control groups existed only for minor neurologic dysfunctions. The conclusion reached was that the main danger of breech presentation lies in the associated complications of the pregnancy rather than the mode of delivery. When examining the long-term neuro-

logic development in children born as breeches, the effect of prematurity and birth weight on the central nervous system must be considered before etiologic conclusions implicating trauma at birth are reached.The final word on this problem has not yet been established.

5. Damage resulting from rough handling during the delivery.
   a. Fractures of the neck, humerus, clavicle, or femur.
   b. Cervical and brachial plexus paralyses.
   c. Rupture of the liver caused by grasping the baby too tightly around the abdomen while extracting it.
   d. Damage to fetal adrenal glands.
   e. Injury to spinal cord.
   f. Traumatized pharynx caused by the obstetrician putting his finger in the baby's mouth to aid delivery.
   g. Damage to abdominal organs. Baby should be grasped by the hips and not the trunk.
6. Size of the baby.
   a. Large babies, over 8 pounds, may be too big for the pelvis.
   b. Premature babies have small bodies in relation to their heads. The little breech is not a good dilator and fails to make room for the head.
7. Rupture of membranes. It has been shown that the fetal mortality is significantly higher if the interval from rupture of the membranes to delivery is prolonged.

INVESTIGATION OF BREECH PRESENTATION AT TERM

Accessory Factors

These increase the risk and include (1) elderly primigravida, (2) precious baby, (3) history of infertility, (4) intrauterine growth retardation, (5) postterm pregnancy, (6) toxemia of pregnancy, (7) diabetes, and (8) uterine myoma.

Radiologic Examination

1. To assess the size and shape of the maternal pelvis. Bad prognostic features are:
   a. Interspinous diameter less than 9.0 cm.
   b. Foreward jutting of the sacrum.
   c. A narrow subpubic arch.
2. To confirm the presentation.

3. To diagnose the type of breech presentation—frank, complete, or footling.
4. To discover congenital anomalies such as anencephaly and hydrocephaly.
5. To rule out hyperextension of the fetal head.

Ultrasonic Examination

1. Confirm the presentation.
2. Discover fetal anomalies.
3. Measure the biparietal diameter of the fetal head and the abdominal and thoracic girth.
4. Compare the biparietal diameter of the fetal head and the measurements of the maternal pelvis.
5. Localize the placenta and rule out placenta previa.

Breech Score of Zatuchini and Andros

At the time of admittance to the labor ward of the patient with a breech presentation, a decision must be made whether a trial of labor is indicated or whether elective cesarean section is to be performed. The breech score is a numerical summary of several important parameters. While this index does not include all the factors which must be taken into consideration, while it is not the final word, and although it is no substitute for clinical judgment, it is a valuable piece of information and is helpful in evaluating the situation.

	0 Points	1 Point	2 Points
Parity	Primigrav	Multip	
Gestational age	39 weeks or more	38 weeks	37 weeks or less
Estimated fetal weight	>8 lb >3630 g	7 to 8 lb 3176—3630 g	<7 lb <3176 g
Previous breech>2500 g	None	1	2 or more
Cervical dilatation on admission by vaginal examination	2 cm or less	3 cm	4 cm or more
Station on admission	−3 or higher	−2	−1 or lower

There is statistical evidence to the effect that scores of 3 or less are associated with a high incidence of fetal morbidity, that prolonged labor is frequent, and that the rate of cesarean section is elevated. Thus, low scores are ominous and of great prognostic value. High scores, on the other hand, are less significant, are no guarantee of successful delivery, and are not a reason for complacency. It is suggested that a score of 3 or less is an indication for cesarean section.

MANAGEMENT OF BREECH PRESENTATION DURING LATE PREGNANCY

External Version

There has long been disagreement as to the advisability of external version during pregnancy. However, because of the dangers to the fetus of vaginal delivery in some cases, and the resultant high incidence of elective cesarean section, there has been a renewed interest in the use of external cephalic version as a means of obviating these problems. (See Chapter 30 for technique.) The procedure must be performed gently, without excessive force, since there is the risk of placental separation or damage to the fetus. Version may be unsuccessful and the procedure abandoned. In those cases where the presentation has been changed to cephalic most fetuses will remain in the new position, but in some instances recurrence to the original presentation takes place. Before attempting external version one must be certain of the position to avoid turning a cephalic presentation to a breech.

The ideal time for version has been considered to be at 32 to 34 weeks of gestation. At this stage of pregnancy the fetus is relatively small and the amniotic fluid abundant, making the procedure easier than at later periods of gestation. However, a number of babies presenting by the breech at 32 to 34 weeks will turn spontaneously to a cephalic presentation if left alone, and version at this stage will have been unnecessary. Furthermore, in a certain percentage of cases where the version at 32 to 34 weeks has been successful, return to the original breech presentation will take place, and the procedure will have been useless.

Delay of external cephalic version to after 37 weeks of gestation has advantages: (1) Fewer procedures are necessary because spontaneous version will occur in a number of cases, even in late pregnancy. (2) Reversion to the original presentation is rare. (3) Should fetal complications develop during the procedure that necessitate immediate delivery, the child will be mature. (4) Contraindications to external cephalic version, such as intrauterine growth retardation, may become evident only in the later stage of the pregnancy.

Unfortunately, because of the larger size of the infant, the relatively smaller amount of amniotic fluid, and the less relaxed state of the myometrium, external cephalic version may be more difficult to accomplish in later, as compared with earlier, stages of gestation. However, the use of a uterine relaxant has made external version possible even at an advanced stage of pregnancy. (See Chapter 30 for technique.)

On the other hand, because (1) fetal death has occurred during or following external version, (2) many breeches will change spontaneously to cephalic presentations, (3) experience in management of breech deliveries must be obtained so that proper care can be taken of those cases that come to labor in the breech presentation, and (4) the more frequent use of cesarean section has reduced perinatal mortality and morbidity, many obstetricians believe that external version is unnecessary and inadvisable.

MANAGEMENT OF DELIVERY OF BREECH PRESENTATION

Classification of Breech Births

Vaginal Delivery

1. *Spontaneous breech delivery:* The entire infant is expelled by the natural forces of the mother, with no assistance other than support of the baby as it is being born.
2. *Assisted breech (or partial breech extraction):* The infant is delivered by the natural forces as far as the umbilicus. The remainder of the baby is extracted by the attendant. In normal cases we believe this to be the best method.
3. *Total breech extraction:* The entire body of the infant is extracted by the attendant.

Cesarean Section
The rate is around 50 percent. It must be pointed out that delivery of the breech by cesarean section takes skill. Infants may be injured during the procedure. The incision must be adequate in length so there is no difficulty with the head. If the lower uterine segment is not well developed, as is often the case in preterm situations, a low vertical incision, which can be extended easily, may be preferable.

Elective Cesarean Section
The following factors are unfavorable for safe vaginal delivery, and cesarean section may be best.

1. Presence of significant relative factors, e.g., history of infertility.
2. Elderly primigravida.

3. Gravidas with poor obstetric histories, e.g., a difficult delivery or a damaged baby.
4. Contracted, borderline, or abnormal pelvis.
5. Chronic fetal distress, including intrauterine growth retardation, diabetes mellitus, and hypertensive disorders.
6. Premature rupture of the membranes.
7. Placenta previa of any degree.
8. Prolapse of the umbilical cord, especially in footling breeches.
9. Breech score of 3 or less.
10. Large baby.
   a. Over 3800 g, estimated by clinical examination and ultrasonography.
   b. Biparietal diameter over 9.5 cm measured by ultrasonography.
11. Hyperextension of the fetal head.
12. Footling breech. The limbs and pelvis of the footling breech deliver easily, but do not dilate the maternal soft parts sufficiently to make room for the aftercoming head. This may make delivery of the head difficult, especially in premature infants.
13. Premature infant. Advances in pediatric care have reached the point where a baby weighing 1000 g, if delivered without trauma or hypoxia in a center for high-risk obstetrics, has an 80 percent chance of survival. At 1500 g the rate of survival is 88 percent, and at over 2000 g it is 99 percent. Even babies weighing less than 1000 g have been saved. In order to obviate the risks of hypoxia during labor, the danger of entrapment of the aftercoming head, and the risk of prolapse of the umbilical cord, cesarean section may be a valid method of avoiding these difficulties and of improving results. In many centers the belief has evolved that strong consideration be given to delivering all preterm babies presenting as a breech by cesarean section. This concept may be correct, but there is, as yet, no scientific proof that the outcome of those breech babies delivered by cesarean section is better than that of children born per vaginam. Effer and his group concluded, on the basis of a large study, that:

> . . . there is not enough evidence to support the recommendation that cesarean section be carried out for breech presentation when the infant weighs less than 1500 g. When pregnancy is less than 28 weeks or the estimated weight of the infant is less than 1000 g, neither the method of delivery nor the presentation is a significant determinant of outcome. The prematurity itself, with all its accompanying patho-

physiology, is so overwhelming that maneuvers involving method of delivery do not alter outcome. We can neither recommend cesarean section nor state that it should not be done.

In most cases the lower uterine segment is not well formed, and a large vertical incision into the body is necessary. To have a trapped head at cesarean section is no better than the same complication during vaginal delivery. The risks to the mother of a difficult cesarean section in the poorly formed lower uterine segment prior to 28 weeks has yet to be determined.

Because spontaneous version may occur even in late pregnancy, cesarean section should not be performed until the onset of labor.

How best to manage the delivery of a preterm breech has not yet been established.

Routine Cesarean Section

Because no clinical, radiologic, or ultrasonic assessment can guarantee a safe and easy birth of the aftercoming head, many obstetricians believe that all infants presenting by the breech should be delivered by cesarean section. Today many infants in breech presentation are delivered abdominally without a trial of labor.

It is clear that cesarean section in both the short and long run (including repeat cesarean section) is not as safe for the mother as vaginal delivery. The current maternal morbidity associated with cesarean section is between 25 and 40 percent; some of the complications are serious.

Furthermore, definite proof of the superiority of cesarean section over vaginal delivery is difficult to obtain. In an unselected group of breech deliveries there seems to be great benefit from cesarean section. In a select group, however, the advantage appears to be less clear.

It is evident that, in cases where the fetus is normal, cesarean section will reduce markedly, if not eliminate entirely, fetal death during delivery. At the same time there is evidence that, with proper selection of cases and meticulous management during labor, and as long as indications for abdominal delivery are wide, and include all unfavorable situations of even the mildest degree, many term breeches can be delivered safely per vaginam.

The controversy as to how to deliver breeches has not been settled.

Trial of Labor

Criteria. The criteria, for consideration of vaginal delivery are:

1. Frank breech
2. Gestational age of 36 to 42 weeks

3. Estimated fetal weight between 2500 and 3800 g
4. Fetal biparietal diameter of less than 9.5 cm measured by ultrasonography
5. Flexed fetal head
6. Adequate maternal pelvis, determined by x-ray pelvimetry
7. No maternal or fetal indication for cesarean section
8. Breech score of 4 or more

Conditions. The trial of labor is carried on under the following conditions, with the understanding that any deviation from the normal is an indication for cesarean section.

1. The fetal heart rate is monitored continuously.
2. The progress of labor is observed meticulously.
3. Progressive cervical dilatation must take place.
4. Adequate descent of the breech must occur.
5. No heroic vaginal procedures are performed.
6. When progress is slow there is a strong probability that the baby is large, and cesarean section should be performed.
7. The use of oxytocin in association with breech presentation is a controversial subject. Labor has been induced with success in cases of premature rupture of the membranes where the criteria for vaginal delivery have been met. Some obstetricians believe that augmentation of labor by infusion of oxytocin is permissible, even indicated, for prolonged latent or active phase cervical dilatation. However, the association of dysfunctional labor and breech presentation is often an ominous sign suggesting disproportion, and stimulation by oxytocin may be dangerous. In such cases cesarean section is the preferable treatment.
8. The patient must be prepared and ready for cesarean section. The organization of the delivery room suite, the nurses, the anesthetist, and the obstetrician must allow the immediate performance of cesarean section if the need arises.

Management of Labor and Delivery in the Progressing Case

First Stage of Labor

1. Because most breech presentations progress to successful vaginal delivery, observant expectancy, supportive therapy, and absence of interference are the procedures of choice.
2. The patient is best in bed.
3. It is best to maintain intact membranes until the cervical dilatation is far advanced. Too frequent vaginal or rectal examina-

tions, or any procedure that might contribute to premature rupture of the bag of waters, should be avoided.
4. When the membranes do rupture, vaginal examination is done to rule out prolapse of the umbilical cord and to determine the exact condition of the cervix.
5. Meconium is no cause for alarm as long as the fetal heart is normal.
6. An intravenous infusion of crystalloid solution (normal saline or Ringer lactate) should be instituted.

Second Stage of Labor

Position for Delivery. Once the cervix is fully dilated, the patient is placed on the delivery table. The firmness of the table and handbars that the patient uses to brace herself increases the effectiveness of the bearing-down efforts and so expedites progress.

When the breech begins to distend the perineum, the patient is placed in the lithotomy position, with the legs in stirrups and the buttocks extending slightly past the end of the table. This is the best position in which to assist the birth and to handle complications.

During a contraction the pressure of the presenting part on the perineum stimulates the patient to move up the table and out of position. Shoulder braces are invaluable in preventing this.

An assistant should be scrubbed and gowned for every delivery.

The patient's bladder is catheterized.

Intravenous Infusion. It is important for successful delivery of a breech presentation that good uterine contractions continue and that the patient retain the ability to bear down, and does so. Should the contractions become weak or irregular during the actual delivery, oxytocin can be added quickly to the infusion, to stimulate the uterus to more effective activity.

Assisted Breech. The fetal heart is checked frequently. As long as the baby is in good condition, spontaneous delivery is awaited. Premature traction on the baby, especially between contractions, must be avoided, since it can lead to deflexion of the head and extension of the arms above or behind the head. It is important that the patient bear down with each contraction, and she must be encouraged to do so. Once the body has been born, the head is out of the upper contracting part of the uterus and in the lower segment, the cervix, or the upper vagina. Since these organs do not have the power to expel the head, its descent and delivery must be effected by the voluntary action of the abdominal muscles, with the attendant exerting suprapubic pressure. Fetal salvage is increased by calmness and slowness rather than by agitation and speed.

Our experience has been that in normally progressing cases the best results are obtained by a policy of:

1. No interference (except episiotomy) until the body is born to the umbilicus. This permits the cervix to become not only fully dilated but also paralyzed, an important factor in minimizing dystocia with the aftercoming head.
2. Hard bearing down by the mother during contractions.
3. The maintenance of suprapubic pressure during descent to aid delivery and to keep the head in flexion.

There are good reasons for using this technique:

1. It has proved successful.
2. It is safe. There is less trauma to the baby.
3. Flexion of the head is maintained.
4. The danger of extension of the arms above the head is reduced.
5. There is less chance of the cervix clamping down around the baby's head or neck.

Anesthesia. A combination of local and general anesthesia is employed. Pudendal block or perineal infiltration permits episiotomy without pain and facilitates delivery by relaxing the muscles. In addition, with each contraction the patient takes several breaths of an anesthetic vapor. This acts as an analgesic, eases the pain, and helps her to bear down more efficiently. Actual general anesthesia is not instituted until the baby is born to the umbilicus.

We have used epidural anesthesia with success. The drawback is that once the perineal dose takes effect, the reflex stimulation from pressure of the presenting part on the perineum may be reduced or removed and the patient's desire to bear down with each contraction lost. This unwanted effect can be obviated by omitting the perineal dose and using local anesthesia for the episiotomy. In this way the analgesic value of the epidural dose during labor is maintained without loss of the perineal reflex during the delivery.

Necessary Equipment. The procedure requires that certain equipment be at hand.

1. A warm, dry towel to be wrapped around the baby's body as soon as it is sufficiently born. The purposes of this are:
   a. To reduce the stimulating effect of cold air on the baby in the hope that respiration does not begin while the head is in the pelvis, resulting in aspiration of amniotic fluid or vaginal contents

   b. To make it easier to hold the slippery baby
2. Piper forceps for the aftercoming head, if it does not deliver easily with assistance
3. Equipment for resuscitation of the infant, ready for immediate use

Episiotomy. Since in many cases the breech dilates the perineum insufficiently to allow easy passage of the head, an adequate episiotomy is essential. It is safer to make a big episiotomy to avoid having to enlarge it while occupied with delivery of the head. A mediolateral incision is preferred. The perineotomy must be done at the optimum time—e.g., before the breech crowns or one is faced with the need for delivering the infant and making the incision simultaneously. On the other hand, if the incision is made too soon the blood loss can be excessive. Hence the episiotomy should be performed just before the buttocks crown or when the attendant feels that their birth will occur with the next one or two contractions.

Delivery of Breech

1. The patient is encouraged to bear down with the contractions but must rest between them.
2. When the buttocks are ready to crown, a wide mediolateral episiotomy is made and hemostasis secured.
3. As long as there is no fetal or maternal distress, spontaneous delivery to the umbilicus is awaited. Up to this point there is no urgency, and the operator should not interfere.
4. Once the umbilicus has been delivered, time becomes an important factor, and the remainder of the birth is expedited gently and skillfully. A free airway to the mouth should be available within 3 to 5 minutes to obviate anoxic brain damage.
5. The legs usually deliver spontaneously; if not they are easily extracted.
6. The baby is covered with a warm towel, and the body is supported.
7. A loop of umbilical cord is pulled down (Fig. 10) to minimize traction on it in case it is caught between the head and the pelvic wall. At the same time it is palpated for pulsations.
8. If a general anesthetic is to be used, the patient is put to sleep at this time.

Delivery of Shoulders and Arms

1. The assistant exerts suprapubic pressure on the head to maintain its flexion.
2. The operator depresses the buttocks and delivers the body to the anterior scapula so that the anterior shoulder comes under the symphysis.
3. To deliver the anterior arm the accoucheur passes his hand up the baby's back, over the shoulder, and down the chest, thus sweeping the arm and hand out under the pubis with his finger (Fig. 11A).
4. The baby is raised so that the posterior scapula and then the posterior arm are born over the perineum by the same maneuver (Fig. 11B).
5. Some obstetricians deliver the posterior arm first.

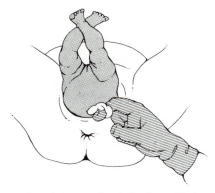

Figure 10. Delivery of cord. Loop of umbilical cord being pulled down.

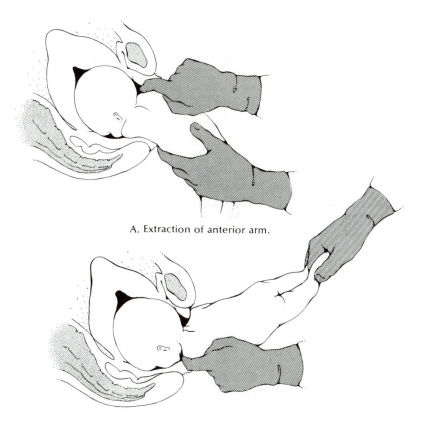

A. Extraction of anterior arm.

B. Extraction of posterior arm.

Figure 11. Delivery of arms and shoulders.

Delivery of Head

1. In almost every case the back turns anteriorly spontaneously. This must be encouraged so that the head rotates the occiput to the pubis and the face toward the sacrum. Rarely, there is a tendency for the back to turn posteriorly. The obstetrician must counteract this and rotate the back anteriorly to prevent the head's rotating face to pubis, a serious and always avoidable complication.

2. Once the back has rotated anteriorly and the fetal head is in the anteroposterior diameter of the pelvis, the body is lowered so that the occiput appears under the symphysis and the nape of the neck pivots there (Fig. 12A).

3. At the same time the assistant maintains suprapubic pressure to guide the head through the pelvis and to keep it flexed.

4. The body is then raised gently so that there is slight extension at the neck.

5. Then by further suprapubic pressure (Kristellar maneuver) the head is delivered in flexion—the chin, mouth, nose, forehead, bregma, and vertex being born, in that order, over the perineum (Fig. 12B).

6. The speed of delivery of the aftercoming head must be considered. The rapid passage of the head through the pelvis causes sudden compression and decompression of the cranial contents. In the extreme, the ligaments of the brain tear, leading to hemorrhage, cerebral damage, and death. On the other hand, too slow delivery of the head results in asphyxia, which may also be fatal. Experience teaches the middle road: slow enough to prevent injury to the brain and sufficiently rapid to avoid asphyxia.

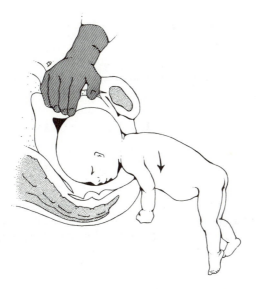

A. Body lowered so that nape of neck is in the subpubic angle. Assistant maintains flexion of the head.

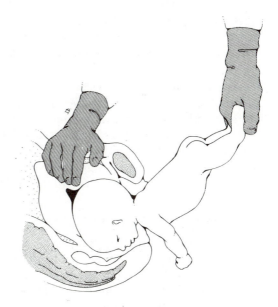

B. Kristellar maneuver: head born in flexion.

Figure 12. Delivery of head.

ARREST IN BREECH PRESENTATION

Most babies who present by the breech are born spontaneously or with the help of, but not interference from, the attendant. The Kristellar maneuver (suprapubic pressure) is all that is needed to deliver the aftercoming head. However, progress may cease and active interference then becomes mandatory. Arrest may take place at the head, neck, shoulders and arms, or buttocks.

Arrest of the Head

Sometimes the body, shoulders, and arms are born, but the bearing-down efforts of the mother and the Kristellar maneuver are not successful in delivering the head. In cases where the head is arrested, several measures are available to extract it.

Wigand-Martin Maneuver

The body of the baby is placed on the arm of the operator, with the middle finger of the hand of that arm placed in the baby's mouth and the index and ring fingers on the malar bones (Fig. 13A). The purpose of the finger in the mouth is not for traction but to encourage and maintain flexion. With the other hand the obstetrician exerts suprapubic pressure on the head through the mother's abdomen.

Mauriceau-Smellie-Veit Maneuver

The position is the same as the Wigand-Martin, with one finger in the baby's mouth and two on the malar bones. The difference is that the accoucheur places his other hand astride the baby's shoulders and produces traction in this way (Fig. 13B). The efficiency of this procedure is increased by an assistant's applying suprapubic pressure on the fetal head while the operator is performing the Mauriceau maneuver.

Piper Forceps on the Aftercoming Head

1. The baby's feet are grasped by an assistant, and the body is raised (Fig. 13C). Care must be taken not to elevate the body too much for fear of damage to the sternomastoid muscles. A good way to keep the arms out of the way is to use a folded towel as described by Savage.
2. The right hand is placed in the vagina, and the left forceps blade is guided into place over the parietal bone.
3. The right blade is then applied using the left hand as a guide.
4. The forceps are locked. The blades fit along the occipitomental diameter, one over each ear.

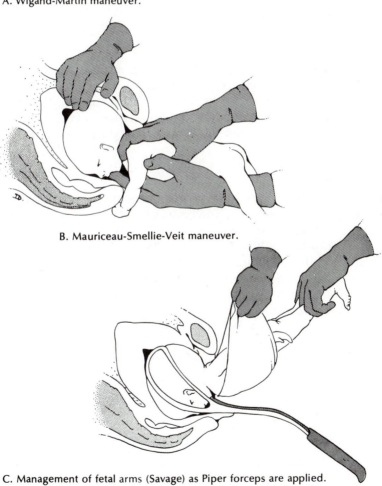

A. Wigand-Martin maneuver.

B. Mauriceau-Smellie-Veit maneuver.

C. Management of fetal arms (Savage) as Piper forceps are applied.

Figure 13. Different maneuvers for arrest of head.

5. With the exception of simple suprapubic pressure, the best method of delivering the aftercoming head is by the use of the Piper forceps. In contrast to those maneuvers in which traction on the head is effected through the neck, the forceps exert traction directly on the head, thereby avoiding damage to structures in the baby's neck.

6. Traction is made and the head extracted slowly (see Chapter 29).This operation should be performed only when the head is in the pelvis. Any type of forceps can be used to deliver the aftercoming head. The Piper forceps have a double curve in the blades and in the shanks; the shanks are long, and the handles are depressed below the arch of the shanks. This instrument should be employed whenever possible, since it is easier to use and more efficient than regular forceps.

Airway

When there is delay in delivery of the head and one is waiting for help or instruments, an ordinary vaginal retractor can be used temporarily to clear an airway in the vagina to the baby's mouth (Fig. 14). The retractor is placed in the vagina and pressure exerted posteriorly. The vaginal contents are sponged out so that air can get to the baby should it breathe.

Chin to Pubis Rotation

Anterior rotation of the chin is rare and occurs usually as part of posterior rotation of the back. The preferred management is as follows: (1) Institute deep anesthesia. (2) Cease all traction. (3) Dislodge the chin from behind the pubis. (4) Rotate the face posteriorly and the back anteriorly. (5) Flex the chin. (6) Effect engagement by suprapubic pressure. (7) Deliver the head with Piper forceps.

When this technique fails, the Prague maneuver (Fig. 15) may be used. Here the fingers are placed over the shoulders, and outward and upward traction is made. The legs are grasped with the other hand, and the body is swung over the mother's abdomen. By this procedure the occiput is born over the perineum. Since this method carries with it the danger of overstretching or breaking the neck of the infant, it is used rarely.

Embryotomy

When delivery of the head is not accomplished within reasonable time, the baby may die. If it does perish the mother's welfare alone should be considered. To save her from needless injury, reduction of the size of the child's head by perforation of the skull is preferable to its extraction by brute force.

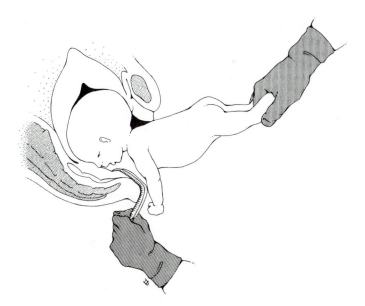

Figure 14. Vaginal retractor providing airway to the baby's mouth and nose.

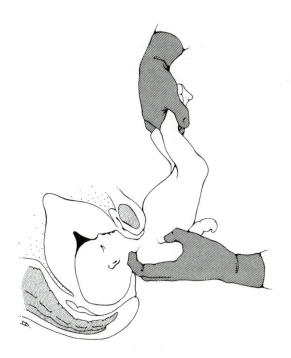

Figure 15. Prague maneuver.

Arrest of the Neck

Occasionally the cervix, which has opened sufficiently to allow the trunk and shoulders to be born, clamps down around the baby's neck, trapping the head in the uterus. The possibility of this happening is greater with the premature delivery, where the body has not yet developed its adipose tissue and is a poor dilating wedge. This dangerous situation calls for rapid action to break the spasm of the previously dilated cervix. This is accomplished by a single bold incision of the cervix with the scissors. The resultant relaxation of the spasm permits the head to be born.

Arrest of the Shoulders and Arms

Extended Arms. The arms are simply extended over the baby's head (Fig. 16A).

Nuchal Arms. There is extension at the shoulder and flexion at the elbow so that the forearm is trapped behind the fetal head (Fig. 16B). One or both arms may be affected.

Prophylaxis
One method of reducing the incidence of this complication is to resist the temptation of pulling on the baby's legs to speed delivery, especially when the uterus is in a relaxed state.

Simple Extraction
When this problem occurs an attempt should be made first to deliver the arms by sweeping them over the chest in the usual way. This succeeds in most cases of simple extension and in some instances of nuchal arms when the upper limb is not jammed tightly behind the head.

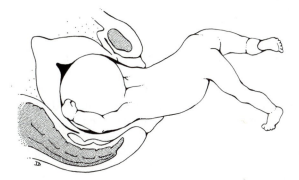

A. Arm extended above the head.

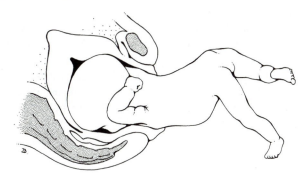

B. Nuchal arm.

Figure 16. Extended and nuchal arms.

Rotation of Body

If extraction fails in the case of a nuchal arm, the baby's body is rotated in the direction to which the hand is pointing (Fig. 16C). This dislodges the arm from behind the head and its delivery is then usually possible as described above (Fig. 16D). If both arms are nuchal, the body is rotated in one direction to free the first arm, which is then extracted, and then in the opposite direction to free the other arm.

Fracture

In the rare instance when rotation fails, the humerus or clavicle must be fractured. This can be done directly, or it can be effected by simply pulling on the arm until it breaks. Once this occurs delivery can be accomplished. Since the fracture usually heals rapidly and well, and since the choice may be between a dead baby and a broken arm, extreme measures are justified.

Failure of Descent of the Breech

Etiology

In any situation, the size of the passenger, the capacity of the pelvis, the dilatability of the maternal soft tissues, and the character of the uterine contractions all play a part in determining whether spontaneous delivery takes place. In frank breech presentation there is an added factor. The splinting effect of the baby's legs across its abdomen can reduce the maneuverability of the fetus to such an extent that progress is arrested.

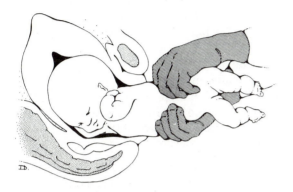

C. Nuchal arm: rotation of the trunk of the child 90° in the direction in which the hand is pointing.

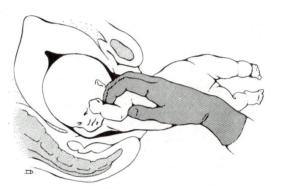

D. Nuchal arm: hand introduced into the uterus to flex and bring down the nuchal arm.

Figure 16. (cont.) Extended and nuchal arms.

Disproportion

In the presence of good uterine contractions, nondescent of the breech is an indication, not for hasty interference, but for the most careful reassessment. Keeping in mind the fact that one of the causes of breech presentation is a large head that cannot engage easily, the accoucheur must be assured, not of the general capacity of the pelvis, but of its adequacy with respect to that particular baby. More and more evidence is appearing in the literature that when a breech fails to descend, in spite of good contractions, disproportion is present and cesarean section must be seriously considered. If, within 30 minutes of full cervical dilatation, the breech does not descend and distend the perineum to the point where the anus of the baby is visible at the introitus, it is safer to deliver the baby by cesarean section. This is so regardless of the reason for the nondescent.

Decomposition

Flexed Breech. If cesarean section cannot be performed, progress and descent can be expedited by reducing the bulk of the breech, an operation known as decomposition. This is done by bringing down the legs, both whenever possible. When there is flexion at the hips and the knees, the feet can be reached easily. The hand is placed in the uterus, the membranes are ruptured, and a foot is grasped and brought down (Fig. 17A). Be sure it is not a hand. The same is done with the other foot. The position has been changed to a footling breech, and labor proceeds.

Frank Breech: Pinard Maneuver. If the breech is frank (flexion at the hips, extension at the knees), it may be impossible to reach the feet, as they are high in the uterus, near the baby's face. In such a situation, and when cesarean section cannot be carried out, the Pinard maneuver is performed under anesthesia (Figs. 17B and C). With a hand in the uterus, pressure is made by the fingers against the popliteal fossa in a backward and outward direction. This brings about sufficient flexion of the knee so that the foot can be grasped and delivered. When possible both feet should be brought down. Unless there are urgent indications for immediate extraction of the infant, labor is allowed to carry on as for a footling breech.

BREECH EXTRACTION

This operation is the immediate vaginal extraction of the baby when signs of fetal distress demand delivery without delay.

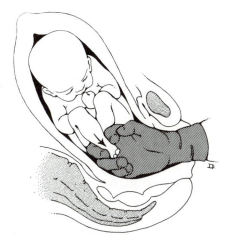

A. Decomposition of breech: bringing down a foot and leg.

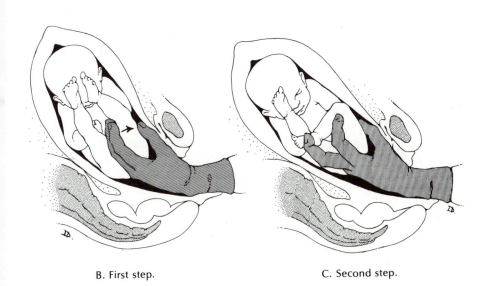

B. First step.   C. Second step.

B and C. Pinard maneuver.

Figure 17. Breaking up the breech.

Prerequisites

There are certain conditions that must be present before this procedure may be performed. (1) The pelvis must be ample, with no disproportion. (2) The cervix must be fully dilated. (3) The bladder and rectum should be empty. (4) Expert and deep anesthesia is essential. (5) Good assistance is mandatory.

Procedure

The patient is placed in the lithotomy position, the bladder catheterized, and anesthesia administered. As described in a previous section, the breech is decomposed and the legs are brought down. The feet are pulled down if the breech is complete; the Pinard maneuver is used if the breech is frank. Instead of the patient going on to spontaneous delivery, the baby is extracted rapidly. Traction from below is substituted for uterine contractions from above, but the maneuvers for delivery of the shoulders, arms, and head are those already set forth in the management of arrested cases.

While expert and experienced obstetricians have reported good results with routine breech extraction as soon as the cervix is fully dilated, we believe that in the hands of the average doctor this operation is hazardous for both mother and child. We feel that it should be carried out only in urgent situations when cesarean section cannot be performed quickly and the baby must be delivered immediately.

HYPEREXTENSION OF THE FETAL HEAD

Hyperextension of the fetal head (Fig. 18) is seen most commonly in face presentation but also occurs with transverse lie and breech presentation. In the latter it is a serious problem.

Etiology

1. Spasm or congenital shortening of the extensor muscles of the neck
2. Umbilical cord around the neck
3. Congenital tumors of the fetal neck
4. Fetal malformations
5. Uterine anomalies
6. Tumors in the placental site

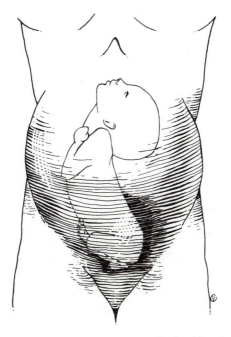

Figure 18. Hyperextension of the fetal head.

Diagnosis

The diagnosis is made by x-ray examination; the appearance is characteristic. When the head presents it is that of a face presentation. When the breech presents the appearance has been described as a "star-gazing breech." In transverse lie the condition is seen as a "flying fetus."

Fetal Danger

There is a definite risk of damage to the lower cervical spinal cord of the fetus during vaginal delivery. The mechanisms by which the injury is caused include (1) excessive longitudinal stretching of the spinal cord, (2) extreme flexion of the neck during delivery, and (3) marked torsion. The resulting lesion is partial or complete laceration of the cervical spinal cord, occasional tears in the dura, and epidural hemorrhage. The latter is the most common manifestation, and is associated with varying degrees of damage to the cord, brain stem, nerve roots, and meninges. Dislocation or fracture of the vertebrae is rare. In the vast majority of cases the injury is caused by the sudden flexion of the head as it descends through the vagina. However, occasionally the damage may occur during pregnancy as a result of the malposition of the fetus.

Fetal Prognosis

In a collected series of 73 cases the perinatal mortality rate was 13.7 percent in babies delivered vaginally in contrast to no deaths in those born by cesarean section. Medullary or vertebral injury occurred in 20.6 percent of babies born per vaginam and in 5.7 percent delivered by cesarean section. Meningeal hemorrhage was found in 6.9 percent of children born vaginally, while none was noted following cesarean section.

In another series of 814 breech presentations there were 33 hyperextended heads, an incidence of 7.4 percent. All 33 infants survived. Follow-up for 2 to 4 years revealed neurologic sequellae in 5 of the 26 children born vaginally, but none in the 7 delivered by cesarean section.

BIBLIOGRAPHY

Collea JV, Chein C, Quilligan EJ: The randomized management of term frank breech presentation: A study of 208 cases. Am J Obstet Gynecol 137:235, 1980

Collea JV: The intrapartum management of breech presentation. Clin Perinatol 8:173, 1981

Cox C, Kendall AC, Hommers M: Changed prognosis of breech-presenting low birthweight infants. Brit J Obstet Gynaecol 89:881, 1982

Effer SB, Saigal S, Rand C, et al: Effect of delivery method on outcomes in the very low-birth weight breech infant: Is the improved survival related to cesarean section or other perinatal care maneuvers? Am J Obstet Gynecol 145:123, 1983

Faber-Nijholt R, Huisjes HJ, Touwen BCL, Fidler VJ: Neurological follow-up of 281 children born in breech presentation: A controlled study. Brit Med J 286:9, 1983

Fall O, Nilsson BA: External cephalic version in breech presentation under tocolysis. Obstet Gynecol 53:712, 1979

Gimovsky ML, Wallace RL, Schiffrin BS, Paul RH: Randomized management of the nonfrank breech presentation at term: A preliminary report. Am J Obstet Gynecol 146:34, 1983

Green JE, McLean F, Smith LP, Usher R: Has an increased cesarean section rate for term breech delivery reduced the incidence of birth asphyxia, trauma, and death? Am J Obstet Gynecol 143:643, 1982

Hofmeyr GJ: Effect of external cephalic version in late pregnancy on breech presentation and cesarean section: A controlled trial. Brit J Obstet Gynaecol 90:392, 1983

Ridley WJ, Jackson P, Stewart JH, Boyle P: Role of antenatal radiography in the managenent of breech deliveries. Brit J Obstet Gynaecol 89:342, 1982

Westgren M, Grundsell I, Ingemarsson A, et al: Hyperextension of the fetal head in breech presentation: A study with long-term follow-up. Brit J Obstet Gynaecol 88:101, 1981

Woods JR: Effects of low-birth-weight breech delivery on neonatal mortality. Obstet Gynecol 53:735, 1979

Transverse Lie

GENERAL CONSIDERATIONS

Definition

When the long axes of mother and fetus are at right angles to one another, a transverse lie is present. Because the shoulder is placed so frequently in the brim of the inlet, this malposition is often referred to as the shoulder presentation. The baby may lie directly across the maternal abdomen (Fig. 1), or it may lie obliquely with the head or breech in the iliac fossa (Figs. 2A and B). Usually the breech is at a higher level than the head. The denominator is the scapula (Sc); the situation of the head determines whether the position is left or right, and that of the back indicates whether it is anterior or posterior. Thus LScP means that the lie is transverse, the head is on the mother's left side, and the baby's back is posterior. The part which actually lies over the pelvic brim may be the shoulder, back, abdomen, ribs, or flank.

Incidence

The incidence of transverse lie is around 1:500. This is a serious malposition whose management must not be left to nature.

Etiology

Anything that prevents engagement of the head or the breech may predispose to transverse lie. This abnormality is more common in multiparas than primigravidas because of the laxness of the uterine and abdominal muscles. Included are such factors as placenta previa; obstructing neoplasm; multiple pregnancies; fetal anomalies; polyhy-

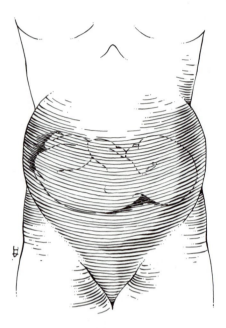

Figure 1. Transverse lie: LScP.

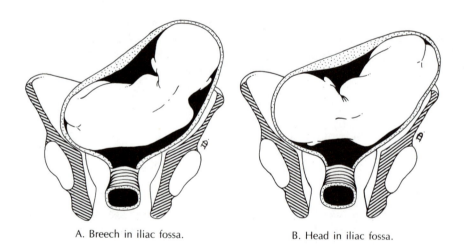

A. Breech in iliac fossa.   B. Head in iliac fossa.

Figure 2. Oblique lie.

dramnios; prematurity; fetopelvic disproportion; uterine abnormalities such as uterus subseptus, uterus arcuatus, and uterus bicornis; and contracted pelvis. In many instances no etiologic factor can be determined, and we assume that the malposition is accidental. The head happens to be out of the lower uterine segment when labor starts, and the shoulder is pushed into the pelvic brim.

DIAGNOSIS OF POSITION: TRANSVERSE LIE

Abdominal Examination

1. The appearance of the abdomen is asymmetrical.
2. The long axis of the fetus is across the mother's abdomen.
3. The uterine fundus is lower than expected for the period of gestation. It has been described as a squat uterus. Its upper limit is near the umbilicus, and it is wider than usual.
4. Palpation of the upper and lower poles of the uterus reveals neither the head nor the breech.
5. The head can be felt in one maternal flank.
6. The buttocks are on the other side.

Fetal Heart

The fetal heart is heard best below the umbilicus and has no diagnostic significance regarding position.

Vaginal Examination

The most important finding is a negative one; neither the head nor the breech can be felt by the examining finger. The presenting part is high. In some cases one may actually feel the shoulder, a hand, the rib cage, or the back. Because of the poor fit of the presenting part to the pelvis the bag of waters may hang into the vagina.

Ultrasonography

Ultrasonic examination will confirm the diagnosis and can detect certain abnormalities in the fetus, such as hydrocephaly and anencephaly.

X-ray

When ultrasonography is unavailable, the fetal presentation can be established by a flat plate of the abdomen.

MECHANISM OF LABOR: TRANSVERSE LIE

A persistent transverse lie cannot deliver spontaneously, and if uncorrected impaction takes place (Fig. 3A). The shoulder is jammed into the pelvis, the head and breech stay above the inlet, the neck becomes stretched, and progress is arrested. Transverse lies must never be left to nature.

Spontaneous Version

Spontaneous version takes place occasionally, more often with oblique than with transverse lies. Before or shortly after the onset of labor, the lie changes to a longitudinal one (cephalic or breech), and labor proceeds in the new position. Unfortunately, the chance of spontaneous version occurring is small, too small to warrant more than a very short delay in instituting corrective measures.

Neglected Transverse Lie

Neglected transverse lie results from misdiagnosis or improper treatment. At first the contractions are of poor quality and the cervix dilates slowly. Because of the irregularity of the presenting part, the membranes rupture early and the amniotic fluid escapes rapidly. As the labor pains become stronger the fetal shoulder is forced into the pelvis, the uterus molds itself around the baby, a state of impaction ensues, and progress is halted. From this impasse there is one of two outcomes:

1. *Uterine rupture*: Labor goes on. The upper part of the uterus becomes shorter and thicker, while the lower segment becomes progressively more stretched and thinned until it ruptures.
2. *Uterine inertia*: The uterus becomes exhausted and the contractions cease. Intrauterine sepsis sets in, and may be followed by generalized infection.

In either event, fetal death is certain and maternal mortality possible. Transverse lies must not be neglected!

Complications

Because the presenting part does not fill the inlet, the membranes tend to rupture early and may be followed by prolapse of a fetal arm or the umbilical cord (Figs. 3B and C). Both are serious complications necessitating immediate action.

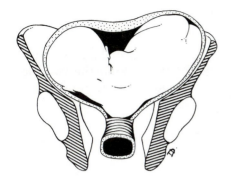

A. Impacted shoulder.

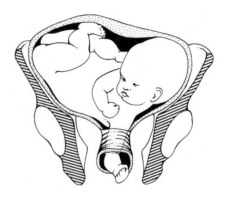

B. Prolapsed arm.

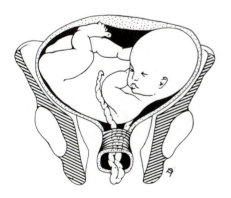

C. Prolapsed umbilical cord.

Figure 3. Complications.

PROGNOSIS: TRANSVERSE LIE

Prognosis depends upon the management. With early diagnosis and proper treatment the outcome is favorable. Neglect leads to the death of almost all infants and puts the mother in serious danger.

MANAGEMENT OF TRANSVERSE LIE

Management Before Labor

1. Careful abdominal, pelvic, ultrasonographic, and, if necessary, radiologic examinations are performed to confirm the diagnosis and to rule out fetal and pelvic abnormalities.
2. External version to a breech or preferably a cephalic presentation should be attempted. This may have to be repeated as there is a tendency for the transverse lie to recur.
3. Elective cesarean section is indicated where conditions are incompatible with safe vaginal delivery. This includes such complications as placenta previa or fetopelvic disproportion.
4. In other cases the onset of labor is awaited, as there is a chance that the malposition will correct itself.

Management During Early Labor

In early labor external version should be attempted, and if successful the new presentation is maintained by a tight abdominal binder until it is fixed in the pelvis.

Management of Patient in Good Labor: Persistent Transverse Lie

Cesarean Section
Cesarean section is the treatment of choice. It is safest for both mother and child. In some instances extraction of the infant through a transverse lower segment incision may be difficult, and a vertical incision in the lower segment, which can be extended upward if necessary, is preferred by many obstetricians.

Internal Podalic Version and Extraction
This is a dangerous procedure for fetus and mother, especially if the membranes have been ruptured for some time and the amniotic fluid has drained away. The use of podalic version and extraction—turning the baby to a footling breech and delivering it as such (see Chapter 30

for technique of internal podalic version)—is considered only in the following situations:

1. When the baby is premature, to the degree of nonviability, and the risk to the mother of cesarean section is not justified
2. Delivery of a second twin
3. When the patient is admitted to hospital with the membranes intact, the cervix fully dilated, and cesarean section cannot be performed immediately

Management of Neglected Transverse Lie

The following conditions are present:

1. There has been prolonged labor.
2. The membranes have been ruptured for a long time.
3. The lower uterine segment is stretched and thin.
4. Intrauterine infection is present.
5. Fetal impaction has taken place.
6. The cord, arm, or both have prolapsed.
7. The baby is dead.

Management under these circumstances is difficult.

1. Cesarean section and intensive therapy with antibiotics are carried out even if the baby is dead.
2. If infection is severe and widespread, hysterectomy may be necessary following the cesarean section.
3. Internal podalic version and extraction may be considered if cesarean is not feasible. This procedure is attended by a grave risk of uterine rupture.
4. In desperate situations a destructive operation can be performed on the child. Decapitation is carried out, the trunk is delivered, and then the head is extracted by forceps.

CONCLUSION

Transverse lies at term, after failure of external version, are treated best by cesarean section. They must never be neglected or left to nature.

Compound Presentations

20

PROLAPSE OF HAND AND ARM OR FOOT AND LEG

Definition

A presentation is compound when there is prolapse of one or more of the limbs along with the head or the breech, both entering the pelvis at the same time. Footling breech or shoulder presentations are not included in this group. Associated prolapse of the umbilical cord occurs in 15 to 20 percent.

Incidence

Easily detectable compound presentations occur probably once in 500 to 1000 confinements. It is impossible to establish the exact incidence because:

1. Spontaneous correction occurs frequently, and examination late in labor cannot provide the diagnosis.
2. Minor degrees of prolapse are detected only by early and careful vaginal examination.

Classification of Compound Presentation

1. Cephalic presentation with prolapse of:
   a. Upper limb (arm-hand), one or both:
   b. Lower limb (leg-foot), one or both:
   c. Arm and leg together
2. Breech presentation with prolapse of the hand or arm

By far the most frequent combination is that of the head with the hand (Fig. 1) or arm. In contrast, the head-foot and breech-arm groups are uncommon, about equally so. Prolapse of both hand and foot alongside the head is rare. All combinations may be complicated by prolapse of the umbilical cord, which then becomes the major problem.

Etiology

The etiology of compound presentation includes all conditions that prevent complete filling and occlusion of the pelvic inlet by the presenting part. The most common causal factor is prematurity. Others include high presenting part with ruptured membranes, multiparity, contracted pelvis, and twins.

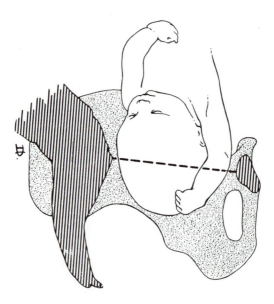

Figure 1. Compound presentation: head and hand.

Diagnosis

The condition is suspected when:

1. There is delay of progress in the active phase of labor.
2. Engagement fails to occur.
3. The fetal head remains high and deviated from the midline during labor, especially after the membranes rupture.

Diagnosis is made by vaginal or rectal examination. In many cases the condition is not noted until labor is well advanced and the cervix fully dilated.

Prognosis

In the past authors suggested a poor prognosis for the child. However, the increased incidence of prematurity and associated prolapse of the cord make it difficult to evaluate accurately the danger to the fetus of uncomplicated prolapse of the hand or foot.

Because of the historically high fetal mortality associated with compound presentations, active therapy (repositioning of the prolapsed part or version and extraction) was the most popular method of management. Recent studies have shown that the high fetal and maternal death rates resulted from overzealous treatment and not from the compound presentation itself. With conservative management the results should be no worse than with other presentations.

Mechanism of Labor

The mechanism of labor is that of the main presenting part. Because the diameter is increased, the chance of arrested progress is greater. In many cases labor is not obstructed, and the leading part is brought down to the outlet. If dystocia occurs, the baby remains high and operative treatment is needed.

MANAGEMENT OF COMPOUND PRESENTATIONS

In choosing the therapeutic procedure, these factors are considered:

1. Presentation
2. Presence or absence of cord prolapse
3. State of the cervix
4. Condition of the membranes
5. Condition and size of the baby
6. Presence of twins

Progressing Case

The best treatment for compound presentations (in the absence of complications such as prolapse of the cord) is masterful inactivity. In most cases, as the cervix becomes fully dilated and the presenting part descends, the prolapsed arm or leg rises out of the pelvis, allowing labor to proceed normally. Hence, as long as progress is being made there should be no interference.

Arrest of Progress

1. *Reposition of the prolapsed part:* In a normal pelvis if progress is arrested the arm or leg should be replaced, under anesthesia, and the head pushed into the pelvis. If the head is low in the pelvis and the cervix fully dilated, the head is extracted with forceps. High forceps must never be used.
2. *Cesarean section:* If there is cephalopelvic disproportion, if reposition is not feasible or is unsuccessful, or if there is some other condition that militates against vaginal delivery, cesarean section should be performed.
3. *Internal podalic version and extraction:* This procedure carries with it the danger of uterine rupture and fetal death. Hence it should not be used in the management of uncomplicated compound presentations. An exception is made in the case of a second twin.

Prolapse of the Cord

In 13 to 23 percent the compound presentation is complicated by prolapse of the umbilical cord. This then becomes the major and urgent problem, and treatment is directed primarily to it (see Chapter 21).

21

The Umbilical Cord

THE NORMAL UMBILICAL CORD

The umbilical cord links the fetus to the placenta and is the fetal life-line. The cord is between 30 and 60 cm in length, the average being 50 cm. It is covered on the outside by the amnion, which blends with the fetal skin at the umbilicus. On the inside of the cord is the thick myx-omatous Wharton jelly. Through the jelly, and protected by it, run the umbilical vessels, one vein and two arteries, in a spiral arrangement. The circulation is the reverse of the adult in that the vein carries oxy-genated blood to the fetus, while the arteries bring venous blood back to the placenta.

The fetal surface of the placenta is covered by amniotic membrane, under which course the large blood vessels, branches of the umbilical vein and arteries. Normally the cord inserts into the center of the pla-centa.

ABNORMALITIES OF THE UMBILICAL CORD

Length

On record are cords as short as 0 cm and as long as 104 cm.

1. A short cord may result in delay in descent of the fetus, fetal distress, separation of the placenta from the wall of the uterus, inversion of the uterus, and rupture leading to hemorrhage and possible fetal exsanguination.
2. A long cord is subject to entanglement, knotting, encirclement of the fetus, and prolapse.

3. When the cord is absent the fetus is attached directly to the placenta at the umbilicus. Omphalocele is always present.
4. It appears that the length of the umbilical cord is determined, at least partly, by the amount of amniotic fluid present in the first and second trimesters of pregnancy, and on the mobility of the fetus. If there is oligohydramnios, amniotic bands, or limitation of fetal movement for any reason, the umbilical cord will not develop to an average length.

Single Umbilical Artery

This occurs in 1 percent of single births and in 7 to 14 percent of multiple pregnancies. The condition is associated with a high rate of congenital fetal anomalies.

Battledore Placenta

Instead of being at the center, the cord is inserted at the margin of the placental disc. This condition has no known clinical significance.

Velamentous Insertion

In this case the vessels of the cord break up into branches before reaching the placenta, so that the cord inserts into the membranes rather than the placental disc. The result is that large vessels course under the membrane and are unprotected by Wharton jelly.

Vasa Previa

In this situation the velamentous vessels lie over the cervix, in front of the presenting part. Rupture leads to fetal bleeding, which may be fatal. The clinical picture is similar to placenta previa.

Hematoma

Rupture of the umbilical cord may lead to a hematoma. This is a serious complication, being associated with a high rate of fetal death. The hemorrhage into the cord and subsequent hematoma compress the vessels of the cord, causing fetal anoxia.

Angiomyxoma

Angiomyxomatous tumors of the umbilical cord are rare, only 12 cases having been reported. Two were associated with fetal death. There is often an associated myomatous degeneration of Wharton jelly. These tumors do not metastasize, and do not usually cause significant vascular obstruction. If the latter does occur it may lead to intrauterine hypoxia and fetal death.

CORD ENTANGLEMENTS

The most common variety of cord entanglement is the umbilical cord around the fetal neck. Four coils have been seen from time to time and as many as nine have been reported. A single loop of cord around the neck is present in 21 percent of deliveries. Two loops are present in 2.5 percent, and three loops in 0.2 percent of normal cases.

During pregnancy trouble is unusual. Sometimes as the fetus descends during labor the coils tighten sufficiently to reduce the flow of blood through the cord, thus causing fetal anoxia.

Only rarely are cord entanglements responsible for fetal or neonatal death. However, abnormalities of the fetal heart rate, meconium-stained amniotic fluid, and babies requiring resuscitation are seen more often when there is an entanglement of the cord. Significantly lower Apgar scores have been reported.

KNOTS OF THE CORD

True Knot

Occasionally a true knot of the umbilical cord is noted after delivery. This complication can occur when there is a long cord, large amounts of amniotic fluid, a small infant, monoamniotic twins, or an overactive fetus or as a result of external version. In many instances the knot is formed when a loop of cord is slipped over the infant's head or shoulders during delivery.

Rarely is the knot pulled tightly enough to cause the death of the fetus from restriction of the circulation in the cord. The umbilical vessels, protected by the thick myxomatous Wharton jelly, are rarely occluded completely. The fetal mortality associated with true knots of the umbilical cord is low. In these cases there is flattening or dissipation of Wharton jelly and venous congestion distal to the knot, as well as partially or completely occlusive vascular thrombi.

False Knots

The blood vessels are longer than the cord. Often they are folded on themselves and produce nodulations on the surface of the cord. These have been termed false knots.

PROLAPSE OF THE UMBILICAL CORD

In this situation the umbilical cord lies beside or below the presenting part. Although an infrequent complication—less than 1 percent (0.3 to 0.6 percent)—its significance is disproportionately great because of the high fetal mortality rate and the increased maternal hazard from the operative procedures used in treatment.

Compression of the umbilical cord between the presenting part and the maternal pelvis reduces or cuts off the blood supply to the fetus, and if uncorrected leads to death of the baby.

Classification of Prolapsed Cord

1. *Umbilical cord presentation.* The membranes are intact.
2. *Umbilical cord prolapse.* The membranes are ruptured. The cord may occupy three positions (Fig. 1):
   a. It may lie beside the presenting part at the inlet. Such an occult prolapse may be more common than is generally accepted. It could kill a baby during labor without leaving a trace of evidence at vaginal delivery.
   b. It may descend into the vagina.
   c. It may pass through the introitus and out of the vagina.

Etiology

Whenever the presenting part does not fit closely and fails to fill the inlet of the pelvis, danger of prolapse of the umbilical cord exists. Compound presentation and rupture of the bag of waters when the presenting part is not in the pelvis increase the risk.

Fetal Etiology

1. *Abnormal presentation*: Abnormal presentation occurs in almost half the cases of prolapse of the cord. Since 95 percent of all presentations are cephalic, the greatest number of prolapsed cords occur when the head leads the way. The highest relative incidence, however, is in the following order: (1) transverse lie; (2) breech presentation, especially the footling variety; and (3) cephalic presentation.
2. *Prematurity:* Two factors play a part in the failure to fill the inlet: (1) the smallness of the presenting part, and (2) the frequency of abnormal positions in premature labors. The fetal mortality is high. One reason for this is that small babies withstand trauma and anoxia badly. The second is the reluctance to

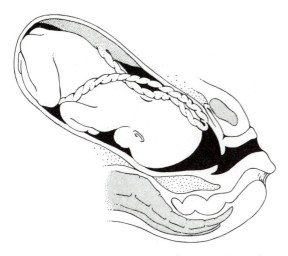

A. Cord prolapsed at the inlet.

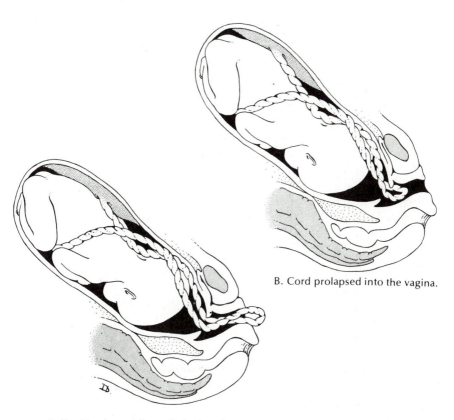

B. Cord prolapsed into the vagina.

C. Cord prolapsed through the introitus.

Figure 1. Prolapsed umbilical cord.

submit the mother to a major operation when the chance of saving the baby is almost nil.

3. *Multiple pregnancy:* The factors involved here include failure of good adaptation of the presenting part to the pelvis, greater frequency of abnormal presentation, polyhydramnios, and rupture of the membranes of the second twin when it is still unengaged.

4. *Polyhydramnios:* When the membranes rupture, the large amount of fluid pours out and the cord may be washed down.

Maternal and Obstetric Etiology

1. *Cephalopelvic disproportion:* Disproportion between pelvis and baby causes failure of engagement, and rupture of the membranes may be attended by prolapse of the cord.

2. *High presenting part:* Temporary delay of engagement may occur even in the normal pelvis, especially in multiparas. Should the membranes rupture during this period, the cord may come down.

Cord and Placental Etiology

1. *Long cord:* The longer the umbilical cord the easier it is for it to prolapse.

2. *Low-lying placenta:* When the placenta is located near the cervix it hinders engagement. In addition, insertion of the cord is nearer the cervix.

Iatrogenic Etiology

One-third of prolapses of the cord are produced during obstetric procedures.

1. Artificial rupture of the membranes. When the head is high, or when there is an abnormal presentation, rupture of the membranes may be attended by prolapse of the cord.

2. Disengaging the head. Elevation of the head out of the pelvis to facilitate rotation.

3. Flexion of an extended head.

4. Version and extraction.

5. Insertion of a bag (rarely used today).

Diagnosis: Prolapse of the Cord

The diagnosis of prolapse of the cord is made in two ways: (1) seeing the cord outside the vulva, and (2) feeling the cord on vaginal examination. Since the fetal mortality is high once the cord has protruded through the introitus, means of earlier diagnosis must be sought.

Vaginal Examination
Vaginal examination should be performed:

1. When there is unexplained fetal distress, and especially if the presenting part is not well engaged. Unfortunately fetal distress may be a late sign.
2. When the membranes rupture with a high presenting part.
3. In all cases of malpresentation when the membranes rupture.
4. When the baby is markedly premature.
5. In cases of twins.

Prognosis: Prolapse of the Cord

Labor
Labor is not affected by the prolapsed cord.

Mother
Maternal danger is caused only by traumatic attempts to save the child.

Fetus
The uncorrected perinatal mortality is around 35 percent. The baby's chances depend on the degree and duration of the compression of the cord and the interval between diagnosis and delivery. The fetal results depend upon the following factors:

1. The better the condition of the baby at the time of diagnosis, the greater its chance of survival. A strongly pulsating cord is a sign of hope, while a cord with a weak pulse is an ill omen.
2. The sooner the baby is delivered after the cord comes down, the better are the results. Delay of over 30 minutes increases the fetal mortality four times.
3. The more mature the fetus, the greater is its ability to withstand traumatic processes.
4. The less traumatic the actual delivery of the child, the better is the prognosis for mother and baby.
5. The fetal mortality increases as the interval between rupture of the membranes and delivery increases.

Management of Prolapsed Cord

No Interference
The prolapsed cord is ignored and labor allowed to proceed under the following conditions:

1. When the baby is dead

2. When the baby is known to be abnormal (e.g., anencephaly)
3. When the fetus is so premature that it has no chance of survival. There is no point in subjecting the mother to needless risk.

Temporary Measures

Immediate delivery of the infant is, of course, the optimal treatment. In those cases, however, where a delay is unavoidable, measures to lessen compression of the umbilical cord and to improve the condition of the baby include the following:

1. The attendant places a hand in the vagina and pushes the presenting part up and away from the cord. At the same time preparations are made for delivery.
2. The patient is placed in the knee-chest or Trendelenburg position, with the hips elevated and the head low.
3. The woman is given oxygen by mask.
4. The fetal heart is checked carefully and often.
5. Vaginal examination is made to ascertain presentation, cervical dilatation, station of the presenting part, and condition of the cord.
6. Because it is difficult to reduce pressure on the umbilical cord as long as strong uterine contractions go on, a tocolytic drug (e.g., ritodrine or isoxsuprine) can be given in an intravenous infusion. A recommended dose of ritodrine is to administer 267 to 400 μg per minute (40 to 60 drops of a solution containing 50 mg in 500 ml of crystalloid solution) according to the effect on the uterus, and with monitoring of the maternal pulse and blood pressure and fetal heart rate.

Cervix Fully Dilated

When the cervix is fully dilated these measures are carried out with these presentations:

1. Cephalic presentation, head low in the pelvis: Extraction by forceps.
2. In other situations cesarean section is the best treatment if it can be performed without delay.
3. If cesarean section cannot be carried out immediately the following procedures are indicated:
   a. Cephalic presentation, head high: Internal podalic version and extraction as a breech. There is the danger of rupturing the uterus, but since this is a desperate attempt to save the child, the chance is taken.
   b. Breech presentation: Extraction as a footling breech.
   c. Transverse lie: Internal podalic version to a footling breech and immediate extraction.

Cervix Incompletely Dilated

When the cervix is incompletely dilated, these measures are carried out:

1. Cesarean section is the treatment of choice as long as the child is mature and in good condition. The fetal results with cesarean section are far superior to other methods of delivery. The danger to the mother is considerably less than forceful delivery through an undilated cervix. While preparations for surgery are being made, the measures previously described for reducing compression of the cord are carried out.
2. Reposition of the cord may be attempted if cesarean section cannot be performed. The cord is carried up into the uterus, and the presenting part is pushed down into the pelvis and held there. Reposition of the cord is successful occasionally, but in most cases valuable time is lost in attempting it.
3. These measures failing, the mother is kept in the Trendelenburg position in the hope that pressure is kept off the cord so that the child survives until the cervix is dilated enough to enable delivery.
4. Manual dilatation of the cervix, cervical incisions, and other forceful methods of opening the cervix are almost never justified. Their success is small, and the risk to the mother is great.

Prophylaxis

Obstetric manipulations that encourage premature rupture of the membranes (such as artificial rupture of the membranes when the leading part is unengaged or when there is a malpresentation) and that increase the incidence of prolapse of the umbilical cord should be avoided. Patients whose membranes rupture at home, either before or during labor, should be admitted to hospital.

BIBLIOGRAPHY

Clare NM, Hayashi R, Khodr G: Intrauterine death from umbilical cord hematoma. Arch Pathol Lab Med 103:46, 1979

Fortune DW, Östöor AG: Angiomyxomas of the umbilical cord. Obstet Gynecol 55:375, 1980

Katz Z, Lancet M, Borenstein R: Management of labor with umbilical cord prolapse. Am J Obstet Gynecol 142:239, 1982

22

Shoulder Dystocia

GENERAL CONSIDERATIONS

Definition

True shoulder dystocia refers to the following situation: The presentation is cephalic; the head has been born, but the shoulders cannot be delivered by the usual methods. There is no other cause for the difficulty.

Incidence

The general incidence is less than 1 percent (0.15 to 0.2 percent). In babies weighing over 4000 g the incidence is 1.6 percent.

Etiology

Shoulder dystocia is associated with: (1) maternal obesity, (2) excessive weight gain, (3) oversized infants, (4) history of large siblings, and (5) maternal diabetes.

MECHANISM OF THE SHOULDERS

Normal Mechanism

In most cases the shoulders enter the pelvis in an oblique diameter. As labor progresses the shoulders descend and, under the rifling effect of the birth canal, rotate the bisacromial diameter toward the anteroposterior diameter of the pelvis. By this mechanism the anterior shoulder comes under the pubic symphysis a little to the side of the midline and is then delivered.

Mechanism in Shoulder Dystocia

Impaction of the shoulders is favored when they attempt to enter the pelvis with the bisacromial diameter in the anteroposterior diameter of the inlet (Fig. 1), instead of utilizing one of the oblique diameters. Rarely do both shoulders impact above the pelvic brim. Usually the posterior shoulder can negotiate its way past the sacral promontory, but the anterior one becomes arrested against the pubic symphysis. Some authors restrict the definition of shoulder dystocia to cases where the shoulders try to enter the pelvis with their bisacromial diameter in the anteroposterior diameter of the inlet.

Causes of Dystocia After Birth of the Head

1. Short umbilical cord
2. Abdominal or thoracic enlargement of the infant (anasarca, monsters, neoplasms)
3. Locked or conjoined twins
4. Uterine constriction ring
5. True shoulder dystocia

EFFECTS OF SHOULDER DYSTOCIA

Effects on the Fetus

With each uterine contraction large amounts of blood are transferred from the baby's trunk to its head. The angulation of the neck and the compression of the chest, which interfere with cardiac function, impair the venous return. The intracranial vascular system of the fetus cannot compensate for the excessive intravascular pressure. Under these conditions anoxia develops and may be accompanied by hemorrhagic effusions. If this condition persists too long the baby suffers irreparable brain damage. It may die during the attempts at delivery or in the neonatal period.

Complications

1. Fetal
   a. Death, intrapartum or neonatal.

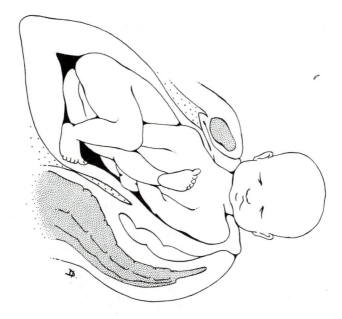

Figure 1. Shoulder dystocia: bisacromial diameter in the anteroposterior diameter of the pelvis.

    b. Immediate birth injuries, such as brachial plexus palsy and fractured clavicle, occur in 20 percent.

    c. Late neuropsychiatric abnormalities are seen in 30 percent of survivors.

2. Maternal

    a. Lacerations of the birth canal.

    b. Rupture of the uterus.

    c. Hemorrhage.

CLINICAL PICTURE

The clinical picture has been described by Morris:

> The delivery of the head with or without forceps may have been quite easy, but more commonly there has been a little difficulty in completing the extension of the head. The hairy scalp slides out with reluctance. When the forehead has appeared it is necessary to press back the perineum to deliver the face. Fat cheeks eventually emerge. A double chin has to be hooked over the posterior vulval commissure, to which it remains tightly opposed. Restitution seldom occurs spontaneously, for the head seems incapable of movement as a result of friction with the girdle of contact of the vulva. On the other hand, gentle manipulation of the head sometimes results in a sudden 90 degree restitution as the head adjusts itself without descent to the anteroposterior position of the shoulders.
>
> Time passes. The child's head becomes suffused. It endeavors unsuccessfully to breathe. Abdominal efforts by the mother or by her attendants produce no advance; gentle head traction is equally unavailing.
>
> Usually equanimity forsakes the attendants. They push, they pull. Alarm increases. Eventually
>
>   By greater strength of muscle
>
>   Or by some infernal juggle
>
> the difficulty appears to be overcome, and the shoulders and trunk of a goodly child are delivered. The pallor of its body contrasts with the plum-colored cyanosis of the face, and the small quantity of freshly expelled meconium about the buttocks. It dawns upon the attendants that their anxiety was not ill-founded, the baby lies limp and voiceless, and too often remains so despite all efforts at resuscitation.

DIAGNOSIS

Diagnosis can be made only after the head has been delivered. Certain signs then appear:

1. There is a definite recoil of the head back against the perineum.
2. Restitution rarely takes place spontaneously. Because of the friction with the vulva, the head seems incapable of movement.
3. The problem is usually recognized when traction from below and pressure from above fail to deliver the child.
4. Vaginal examination is made to rule out other causes of difficulty, as listed above under "Causes of Dystocia After Birth of the Head."

Prophylaxis

While this complication cannot be prevented, the results can be improved by recognizing the situations in which it occurs and by insisting on expert obstetric care for these patients. Warning signs of macrosomia include prolonged labor and failure of proper descent of the head in the second stage of labor

It has been suggested that when the transthoracic and abdominal diameters of the fetus are found, by ultrasonography, to be larger than the fetal biparietal diameter, shoulder dystocia may be anticipated. One study has shown that neonates experiencing shoulder dystocia had significantly greater shoulder-to-head and chest-to-head disproportions than did macrosomic infants delivered by cesarean section for failure to progress during labor or macrosomic infants delivered vaginally without shoulder dystocia.

MANAGEMENT OF SHOULDER DYSTOCIA

Accessory Measures

1. Anesthesia is administered, or if already in progress it should be deepened; complete muscle relaxation is of great value. Time is precious, and while the anesthesia is being given the operator must act.
2. The respiratory tract is cleared of mucus and debris to provide a clear airway.
3. Vaginal examination of the infant and the pelvis is made to rule out the other complications that prevent descent of the body: short umbilical cord, locked or conjoined twins, enlargement of abdomen or thorax, and uterine constriction ring.
4. An episiotomy, preferably mediolateral and large, is made to make room and to prevent tears into the rectum.

Basic Method of Delivery of Shoulders

Gentle backward traction is made on the delivered head, without forced rotation and without excessive angulation (Fig. 2A). At the same time the patient is told to bear down, if she is awake; if she is asleep, pressure on the fundus is made by an assistant at the same time that traction is being exerted on the head. The traction must be smooth and continuous, and sudden jerks avoided. The duration of these efforts should rarely exceed 4 to 5 seconds. If the cause of the difficulty is merely the friction of large shoulders in the oblique or transverse diameters, these simple measures almost always produce advancement. One or two efforts, however, are sufficient. If they fail, this method of delivery should be abandoned.

OPERATIVE METHODS OF TREATING SHOULDER DYSTOCIA

Delivery of Anterior Shoulder

1. The hand is placed deeply in the vagina behind the anterior shoulder.
2. With the next contraction the axis of the shoulders is rotated into an oblique diameter of the pelvis (Fig. 2B).
3. Firm traction is made on the head, deflecting it toward the floor.
4. Suprapubic pressure is exerted; this usually succeeds in bringing the anterior shoulder into and through the pelvis.
5. Sometimes the extraction may be furthered by the operator's hooking a forefinger under the axilla.

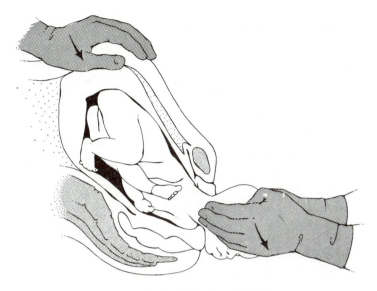

A. Basic method of delivering shoulders.

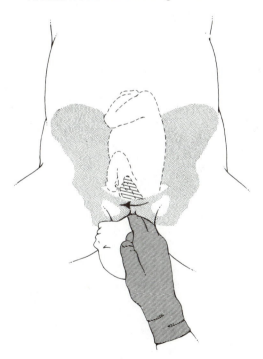

B. Shoulder dystocia: rotation of bisacromial diameter from anteroposterior diameter pelvis into the oblique.

Figure 2. Delivery of anterior shoulder.

Extraction of Posterior Shoulder and Arm

1. The hand of the obstetrician is placed deeply into the vagina along the curvature of the sacrum and behind the posterior shoulder of the fetus. If the back of the fetus is towards the physician's right side, the left hand is used. If the back is towards the doctor's left, the right hand is preferred (Fig. 3A).
2. The antecubital fossa of the posterior arm is located and, using the pressure of a finger, an attempt is made to flex the arm in a fashion similar to the Pinard maneuver in a breech extraction.
3. The forearm is swept across the chest and face, the hand is seized, and the arm extracted (Fig. 3B).
4. Once this is accomplished the anterior shoulder delivers as well in the majority of cases. If it does not, the body is rotated 180° so that the anterior shoulder is now posterior. It is then extracted by the same maneuver.

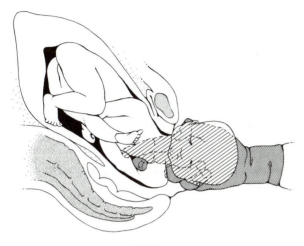

A. First step.

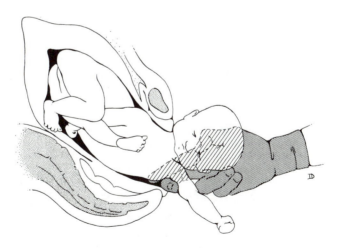

B. Second step.

Figure 3. Extraction of posterior shoulder and arm.

Screw Principle of Woods

1. The position of the head is LOT. This technique is not possible until the posterior shoulder has passed the spines.
2. Downward pressure is made on the baby's buttocks through the mother's abdomen by the operator's hand (Fig. 4A).
3. Two fingers of the left hand are placed on the anterior aspect of the posterior shoulder. Pressure is made against the shoulder so that it moves counterclockwise, the posterior aspect leading the way (Fig. 4B). It is turned 180°, past 12 o'clock. In this way the posterior shoulder is delivered under the pubic arc. The head has turned from LOT to ROT.
4. The posterior shoulder has been delivered, and the anterior shoulder is now posterior.
5. Pressure is again made on the baby's buttocks in a downward direction.
6. At the same time two fingers are placed against the anterior aspect of the newly posterior shoulder. By pressure against the shoulder, it is moved in a clockwise direction, the posterior aspect leading the way (Fig. 4C). It is turned 180°, past 12 o'clock, and the posterior shoulder is again delivered (Fig. 4D). The head rotates from ROT to LOT.

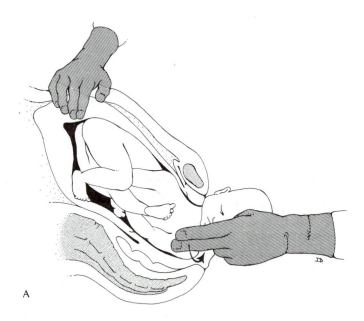

A

Figure 4. Screw principle of Woods. A through D represent steps one through four in this maneuver.

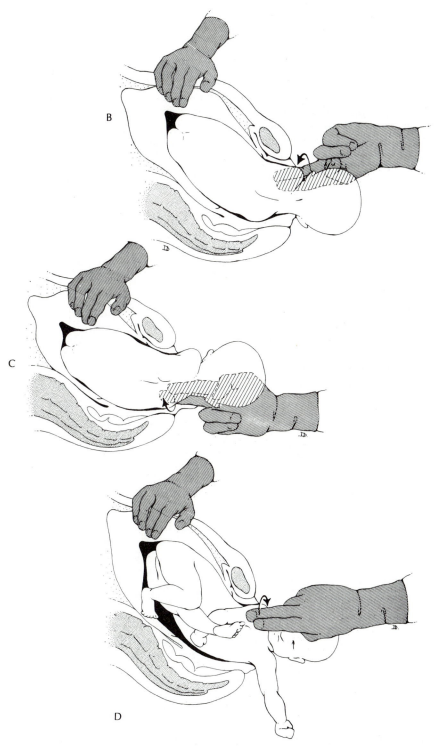

Figure 4. (cont.) Screw principle of Woods.

BIBLIOGRAPHY

Benedetti TJ, Gabbe SG: Shoulder dystocia. Obstet Gynecol 52:526, 1978

Benedetti TJ: Managing shoulder dystocia. Contemp OB/GYN 14:33, 1979

Hopwood HG: Shoulder dystocia: Fifteen years experience in a community hospital. Am J Obstet Gynecol 144:162, 1982

Modanlou HD, Komatsu G, Dorchester W, et al: Large-for-gestational neonates: Anthropometric reasons for shoulder dystocia. Obstet Gynecol 60:417, 1982

Morris WIC: Shoulder dystocia. J Obstet Gynaecol Brit Emp 62:302, 1955

Resnik R: Management of shoulder girdle dystocia. Clin Obstet Gynecol 23:559, 1980

Multiple Pregnancy

23

INCIDENCE

Hellin's law propounds the following rates of multiple pregnancy:

Twins	1:89
Triplets	$1:89^2$
Quadruplets	$1:83^3$
Quintuplets	$1:89^4$

Another way of expressing the approximate incidence is:

Twins	1:100
Triplets	1:10,000
Quadruplets	1:750,000

The etiology of multiple pregnancy is unknown in most cases. Excessive gonadotropic stimulation leading to superovulation is a factor in dizygous twinning. A tendency to plural births does run in families, more often on the maternal side.

An American survey noted that the mean birthweight and duration of pregnancy for the single fetus was 3377 g and 280.5 days, for twins 2395 g each and 261.6 days, and for triplets 1818 g each and 246.8 days. For a comparable period of gestation the mean weight of a singleton is 200 to 800 g greater than that of a twin.

TWIN PREGNANCY

Dizygous: Double Ovum

About 75 percent of twins are binovular (Figs. 1A and 1B). Two fetuses develop from the fertilization of two ova liberated during the same menstrual cycle. The incidence of double ovum twins is influenced by heredity, race, maternal age, and parity. Each twin has its own placenta, chorion, and amniotic sac. When the ova are implanted near each other, the two placentas may seem to fuse. The circulations, however, remain completely separate. These children are fraternal twins. They resemble each other only to the extent that siblings of the same age would. They may be of different sex and sometimes look entirely dissimilar. Weinberg's rule states that the number of dizygous twins in any population is twice the number of twins of different sex; the remainder are monozygous. Dizygous twinning is the result of multiple ovulation, which may be caused by high levels of gonadotropic hormones overstimulating the ovary. The artificial induction of ovulation by clomiphene or gonadotropins increases the chance of multiple pregnancy.

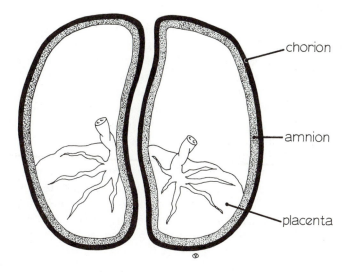

A. Separate dichorionic diamniotic placentae.

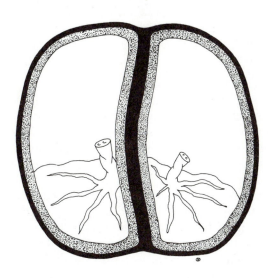

B. Fused dichorionic diamniotic placentae.

Figure 1. Placenta and membranes in twin pregnancy.

Monozygous: Single Ovum

Some 25 percent of twins are uniovular; these are identical, or true, twins. They represent complete cleavage of the blastodermic vesicle. There is one egg fertilized by a single sperm, and therefore the offspring arise from the same germ plasm. The frequency of single ovum twinning is independent of heredity, race, maternal age, and parity. These children are always of the same sex and look alike. Incomplete division results in anything from conjoined twins to double monsters. There is one placenta, one chorion, and two amniotic sacs. The blood circulations of the twins intercommunicate in the common placenta. In some cases a stronger twin monopolizes the circulation, which results in poor development of the other fetus. The undersized member tends to remain inferior into adult life. The smaller twin does not catch up to the larger in weight, length, head circumference, or the scores of intelligence tests. It is possible that the inability of the placenta to transmit adequate amounts of nutrition to the smaller twin leads to a cellular deficit that may restrict the final growth potential. The survival rate of both monozygotic twins is some 10 percent lower than the dizygotic variety. The incidence of congenital anomalies in monozygotic twins is greater than in dizygotic twins. The twins may have the same malformation.

The incidence of monozygous twinning is constant throughout the world. The explanation for or the cause of this event is not known. What seems to be true is that the time when the unknown factor acts influences how the development of the fertilized ovum will proceed.

1. *Dichorionic diamniotic twins:* In this case the division occurs at the blastomere stage, no later than 2 to 3 days after fertilization. The inner cell mass has not yet been delineated. Separate embryos develop, undistinguishable at birth from dizygous twins. Each twin has its own chorion, amnion, and placenta. The latter may be separate or fused depending on the site of implantation (Figs. 1A and 1B).
2. *Monochorionic diamniotic twins:* The split takes place at the blastocyst stage between 4 and 6 days. The inner cell mass, which has been formed, divides in two. The placenta has one chorion, but two amnions. Each twin lies in its own sac (Fig. 1C).
3. *Monochorionic monoamniotic twins:* The division takes place in the primitive germ disc at between 7 and 13 days. The amnion has already formed. The twins lie in the same amniotic sac. Monoamniotic twins are rare (Fig. 1D).

   Because the fetuses are not separated by membranes, there is a great possiblility of knotting, tangling, and strangulation of the umbilical cords. The resultant anoxia may lead to fetal

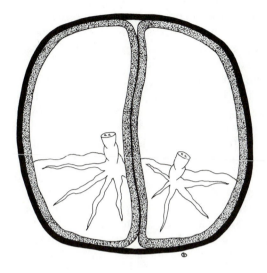

C. Monochorionic diamniotic placentae.

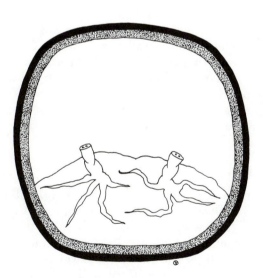

D. Monochorionic monoamniotic placentae.

Figure 1. (cont.) Placenta and membranes in twin pregnancy.

death. The prognosis for monoamniotic twins is poor; in only 50 percent of cases do both infants survive. If, after the birth of the first baby, the umbilical cord is observed to be knotted or twisted, or if there is no second bag of waters, the other twin should be delivered without delay.

The diagnosis of monoamniotic twins during pregnancy is difficult. It has been suggested that the finding of a variable deceleration pattern during a nonstress test in a twin gestation is suggestive of the possibility of cord entanglement and monoamniotic twins. Examination by ultrasonography and amniography should be carried out to establish the diagnosis. If monoamniotic twins are present, immediate delivery must be considered.

4. *Conjoined twins—monochorionic monoamniotic:* After the primitive streak of the embryo has appeared and the cells of the germ disc have assumed an axial arrangement (around 14 days), complete separation does not occur, and conjoined twins can develop.

Placentas of Twins

The only time that twins can be proved to be fraternal is when they are of different sexes. Identical twins may have one or two chorionic sacs, but only when there is a single chorionic sac can identicity be proved. Thus twins with one chorion are always identical. Twins of the same sex with two chorionic sacs may be identical or fraternal, and no examination of the placenta or membranes can establish the true status. In 80 percent of twins, zygosity can be shown at birth by examination of the placental membranes. In the remainder, study of the blood types and morphologic features of the infants will be necessary.

Twin Transfusion Syndrome

This occurs in monozygous twins with a single placenta in which arteriovenous fistulization leads to a parabiotic relationship. The donor twin is anemic (as low as 8 g of hemoglobin), while the recipient is plethoric (hemoglobin as high as 27 g) and is in danger of developing neonatal cardiac failure. The difference in weight is as much as 1000 g. The smaller twin may be associated with oligohydramnios; polyhydramnios is more common in the larger infant. The placenta of the donor twin is pale and swollen or atrophied; that of the recipient is large and congested.

Management includes (1) exchange transfusion, (2) venesection of the recipient, (3) treatment of hypoglycemia. Neonatal mortality has been reported to be as high as 70 percent.

Superfetation

Superfetation has been defined as the development of a second fertilized ovum within a uterus that already contains a developing conceptus fertilized in a previous cycle. There is doubt that superfetation takes place because:

1. The rapid development of the corpus luteum inhibits further ovulation.
2. The cervical canal is occluded by a plug of mucus that acts as a barrier to the ascent of sperm into the uterus.
3. By the 14th week of pregnancy the uterine cavity is obliterated by the enlarging fetal sac, making passage of sperm unlikely. However, a few cases have been reported in which the possibility of superfetation exists, and the belief that the condition is impossible cannot be proved.

Superfecundation

Superfecundation has been defined as the condition in which two or more ova belonging to or originating during the same period of ovulation are fertilized by sperm from coitus practiced at different times by the same or another male. It is difficult to prove the existence of superfecundation and difficult to prove that it is impossible.

DIAGNOSIS OF MULTIPLE PREGNANCY

1. Suggestive findings:
   a. Familial history.
   b. The uterus and abdomen seem larger than expected for the period of amenorrhea.
   c. Uterine growth is more rapid than normal.
   d. There is unexplainably excessive weight gain.
2. Positive signs:
   a. Palpation of two heads or two breeches.
   b. Two fetal hearts auscultated at the same time by two observers and differing in rate by at least 10 beats per minute.
   c. X-ray of the abdomen shows two skeletons. These may appear by the 18th week or sooner, but a second skeleton cannot be ruled out until the 25th week.
   d. Ultrasonography demonstrates the presence of two or more fetal skulls.
3. The diagnosis of twins is not easy unless there is a high index of suspicion. The frequency of preterm labor makes the diagnosis before the onset of labor even less frequent.

EFFECTS OF MULTIPLE PREGNANCY

Maternal Effects

1. Because the volume of the intrauterine contents is large, symptoms ranging from discomfort to actual abdominal pain are frequent. Pressure against the diaphragm leads to dyspnea.
2. The mechanical and metabolic loads increase with the multiplicity of the pregnancy.
3. Polyhydramnios, an excessive amount of amniotic fluid, is more common than in single pregnancies.
4. The incidence of preeclampsia is increased.
5. Anemia is prevalent.
6. Excessive weight gain occurs for several reasons, including overeating, water retention, the presence of more than one fetus, and polyhydramnios.
7. Complaints of fetal overactivity are frequent.

Fetal Effects

1. While the individual child is smaller than average, the combined weight of the babies is larger than that of a single child. One twin may be 50 to 1000 g heavier than the other. In half the cases the children are of term size. In one-eighth of pregnancies both babies are under 1500 g. The remaining three-eighths are between 1500 and 2500 g.
2. The combination of small babies and large amounts of amniotic fluid leads to an increased incidence of malpresentation.
3. Fetal mortality is increased in twin pregnancy to four times that of singletons. The gross mortality varies from 9 to 14 percent. While malpresentations and congenital abnormalities play a part, the major cause of death is prematurity. Birth weight is an important factor. The survival rate of twins born after 36 weeks gestation is several times higher than that of twins born before this period.
4. The risk to the second twin is greater than to the first. Reasons for this include:
   a. Greater incidence of operative deliveries.
   b. Too long an interval between the birth of the first and second twins.
   c. Reduction of the uterine capacity after the birth of the first baby: This may alter the placental hemodynamics and result in fetal anoxia.

    d. The second twin occupies a less favorable position in the actively contracting upper uterine segment.

    e. There is an increased incidence of malpresentation in the second twin.

5. The least possible delay should be permitted between delivery of the children. After the first is born it may be wise to give the mother oxygen to breathe in an effort to prevent anoxia of the second twin. The greater loss of the second twin is the result of death in the neonatal period rather than before or during labor.

6. Congenital malformations are more common in twins than in singletons.

7. Kurtz found that in no set of triplets did the combined weight reach 7500 g, indicating that triplets average under 2500 g. The second and third babies have a higher mortality than the first.

Effects on Labor

1. Overstretching of the uterus by the large combined weights of the babies, two placentas, and copious amniotic fluid, leads to the following:
   a. Preterm labor occurs, on the average, 3 weeks before term.
   b. Early rupture of the membranes is frequent and is one cause of premature labor.
   c. Most twin labors are satisfactory. Sometimes the over-lengthened uterine muscles produce weak and inefficient contractions, resulting in slow progress.
   d. The increased incidence and danger of postpartum hemorrhage must be kept in mind.
   e. Malpresentations are common.
   f. Umbilical cord prolapse is caused by rupture of the membranes with the gushing out of large amounts of fluid, especially with the second twin.
   g. Multiple pregnancy accelerates the problem of cervical incompetence and can result in effacement and dilatation as early as the first trimester.
2. In 80 percent of cases the second twin is born within 30 minutes of the first.
3. The two babies are born first and then the two placentas.
4. The combinations of presentations (Fig. 2) are, in descending order of frequency:
   a. Two vertices (most common and most favorable presentation)
   b. Vertex and breech
   c. Two breeches
   d. Vertex and transverse lie
   e. Breech and transverse lie
   f. Both in the transverse lie

MANAGEMENT OF MULTIPLE PREGNANCY

Management During Pregnancy

Early diagnosis enables the parents to make preparations for more than one child and alerts the doctor to the problems of multiple pregnancy. The two main complications, premature labor and preeclampsia, call for special care during the prenatal period.

1. The patient should cease outside work by 24 weeks. She needs frequent rest periods.
2. Travel is restricted, since the probability of early labor is strong.

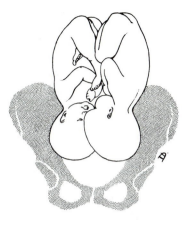

A. Two vertexes.

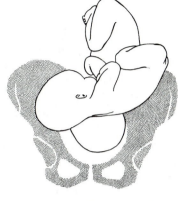

D. Vertex and transverse lie.

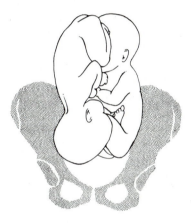

B. Vertex and breech.

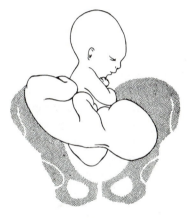

E. Breech and transverse lie.

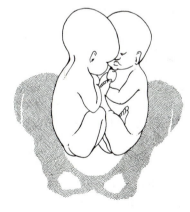

C. Two breeches.

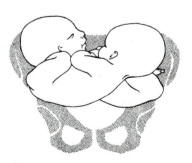

F. Two transverse lies.

Figure 2. Twin presentations.

3. Coitus is forbidden during the last 3 months.

4. It is believed that one reason for preterm labor is the inability of the cervix to contain the enlarging products of conception. If at any time the cervix becomes effaced and open, the patient should be put to bed.

5. Prenatal visits are made more often so that the presence of toxemia can be noted as soon as possible.

6. Bed rest: Since the greatest cause of fetal mortality in multiple pregnancy is preterm labor, the maintenance of the pregnancy to 36 or 37 weeks is desirable. Many obstetricians believe that bed rest, at home or in hospital, helps to achieve this goal. Rest in bed during pregnancy has two main effects: it delays the onset of labor by taking pressure off the cervix, and it promotes intrauterine fetal development; multiple gestation may represent a form of intrauterine growth retardation. The period of bed rest, with rising for meals and use of the bathroom, is from the 28th to the 36th or 37th week. Once the babies have attained a good size the patient may resume her activities gradually.

7. Ultrasonography: The highest rate of perinatal mortality occurs in those pregnancies that terminate before the 30th week of gestation. It may be that bed rest instituted at 28 weeks is too late for these cases. Because the early diagnosis of multiple pregnancy is so important, it has been suggested that ultrasonographic screening be carried out on all pregnant women at 20 weeks.

Management During Labor

1. Accurate diagnosis of the presentations is essential. Ultrasonic or x-ray examination is used when needed.

2. Sedatives and analgesics are administered with care, since small babies are susceptible to drugs that depress the vital centers.

3. The higher incidence of postpartum hemorrhage calls for precautionary measures, even to the extent of having cross-matched blood available, especially if the mother is anemic.

4. Watchful expectancy is the procedure of choice during labor. The best results are obtained when the least interference is employed.

5. When delivery is near, the patient is placed on the delivery table and an intravenous infusion of crystalloid is started. This precautionary measure has two uses: (a) Should uterine atony occur, either before or after the birth of the baby, oxytocin can be added to the solution to stimulate the myometrium. (b) If

postpartum hemorrhage does take place, the route for the administration of fluids or blood is available immediately.

6. The first baby is delivered in the usual way, as if it were a single pregnancy.

7. The umbilical cord must be clamped doubly. This is to prevent the second baby from bleeding through the cord of the first in uniovular twins, in whom the placental circulations communicate.

8. Intravenous egometrine should not be given before birth of the second twin is complete. The strong contraction that results may be dangerous to the baby still in utero, especially if it is placed badly.

9. Careful examination is made to determine the position and station of the second baby. If the vertex or breech is in or over the inlet and the uterus is contracting, the membranes should be ruptured artificially, care being taken that the cord does not prolapse. If uterine inertia has set in, an oxytocin drip may be given to reestablish uterine contractions; when this has been achieved, amniotomy is performed. The presenting part is guided into the pelvis by the vaginal hand. If necessary, pressure is made on the fundus with the other hand. Since the first baby has already dilated the birth canal, the second one descends rapidly to the pelvic floor.

10. Once the presenting part is on the perineum it is delivered spontaneously or by simple operative measures.

11. If the presentation is abnormal, if fetal or maternal distress supervenes, or if spontaneous delivery of the second twin has not taken place within 15 minutes, operative interference is considered, since the risk to the second baby increases with time. The second baby should be extracted as a breech if it so presents, and by version and extraction if it is a cephalic presentation or transverse lie. We do not believe in routine version and extraction for normal positions.

12. The sudden reduction of the intrauterine contents by delivery of the first twin may lead to premature separation of the placenta, endangering the second baby.

13. The placentas are delivered after both twins have been born.

14. Cesarean section is never performed when the presence of twins is the sole indication. The reason for operative delivery is some accompanying complication, such as toxemia of pregnancy, antepartum hemorrhage (placenta previa and abruptio placentae), transverse lie, or prolapse of the umbilical cord. Twin pregnancy does not impose a special threat to the integrity of a preexisting low transverse cesarean scar. It is not nec-

essary to schedule a repeat cesarean any earlier for a twin pregnancy than for a singleton.

15. Cesarean section for second twin: There has developed a trend to deliver by cesarean section all second twins that are in a non-cephalic presentation. Reported results do not support this concept. We believe that vaginal delivery is preferable. However, there are situations where vaginal delivery of the second twin cannot be effected promptly, and, in such cases, cesarean section should be considered. Included here are separation of the placenta, contracted cervix, prolapse of the umbilical cord, and fetal distress. The reported incidence of fetal loss of the second twin born by cesarean section is around 20 percent.

TRIPLET AND QUADRUPLET PREGNANCY

In the past, multiple pregnancy involving more than two infants was rare, but the inducers of ovulation, such as clomiphene citrate and especially gonadotropins, have increased the incidence of plural births significantly.

During pregnancy the main problems, outside of the large intrauterine volume, are anemia, pregnancy-induced hypertension, and intrauterine growth retardation.

The prime cause of relatively high fetal loss is preterm labor, often preceded by spontaneous rupture of the membranes. Delivery occurs before 37 weeks in over 90 percent of cases.

Most of the first infants present by the head. In triplets malpresentation is more common for the second and third babies. The mean weight is 1900 g for boys and 1770 g for girls. The fetal mortality is around 30 percent.

The prognosis for fetal survival was associated with several factors:

1. It was higher in older mothers.
2. Female infants did better than males.
3. The second and third infants fared worse than the first.
4. Fetuses presenting by the breech had a higher perinatal mortality rate, independent of birth order.
5. Parity did not have much effect on fetal survival.
6. The maturity of the infants at birth had more importance than the weight.

Management

1. Early diagnosis is essential. Ultrasonography should be performed by 6 to 8 weeks in all pregnancies resulting from

ovulations induced by gonadotropins or clomiphene, and whenever multifetal pregnancy is suspected. The most reliable means of diagnosis is by x-ray during the late second and third trimesters.

2. Prolongation of the pregnancy: Bed rest is advised as soon as the diagnosis is made, and hospitalization by 28 to 30 weeks, or with the development of complications. Bed rest delays the onset of labor and improves the placental blood flow. Hospitalization makes it possible to provide immediate medical treatment should preterm labor commence.

3. Fetal growth is monitored every 3 weeks by ultrasonography.

4. Nonstress tests are performed weekly while the patient is in hospital to determine fetal well-being.

5. The cervix is examined weekly for silent effacement and dilatation.

6. Tocolysis: Oral ritodrine or isoxsuprine in a dose of 30 mg twice daily has been used, starting at 28 to 30 weeks, to obviate the onset of labor. If preterm contractions do begin, the drugs are given by intravenous infusion.

7. Cerclage of the cervix has been tried when painless dilatation occurred. However, there is no good evidence that it is of benefit.

8. Pulmonary maturity: Betamethasone may be given to stimulate the fetal lungs to mature and to prevent the development of the respiratory distress syndrome after birth. The dose is 12 mg intramuscularly, repeated in 12 hours, and then weekly until fetal pulmonary maturity is achieved.

9. Depo-hydroxyprogesterone caproate, 500 mg twice a week, given intramuscularly to the mother, from the middle of the second trimester to delivery or fetal maturity has been used, and success claimed. However, the evidence is tenuous.

10. Mode of delivery: Some experienced obstetricians believe that, after 34 weeks of gestation, it is reasonable to allow vaginal delivery of uncomplicated triplets, and reserve cesarean section for complications such as dysfunctional labor, malpresentation of the first fetus, and medical or obstetric complications. However, when there are three or more fetuses, in only one-third of cases will they all present by the head. Some authorities feel, therefore, that cesarean section is preferable, because delivery and neonatal care involve so many additional physicians and nurses to care for the babies, that careful planning is essential. The procedure is carried out at 34 to 36 weeks, in a hospital with an excellent neonatal intensive care nursery. The poor prognosis for triplets delivered as breeches suggests that cesarean section may be a preferred

way to deliver these babies. It may also be safer for the mother because it eliminates the risks of manipulations in the overdistended uterus.

LOCKING OF TWINS

Locking of twins is the situation in which one baby impedes the descent and delivery of the other. The problem is more common in primigravidas. Small babies are more likely to lock than large ones. This complication is so rare that most obstetricians never see a case. There are four varieties:

1. *Collision:* The contact of any fetal parts of one twin with those of its co-twin, preventing the engagement of either (Fig. 3A).
2. *Impaction:* The indentation of any fetal parts of one twin onto the surface of its co-twin, permitting partial engagement of both simultaneously (Fig. 3B).
3. *Compaction:* The simultaneous full engagement of the leading fetal poles of both twins, thus filling the true pelvic cavity and thereby preventing further descent or disengagement of either twin.
4. *Interlocking:* The intimate adhesion of the inferior surface of a twin's chin with that of its co-twin above or below the pelvic inlet (Fig. 3C). If this occurs within the true pelvis, compaction results.

There are four main categories of locked twins.

1. Breech-vertex (most common)
2. Vertex-vertex
3. Vertex-transverse lie
4. Breech-breech

Interlocking is a rare condition. The incidence is 1 per 1000 twin gestations. However, in the situation in which both twins occupy longitudinal lies, when the fetal poles are opposite to each other, and when the first presents as a breech, the incidence is 1 per 100 cases.

In interlocking the first infant presents as a breech and the second is cephalic. Interlocking takes place between the chins. The first child delivers uneventfully until the scapula is born. The interlocking makes further descent impossible. Unless the condition is corrected rapidly, the first child will die of asphyxia.

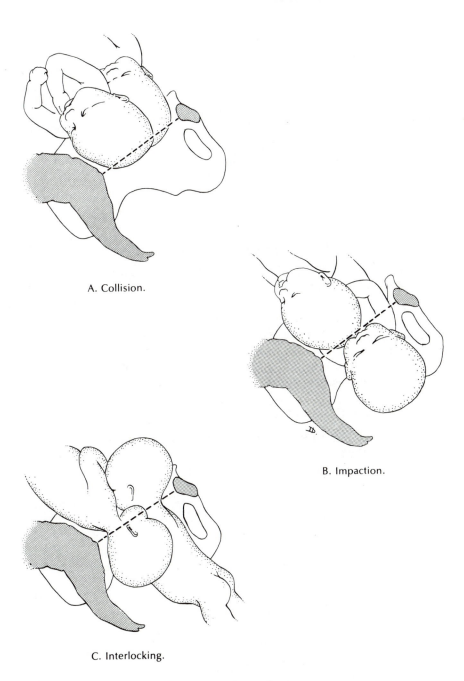

A. Collision.

B. Impaction.

C. Interlocking.

Figure 3. Locking of twins.

Diagnosis and Prevention

Early diagnosis is rare. True locking occurs only in the second stage of labor and treatment must be instituted before the condition progresses to the point of irreversibility. The following are recommended:

1. An x-ray is taken for every twin gestation during labor.
2. If twin A is presenting as a breech and twin B by the head, the x-ray is repeated after 2 hours of active labor.
3. If there is collision of the twins or suspicion of interlocking, cesarean section should be performed.

Management

Management of Collision, Impaction, Compaction

1. Strong traction and fundal pressure must be avoided.
2. In general, an attempt is made under deep anesthesia to push the second twin out of the way and out of the pelvis before traction is applied to the first twin and its delivery effected.
3. The second twin is delivered in the usual way.
4. If this method fails and the babies are alive, cesarean section is performed.
5. Embryotomy is a last resort.

Management of Chin to Chin Interlocking

1. Under anesthesia an attempt is made to unlock the chins, so that the second twin can be pushed out of the way, enabling the first to be born. Traction on the first twin must be avoided as this aggravates the problem.
2. If this does not succeed within a short time, the first baby dies from asphyxia and the trauma of the manipulations.
   Efforts are then concentrated on saving the second twin. The locking is broken up by decapitating the first twin.
   a. A couple of strong sutures are placed in the head of the first twin.
   b. Decapitation is performed, the incision being made below the level of the sutures.
   c. The trunk of the first twin is delivered.
   d. The second twin is delivered.
   e. Traction is made on the sutures to fix the head of the first twin so that forceps can be applied and the head extracted.
3. Cesarean section is contraindicated. It would entail pulling the body of the first twin, which is outside of the vulva, back through

the vagina, uterus, and peritoneal cavity. This would carry with it grave danger to the mother of peritonitis and general sepsis when there is nothing to gain by this procedure.

Prognosis

The maternal prognosis is good, but fetal prognosis is bad. The perinatal mortality is between 40 and 50 percent. As many as 60 to 70 percent of the deaths are in the first twin, and half of these result from embryotomy.

CONJOINED TWINS

Conjoined twins are uniovular twins in whom the embryonic area failed to split completely and the two individuals remain attached. Siamese twins are one variety.

Incidence

The incidence is from 1:100,000 to 1:50,000 births. In twin gestation the incidence is from 1:900 to 1:650. Most are female.

Etiology

Because these fetuses originate from a single ovum they are monovular, monozygotic, and monoamniotic, with the same sex and chromosomal pattern. The basic defect is thought to be an incomplete, delayed fission of the inner cell mass, which takes place after the 14th day following fertilization. The precise etiology of conjoined twins is not known, but the same influences are responsible as those that cause monozygotic twinning.

Classification

The numerous types of conjoined twins fall into two main groups:

1. Diplopagus *(Duplicatas completa)*: In this group there is equal or nearly equal and symmetrical duplication of structures.
2. Heteropagus *(Duplicatas incompleta)*: In this group only part of the anatomic structure of the fetus is duplicated. One component is smaller and dependent on the other.

The most frequently encountered types include:

1. Thoracopagus—joined at the chest: 40 percent.
2. Xiphopagus or omphalopagus—joined at the anterior abdominal wall from the xiphisternum to the level of the umbilicus: percent.
3. Pyopagus—joined at the buttocks: 18 percent.
4. Ischiopagus—joined at the ischium: 6 percent.
5. Craniopagus—joined at the head: 2 percent.

Diagnosis

The antepartum diagnosis of conjoined twins is important in that it will:

1. Minimize maternal trauma and morbidity.
2. Improve the rate of survival of the fetus or fetuses.
3. Enable a plan for delivery to be made.
4. Provide time to assemble pediatric and surgical teams.
5. Prepare the parents.

Regrettably, it is rare for conjoined twins to be discovered prior to the time of delivery. Most cases are diagnosed only in the second stage of labor, when obstruction has taken place.

In all multiple pregnancies the possiblility of conjoined twins should be considered and investigated. Suspicion provoking factors include:

1. Polyhydramnios is found in 50 percent of cases of conjoined twins.
2. The finding of a single fetal heart in a multiple pregnancy.
3. A lack of engagement when the lie is longitudinal.
4. A similar parallel lie (vertex-vertex, breech-breech).
5. An abnormal fetal attitude.

Methods of Diagnosis

1. Ultrasonography. Diagnostic criteria include:
   a. Demonstration of a continuous nonseparated external skin contour.
   b. The body parts of the twins are on the same level and imaged in the same sonar plane.
   c. There is no change in the relative positions of the twins to one another on successive scans.
   d. Recognition of a face-to-face relationship in the case of thoracopagus twins.
   e. The demonstration of a single placenta. Real-time scanning is of value in assessing fetal movement and in identifying individual structures, such as the heart.

2. X-ray. Diagnostic criteria include:
   a. The fetal heads are at the same level and in the same body plane.
   b. The spines are in unusually close proximity.
   c. The spines are extended.
   d. The fetuses do not change position relative to each other after movement, manipulation, or the passage of time. Unless there is a bony fusion the radiographic diagnosis is unreliable, and radiography has been largely replaced by ultrasonography.
3. Amniography. The injection of a radioopaque dye into the amniotic cavity followed by radiologic examination should be carried out when conjoined twinning is suspected from ultrasonic or radiographic study.
   a. The presence of a soft tissue union will be confirmed and the extent and nature of the attachment evaluated. This information will help determine the mode of delivery.
   b. Valuable data are provided regarding the likelihood of fetal survival and the possibility of surgical separation.
   c. Associated anomalies of the neural tube, the abdominal wall, and the gastrointestinal tract may be detected.
4. During labor. When, in a twin pregnancy, dystocia develops, one should consider the possibilities of conjoined twins, locked twins, or congenital anomalies. Since conjoined twins always develop within a single amniotic sac, palpation of a second sac after the rupture of the first will rule out conjoined twins. On the other hand, multiple fetal limbs close to each other, failure of traction to deliver the first twin in the second stage of labor, and inability to move one twin without moving the other all suggest conjoined twins. When vaginal examination reveals a bridge of tissue betwen the fetuses, the diagnosis is confirmed.

Management

The decision as to whether delivery should proceed per vaginam or by cesarean section is based on the following factors:

1. The possibility of the infant's survival: In most cases this cannot be predicted accurately. However, when serious anomalies, such as anencephaly, are present, the answer is clear. More accurate methods of diagnosis and improved surgical techniques and care have increased the chances for survival of conjoined twins as separate individuals. In all cases, therefore, the welfare of the children is of paramount importance.
2. The size of the infants: In most reported cases the combined

weight is less than 5000 g; often the combined weight does not exceed that of a normal infant. The small size is the result of the frequent occurrence of preterm labor and delivery.

3. The extent and location of the union: In many cases the union is sufficiently flexible that enough movement is possible to allow vaginal delivery with or without manipulation or by forceps. Extensive bony fusion may preclude movement and vaginal delivery is impossible.

4. Fetal presentation: Abnormal presentations, such as breech and transverse lie, occur frequently.

5. The possibility of surgical separation.

6. The attitudes of the parents.

Method of Delivery

1. Cesarean section: This procedure offers the best chance for fetal survival, obviates damage to the mother by a difficult vaginal delivery, and is considered to be the method of choice for delivery when the diagnosis of conjoined twins has been made during the pregnancy. Elective cesarean section is performed when fetal maturity has been attained. Even in cases of fetal death, especially when the fetuses are large, cesarean section is advisable to avoid maternal injury. At cesarean section, a lower segment vertical incision, that can be extended upward easily if necessary, is preferable so that maximum exposure can be achieved.

2. Vaginal delivery: If the pregnancy is well before term, the babies are small, the point and type of union permit mobility, and if the infants are dead, vaginal delivery can be effected without serious injury to the mother. However, dystocia is common and manipulations such as forceps extraction or traction on the head, legs, or buttocks are necessary.

3. Destructive operations: When part of the fetus has been born, and complete delivery is not possible, a destructive operation becomes the only alternative. Such procedures include evisceration and amputation of parts of the body.

FETUS PAPYRACEUS

This is a rare condition, the reported incidence being 1:12,000 live births and 1:184 twin pregnancies.

The mechanism of papyraceus formation involves the death and compression of one twin resulting in a small, underdeveloped, and wafer-thin body that resembles old parchment. Most of the fetal deaths occur in the second trimester, rarely in the third. The etiology is un-known.

The diagnosis is usually made during labor or after delivery of the papyraceus. Antepartum diagnosis is rare. When there is suspicion that a twin pregnancy is not progressing properly, the diagnosis can be made by serial ultrasonic examinations that show evidence of fetal death.

In most cases the presence of the papyraceus has little effect on the mother or the viable fetus. In rare cases the dead fetus may obstruct labor, making cesarean section necessary. Postpartum hemorrhage and infection caused by the retention of the dead fetus have been reported. Congenital anomalies may occur in the surviving fetus, as well as a serious disorder of the skin, known as aplasia cutis congenita.

BIBLIOGRAPHY

Acker D, Lieberman M, Holbrook RH, et al: Delivery of the second twin. Obstet Gynecol 59:710, 1982

Evrard JR, Gold EM: Cesarean section for delivery of the second twin. Obstet Gynecol 57:581, 1981

Galea P, Scott JM, Goel KM: Feto-fetal transfusion syndrome. Arch Dis Child 57:781, 1982

Harper RG, Kenigsberg K, Sia CG, et al: Xiphopagus conjoined twins: A 300-year review of the obstetric, morphopathologic, neonatal, and surgical parameters. Am J Obstet Gynecol 137:617, 1980

Hawrylyshyn PA, Barkin M, Bernstein A, Papsin FR: Twin pregnancies—a continuing perinatal challenge. Obstet Gynecol 59:463, 1982

Holcberg G, Biale Y, Lewenthal H, Insler V: Outcome of pregnancy in 31 triplet gestations. Obstet Gynecol 59:473, 1982

Itzkowic D: Surgery of 59 triplet pregnancies. Brit J Obstet Gynaecol 86:23, 1979

Loucopoulos A, Jewelewicz R: Management of multifetal pregnancies: Sixteen years' experience at the Sloane Hospital for Women. Am J Obstet Gynecol 143:902, 1982

Nissen ED: Collision, impaction, compaction, and interlocking. Obstet Gynecol 11:514, 1958

Quigley JK: Monoamniotic twin pregnancy: Am J Obstet Gynecol 29:354, 1935

Ron-El R, Caspi E, Schreyer P, et al: Triplet and quadruplet pregnancies and management. Obstet Gynecol 57:458, 1981

Shennan AT, Milligan JE, Yeung PK: Successful management of quadruplet pregnancy in a perinatal unit. Can Med Assoc J 121:741, 1979

24

Obstetric Forceps

The obstetric forceps, invented by Peter Chamberlen at the beginning of the seventeenth century, is an instrument designed for extraction of the fetal head. While many varieties of forceps have been described, the basic design and purpose remain unchanged.

PARTS OF THE FORCEPS

1. There are *handles* by which to grip the forceps.
2. *The lock* holds the forceps together. It is so constructed that the right one fits on over the left. For this reason, unless the particular situation necessitates doing otherwise, the left blade should be applied first. The main types of lock are:
   a. *The English lock* (e.g., Simpson forceps) has a shoulder and flange in each shank which fit into each other (Fig. lA). Articulation is fixed at a given point.
   b. *The French lock* (e.g., Tarnier and De Wees) has a pinion and screw (Fig. 1B). The left shank bears a pivot fitting into a notch on the right shank. After articulation the pivot is tightened by screwing it home.
   c. *The sliding lock* (e.g., Kjelland) is built into the left blade only (Fig. 1C). The right blade fits into the lock, but articulation is not fixed. This type of lock is useful when application is not perfect, as when the head is asynclitic.

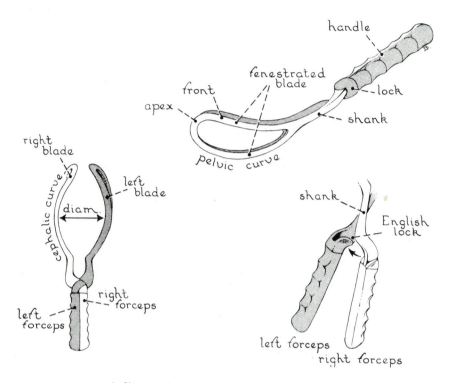

A. Simpson forceps showing the various parts.

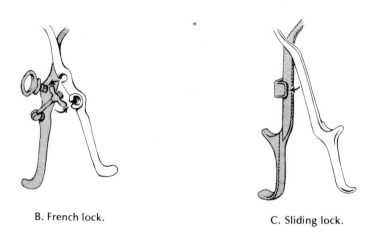

B. French lock.

C. Sliding lock.

Figure 1. Obstetric forceps.

3. *The shank* connects the handle and the blade. A short-shanked instrument is satisfactory when the fetal head is low in the pelvis. When the head has not reached the perineum a longer shank is needed.

4. *The blades,* which enclose the head, may be solid or fenestrated. They are designed to grasp the head firmly but without excessive compression. The solid blades may cause less trauma, but the fenestrated blades are lighter, grip the fetal head better, and are less likely to slip. The edges are smooth to reduce damage to the soft tissues.

5. *Forceps are right or left* depending on the side of the maternal pelvis to which they are applied. Since most forceps cross at the lock, the handle of the right forceps is held in the operator's right hand and fits the right side of the pelvis. The left blade fits the left side of the maternal pelvis, and its handle is held in the left hand of the operator.

6. *The front* of the forceps is the concave side.

7. *The apex* is the tips of the blades.

8. *The diameter* is the widest distance between the blades. It measures about 7.5 cm.

9. The forceps have two curves:

    a. *The cephalic curve* fits the shape of the baby's head and reduces the danger of compression.

    b. *The pelvic curve* follows the direction of the birth canal. It makes application and extraction easier, and decreases damage to the maternal tissues.

TYPES OF FORCEPS

There are many general-duty forceps and several with specialized functions (Figs. 2 and 3). We believe that the new obstetrician should learn to use one instrument well, so that he becomes thoroughly at home with it. Once he has achieved this experience he must try other instruments, so that he has several familiar types at his command.

1. *Simpson forceps:* This is the common forceps. It has a cephalic and a pelvic curve. The shank is straight. The lock is of the English variety. This is a good general-duty forceps and is used widely and successfully for all obstetric forceps operations.
2. *DeLee forceps:* This is the Simpson forceps with a few minor modifications. The shank is a little longer to keep the handle away from the anus. The handle is changed to secure lightness, a better grip, and ease of cleaning.
3. *Tucker-McLane forceps:* The blades are solid.
4. *Kjelland forceps:* The pelvic curve is almost nonexistent, making the instrument ideal for rotating the fetal head. Rotation can be accomplished simply by twisting the closed handles instead of sweeping them through a wide arc, as is necessary when using forceps with a deep pelvic curve. The sliding lock makes the locking of the blades easier. Delivery can be accomplished with the same instrument: no reapplication is needed.
5. *Barton forceps:* The construction is such that an exact cephalic application can be made without disturbing the relationship of the head to the pelvis. The blades are joined to the shank at an angle of 135°. The posterior blade is attached to the shank in a fixed manner. The anterior blade is hinged at its junction to the shank, allowing movement through 45°. This feature, plus the sliding lock, allows the blades to be locked even when there is marked asynclitism. This is a good forceps for rotation of a head in transverse arrest.
6. *Piper forceps:* The blade of this forceps is similar to that of the Simpson forceps. The shank has been lengthened and curved downward so that the handles are lower than the blades. Thus the forceps has a double pelvic curve, which facilitates application to the aftercoming head in breech presentations.
7. *DeWees forceps:* The blades are standard. The handles are modified so that an axis-traction bar can be attached.
8. *Axis-traction forceps:* These are forceps specially designed so that a traction apparatus can be attached either to the blades at the bases of the fenestrae (Tarnier and Milne-Murray) or to the handles (DeWees). The traction bar is attached to the forceps by

a series of joints, which has the effect of a universal joint. The forceps are applied to the head in the usual way, and the traction apparatus is attached. The baby's head is then extracted by pulling only on the traction bar. The advantages of this technique are:

a. The line of traction is in the axis of the birth canal.
b. The universal joint permits the blades to rotate with the head and thus to follow the natural rotation of the head as it accommodates itself to the maternal pelvis in its descent.
c. Axis traction was of value in difficult high and midforceps deliveries. Since in modern obstetrics we try to eliminate these traumatic operations, axis traction is needed rarely today.

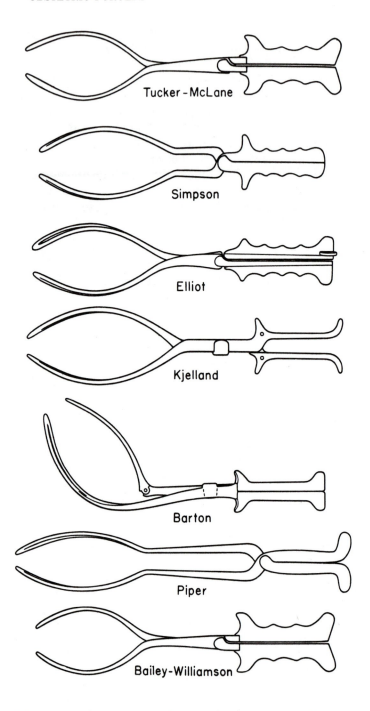

Figure 2. Front view of some commonly used forceps. (*From Douglas and Stromme. Operative Obstetrics, 4th ed., 1982. Courtesy of Appleton-Century-Crofts.*)

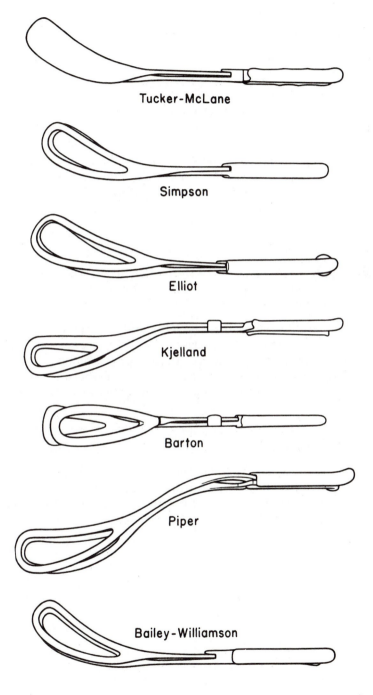

Figure 3. Lateral view of some commonly used forceps. (*From Douglas and Stromme. Operative Obstetrics, 4th ed., 1982. Courtesy of Appleton–Century–Crofts.*)

APPLICATION OF FORCEPS

Cephalic Application

A cephalic application is made to fit the baby's head (Fig. 4A). An ideal cephalic application in occipitoanterior positions is biparietal, along the occipitomental diameter, with the fenestrae including the parietal bosses and the tips lying over the cheeks. The concave edges should point to the denominator and the convex edges toward the face.

With this application, pressure on the head causes the least damage. If the forceps are applied so that one blade lies over the face and the other over the occiput, a relatively small degree of compression may cause tentorial tears and intracranial hemorrhage.

Pelvic Application

A pelvic application is made to fit the maternal pelvis (Fig. 4B), regardless of how the forceps grip the fetal head. The best pelvic application is achieved when:

1. The left blade is next to the left side of the pelvis.
2. The right blade is on the right side of the pelvis.
3. The concave margin is near the symphysis pubis.
4. The convex margin is in the hollow of the sacrum.
5. The diameter of the forceps is in the transverse diameter of the pelvis.

Perfect Application

A perfect application (Fig. 4C) is achieved when both the cephalic and pelvic requirements have been fulfilled. When the occiput has rotated under the symphysis pubis and the sagittal suture is in the anteroposterior diameter, an ideal application is possible.

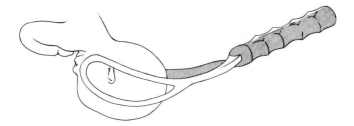

A. Cephalic application.

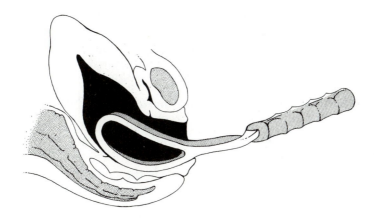

B. Pelvic application.

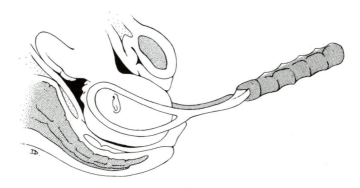

C. Perfect application.

Figure 4. Application of forceps.

FUNCTIONS OF OBSTETRIC FORCEPS

Of the six original uses of forceps—traction, rotation, compression, dilatation, leverage, irritation—only traction and rotation are acceptable today. Compression of the head may be an unavoidable accompaniment but is never a function of forceps.

Traction

In other than expert hands the use of forceps should be restricted to that of traction (Fig. 5A). The direction of traction must be along the pelvic curvature, and as the station changes during descent so does the line of traction. The direction of pull should be perpendicular to the plane of the level at which it is being applied. The higher the level, the more posterior the line of traction.

Rotation of Head from Posterior or Transverse Positions

An important principle must be remembered when using the forceps for rotation. The handles should be swung through a wide arc in order to reduce the arc of the blades (Figs. 5B and C). This lowers the incidence and extent of vaginal lacerations and at the same time makes the operation easier.

CLASSIFICATION OF FORCEPS OPERATIONS

Low Forceps

Low forceps is the application of forceps after the head has become visible, the skull (not the caput) has reached the perineal floor, and the sagittal suture is in or near the anteroposterior diameter of the pelvis. The station is $+3$.

Midforceps

Midforceps is the application of forceps before the criteria of low forceps have been met but after engagement has taken place. The biparietal diameter has passed through the inlet and the lowest part of the skull has reached the level of the ischial spines. The station is 0 to $+2$. Frequently rotation is not complete. This can be a difficult operation, even for the experienced obstetrician.

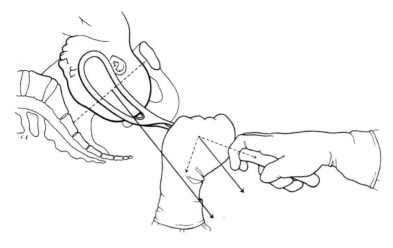

A. Traction with forceps.

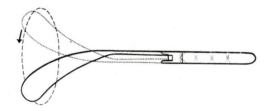

B. Rotation with forceps, incorrect technique.

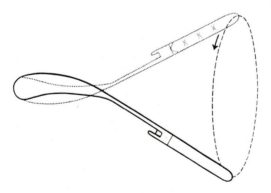

C. Rotation with forceps, correct technique.

Figure 5. Traction and rotation with forceps. (*From Douglas and Stromme. Operative Obstetrics, 4th ed., 1982. Courtesy of Appleton-Century-Crofts.*)

High Forceps

The head has entered the pelvis but is not engaged. The widest diameter has not passed through the inlet, and the bony presenting part has not reached the level of the ischial spines. The danger of damage to both baby and mother is great, and this operation is rarely carried out.

Floating Forceps

The whole fetal head is above the pelvic brim. This procedure is not performed today, having been superseded by cesarean section.

Summary

The average case fits nicely into these categories. However, when there is extreme molding, marked asynclitism, large caput succedaneum, attitude of extension, or abnormal pelvis, errors are often made in thinking that the station is lower than it really is. The operator believes he is about to perform a midforceps operation and finds himself doing a high forceps.

ACOG Classification

In 1964 the Executive Board of the American College of Obstetricians and Gynecologists adopted the following classification of forceps deliveries (Fig. 6).

Outlet Forceps. The application of forceps when the scalp is or has been visible at the introitus without separating the labia, the skull has reached the pelvic floor, and the sagittal suture is in the anteroposterior diameter of the pelvis.

Midforceps. The application of forceps when the head is engaged but the conditions for outlet forceps have not been met. In the context of this term, any forceps delivery requiring artificial rotation, regardless of the station from which extraction is begun, shall be designated a midforceps delivery. The term low midforceps is disapproved. A record shall be made of the position and station of the head when the delivery is begun. In addition, a description of the various maneuvers and of any difficulties encountered in the application of the forceps and in the extraction of the infant shall be recorded.

High Forceps. The application of forceps at any time prior to full engagement of the head. High forceps delivery is almost never justified.

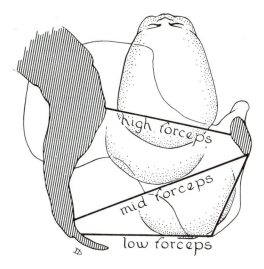

Figure 6. Classification of forceps operations according to station.

CONDITIONS AND PREREQUISITES

Before obstetric forceps may be used safely certain conditions, requirements, or prerequisites must be present.

1. An adequate pelvis with no disproportion is an absolute condition. Failure to observe this rule may lead to disaster for fetus and mother.
2. There must be no serious bony or soft tissue obstruction, such as presenting ovarian cysts or uterine fibromyomas.
3. The fetal head must be engaged so that the bony skull (not the caput succedaneum) is at least at the level of the ischial spines. In modern times forceps are not employed unless the station is +1, +2, or lower.
4. The cervix must be completely dilated and retracted. Disregard for this rule leads to tears of the cervix, hemorrhage, and possible "failed forceps."
5. Accurate diagnosis of position and station is essential.
6. The membranes should be ruptured. If they are not there is increased chance of the blades slipping, and there is danger of pulling the placenta away from the uterine wall. If the bag of waters is intact it should be broken. Frequently this results in better labor and progress, so that the need for forceps is obviated.

7. The patient is placed on a good delivery table, with her legs in stirrups and her buttocks well down and a little past the end of the table.
8. Some form of anesthesia—general, conduction, or local—should be used. This achieves both relaxation and relief of pain.
9. The bladder must be emptied by using a rubber catheter before the forceps are applied. An empty bladder occupies less space than a full one and is less liable to injury.
10. The rectum should be empty. This is usually already accomplished by an enema earlier in labor.
11. The operation is performed under strictly aseptic conditions.

INDICATIONS FOR USE OF FORCEPS

Fetal Distress

Signs that suggest the baby is suffering from lack of oxygen include:

1. Irregular fetal heart beat
2. Bradycardia, under 100 beats per minute, between uterine contractions
3. Late decelerations of the fetal heart rate
4. Rapid fetal heart—more than 160 beats per minute
5. Passage of meconium in cephalic presentations

Once fetal distress has developed the baby must be delivered immediately, providing the prerequisites have been met.

The more serious signs are irregularity and slowness of the fetal heart. Prolapse of the umbilical cord may be in the background. Occasionally a loop of cord around the baby's neck tightens as the fetus descends; the flow of blood through the cord is reduced, and hypoxia or anoxia results, with bradycardia as a clinical sign. Often babies who demonstrate intrauterine bradycardia or pass meconium are born in good condition and remain so. Thus when signs of distress are present and delivery can be expedited by an easy low forceps delivery, this should be done immediately. On the other hand, in the panicky attempt to save a baby with possible anoxia one should beware of damaging it or even killing it by a difficult, traumatic, and sometimes needless forceps extraction.

Maternal Conditions

1. Maternal distress or exhaustion
2. Maternal disease

An extraction of the baby for maternal reasons is justified if the risk to mother and child is less than that of waiting for spontaneous delivery.

Maternal distress or exhaustion is shown by dehydration, concentrated urine, and pulse and temperature above 100. These patients are not in shock, they are simply becoming exhausted.

When there is maternal disease—cardiac disease, tuberculosis, toxemia, or any debilitating condition—forceps can be used to shorten the second stage and obviate the need for prolonged bearing-down efforts by the patient.

It is essential in these situations that the forceps delivery be easy. The patient is not helped by a difficult forceps extraction with attendant lacerations and hemorrhage.

Failure of Progress in the Second Stage

1. Failure of descent
2. Failure of internal rotation

Providing the conditions for the use of forceps have been met, lack of advancement in the presence of good uterine contractions for 1 hour in a multipara or 2 hours in a primigravida is an indication for assessment of the situation and consideration of delivery by forceps. The limit to the length of the second stage was established because the rates of fetal (and maternal as well) morbidity rose when the second stage of labor was prolonged. However, under modern conditions provided by continuous electronic fetal monitoring, when a more accurate assessment of the condition of the infant is possible, it is permissible to extend the length of the second stage of labor beyond 2 hours if there is hope of progress and the baby and mother are in good condition.

Situations that predispose to arrest of progress include:

1. Poor uterine contractions
2. Minor degrees of relative disproportion caused by such conditions as a large baby or prominent ischial spines
3. Abnormal fetal position such as posterior position of the occiput or attitudes of extension
4. A rigid perineum, which the advancing head cannot thin out
5. Diastasis of the rectus abdominis muscle, which reduces the efficiency of the bearing-down effects of the patient
6. A lax pelvic floor, which inhibits proper rotation of the head

Elective Outlet Forceps: Prophylactic Forceps

This procedure is prophylactic in that it is designed to prevent fetal asphyxia and death and to reduce injury and needless suffering of the mother. It is done in conjunction with early episiotomy. The reasoning is:

1. It is better to do the episiotomy before the tissues are over-stretched. This may reduce the incidence of relaxation of the perineum and pelvic floor and of prolapse of the uterus in later life.
2. It saves the mother a period of bearing down and may prevent painful hemorrhoids.
3. The extraction of the baby with outlet forceps is less damaging than prolonged pounding of the head on the perineum.

In a study by the Collaborative Perinatal Project the offspring of 30,000 gravidas, delivered spontaneously or by low forceps, were followed to 4 years of age. The data showed that, when compared with infants born spontaneously, the incidence of neonatal death or subsequent neurologic impairment was no higher in those born by low forceps. These findings suggest that the procedure is safe. Whether the operation is "protective" to the infant is less certain.

Optimum Time to Use Forceps

The indications, conditions, and time limits, as detailed previously, cannot be considered rigid and unchangeable. The attendant must at all times exercise his prerogative to modify the indications to suit the situation at hand. Sometimes interference is carried out sooner than usual, while in other instances more time is allowed before operative measures are instituted.

Once fetal distress is present, interference is mandatory. However, rather than waiting for marked bradycardia with subsequent desperate activity by the obstetrician, it is better to extract the infant while it is still in good condition and better able to stand the trauma of the operation and anesthesia. In cases of prolonged labor with slow advance, for example, the possibility of fetal distress should be anticipated.

Maternal distress is a definite indication for operative delivery. One should not permit the patient to become completely exhausted before offering assistance.

The rule to wait until progress in the second stage has ceased for 1 hour in a multipara and 2 hours in a primipara is not absolute. Often the attendant can decide much sooner whether there is hope for advancement. For instance, when the head is on the perineum there is no justification in running out the clock when an episiotomy or low forceps would be of assistance to the fetus, the mother, and the perineum.

The best time to use forceps is a matter of judgment. One should not resort to operative delivery needlessly or too quickly. On the other hand, one must not wait so long that the life of the baby and the health of the mother are jeopardized.

CONTRAINDICATIONS TO USE OF FORCEPS

1. Absence of a proper indication
2. Incompletely dilated cervix
3. Marked cephalopelvic disproportion
4. Unengaged fetal head
5. Lack of experience on the part of the operator

DANGERS OF FORCEPS

Maternal Dangers

1. Lacerations of vulva, vagina, cervix, and extension of episiotomy
2. Rupture of the uterus
3. Hemorrhage from lacerations and uterine atony
4. Injury to bladder and/or rectum
5. Infection of genital tract
6. Atony of bladder leading to urinary infection
7. Fracture of coccyx

Fetal Dangers

1. Cephalhematoma
2. Brain damage and intracranial hemorrhage
3. General depression and asphyxia
4. Late neurologic sequelae
5. Fracture of skull
6. Facial paralysis
7. Brachial palsy
8. Bruising
9. Cord compression
10. Death

Serious injuries to the fetus delivered by forceps consist mainly of damage to the falx cerebri, the tentorium cerebelli, and the associated venous sinuses and other vessels. Lacerations are caused by excessive force and excessive compression. These injuries are associated mainly with deliveries from the midpelvis or higher. The dangers are especially great when (1) the forceps are applied in other than the biparietal diameter, (2) the fetal head is drawn through the least favorable diameters of the pelvis, (3) forceful rotation is made at the wrong level of the pelvis, (4) excessive force is used in other than the correct line of the axis of the pelvis.

MIDPELVIC ARREST: FORCEPS OR CESAREAN SECTION

Midpelvic arrest is one of the major problems encountered in the labor room. When the fetal head is out of the pelvis, the obvious solution is cesarean section. However, once the head is in the pelvis, a difficult decision has to be made—to allow labor to go on, to effect delivery by midforceps, or to perform cesarean section. The obstetrician is faced with the concept of a balance between the morbidity of the mother and that of the fetus. After a prolonged second stage of labor the risk of cesarean section is primarily to the mother; the major danger of midforceps is to the infant, although damage to the maternal pelvis can occur.

Current obstetric practice is likely to discourage the use of midforceps for delivery of patients whose second stage of labor is prolonged. There are a number of reasons for this, some justified, others not yet established.

1. The prolonged second stage of labor no longer has the ominous prognosis with which it used to be associated. The use of continuous electronic fetal heart rate monitoring has decreased the danger to the infant. As long as the mother and fetus appear to be well, the second stage may go on for longer than 2 hours if there is hope of progress.
2. The proper augmentation of desultory labor by an infusion of oxytocin obviates the need for interference in many cases.
3. The danger of injury to the baby of midforceps is greater than with cesarean section. It should be noted, however, that some 90 percent of fetal trauma occurring as a result of midforceps deliveries took place in operations that were described by the operator as "difficult," or where the presenting part had descended only to the level of the ischial spines. A common reason for delivery by forceps is fetal distress. It is probable that at least part of the cause of the neonatal morbidity associated with midforceps rests with the indication for the operation, as well as the procedure itself. Other conditions in this area include cephalopelvic disproportion, prolonged labor, and excessive anesthesia. In such situations it may be prudent to avoid using midforceps.
4. The effect of midforceps on the infant's long-term neuropsychiatric potential is unclear. Two groups of investigators, analyzing

the statistics from the Collaborative Perinatal Project, have come to diametrically opposing conclusions. Until there are prospective, randomized studies, with long-term follow-up, comparing the midforceps operation to cesarean section, it cannot be concluded that the replacement of all midforceps procedures by cesarean section is the optimal method to prevent the adverse neuropsychiatric sequelae reported currently in infants delivered by midforceps.

5. Maternal mortality from cesarean section has declined, although the rates of morbidity remain high.
6. Vaginal delivery following cesarean section is safe in selected cases, so the rate of repeat cesarean section can be reduced.
7. Training physicians in the art of delivery by forceps has become difficult to carry out. In contrast to the skill required to perform a midforceps operation successfully and safely, cesarean section is a straightforward procedure.

Should, therefore, midforceps even be used? Some maintain that the danger of both obvious and hidden damage is too great, and that this procedure must be replaced by cesarean section. In opposition to this view is the belief that, while the heavy traction of the past is no longer acceptable, the easy midforceps operation is safe and has fewer complications than cesarean section.

Providing there is no cephalopelvic disproportion, midforceps when performed properly by competent hands and on correct indications need not be mutilating to the mother nor impose undue hazard on the fetus. When the head is engaged deeply, with the biparietal diameter at the level of the ischial spines and the station at +2, midforceps is the procedure of choice, especially when uterine inertia or maternal fatigue results in arrest in the second stage. The midforceps operation is an important part of obstetrics.

FAILED FORCEPS OR CATASTROPHIC SUCCESS

An attempt to deliver the child by forceps may fail completely; or it may produce a damaged or dead baby and leave the mother with a lacerated pelvis. Pitfalls that contribute to making a wrong decision include the following:

1. Misunderstanding the significance and the relationship of station and the level of the biparietal diameter. Station zero means that the presenting part has reached the level of the ischial spines. In most women when the station is zero the biparietal diameter is at or just through the pelvic inlet. Thus when forceps

are applied at station zero, the essence of the procedure lies, not in extracting the presenting part from the midpelvis, but in dragging the biparietal diameter all the way from the inlet, through the midpelvis and the outlet. This is a difficult and potentially dangerous procedure. On the other hand, when the station is + 2 and the biparietal diameter is at or below the spines, a midforceps operation is often easy and safe. Hence we must always consider both the station of the presenting part and the level of the biparietal diameter.

2. Unrecognized disproportion, caused by:
   a. Small or abnormal pelvis.
   b. Large baby. This is the most treacherous of all situations, especially in a multipara who had a normal delivery previously. An anticipated easy birth turns into the nightmare of a difficult forceps extraction, vaginal and cervical lacerations, postpartum hemorrhage, and too often a damaged or dead infant. Whenever progress has ceased, the size of the baby must be reassessed before any action is taken.

3. Misdiagnosis of station.
   a. Rectal examination may be adequate for the management of normal labor, but it is inaccurate and unreliable and leads to serious errors when a problem exists. In such cases careful, sterile vaginal examination is mandatory before a decision is made.
   b. Caput succedaneum (edema of the scalp). In prolonged labor the caput may be 1 to 2 cm thick, and hence the bony skull is at a correspondingly higher level in the pelvis. It is important to ascertain the station of the skull and not the edematous scalp. A large caput indicates strong contractions, great resistance, or both. A small or absent caput suggests that the contractions and/or the resistance of the pelvic tissues are weak.
   c. Molding. Excessive molding makes the head pointed by lengthening its long axis: therefore the biparietal diameter is at a greater distance from the leading part of the skull. In such situations engagement may not have taken place when the station is zero. Not only is the forceps operation difficult, but the pressure of the instrument on a brain already under stress increases the risk of permanent damage. Extreme molding is a sign of trouble.

4. Misdiagnosis of position. In descending order of importance, the steps in the use of forceps are diagnosis of position, application, and traction. It is obvious that if the exact position of the fetal

head is not known the forceps cannot be applied correctly. Difficulty in applying forceps demands a complete reevaluation of the situation and not forceful delivery. Whenever labor ceases to advance, the possibility of an abnormal position or a malpresentation (such as brow) must be kept in mind.

5. Incorrect diagnosis of cervical dilatation. Often the patient thought to be ready for delivery is found during the final vaginal examination to have an incompletely dilated cervix. Except in the rarest situation, forceps must not be applied through a cervix that is not open fully. This may be a sign of disproportion, and forceful vaginal delivery leads to catastrophe. If there is no disproportion and the mother and fetus are in good condition, labor should proceed until sufficient advancement has been made. If there is disproportion or fetal distress, cesarean section is indicated.

6. Misdiagnosis of inefficient uterine action. The erroneous assumption that the lack of progress is the result of poor contractions leads to trouble in two ways: (1) Forceps are applied too soon. (2) An oxytocin infusion may dilate the cervix and jam the fetal head into the pelvis just far enough to encourage the performance of a misguided forceps extraction.

7. A constriction ring is a localized area of myometrial spasm that grips the fetus tightly and prevents descent, either spontaneously or by forceps.

8. Premature interference. This involves the use of forceps either before the patient is ready and the prerequisites are fulfilled, or when there are no valid indications. The factors here are:
   a. An impatient doctor
   b. Pressure from the patient and her family to do something
   c. Anesthesia administered too soon because of (1) error in deciding how far advanced in labor the patient is, (2) fear of precipitate delivery, and (3) a rambunctious patient

9. Indecision and stubbornness.
   a. The doctor does not make up his mind and waits too long; by the time he decides to act, the baby and mother are already in bad shape.
   b. Stubbornness is of two kinds. In the first place is the doctor who simply cannot admit to an error in judgment and proceeds to compound it. In the second situation is the doctor who refuses to obtain consultation.
   c. A treacherous problem occurs when small advancement does take place. This encourages the accoucheur to go on when cesarean section would be preferable.

TRIAL FORCEPS AND FAILED FORCEPS

Once a decision has been made to attempt delivery by means of forceps, one of several outcomes is possible.

1. Final vaginal examination reveals an unfavorable situation or the presence of unexpected disproportion, and vaginal delivery is abandoned in favor of cesarean section or a further trial of labor.
2. An easy, atraumatic operation produces a healthy child.
3. An excessively forceful, difficult, and ill-advised procedure is carried out, and a damaged or dead infant is born.
4. Failed forceps fall into two categories.
   a. Failure of application. The forceps cannot be applied properly to the fetal head.
   b. Failure of extraction. The forceps are applied, but despite an all-out effort delivery cannot be accomplished. By the time the attempt is stopped the baby may be injured.

   Causes of failed forceps include: (1) disproportion, (2) malposition, (3) cervix not fully dilated, (4) constriction ring, and (5) premature interference.
5. Trial forceps. The principle of trial forceps postulates that after successful application has been achieved gentle traction is made. Should the head come down easily, the operation is continued and the baby delivered. If, on the other hand, the operator feels that an undue amount of force would be required to extract the head, the forceps are removed and cesarean section is carried out. In order to avoid delay, all preparations for cesarean should be made before the vaginal delivery is attempted. To a degree, every forceps delivery is a trial. Of course, if there is obvious disproportion a trial of forceps is contraindicated.

VACUUM EXTRACTOR

In 1964 James Yonge had described the use of a cupping glass on the fetal scalp to assist the delivery of the fetal head. Saemann and Arnott each reported the use of vacuum instruments in 1829. James Y. Simpson demonstrated the use of a vacuum extractor in 1848. The modern apparatus was made by Malmstrom in 1954, and the modified instrument, now in general use, was developed in 1957.

The modern instrument consists of an all metal cup of four sizes— 30, 40, 50, and 60 mm in diameter. The largest diameter is in the interior of the cup. A rubber tube extends from the cup to a pump, which creates the suction. Attached to the cup and inside the tubing is a chain by which traction on the cup is effected. The scalp is drawn into the cup (Fig. 7), and an artificial caput succedaneum is formed. A dusky ring remains after the cup is removed; this is gone by the time the baby leaves the hospital.

Indications

The indications are much the same as those for forceps. The vacuum extractor cannot be used for face presentations, nor on the aftercoming head in breeches.

1. Second stage of labor
   a. Maternal exhaustion or disease (e.g., heart)
   b. Fetal distress
   c. Failure of descent or rotation
   d. Elective outlet application
2. First stage of labor
   a. Inertic labor
   b. Fetal distress

Contraindications

1. Absolute
   a. Cephalopelvic disproportion
   b. Face presentation
   c. Aftercoming head in a breech
2. Relative
   a. Partially dilated cervix. While it is preferable for the cervix to be fully dilated, the vacuum extractor can be used when the cervix is incompletely dilated with little or no injury to fetus or mother. In properly selected cases cesarean section can be avoided.

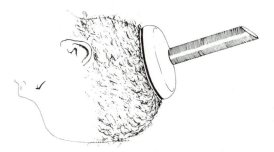

Figure 7. Vacuum extractor in place.

   b. Unengaged head. Under ideal conditions the extractor should not be used when the head is high. However, in some cases of fetal distress the delivery can be effected more quickly by the vacuum extractor than by cesarean section.

   c. Premature infants can be delivered by the vacuum extractor, but it is safer not to do so.

   d. Congenital anomalies, such as hydrocephalus, make it difficult and traumatic to effect delivery by vacuum extraction.

   e. Dead fetus. Suction and traction are not efficient in this case.

Advantages

1. Some 18 lb of traction can be applied with only 1/20 the rise in intracranial pressure resulting from the use of forceps.
2. The vacuum extractor can be used before cervical dilatation is complete.
3. The vacuum extractor does not encroach on the space in the pelvis, reducing the incidence of damage to maternal tissues.
4. The fetal head is not fixed by the application so it can go through the rotations that the configurations of the birth canal require.The fetal head is allowed to find the path of least resistance.
5. While it is safest to use the vacuum extractor when the head is well engaged, it can be applied to the head at a station inaccessible to forceps.

Application

The cervix should be dilated to at least 4 cm. The patient is positioned and prepared just as for a forceps delivery. The largest cup that fits is used. The lubricated cup is placed on the fetal head, over the posterior fontanelle and as close to the occiput as possible. The knob on the cup should point to the posterior fontanelle. Slowly the negative pressure is pumped up until it reaches 0.7 to 0.8 kg/cm². This takes 8 to 10 minutes. The apparatus is now ready for traction (Fig. 8). As the development of the vacuum progresses, an artificial caput succedaneum, called a "chignon," is formed.

Forces

The vacuum extractor exerts four types of force on the fetal scalp.

1. Negative outward suction from the vacuum itself.
2. Downward force from the traction.
3. A circular force if rotation takes place.

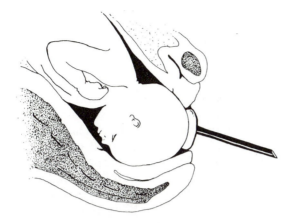

A. Traction outward and posteriorly.

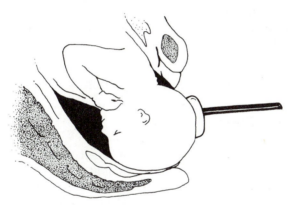

B. Traction outward and horizontally.

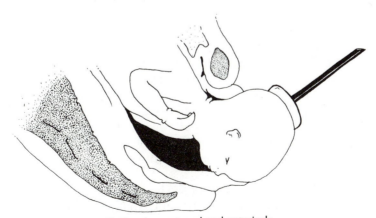

C. Traction outward and anteriorly.

Figure 8. Vacuum extractor traction.

351

4. A shearing force occurs when the direction of traction is not perpendicular to the surface of the scalp.

Delivery

If the uterine contractions are weak, an oxytocin drip can be used. A series of tractions synchronized with the labor pains are applied, the right hand pulling the chain-tube, while the left hand presses the traction cup and the fetal head posteriorly against the sacrum. This produces a force in the direction of the birth canal. The total extraction time takes about 15 minutes, or five to ten tractions during uterine contractions. If the cervix is not fully dilated it may take longer. The upper time limit is 30 minutes (rarely 45) to prevent damage to the baby. If delivery is not accomplished during this time, the case is considered unsuitable for vaginal delivery and cesarean section is performed. After delivery the vacuum is released and the cup removed. The large artificial caput disappears in about 10 minutes, and by the end of a week only a slight circular area of redness is seen.

Safeguards in the Use of Vacuum Extraction

1. Cephalic presentation, preferably well fixed.
2. No cephalopelvic disproportion.
3. The membranes must be ruptured.
4. Cervical dilatation must be sufficient to admit the cup. The larger cup is safer and more efficient.
5. The cup is placed as near to the occiput as possible.
6. Negative vacuum pressure must not exceed 0.7 to 0.8 kg/cm^2.
7. The cup should not remain on the fetal scalp for longer than 45 minutes. The shorter the time, the less the danger of damage to the fetal scalp.
8. Traction should be maintained at right angles to the application of the cup. The possibility of damage to the scalp is increased by diagonal or shearing forces and rocking motions.
9. Traction is exerted concomitantly with the uterine contractions and the maternal expulsive efforts.
10. When insufficient time is allowed for the development of the caput within the cup there is the risk of the cup's "popping off." This accident causes tearing of the fetal scalp and should be avoided.
11. Rotation of malpositions of the head should be allowed to take place spontaneously as traction is applied. Attempts to rotate the head by turning the cup leads to avulsion injuries.
12. If advancement is not evident after three to four pulls, the pro-

cedure should be discontinued, the situation reevaluated, and a different method of delivery considered.

Complications

Maternal. The incidence is low. Small lacerations of the vagina and cervix are a little more common than with spontaneous birth.

Fetal. These are similar to those that occur with forceps and include:

1. The formation of a pronounced caput succedaneum is an integral part of the procedure and is seen in almost all cases. As a rule the caput disappears in a few hours.
2. Abrasions, necrosis, and ulceration of the scalp at the site of application of the cup, probably as a result of the instrument's being left on too long or of improper traction. These are treated by gentle cleansing and antibiotic ointments. The skin at the site of the suction must be handled carefully to avoid rubbing off of the friable superficial layer. These areas heal without residual effects.
3. Cephalhematoma. This occurs in 10 to 15 percent of cases, and is higher than that reported for spontaneous births and deliveries by forceps. Serious difficulties are rare and the prognosis is good.
4. Subaponeurotic or subgaleal hemorrhage may occur from beneath the galea aponeurotica layer of the scalp. Sometimes it is not evident until a couple of days after birth. The bleeding may be massive and life threatening because the subaponeurotic space is continuous across the cranium without periosteal attachments. A hematoma in this space can dissect across the cranial vault, elevating part or all of the scalp.
5. Postnatal asphyxia.
6. Cerebral irritation related to the number of pulls, which seems to increase after five or six tractions.
7. Intracranial hemorrhage and/or signs of cerebral irritation are seen in around 2.5 percent of babies delivered by vacuum extraction. Many of these cases are associated with prolonged labor. Long-term studies have shown few, if any, permanent effects.
8. Retinal hemorrhage does occur more frequently than with spontaneous births or deliveries by forceps. The clinical significance of retinal hemorrhage following vacuum extraction is unclear. There seems to be no residual damage.

BIBLIOGRAPHY

Bowes WA, Bowes C: Current role of the midforceps operation. Clin Obstet Gynecol 23:549, 1980

Healy DL, Quinn MA, Pepperell RJ: Rotational delivery of the fetus: Kielland's forceps and two other methods compared. Brit J Obstet Gynaecol, 89:501, 1982

Ingardia CJ, Cetrulo CL: Forceps—use and abuse. Clin Perinatol 8:63, 1981

Kadar N, Romero R: Prognosis for future childbearing after midcavity instrumental deliveries in primigravidas. Obstet Gynecol 62:166, 1983

Kappy KA; Vacuum extractor. Clin Perinatol 8:79, 1981

Plauché WC: Fetal cranial injuries related to delivery with the Malmström vacuum extractor. Obstet Gynecol 53:750, 1979

Varner MW: Neuropsychiatric sequelae of midforceps deliveries. Clin Perinatol 10:455, 1983

25

Anterior Positions of the Occiput: Delivery by Forceps

LOW FORCEPS DELIVERY: OCCIPUT ANTERIOR

In order to prevent the omission of essential steps, the obstetrician should train himself to perform forceps operations with a definite routine in mind. After a time these procedures become automatic. The exact details of application are described here and are not repeated in succeeding sections.

Preparations

1. The conditions and indications are rechecked to be certain that the correct procedure is being carried out.
2. The patient is placed on the delivery table with the legs in stirrups and the buttocks a little past the lower end of the table (see Chapter 11, Fig. 3C).
3. The vulva, upper thighs, and lower abdomen are cleansed thoroughly.
4. If spinal or epidural anesthesia is to be used, it should have been administered by this time. If local anesthesia has been chosen, the injection is made. If general anesthesia is employed, it is administered at this point.

Orientation

Vaginal Examination

Vaginal examination (Fig. 1A) is made to diagnose accurately the position and station of the head, whether there is flexion or extension, and the presence of synclitism or asynclitism. Since this is a low forceps procedure for occipitoanterior position, the following conditions are present:

1. The presentation is cephalic.
2. The sagittal suture is in the anteroposterior diameter of the pelvis.
3. The occiput and posterior fontanelle are next to the pubis.
4. The face and bregma are in the hollow of the sacrum.
5. The station is +2 to +3.

Orientation and Desired Application

The locked forceps are positioned outside the vagina in front of the perineum in the way they are to be when applied to the fetal head in the pelvis (Fig. 1B and C). By this simple procedure the operator fixes in his mind exactly how and where each blade should fit. In the occipitoanterior position both a perfect cephalic and an ideal pelvic application are possible (Fig. 1).

1. With the cephalic application:
   a. The blades are over the parietal bones in an occipitomental application.
   b. The front of the forceps (concave edges) point to the denominator (occiput).
   c. The convex edges point to the face.
2. With the pelvic application:
   a. The left blade is next to the left sidewall of the pelvis and the right blade near the right sidewall.
   b. The concave edges point to the pubis.
   c. The convex edges point to the sacrum.
   d. The diameter of the forceps is in the transverse diameter of the pelvis.

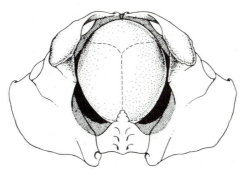

Figure 1A. Occiput anterior (OA).

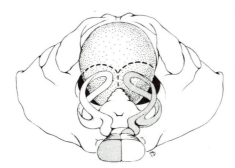

Figure 1B. Low forceps, Simpson. Orientation.

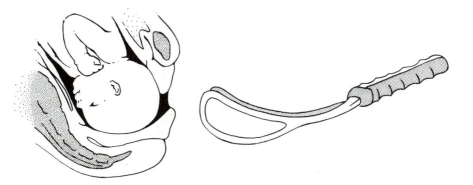

Figure 1C. Low forceps, Simpson. Orientation.

Application of Left Forceps

1. The left blade is inserted first. The handle is held by the thumb and the first two fingers of the left hand. At first the forceps is in an almost vertical position, with the handle near the mother's right groin (Fig. 2A).
2. The fingers of the right hand are placed in the vagina between the fetal head and the left vaginal wall.
3. The left blade is inserted gently into the vagina at about 5 o'clock, between the fingers and the fetal head.
4. The handle is lowered slowly to the horizontal and toward the midline; at the same time the blade is moved up by the vaginal fingers over the left side of the head, giving an occipitomental application. The blade lies between the left parietal bone and the left pelvic wall (Fig. 2B).
5. The fingers are removed and the handle is supported by an assistant, if one is available.

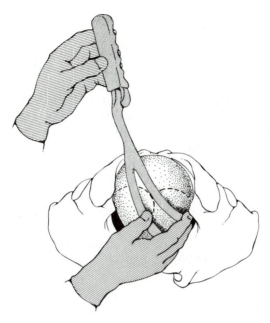

Figure 2A. Insertion of left blade between fetal head and left side of pelvis.

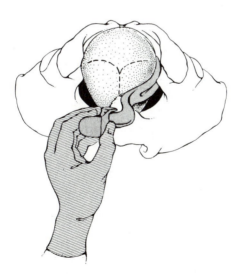

Figure 2B. Handle of left forceps is lowered and the blade moved up over the left parietal bone.

Application of Right Forceps

1. The right forceps is grasped in the right hand and is held in an almost vertical position, with the handle near the mother's left groin.
2. The fingers of the left hand are inserted in the right side of the vagina between the fetal head and the vaginal wall.
3. The right blade is inserted over the left forceps between the fingers and the fetal head, at about 7 o'clock (Fig. 2C).
4. The handle is lowered to the horizontal and toward the midline. At the same time the blade is moved by the vaginal fingers up over the right side of the head to the occipitomental position. The blade fits between the right parietal bone and the right pelvic wall (Fig. 2D).
5. The fingers on the left hand are removed from the vagina, and the forceps are ready for locking.

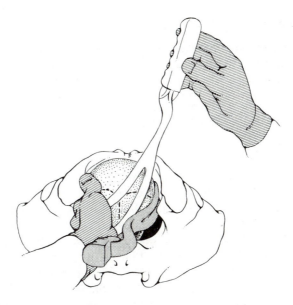

Figure 2C. Insertion of right blade between fetal head and right side of pelvis.

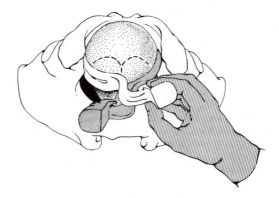

Figure 2D. Handle of right forceps is lowered, and the blade moved up over the right parietal bone.

Locking

When both blades have been applied correctly locking is easy. There should be no difficulty, and the handles must never be forced together (Fig. 3).

Extraction of the Head

Preextraction Reexamination

1. Auscultation of the fetal heart is performed.
2. Vaginal examination is made to be sure that there is nothing between the forceps and the fetal head. This includes umbilical cord, cervix, and membranes.
3. Vaginal examination is performed to check the application. The blades of the forceps must be over the sides of the fetal head in a biparietal application. The left blade should be next to the left side of the pelvis and the right blade on the right side. The concave edges of the forceps should be under the pubis and the convex edges near the sacrum. The diameter of the blades should be in the transverse diameter of the pelvis. Sometimes the blades may be a little off center, with one blade nearer the occiput and the other closer to the face. In such cases the forceps must be unlocked and the blades moved so that the application becomes symmetrical.

Trial Traction

A gentle pull on the forceps ought to bring about a small advancement of the head.

Indications for Complete Reassessment

1. When locking is difficult or impossible.
2. When trial traction fails to advance the head.
3. When vaginal examination reveals an incorrect application. The forceps should be removed and the whole situation reassessed. Reasons for the failure include:
   a. Wrong diagnosis of position.
   b. Incorrect application of forceps.
   c. Cephalopelvic disproportion.
   d. Cervix between the blades and the head.
   e. Uterine constriction ring.

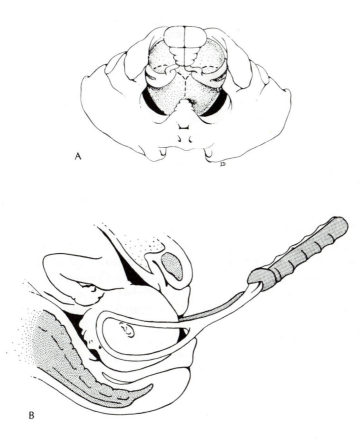

Figure 3. OA: Locking. A and B. Forceps locked in cephalic and pelvic application.

Extraction of the Head

1. The operator sits on a stool and grasps the forceps with both hands, one hand on the handles and the other on the shanks (see Chapter 24, Fig. 5A).
2. The traction must be intermittent, every 1 to 2 minutes and lasting 30 to 40 seconds.
3. Between periods of traction the forceps should be unlocked to relieve the compression of the baby's head. The fetal heart must be checked often.
4. If the patient is under general or spinal anesthesia the uterine contractions are of little help, and, since the patient cannot bear down, the baby is delivered by traction alone or by the assistant exerting pressure on the uterus. On the other hand, if the patient has been given a local or epidural anesthetic, traction should be made during the uterine contractions and with the patient bearing down. The combined effort makes the delivery easier.
5. The direction of traction must follow the birth canal. First the pull should be outward and posteriorly until the occiput comes under the symphysis of the pubis and the nape of the neck pivots in the subpubic angle (Fig. 4A). In performing the Pajot maneuver, the hand on the handles makes traction in an outward direction while the hand on the shanks pulls the head posteriorly.
6. Then the direction is changed to outward and anterior to promote extension of the head. This mimics the course of events in spontaneous birth (Fig. 4B).
7. In all primigravidas and in most multiparas an episiotomy should be made before the baby is extracted and the perineum overstretched.

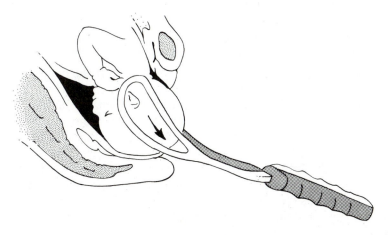

A. Traction is made outward and posteriorly until the nape of the neck is under the pubic symphysis.

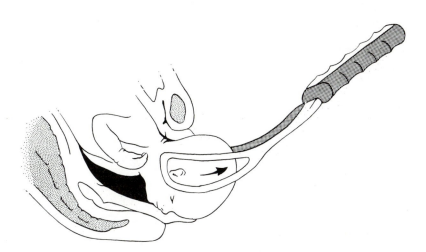

B. The direction of traction is changed to outward and anteriorly to promote extension of the head.

Figure 4. OA: Traction with forceps.

Birth of the Head and Removal of Forceps

Birth of the head and removal of the forceps can be accomplished in two ways:

1. Traction with the forceps is continued, and by a process of extension the forehead, face, and chin are born over the perineum. The forceps are now out of the vagina and slip off the head easily.
2. When the head is crowning, the forceps are removed by a process that is the reverse of their application. First the handle of the right blade is raised toward the mother's left groin and the blade slides around the head and out of the pelvis (Fig. 5A). Then the same is done with the left forceps by raising the handle toward the right groin (Fig. 5B). Once this has been accomplished the head is delivered by the modified Ritgen maneuver. Removing the forceps has the advantage of reducing the circumference of the part passing through the introitus by 0.50 to 0.75 cm.

Lacerations of the vagina, cervix, and uterus must be ruled out by careful examination after all forceps deliveries. If tears are found they are repaired.

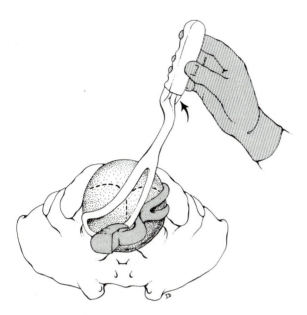

A. Removal of right forceps.

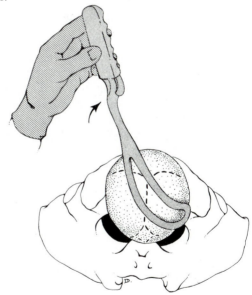

B. Removal of left forceps.

Figure 5. OA: Removal of forceps.

FORCEPS DELIVERY: LOA

Orientation

Vaginal Examination

1. The presentation is cephalic.
2. The sagittal suture is in the right oblique diameter of the pelvis.
3. The posterior fontanelle is in the left anterior quadrant of the pelvis (Fig. 6A).
4. The bregma is in the right posterior quadrant.
5. The station is 0 to +3 in most cases.

Orientation and Desired Application
The aim is for a perfect cephalic application (Fig. 6B).

1. The blades are over the parietal bones in an occipitomental application.
2. The concave edges point to the occiput.
3. The convex edges point to the face.

The pelvic application is not perfect.

1. The diameter of the forceps is in the left oblique diameter of the pelvis.
2. The left blade is in the left posterior quadrant.
3. The right blade is in the right anterior quadrant.
4. The concave edges point anteriorly and to the left.
5. The convex edges point posteriorly and to the right.
6. This can be a low to midforceps, depending on the exact station of the head.

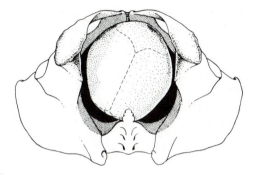

Figure 6A. Left occiput anterior (LOA).

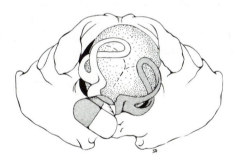

Figure 6B. Low forceps, Simpson. Orientation.

Application of Forceps

1. The left forceps is inserted into the vagina at 5 o'clock so that it lies over the left parietal bone in an occipitomental application and in the left posterolateral quadrant of the pelvis (Fig. 7A).
2. The right blade is inserted into the vagina at 7 o'clock (Fig. 7B).
3. It is then moved anteriorly around the fetal head so that it lies over the right parietal bone in an occipitomental application, and in the right anterior quadrant of the pelvis.
4. The forceps are now locked, and vaginal examination is made to be sure that the application is correct. If not, the forceps are unlocked and the necessary adjustments made (Fig. 7C).
5. The cephalic application is ideal; the pelvic application is not, for the diameter of the blades is in the oblique diameter of the pelvis.

Rotation and Extraction

1. Traction is made in an outward and posterior direction until the occiput comes under the symphysis and the nape of the neck pivots in the subpubic angle.
2. In many cases as traction is being made the head rotates spontaneously from the LOA to the OA position. If this does not occur the operator must rotate the occiput 45° to the anterior at the same time that he is exerting traction (Fig. 7D).
3. Once the nape of the neck pivots in the subpubic angle, the direction is changed from outward and posterior to outward and anterior so that the head is born over the perineum by extension (see Fig. 4B).

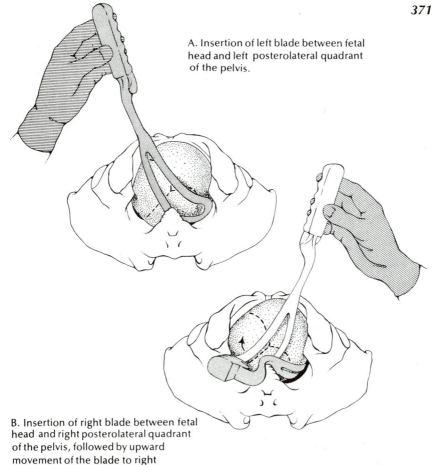

A. Insertion of left blade between fetal head and left posterolateral quadrant of the pelvis.

B. Insertion of right blade between fetal head and right posterolateral quadrant of the pelvis, followed by upward movement of the blade to right anterolateral quadrant of the pelvis.

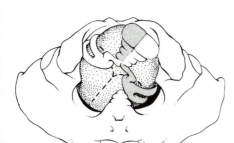

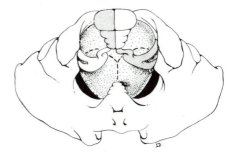

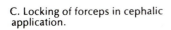

C. Locking of forceps in cephalic application.

D. Head is rotated from LOA to OA. It is now ready for extraction.

Figure 7. LOA: application of forceps.

26

Arrested Transverse Positions of the Occiput

Transverse arrest high in the pelvis is managed best by cesarean section. However, when the head is low and there is no disproportion, vaginal delivery by forceps is preferable. This can be accomplished in two ways: (1) application of forceps in the LOT position, rotation with forceps to OA, followed by extraction—always a midforceps operation; or (2) manual rotation of the head 90° to the occipitoanterior position, LOT to LOA to OA. The head is then extracted with forceps as an occiput anterior. Sometimes the rotation can be carried out only 45°, LOT to LOA. The forceps are applied to the LOA, and rotation and extraction are completed.

FORCEPS ROTATION AND EXTRACTION: LOT

Orientation

Vaginal Examination

1. The presentation is cephalic.
2. The sagittal suture is in the transverse diameter of the pelvis.
3. The posterior fontanelle and occiput are on the left side at 3 o'clock: LOT (Fig. 1A).
4. The bregma and face are on the right side at 9 o'clock.
5. This situation is associated frequently with the military attitude, so the bregma and the posterior fontanelle may be at almost the same level in the pelvis (neither flexion nor extension).
6. The baby's right ear is next to the bladder, and the left one near the rectum.
7. Asynclitism is common, and the sagittal suture may be nearer the pubis (posterior asynclitism) or closer to the sacral promontory (anterior asynclitism).
8. The station in the majority of cases is +1 or +2.
9. Molding and caput succedaneum may obscure the landmarks.

Orientation and Desired Application

1. The aim is for an ideal cephalic application (Figs. 1B and C, 2E).
   a. The front of the forceps (the concave edges) is pointing toward the denominator (the occiput).
   b. The blades are over the parietal bones in an occipitomental application.
2. The pelvic application is not ideal.
   a. The diameter of the blades is in the anteroposterior diameter of the pelvis (instead of the transverse).
   b. The anterior (right) blade is between the pubis and the fetal head (instead of being next to the pelvic side wall).
   c. The posterior (left) blade is between the sacrum and head.
   d. The concave edges of the blades point to the left side of the pelvis.
   e. The convex edges point to the right side.

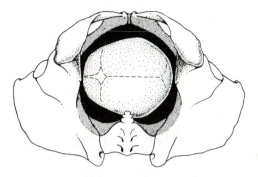

Figure 1A. Left occiput transverse.

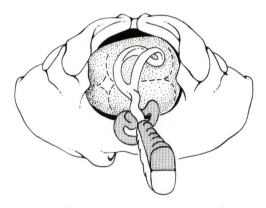

Figure 1B. Midforceps, Simpson. Orientation.

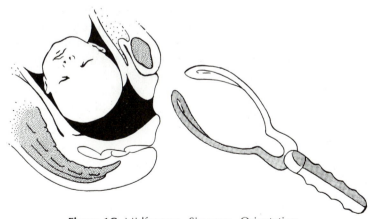

Figure 1C. Midforceps, Simpson. Orientation.

Application of Forceps

We apply the anterior blade first, for two reasons: (1) Any difficulty in application is with the anterior blade. Hence there is no point in placing the posterior blade into the vagina until we are certain that the anterior one can be put in place correctly. (2) The posterior blade occupies space and, if put in first, gets in the way and makes application of the anterior forceps more difficult.

The anterior blade (for LOT it is the right) is inserted into the vagina between the posterior parietal bone (left) and the sacrum (Fig. 2A). The next step is to make the forceps wander around the fetal head into position between the anterior parietal bone (right) and the pubis (Figs. 2B and C). This is accomplished by manipulating the blade with the fingers in the vagina, and the handle with the other hand. There are two ways in which this maneuver can be accomplished:

1. The blade can be moved over the baby's face. With the left hand in the vagina manipulating the blade and the right hand on the handle, the blade is moved over the baby's face into position between the anterior parietal bone and the pubis. The advantage of this method is that the smaller face offers less resistance than the bulky occiput and there is less danger of damaging the maternal tissues. The disadvantage is that should the head move with the forceps the occiput rotates posteriorly.
2. The blade can be moved around the occiput. The right hand is placed in the vagina to manipulate the blade, and the left hand is on the handle. The blade is moved gently around the occiput and into position between the anterior parietal bone and the pubis. The advantage of this method is that should the head turn with the forceps, the occiput moves anteriorly, a desirable effect. The drawback is that the bulkiness and hardness of the occiput makes less room for the blade, and there is greater danger of maternal lacerations than when the blade is wandered around the face.

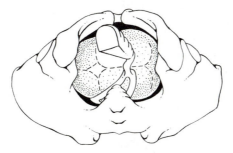

A. Insertion of anterior (right) blade between posterior parietal bone and sacrum.

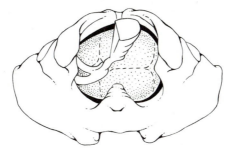

B. The blade is wandered anteriorly so that it lies between the face and the pelvic wall.

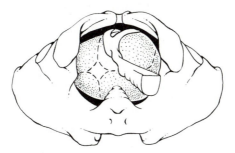

C. The blade is wandered further until it lies between the anterior parietal bone and the pubis.

Figure 2. Forceps application and rotation: LOT to OA.

The posterior blade (for LOT it is the left) is inserted into the vagina between the posterior parietal bone (left) and the sacrum (Fig. 2D). The forceps are locked, and the application is checked to be certain that a good biparietal application has been achieved (Fig. 2E).

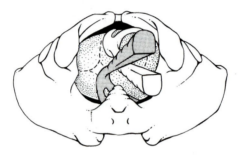

D. The posterior (left) blade is inserted between the posterior parietal bone and the sacrum.

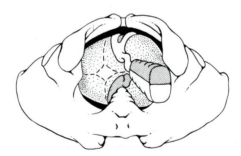

E. LOT: The forceps are locked in a cephalic application.

Figure 2. (cont.) Forceps application and rotation: LOT to OA.

Rotation and Extraction

With the handles making a wide arc the head is rotated 90° to the anterior, LOT to LOA to OA (Fig. 3). Now the occiput is under the pubis, the face is next to the sacrum, and the sagittal suture is in the anteroposterior diameter of the pelvis. The ideal cephalic application has been maintained. The pelvic application is also good, since the diameter of the forceps is in the transverse diameter of the pelvis, the concave edges point to the pubis, the convex edges lie in the hollow of the sacrum, and the sides of the blades lie next to the side walls of the pelvis.

The head is extracted as an occipitoanterior. Traction is outward and posterior until the occiput comes under the pubis and the nape of the neck pivots in the subpubic angle. The direction is then changed to outward and anterior, so that by extension the forehead, face, and chin are born over the perineum.

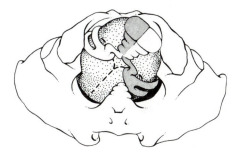

A. LOT to LOA (45°).

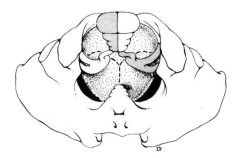

B. LOA to OA (45°). The head is ready for extraction.

Figure 3. Anterior rotation.

MANUAL ROTATION AND FORCEPS EXTRACTION: LOT

1. With the patient in the lithotomy position, the operator stands facing the perineum and inserts the right hand into the vagina. The fetal head is grasped with the four fingers over the posterior parietal (left) bone and the thumb over the anterior parietal (right) bone (Fig. 4A).
2. By pronating the arm, the operator turns the fetal head 90° to the anterior, LOT to LOA to OA (Fig. 4B).
3. Forceps are then applied in the OA position, and the head is extracted as an occiput anterior.
4. ROT is managed in the same way, except that the left hand is used and the rotation is ROT to ROA to OA.

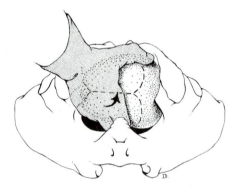

A. Grasping the head with the right hand.

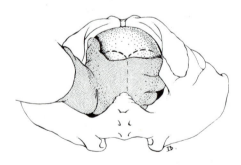

B. LOT to OA (90°).

Figure 4. Manual rotation: LOT to OA.

27

Arrested Posterior Positions of the Occiput

Persistent occipitoposterior arrest high in the pelvis is managed best by cesarean section. However, when the head is low and there is no disproportion, vaginal delivery with forceps should be carried out. There are several techniques for accomplishing this safely.

FORCEPS DELIVERY FACE TO PUBIS: OCCIPUT POSTERIOR

Occasionally the head seems to fit the pelvis better with the occiput posterior. This is so, for example, in some anthropoid pelves. When this is the case and especially when the vertex is at or near the perineum, it is wiser to follow nature's lead and deliver the head to pubis.

Orientation

Vaginal Examination

1. The presentation is cephalic (Fig. 1A).
2. The sagittal suture is in the anteroposterior diameter of the pelvis.
3. The posterior fontanelle and occiput are in the hollow of the sacrum.
4. The bregma and face are anterior, under the pubis.
5. The station is +1 to +3.

Orientation and Desired Application

1. The cephalic application is not perfect but is satisfactory (Figs. 1B and C).
   a. The blades are over the parietal bones in an occipitomental application. The left blade is on the right parietal bone, and the right blade is on the left parietal bone.
   b. The front of the forceps (concave edges) point to the face. In an ideal cephalic application they point to the occiput.
   c. The convex edges point to the occiput. In the ideal application they point to the face.
2. The pelvic application is perfect.
   a. The diameter of the forceps is in the transverse diameter of the pelvis.
   b. The sides of the blades are next to the sidewalls of the pelvis, the left blade near the left side and right blade near the right side.
   c. The concave edges point to the pubis.
   d. The convex edges point to the sacrum.
   e. This may be low to midforceps, depending on the exact station of the head.

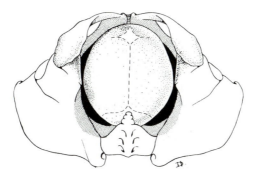

Figure 1A. Occiput posterior.

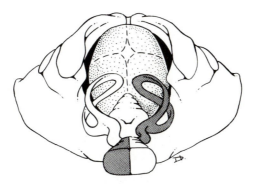

Figure 1B. Simpson forceps. Orientation.

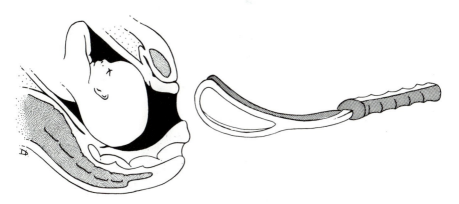

Figure 1C. Simpson forceps. Orientation.

Application of Forceps

1. The left blade is inserted gently into the vagina at about 5 o'clock (Fig. 2A).
2. It is then moved anteriorly so that it lies between the right parietal bone and the left side of the pelvis (Fig. 2B).
3. The right blade is inserted (over the left) into the vagina at about 7 o'clock (Fig. 2B).
4. It is then moved anteriorly so that it fits between the left parietal bone of the fetal head and the right side of the pelvis.
5. The forceps are locked, and vaginal examination is made to be certain that the application is correct and that there are no obstacles to extraction. The application is biparietal. The concave edges of the blades point to the pubis and the fetal face, while the convex edges point to the sacrum and the occiput (Figs. 2C and D).

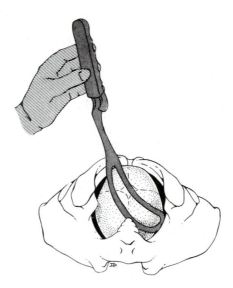

A. Insertion of left blade between fetal head and left side of pelvis.

Figure 2. OP: application of forceps.

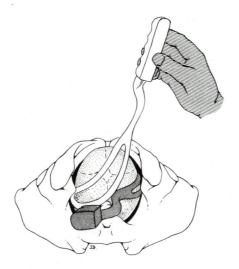

B. Handle of left blade is lowered and the blade moved up over the right parietal bone. Insertion of right blade between fetal head and right side of pelvis.

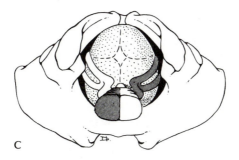

C

C and D. Forceps locked in biparietal application.

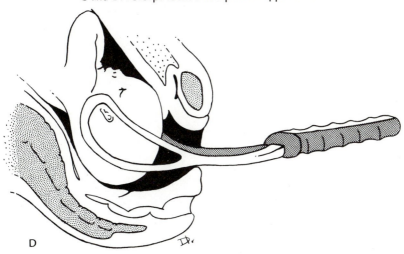

D

Figure 2. (cont.) OP: application of forceps.

Extraction of the Head

1. Traction is made outward and posteriorly until the area between the bregma and the nasion lies under the pubic arch (Fig. 3A).
2. Delivery is by one of two methods:
   a. The direction is changed to outward and anterior (Fig. 3B); as the handles of the forceps are raised, the occiput is born over the perineum by flexion. The forceps then slip off the head.
   b. The direction is changed to outward and anterior until the occiput is on the perineum. The forceps are removed by raising first the right handle toward the left groin so that the blade slips around the head and out of the vagina. Then the left handle is raised toward the right groin so that the left blade slides out. By a modified Ritgen maneuver flexion is increased until the occiput has cleared the perineum completely.
3. The head then falls back in extension; and the nose, face, and chin are delivered under the pubis.
4. If the head cannot be delivered as a posterior presentation without using an excessive amount of force, this method of delivery should be abandoned and an anterior rotation of the occiput carried out.
5. Since the diameter distending the perineum (biparietal, 9.5 cm) is larger than in anterior positions (bitemporal, 8.0 cm), lacerations are more extensive and an adequate episiotomy should be made.

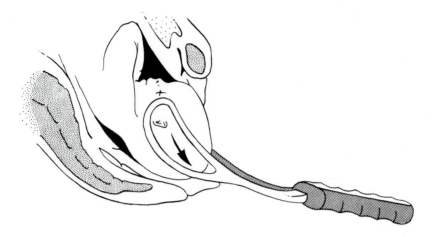

A. Traction is made outward and posteriorly until the area between the bregma and nasion lies under the pubic arch.

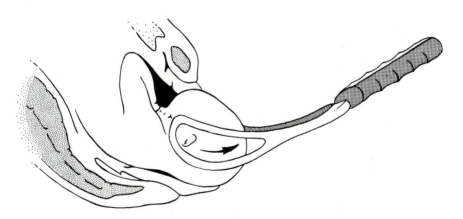

B. Traction is made outward and anteriorly to promote flexion.

Figure 3. Extraction face to pubis, OP.

FORCEPS ROTATION: ROP TO OP AND EXTRACTION FACE TO PUBIS

Orientation

Vaginal Examination

1. The presentation is cephalic.
2. The sagittal suture is in the right oblique diameter of the pelvis.
3. The posterior fontanelle is in the right posterior quadrant of the pelvis (Figs. 4A and 5C).
4. The bregma is in the left anterior quadrant.
5. The station is usually 0 to +2.

Orientation and Desired Application

1. The cephalic application is not perfect but is satisfactory (Fig. 4B).
   a. The blades are over the parietal bones in an occipitomental application. The left blade is on the right parietal bone, and the right blade is on the left parietal bone.
   b. The front of the forceps (concave edges) point to the face. In an ideal cephalic application they point to the occiput.
   c. The convex edges point to the occiput. In the ideal application they point to the face.
2. The pelvic application is oblique.
   a. The diameter of the blades is in the left oblique diameter of the pelvis.
   b. The left blade is in the left posterior quadrant of the pelvis.
   c. The right blade is in the right anterior quadrant.
   d. The concave edges point anteriorly and to the left.
   e. The convex edges are posterior and to the right.

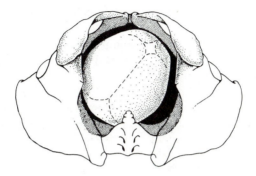

Figure 4A. Right occiput posterior (ROP).

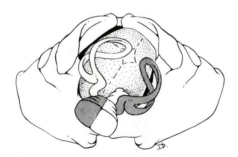

Figure 4B. Midforceps, Simpson. Orientation.

Application of Forceps

1. The left blade is inserted gently into the vagina at about 5 o'clock, so that it lies between the right parietal bone and the left posterolateral wall of the pelvis (Fig. 5A).
2. The right blade is inserted over the left into the vagina at about 7 o'clock (Fig. 5B).
3. It is then moved anteriorly about 90° around the fetal head so that it fits between the left parietal bone and the right anterolateral wall of the pelvis.
4. The forceps are locked, and vaginal examination is performed to make sure that the application is correct. If it is not, the forceps are unlocked and the necessary adjustments made (Fig. 5C).

Rotation and Extraction

1. The head is rotated 45° from ROP to OP, so that the occiput is in the hollow of the sacrum and the face under the pubis (Fig. 5D).
2. Traction is made outward and posteriorly until the area between the bregma and the nasion lies under the pubic arch.
3. The direction is then changed to outward and anterior, and as the handles of the forceps are raised the occiput is born over the perineum by flexion. The forceps are then removed.
4. Details of the technique for extracting the head are included in the previous section dealing with face to pubis delivery.

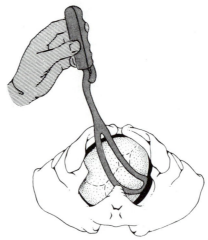

A. Insertion of left blade between fetal head and left posterolateral quadrant of pelvis.

Figure 5. ROP: forceps rotation to OP.

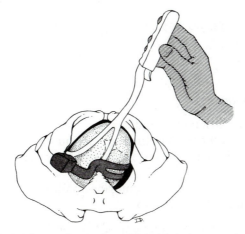

B. Handle of left blade is lowered. Insertion of right blade between fetal head and right posterolateral quadrant of pelvis, followed by upward movement of the blade to right anterolateral quadrant of pelvis.

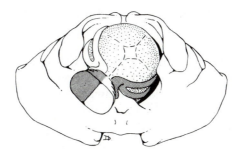

C. Locking of forceps in biparietal application.

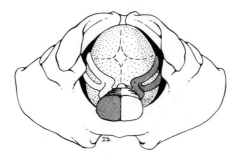

D. Posterior rotation ROP to OP (45°).

Figure 5. (cont.) ROP: forceps rotation to OP.

MANUAL ROTATION TO THE ANTERIOR

Orientation

Vaginal Examination

1. The presentation is cephalic.
2. The sagittal suture is in the right oblique diameter of the pelvis.
3. The posterior fontanelle is in the right posterior quadrant of the pelvis (Fig. 6A).
4. The bregma is in the left anterior quadrant.
5. The station is usually 0 to +2.

Rotation is accomplished by one of two methods: (1) manual rotation of the head and shoulders (the Pomeroy maneuver); or (2) manual rotation of the head.

Pomeroy Maneuver: ROP

1. The operator places his left hand into the posterior part of the vagina between the head and the sacrum and past the fetal head into the uterus, so that the fingertips grasp the anterior shoulder and the head lies in the palm of the hand (Fig. 6B).
2. By pressure upward on the anterior shoulder (as the hand is pronated), the body and head are turned anteriorly (Fig. 6C).

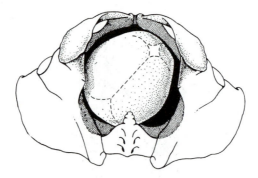

A. Right occiput posterior.

Figure 6. ROP: Pomeroy maneuver.

The advantage of this maneuver is that since the body has been rotated, the head does not slip back to its original position. To ensure against this happening the head may be overrotated, ROP to LOA.

The disadvantage is that the head must be dislodged to the point of disengagement so that the hand can reach the shoulder. There is danger that the umbilical cord may prolapse or that the head may be extended and may not reengage properly.

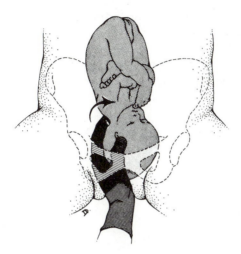

B. Fingers of the left hand are placed behind the anterior shoulder.

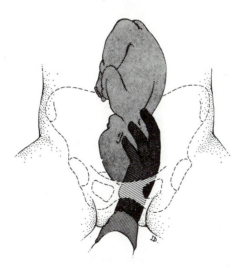

C. Anterior rotation of the shoulders and head, ROP to LOA.

Figure 6. (cont.) ROP: Pomeroy maneuver.

Manual Rotation of Occiput to Anterior: ROP

1. After the patient is anesthetized the operator inserts the left hand in the vagina and grasps the fetal head, placing the thumb on the anterior parietal (left) bone and the fingers on the posterior parietal (right) bone. The left hand is better for ROP and the right for LOP (Figs. 7A and B).
2. First the head is flexed.
3. Then the head is rotated anteriorly to the occiput anterior position by pronating the hand in the vagina: ROP to ROT to ROA to OA (Figs. 7C through E).
4. At the same time the operator turns the body in the identical direction by applying pressure with his other hand on the shoulders or breech through the maternal abdomen.

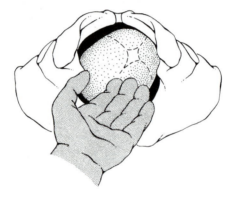

A. Orientation, left hand.

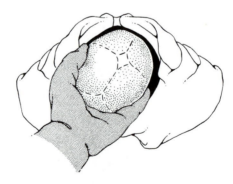

B. Left hand grasps the head; the thumb is on the anterior parietal (left) bone, and the fingers are on the posterior parietal (right) bone.

Figure 7. ROP: manual rotation to OA.

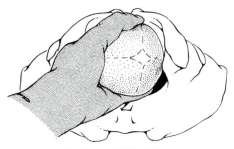

C. ROP to ROT (45°).

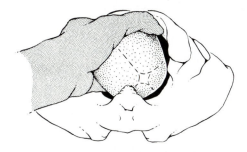

D. Manual rotation using left hand: ROT to ROA (45°).

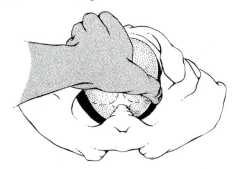

E. Manual rotation using left hand: ROA to OA (45°). Head ready for extraction.

Figure 7. (cont.) ROP: manual rotation to OA.

This method is safe for the baby and for the mother. However, when the fit between baby and pelvis is snug or when the head is impacted, it is difficult to obtain a good grasp of the head and manual rotation may be impossible. Furthermore, the shoulders do not always rotate with the head, and sometimes when the head is released by the operator's hand it returns to the original posterior position. Despite these disadvantages manual rotation is so safe and so free from vaginal tears that it should be tried before resorting to more complicated methods.

Sometimes complete rotation to the OA position is not possible. In such cases forceps are applied to the head in the new position (ROT or ROA), rotation to OA is achieved with the forceps, and the head is extracted.

Delivery

Once manual rotation of the head to the occipitoanterior has been accomplished, two methods of delivery are available: Originally the patient was permitted to awaken from the anesthetic and the onset of labor was awaited, the hope being that spontaneous delivery would take place. Today we believe that, once the indications for interference are present, the baby should be born without delay. Hence manual rotation is followed by extraction with forceps in the new position.

DOUBLE APPLICATION OF FORCEPS: ROP (MODIFIED SCANZONI MANEUVER)

A double application of forceps for the treatment of occipitoposterior positions was performed by Smellie during the eighteenth century. In 1830 Scanzoni revived, improved, and popularized the maneuver, which has since been associated with his name. Bill further modified the operation, and his technique is the one that we use today.

Orientation

Vaginal Examination

1. The presentation is cephalic.
2. The sagittal suture is in the right oblique diameter of the pelvis.
3. The posterior fontanelle is in the right posterior quadrant of the pelvis (Fig. 8A).
4. The bregma is in the left anterior quadrant.
5. The station is usually 0 to +2.

Orientation and Desired Application

1. The cephalic application is not perfect but is satisfactory.
   a. The blades are over the parietal bones in the occipitomental application. The left blade is on the right parietal bone, and the right blade is on the left parietal bone (Figs. 8B and 9C).
   b. The front of the forceps (concave edges) point to the face. In an ideal cephalic application they point to the occiput.
   c. The convex edges point to the occiput. In the ideal application they point to the face.
2. The pelvic application is oblique.
   a. The diameter of the blades is in the left oblique diameter of the pelvis.
   b. The left blade is in the left posterior quadrant of the pelvis.
   c. The right blade is in the right anterior quadrant.
   d. The concave edges point anteriorly and to the left.
   e. The convex edges are posterior and to the right.

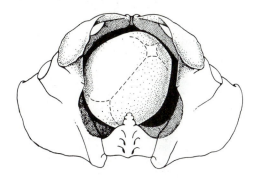

A. ROP orientation.

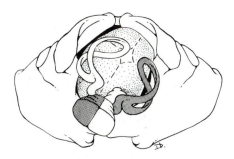

B. Midforceps, Simpson. Orientation.

Figure 8. Scanzoni maneuver.

Application of Forceps

1. The left blade is inserted gently into the vagina at about 5 o'clock, so that it lies between the right parietal bone and the left posterolateral wall of the pelvis (Fig. 9A).
2. The right blade is inserted into the vagina at about 7 o'clock (Fig. 9B).
3. It is then moved anteriorly about 90° around the fetal head so that it fits between the left parietal bone and the right anterolateral wall of the pelvis.
4. The forceps are now locked, and vaginal examination is performed to make sure that the application is correct. If it is not, the forceps are unlocked and the necessary adjustments made (Fig. 9C).

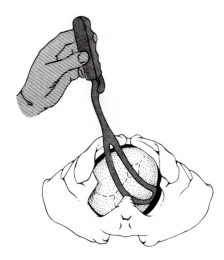

A. Insertion of left blade between fetal head and left posterolateral quadrant of pelvis.

Figure 9. Scanzoni maneuver: application of forceps: ROP.

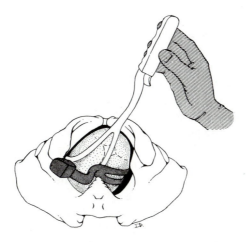

B. Handle of left blade is lowered. Insertion of right blade between fetal head and right posterolateral quadrant of pelvis, followed by upward movement of blade to right anterolateral quadrant of pelvis.

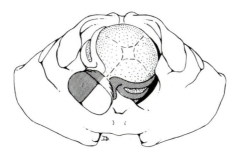

C. Locking of forceps in biparietal application.

Figure 9. (cont.) Scanzoni maneuver: application of forceps: ROP.

Rotation: ROP to OA

1. After the forceps are locked the handles are raised toward the opposite groin, in ROP toward the left groin. This maneuver favors flexion of the head (Fig. 10A).

2. Without traction the handles are carried around in a large circle so that they point first to the left groin (ROP), next toward the left thigh (ROT; Fig. 10B), then toward the left ischial tuberosity (ROA; Fig. 10C), and finally toward the anus and floor (OA; Fig. 10D). With the wide sweep of the handles the blades turn in a small arc and do not deviate from the same axis during the process of rotation. The fetal head turns with the use of very little force on the part of the operator.

3. The rotation is continued until the occiput lies under the symphysis pubis and the sagittal suture is in the anteroposterior diameter of the pelvis. The extent of the rotation is 135°, and the sequence is ROP to ROT to ROA to OA. The relationship of the forceps to the fetal head has not changed, but now the concave edges of the blades are posterior and the convex edges are anterior. The forceps are upside down, and the pelvic curve of the blades is the reverse of the curve of the maternal pelvis. This situation is not suitable for extracting the head, and adjustments are necessary.

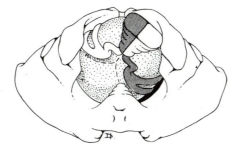

A. ROP: head is flexed by raising the handles of the forceps.

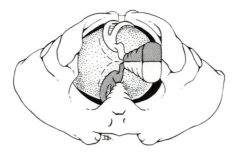

B. Anterior rotation by forceps: ROP to ROT (45°).

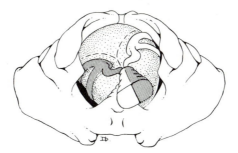

C. ROT to ROA (45°).

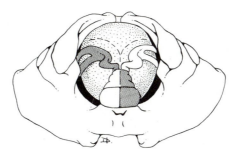

D. ROA to OA (45°).

Figure 10. Scanzoni maneuver. Anterior rotation.

Removal of Forceps

1. Before removing the forceps a small amount of traction is made, not with the idea of delivering the head but simply to fix it in its new position.
2. The forceps are unlocked.
3. The right forceps is removed first by depressing the handle further so that the blade slides around the head and out of the vagina (Fig. 11A).
4. Then the left forceps is removed in the same way (Fig. 11B).

A vaginal examination is performed in the new OA position (Fig. 11C).

1. The sagittal suture is in the anteroposterior diameter of the pelvis.
2. The occiput is under the pubis.
3. The face is near the sacrum.

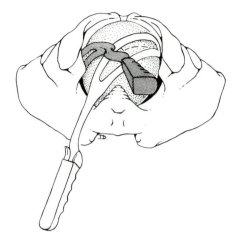

A. Removal of right blade.

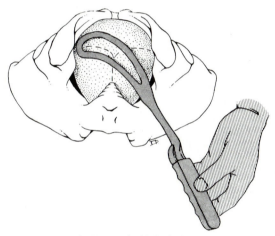

B. Removal of left blade.

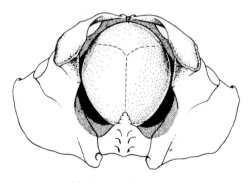

C. New position: OA

Figure 11. Scanzoni maneuver. Removal of forceps.

Reapplication of Forceps

1. The left blade is inserted between the fetal head and the left posterolateral quadrant of the pelvis (Fig. 12A).
2. The handle is lowered to the horizontal and the blade moved
   over the left parietal bone.
3. The right blade is inserted between the fetal head and the right
   posterolateral quadrant of the pelvis (Fig. 12B).
4. The handle is lowered to the horizontal and the blade moved
   over the right parietal bone.
5. The forceps are locked in a biparietal cephalic and pelvic application (Fig. 12C).
6. Then the head is extracted in the usual way.

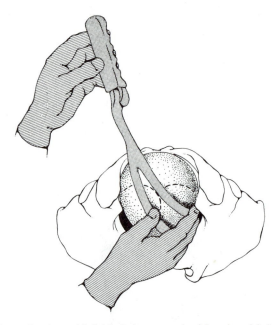

Figure 12A. Reapplication of left blade between fetal head and left side of pelvis.

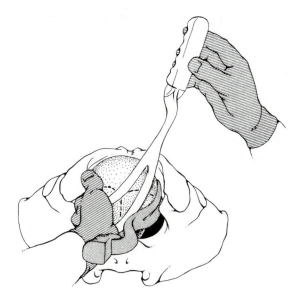

Figure 12B. Reapplication of right blade between fetal head and right side of pelvis.

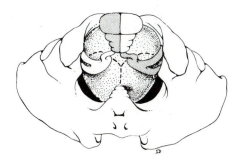

Figure 12C. Locking of forceps in biparietal cephalic and pelvic application.

Alternate Method of Removing and Reapplying Forceps Using Two Sets

At the end of the rotation, the head is in the OA position and the forceps are upside down (Fig. 13A). Occasionally the shoulders do not rotate with the head and there is a tendency for the head to turn back to the ROP position once the forceps are removed. This can be prevented by employing two sets of forceps in the following way:

1. The right blade (upside down) is removed from the left side of the pelvis (Fig. 13B). An assistant holds the original left blade in place preventing the head from turning back.
2. The left blade from the new set is then inserted right side up into the left side of the maternal pelvis in the usual manner (Fig. 13C).

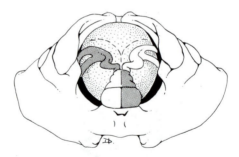

A. New position: OA. Forceps upside down.

Figure 13. Two-forceps maneuver.

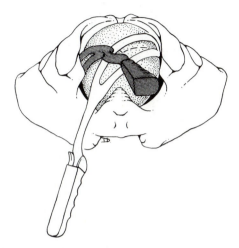

B. Removal of right Simpson forceps from left side of pelvis.

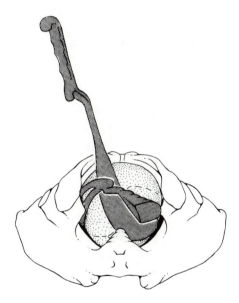

C. Insertion of left Tucker-McLane forceps between fetal head and left side of pelvis. The left Simpson is still in place.

Figure 13. (cont.) Two-forceps maneuver.

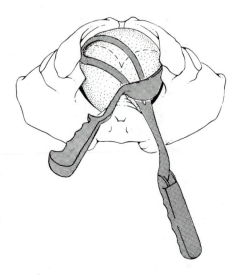

D. Removal of left Simpson forceps from right side of pelvis.

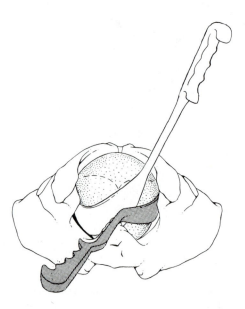

E. Insertion of right Tucker-McLane forceps between fetal head and right side of pelvis.

Figure 13. (cont.) Two-forceps maneuver.

3. The left upside down blade is removed from the right side of the pelvis (Fig. 13D). The head is prevented from turning back by the new left blade, which is held by an assistant.
4. The right blade of the new set is now inserted into the vagina (Fig. 13E).
5. The forceps are now in a correct application and are locked (Fig.13F).
6. Extraction is carried out in the usual way.

The risk of extensive vaginal lacerations, claimed by some authors to be inherent in the Scanzoni maneuver because of the long forceps rotation, has been exaggerated greatly. As long as the operation is performed gently and slowly a minimal amount of damage occurs. Many of the extensive vaginal tears and vesical and rectal fistulas occurred in cases of definite disproportion, where vaginal delivery should never have been carried out.

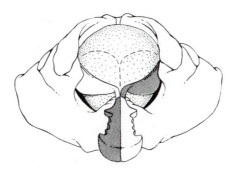

F. Locking of Tucker-McLane forceps in biparietal cephalic and pelvic application.

Figure 13. (cont.) Two-forceps maneuver.

As the following translation of Scanzoni's article reveals, Scanzoni described the rotation of the head only as far as the ROT or ROA position.

> The head stands with the forehead turned toward the front and left so that the sagittal suture passes in the right oblique diameter; the left blade is applied in front of the left sacroiliac synchondrosis, the right behind the right obturator foramen: with this the transverse diameter of the forceps is placed in the left oblique diameter of the pelvis, their concave edges and tips are turned to the anterior circumference of the left lateral hemisphere of the pelvis, and so also with the forehead. An eighth of a circle is now described with the instrument, directed from left to right, whereby the right blade comes to rest under the symphysis and the left in the hollow of the sacrum; and in this way the head is rotated, the earlier standing forehead is moved to the middle of the left lateral wall of the pelvis, and the sagittal suture is placed parallel with the transverse diameter of the pelvis.
>
> Now both blades of the forceps are removed and again applied, so that the left blade comes to lie behind the left obturator foramen, the right in the front of the right sacroiliac ligament, whereupon by the next rotation the occiput is brought completely under the pubic arch.

MAUGHAN MANEUVER: ROP

1. The left forceps blade is placed upside down in the right posterolateral part of the vagina so that it lies over the occiput. The concave side of the blade points posteriorly and the convex side anteriorly (Fig. 14A).
2. The blade is wandered anteriorly so that it sweeps by the occiput, catches the anterior fetal ear, and rotates the ear to a position directly behind the symphysis pubis. The sequence is ROP to ROT (45°). The sagittal suture is now in the transverse diameter of the pelvis (Fig. 14B).
3. The second blade is inserted between the fetal head and the sacrum so that it lies over the posterior ear (Fig. 14C).
4. The forceps are then locked, each blade resting over an ear.
5. The head is rotated slowly 90° so that the occiput is placed behind the symphysis. The sequence is ROT to ROA to OA.
6. The head is then extracted as an occipitoanterior.

This maneuver for rotation of the fetal head is primarily one of a single-forceps blade application, applied upside down to the opposite side of the maternal pelvis (i.e., in right occipitoposterior, the left blade to the right side of the pelvis) in such fashion that, on anterior sliding

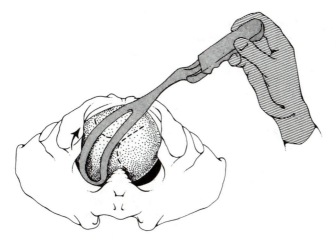

A. ROP. Left forceps blade inserted upside down over the occiput.

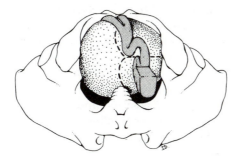

B. Forceps blade moved anteriorly under the pubis; head rotates ROP to ROT.

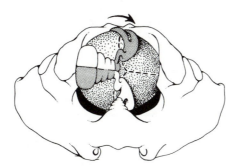

C. Posterior blade inserted between parietal bone and sacrum. Forceps locked in biparietal cephalic application. Arrow shows direction of further rotation ROT to OA.

Figure 14. Maughan maneuver.

movement, it sweeps over the occiput and, catching on the anterior fetal ear, rotates it to a position directly behind the symphysis pubis. The movement of this blade into place is therefore completely in the direction that rotation of the fetal head is intended, without upward displacement of the head.

KEY IN LOCK MANEUVER OF DeLEE

This is a multiple application method. The forceps are applied in the transverse diameter of the pelvis so that each blade lies next to the corresponding side of the maternal pelvis. Since application to the fetal skull is often not ideal, this operation must be performed delicately, with the least possible compression being applied to the baby. The head is pushed up a short distance in the axis of the birth canal and rotated gently, so that the small fontanelle is brought anteriorly about 5°. This is accomplished by sweeping the handles of the forceps through an arc of 10° outside the pelvis. The head is then pulled down in the pelvis, a little less than it was pushed up, to fix it in its new position. The forceps are loosened and returned to the transverse diameter of the pelvis, but the head is maintained in its new position. The head is then pushed up and rotated another 5°. These small rotations are continued until eventually the head is in the anterior position and the front (concave side) of the forceps points properly to the symphysis pubis and also to the fetal occiput. The head is then extracted in the usual way.

28

Arrested Face Presentations

FORCEPS EXTRACTION: MENTUM ANTERIOR

Orientation

Vaginal Examination

1. The presentation is cephalic (Fig. 1A).
2. The long axis of the face is in the anteroposterior diameter of the pelvis.
3. The chin is under the pubic symphysis.
4. The forehead is toward the sacrum.

Orientation and Desired Application

1. The aim is for a biparietal cephalic application (Figs. 1B and 2A).
   a. The front of the forceps (concave edges) points toward the denominator (the chin).
   b. The blades are over the parietal bones in a mentooccipital (reverse occipitomental) application.
2. The pelvic application is correct.
   a. The diameter of the blades is in the transverse diameter of the pelvis.
   b. The sides of the blades are next to the corresponding side walls of the pelvis.
   c. The concave edges point to the pubis.
   d. The convex edges are in the hollow of the sacrum.

Application of Forceps

1. The left blade is inserted into the vagina at about 5 o'clock and is moved around the face slightly until it lies between the right cheek and the left wall of the pelvis.
2. The right blade is inserted into the vagina at about 7 o'clock and is moved around the face until it lies between the left cheek and the right wall of the pelvis.
3. The forceps are locked, and vaginal examination is made to be sure that the application is correct and that no adjustment is necessary (Fig. 2A).

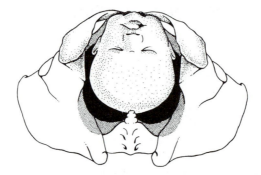

Figure 1A. Face presentation: mentum anterior.

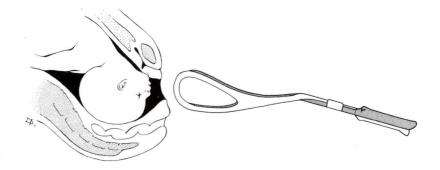

Figure 1B. Face presentation: Kjelland forceps.

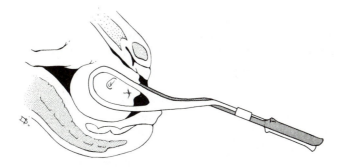

A. Locking of forceps. Beginning traction in the axis of the birth canal.

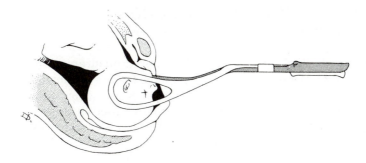

B. Horizontal traction.

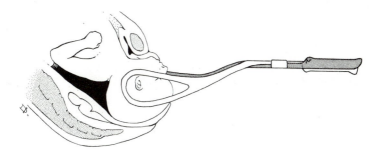

C. Delivery by flexion of the head.

Figure 2. Mentum anterior.

Extraction of the Head

1. The handles of the forceps are depressed toward the floor to deflex the head completely.
2. Traction is made in an outward, horizontal, and slightly posterior direction until the chin appears under the symphysis pubis and the submental region of the neck impinges in the subpubic angle (Fig. 2B).
3. With further descent the face and forehead appear, and the direction of traction is changed to outward and anterior. This brings about both descent and flexion, and the vertex and occiput are born over the perineum (Fig. 2C).
4. Since a large diameter is being born over the perineum, an episiotomy is advisable.

FORCEPS ROTATION AND EXTRACTION: MENTUM POSTERIOR

Because the bulk of the head is in the anterior quadrant of the pelvis, the usual application is not practical and the forceps are applied upside down. Because of their small pelvic curve the Kjelland forceps are valuable for this operation, but any forceps can be used. It must be noted that this operation may be difficult to carry out, and in modern times cesarean section is preferred in most cases.

Orientation

Vaginal Examination

1. The long axis of the face is in the anteroposterior diameter of the pelvis (Fig. 3).
2. The chin is in the hollow of the sacrum.
3. The forehead is under the pubic symphysis.

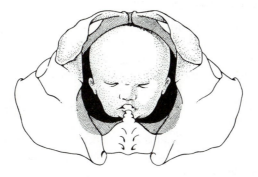

Figure 3. Mentum posterior (MP). Face presentation.

Orientation and Desired Application

1. The cephalic application is biparietal.
   a. The front of the forceps (concave edges) points to the denominator, the chin (Figs. 4A and B).
   b. The blades are over the parietal bones.
2. The pelvic application is upside down.
   a. The diameter of the blades is in the transverse diameter of the pelvis.
   b. The sides of the blades are next to the opposite side walls of the pelvis: left blade next to the right wall, and right blade near the left wall.
   c. The concave edges point to the sacrum.
   d. The convex edges point to the pubis.

Application of Forceps Upside Down

1. The right blade is inserted first. Its handle is grasped by the left hand and is held a little below the vagina and near the mother's right thigh. The convex edge of the blade is anterior.
2. The right blade is inserted into the vagina between the left side of the face and the left wall of the vagina.
3. The left blade is inserted next. Its handle is grasped by the right hand and is held a little below the vagina and near the mother's left thigh. The convex edge is anterior (upside down).
4. The left blade is introduced into the right side of the vagina between the right side of the face and the right pelvic wall.
5. The forceps are locked, and vaginal examination is made to be sure that the application is correct (Fig. 4B).

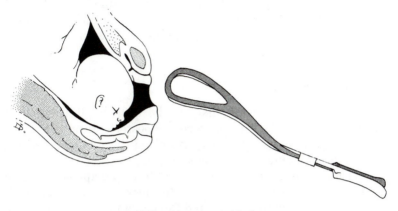

A. Kjelland forceps upside down.

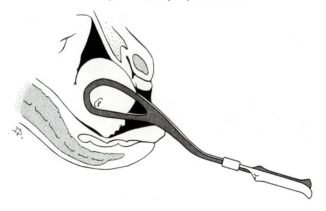

B. Forceps locked, upside down.

Figure 4. MP orientation and application of forceps.

Rotation to Anterior: MP to MA

1. The face is then rotated 180° with the forceps MP to RMP to RMT to RMA to MA. The chin is now under the pubis, and the forehead is in the hollow of the sacrum (Fig. 5).
2. The cephalic application has been maintained.
3. The pelvic application is now right side up, with the concave edges of the forceps next to the pubis and the convex edges near the sacrum.

Extraction of the Head

1. Vaginal examination is made to check the application.
2. Traction is made in an outward and posterior direction until the chin appears under the symphysis and the submental region of the neck impinges in the subpubic angle.
3. With further descent, the face and forehead appear and the direction of traction is changed to outward and anterior. This brings about both descent and flexion, and the vertex and occiput are born over the perineum.
4. Because of the large diameter being delivered, an episiotomy is advisable.

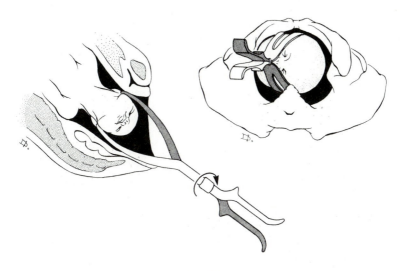

A. MP to RMT.

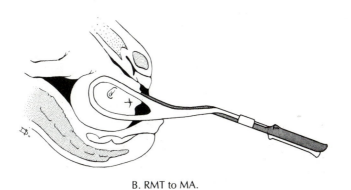

B. RMT to MA.

Figure 5. Anterior rotation with forceps.

29

Breech: Delivery of the Aftercoming Head by Forceps

While any type of forceps can be used for this procedure, the Piper forceps, which was designed especially for this operation, is best. The handles are depressed below the arch of the shanks, the pelvic curve is reduced, and the shanks are long and curved. These features make this instrument easier to apply to the aftercoming head.

FORCEPS DELIVERY

Orientation

Vaginal Examination

1. The long axis of the head is in the anteroposterior diameter of the pelvis.
2. The occiput is anterior.
3. The face is posterior.

Orientation and Desired Application

1. The cephalic application is biparietal and mentooccipital, with the front of the forceps (concave edges) toward the occiput and the convex edges toward the face.
2. The pelvic application is good, with the diameter of the forceps in the transverse diameter of the pelvis, the concave edges pointing toward the pubis and the convex edges toward the sacrum. The sides of the blades are next to the side walls of the pelvis.

Application of Forceps

1. An assistant lifts the baby's body slightly (Fig. 1A), but not too much, for the structures in the neck are damaged by excessive stretching. The lower and upper limbs and the umbilical cord are kept out of the way.
2. The handle of the left blade is grasped in the left hand.
3. The right hand is introduced between the head and the left posterolateral wall of the vagina.
4. The left blade is then inserted between the head and the fingers into a mentooccipital application.
5. The fingers are removed from the vagina, and the handle is steadied by an assistant.
6. The handle of the right blade is grasped with the right hand.
7. The left hand is introduced between the head and the right posterolateral wall of the vagina.
8. The right blade is introduced between the head and the fingers into a mentooccipital application.
9. The fingers are removed from the vagina.
10. The forceps are locked (Fig. 1B), and vaginal examination is made to be certain that the application is correct.

Extraction of the Head

1. Traction is outward and posterior until the nape of the neck is in the subpubic angle.
2. The direction is then changed to outward and anterior, and the face and forehead are born over the perineum in flexion.
3. An episiotomy should be used.

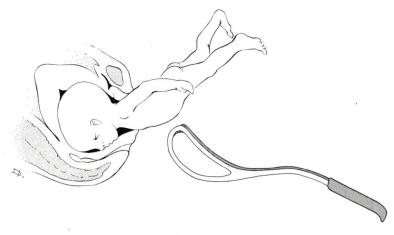

A. Orientation: Piper forceps.

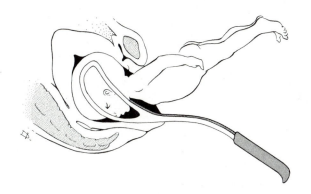

B. Piper forceps locked in cephalic application. Beginning traction.

Figure 1. Breech presentation.

30

Version and Extraction

DEFINITIONS

Version is an operation by which the fetus is turned in utero for the purpose of changing the presentation.

CEPHALIC VERSION   This results in a cephalic presentation.

PODALIC VERSION   This results in a breech.

EXTERNAL VERSION   All manipulations are done through the abdominal wall.

INTERNAL VERSION   The operation is performed with the hand or fingers inside the uterus. In most cases the intrauterine manipulations are furthered by the other hand acting through the abdominal wall.

EXTRACTION   This is the operative and immediate forceful delivery of the child.

EXTERNAL VERSION

Indications

Cephalic version is used to:

1. Turn a breech to a cephalic presentation.
2. Change a transverse lie to a cephalic presentation.

Podalic version is used to turn a transverse lie to a breech presentation. This is done only when cephalic version has failed.

Time of External Version

In the past it was believed that the best time to perform external version was 32 to 34 weeks. At this stage of pregnancy the fetus is relatively small and the amniotic fluid abundant, making the procedure easier to carry out than at later periods of gestation. However, a significant number of babies presenting by the breech will turn spontaneously to a cephalic presentation if left alone and version will have constituted unnecessary interference. Furthermore, in a certain percentage of cases, where the version at 32 to 34 weeks has been accomplished, return to the original breech presentation will take place, and the procedure will have been useless.

Several reports have appeared recently, advising that external version be delayed to 37th week of gestation. It is true that late in pregnancy, because of the larger size of the fetus, the relatively smaller amount of amniotic fluid, and the less relaxed state of the myometrium, external cephalic version may be more difficult to accomplish in later, as compared with earlier, stages of gestation. However, delay of version to 37 weeks has several advantages:

1. Fewer procedures are necessary because spontaneous version will take place in a large number of cases.
2. At this late stage reversion to the original presentation occurs rarely.
3. Contraindications to external cephalic version, such as intrauterine growth retardation, may become evident only in the later stages of pregnancy.
4. Should fetal complications that necessitate immediate delivery occur during the procedure, the child will be mature and able to survive.

A disadvantage of waiting until 37 weeks is that in those patients that go into labor preterm, the opportunity to perform external cephalic version may be missed.

Prerequisites

Certain conditions must be present before external version is attempted:

1. There must be a single pregnancy.
2. Accurate diagnosis of the fetal position is of prime importance.
3. Fetopelvic disproportion should be ruled out.
4. The presenting part must not be deeply engaged.
5. The fetus must be freely movable.

6. There must be intact membranes with a good quantity of amniotic fluid.
7 Uterine relaxation is essential.
8. The maternal abdominal wall must be lax and thin enough to permit manipulations.
9. Ultrasonography should demonstrate: (a) a single fetus; (b) adequate amniotic fluid; (c) no gross fetal anomaly; (d) no nuchal cord (umbilical cord around the neck); (e) no placenta previa.
10. A cardiotocographic nonstress test must be performed, and the result must be reactive (normal) before version is attempted.

Contraindications

1. Multiple pregnancy
2. Gross congenital abnormality of the fetus
3. Intrauterine fetal death
4. Vaginal bleeding in the 3rd trimester
5. Placenta previa
6. Deep engagement of the breech in the pelvis
7. Preterm labor
8. Premature rupture of the membranes
9. Cervical effacement and dilatation of more than 2 cm before 37 weeks of gestation
10. When vaginal delivery is not intended
11. Uterine scars, e.g., previous cesarean section
12. Severe preeclampsia and hypertension
13. Placental insufficiency and intrauterine growth retardation is a relative, not an absolute, contraindication

Dangers

1. Unexplained fetal death may follow version.
2. Fetal bradycardia is noted in many cases immediately following the version, although almost all heart rates return to normal within 3 minutes.
3. The position achieved by the version may be worse than the original one. For example, little has been gained by changing a breech to a brow presentation.
4. There is danger of injury to the umbilical cord and interference with the uteroplacental circulation.
5. There may be prolapse of the umbilical cord.
6. Induction of premature labor may take place.

7. There may be premature separation of the placenta from the uterine wall.
8. Premature rupture of the membranes may occur after version.

Technique

Preparation

1. The patient lies on her back on a firm table with the abdomen uncovered. To help relax the abdominal wall muscles, a pillow is put under the head, and the hips and knees are flexed.
2. Placing the woman in slight Trendelenburg position (hips higher than the shoulders) for 15 to 20 minutes may help dislodge the presenting part and so make the version easier.
3. The bladder should be empty.
4. If the mother's abdomen or the operator's hands are moist, powder should be sprinkled on the abdomen.
5. Diagnosis must be precise. The presentation of the fetus and the location of the placenta are demonstrated by ultrasonography.
6. Anti-D globulin is administered to Rhesus-negative patients.

Anesthesia

There is considerable controversy about the use of an anesthetic agent in the performance of version. There is no doubt that it is easier to perform the operation when the patient is asleep and completely relaxed. On the other hand, it increases the danger of injury. When the patient is awake, her complaints of pain serve as an indication that the manipulations are too vigorous and that it is wise to be more gentle or to stop. At the present time the use of anesthesia is not advised.

Procedure

1. The operator stands at the patient's side.
2. The fetal heart is auscultated every 2 minutes during the procedure. If at any time there is irregularity or a marked change in the rate, the operation is discontinued.
3. One hand is placed on the head and the other on the breech.
4. The presenting part is dislodged from the pelvis (Fig. 1A).
5. The head is moved toward the pelvis and the breech toward the fundus to achieve a transverse lie (Fig. 1B). This position is maintained while the fetal heart is auscultated.
6. If the fetal heart rate is slow or irregular, the baby is turned back to the original position.
7. If the heart is normal the version is continued until the head is over the pelvis and the breech is in the fundus (Fig. 1C).

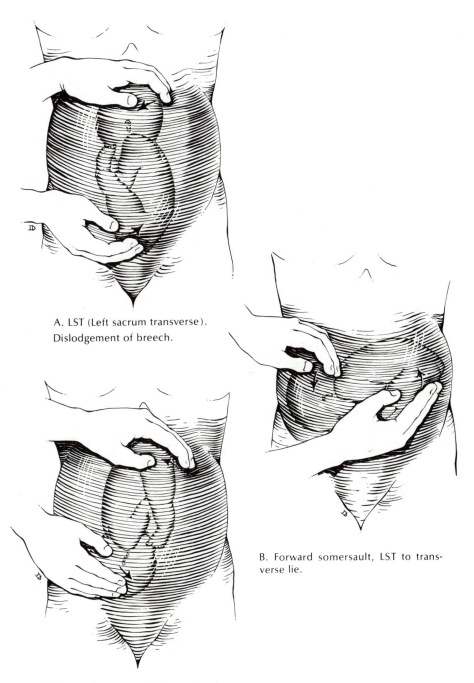

A. LST (Left sacrum transverse).
Dislodgement of breech.

B. Forward somersault, LST to transverse lie.

C. Forward somersault completed, transverse lie to ROT.

Figure 1. External version.

8. If at this point the baby's heart is abnormal, the fetus must be returned to its primary position.
9. After the version is complete and the fetal heart is noted to be normal, the head should be pushed into the pelvis to try and prevent recurrence of the malpresentation. Unfortunately and despite all efforts, this does happen in some cases.
10. Version must never be forced. If the procedure cannot be performed easily and gently, it should be abandoned or postponed.
11. Following completion of the operation (successful or unsuccessful) observation of the fetal heart is continued until a reactive cardiotocogram has been recorded.
12. Each attempt at version must not last longer than 5 minutes, and there should be an interval of at least 3 minutes between attempts.

Direction of Version
The fetus may be turned either forward (face leading the way) or backward (occiput in the lead). It is important that flexion of the head be maintained, and this is easier to accomplish by the backward somersault, but there is greater danger of the legs and feet tangling with the umbilical cord and traumatizing the placenta. Hence, most authorities favor the forward somersault, and advise that, if this fails, attempts at version should be abandoned.

Causes of Failed or Discontinued Version

1. Large fetus and/or small amount of amniotic fluid
2. Fetal bradycardia
3. Maternal obesity
4. Uterine malformation
5. Maternal bleeding
6. Unknown

External Cephalic Version Under Tocolysis
In cases where the myometrium is tense and external version is difficult, beta-mimetic drugs have been used with success to relax the uterus and make the version easier.
The procedure is as follows:

1. The patient is placed in the supine position.
2. An intravenous infusion is set up with lactated Ringer solution.
3. Ritodrine 50 μg, or isoxsuprine 50 μg per minute is infused for 10 to 15 minutes before and during the version.
4. The maternal heart rate and blood pressure are measured every 5 minutes.

5. The fetal heart rate is monitored before, during, and for 60 minutes following the external version.

INTERNAL PODALIC VERSION

Internal version is always podalic. With a hand inside the uterus the feet can be grasped and the baby turned to a footling breech presentation. It is not possible to take hold of the head. Once the feet have been brought through the cervix the version is complete. In most situations where internal podalic version is necessary, immediate extraction of the infant is carried out.

Indications

1. When the situation of the mother or fetus is such that immediate rapid delivery is essential
2. Prolapse of the umbilical cord
3. In compound presentations where the arm is prolapsed below the head and cannot be pushed out of the way
4. Delivery of the second twin if it has not engaged within 30 minutes of the birth of the first
5. Transverse or oblique lie

Prerequisites

1. Accurate diagnosis of position of the child is essential.
2. The child must be alive. There is no point in submitting the mother to a dangerous procedure if the baby is dead.
3. The presenting part should not be deeply engaged.
4. The pelvis must be large enough to permit the passage of the fetal head, i.e., no disproportion.
5. The cervix must be open enough to admit the hand.
6. If extraction is to follow the version, the cervix must be dilated fully.
7. The uterus must not be in tetanus nor be too tightly coapted around the child. The baby must be freely movable.
8. Membranes should be intact or recently ruptured. There must be sufficient amniotic fluid to permit turning.

Contraindications

1. Contracted pelvis with fetopelvic disproportion. It is pointless to perform podalic version if there is not enough room for the head to come through.

2. An incompletely dilated or a rigid cervix.
3. A spastic uterus, which does not relax even under anesthesia. A spastic uterus not only makes version difficult or impossible but increases greatly the danger of uterine rupture.
4. Danger of uterine rupture. When the patient has been in labor for a long time with the lower uterine segment thinned out and with a high retraction ring, any intrauterine manipulations carry a grave danger of uterine rupture.
5. Rupture of the membranes. Once the membranes have been ruptured for a long time (over 1 hour) and the amniotic fluid has drained away, version is difficult, and the attempt carries with it the risk of uterine rupture and fetal death.
6. Uterine scar from previous cesarean section or extensive myomectomy.

Dangers

Maternal Dangers

1. Inherent dangers of deep anesthesia
2. Rupture of the uterus
3. Lacerations of the cervix
4. Abruptio placentae
5. Infection following the intrauterine manipulations

Fetal Dangers

1. Asphyxia from cord prolapse or compression
2. Anesthetic depression, causing asphyxia
3. Asphyxia from placental separation
4. Intracranial damage and hemorrhage
5. General trauma from the difficult procedure

Technique

Preparation

1. The patient is placed in the lithotomy position with the buttocks a little past the end of the table.
2. The bladder is catheterized. The rectum should be empty.
3. An intravenous infusion with a large bore needle is set up.
4. Cross-matched blood should be available.
5. The patient is anesthetized deeply.

Procedure

1. One hand is placed on the uterine fundus to steady the uterus and the baby.
2. The other hand is placed through the cervix into the uterine cavity.
3. When the operator is ready for immediate action, the membranes are ruptured.
4. The fetal head is displaced upward out of the pelvis if the presentation is cephalic.
5. With the intrauterine hand, both feet are grasped if possible (Fig. 2A). If both feet are not attainable, then one foot is grasped. The operator must make sure that he has a foot and not a hand.
6. The feet are pulled slowly toward the pelvic inlet (Fig. 2B).

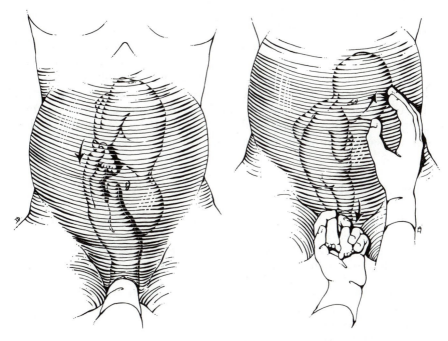

A. Cephalic presentation. Grasping both feet.

B. Downward traction on feet. Upward pressure on head. Cephalic presentation converted to footling breech.

Figure 2. Internal podalic version.

7. With the outer hand the head is pushed gently toward the fundus.
8. When possible the baby should be turned so that the back remains anterior and the head in flexion.
9. When the knees have reached the introitus, version is complete.

EXTRACTION FOLLOWING VERSION

If there is an indication for immediate delivery, and this is so in most cases where internal version is performed, the baby is extracted as a footling breech. This procedure is described in Chapter 18.

CESAREAN SECTION OR VERSION AND EXTRACTION

In the days when cesarean section was fraught with great danger to the mother, version and extraction was employed frequently in the management of various obstetric difficulties. The improvement in surgical techniques, discovery of antibiotics, advances in anesthesia, and availability of blood for transfusion have decreased the fetal and maternal mortality and morbidity associated with abdominal delivery to a point where cesarean section is preferable by far to version and extraction. The use of the latter procedure is limited today to situations of an emergent nature, when immediate delivery of the baby is essential, and cesarean section cannot be carried out.

BIBLIOGRAPHY

Fall O, Nilsson BA: External cephalic version in breech presentation under tocolysis. Obstet Gynecol 53:712, 1979
Fianu S, Vaclavinkova V: External cephalic version in the management of breech presentation with special reference to the placental location. Acta Obstet Gynecol Scand 58:209, 1979
Hofmeyr FJ: Effect of external cephalic version in late pregnancy on breech presentation and caesarean section rate: A controlled trial. Brit J Obstet Gynaecol 90:302, 1983
Van Dorsten JP, Schifrin BS, Wallace RL: Randomized control trial of external cephalic version with tocolysis in late pregnancy. Am J Obstet Gynecol 141:417, 1981

31

Obstetric Analgesia and Anesthesia

Donald C. Oxorn

Pain is one of nature's defense mechanisms, a warning of danger. In pregnancy, it tells the woman that she is having uterine contractions. A painless labor is as treacherous as a silent coronary thrombosis. However, once labor has been diagnosed and proper care instituted, pain has served its purpose; it then becomes appropriate to offer the woman relief. In 1847 Sir James Young Simpson introduced anesthesia into obstetric practice. Intermittently inhaled ether and then chloroform were used to relieve the pains of the final stages of labor and delivery.

Today, obstetric anesthesia has evolved into a complex subspecialty. The physiology and pathophysiology of pregnancy, labor, delivery, and the transition from fetus to neonate, must be fully understood. Only then can the most appropriate form of analgesia and anesthesia be offered to each patient.

CAUSES OF PAIN DURING LABOR

There are a variety of noxious stimuli that lead to the pain of labor. They give rise to subjective discomfort, as well as objective alterations in cardiorespiratory function and the autonomic nervous system.

1. Myometrial hypoxia: Contraction of a muscle during a period of hypoxia causes pain. When uterine relaxation between contractions is insufficient to allow adequate oxygenation, the severity of the pain is increased.
2. Stretching of the cervix: The pain is felt mainly in the back.

3. Pressure on nerve ganglia adjacent to the cervix and vagina.
4. Traction on the tubes, ovaries, and peritoneum.
5. Traction on and stretching of the supporting ligaments.
6. Pressure on the urethra, bladder, and rectum.
7. Distention of the muscles of the pelvic floor and perineum.

INNERVATION OF PELVIC STRUCTURES

Uterus and Cervix

The pain caused by uterine contractions and cervical dilatation is transmitted by way of sensory sympathetic fibers that pass to the spinal cord by way of the posterior roots of the eleventh and twelfth thoracic nerves with some fibers from the tenth thoracic and first lumbar roots. These fibers pass through and are component parts of the uterine and cervical plexus (sometimes called the "ganglion of Frankenhauser"), the inferior hypogastric plexus, the middle hypogastric nerve, the superior hypogastric plexus (commonly known as the "presacral nerve"), and the lumbar and lower thoracic sympathetic chains. The pain of uterine contractions is referred to the corresponding dermatomes.

The motor nerves are also sympathetic, although uterine activity during labor is more dependent on hormonal influences and adequate uterine blood flow. They start in the tenth, eleventh, and twelfth thoracic rami and pass through the aortic, hypogastric, pelvic, and uterine plexuses to terminate in the uterus. In addition there are fibers from the sacral sympathetic chain and parasympathetic branches ("nervi erigentes") that arise from the anterior roots of the sacral nerves.

Vagina, Vulva, and Perineum

The pain resulting from distension of the birth canal, perineum, and vulva is conveyed by afferent fibers of the posterior roots of the second, third, and fourth sacral nerves.

The pudendal nerve is the main supply of the perineum. It arises from the anterior branches of the second, third, and fourth sacral nerves. These join into a single trunk 0.5 to 1.0 cm proximal to the ischial spine. The nerve passes through the greater sciatic foramen, somewhat diagonally across the posterior surface of the sacrospinous ligament, medial to the pudendal vessels, to enter the lesser sciatic foramen. As the nerve passes medial and posterior to the inferior tip of the spine, it enters the pudendal canal and proceeds to the lower edge of the urogenital diaphragm. The nerve is blocked most easily where it lies close to the tip of the ischial spine.

The pudendal nerve divides into three main branches: (1) the inferior hemorrhoidal nerve, (2) the dorsal nerve of the clitoris, and (3) the perineal nerve. The inferior hemorrhoidal nerve supplies the lower rectum, the external sphincter ani, and the skin anterior and lateral to the anus. In 50 percent of cases this nerve arises as a separate branch from the fourth sacral nerve and is not part of the pudendal trunk. In these cases it lies close to the pudendal nerve medial to the ischial spine. The dorsal nerve of the clitoris supplies that organ and the area around it. The perineal nerve is the largest branch. It supplies the superficial structures of the vulva and the skin, fascia, and deep muscles of the perineum.

While the main sensations of pain are carried by the pudendal nerve, a few impulses pass via the posterior femoral cutaneous nerve into the second, third, and fourth sacral nerves, and the ilioinguinal nerve into the first lumbar segment.

The initiation of the painful impulses arises from the aforementioned noxious stimuli. These impulses are modulated peripherally and centrally by both physical and psychologic factors.

PAIN DURING THE STAGES OF LABOR

1. *First stage:* Pain is caused mainly by uterine contractions, thinning of the lower segment of the uterus, and dilatation of the cervix.
2. *Second stage:* Pain results from two sources. The first is the stretching of the vagina, vulva, and perineum; and the second is the contracting myometrium.
3. *Third stage:* Pain is caused by passage of the placenta through the cervix, plus that produced by the uterine contractions.

PHYSIOLOGIC CHANGES

Before discussing the use of anesthesia and analgesia during labor and delivery, it is appropriate to consider the maternal physiologic changes that are present at term.

1. Respiratory system: The body's oxygen consumption is increased. The elevation of the diaphragm secondary to the enlarged uterus compromises the lungs' functional residual capacity, and makes oxygen intake of the lungs less efficient. The upper airways tend to be edematous. These factors together make the mother and fetus more susceptible to periods of hypoxemia, especially when general anesthesia is employed.
2. Cardiovascular system: Blood volume and red cell mass both increase. Hemoglobin concentration tends to fall slightly. The cardiac

output is increased, especially during contractions. Beginning in the second trimester, the mother becomes prone to the supine hypotension syndrome.When the supine posture is assumed, the aorta and inferior vena cava are compressed by the uterus at the pelvic brim, leading to maternal hypotension and decreased uterine perfusion.

3. Gastrointestinal system: Gastric emptying is impaired, the gastroesophageal sphincter is rendered incompetent, and gastric acidity is increased. All these factors render the mother susceptible to pulmonary aspiration of gastric contents.

OBJECTIVES AND METHODS

Mother

1. Relief of pain.
2. By relieving pain the changes of ventilation, circulation, hormonal function that ordinarily accompany pain can be controlled.
3. Freedom from fear.
4. Safe and relatively painless delivery.

Infant

1. To be given a favorable physiologic milieu for delivery
2. To use techniques not associated with fetal depression or poor long-term outcome

Obstetrician

1. More deliberate management of labor
2. Reduction of pressure from patient and relatives to do something prematurely
3. Optimum conditions at delivery

Methods of Achieving Objectives

1. Prenatal training for childbirth, which dissipates fear and tension
2. Sedation by the use of drugs such as barbiturates and tranquilizers
3. Analgesia by narcotics such as morphine and Demerol
4. Anesthesia by a wide variety of techniques: conduction (epidural, spinal), local (nerve block or infiltration), inhalant, and intravenous

Criteria for Ideal Method

The method must ensure that:

1. The health of the mother is not endangered.
2. The newborn should not be depressed at delivery. Most drugs given to the mother cross the placenta and may affect the fetus. Techniques should be chosen which minimize this danger.
3. The technique effectively controls pain.
4. The efficiency of uterine contractions is not decreased. Decrease could cause prolonged labor during the first and second stages and atonic postpartum hemorrhage in the third.
5. The ability of the patient to cooperate intelligently with the medical and nursing staff is maintained.
6. There is no need for operative interference because of the anesthesia.
7. The method is relatively simple to use.

There is no system of anesthesia and analgesia which fulfills all these criteria. Safety to the mother and newborn are of paramount importance.

A widely held belief is that any pharmacologic intervention can only be detrimental to the fetal milieu and should be avoided at all costs. There is increasing evidence to the contrary. The stress of labor leads to increases in maternal catecholamines and maternal hyperventilation. The catecholamines may cause uterine artery vasoconstriction and reduced oxygen delivery to the fetus, whereas hyperventilation impairs the release of oxygen from maternal hemoglobin. Both these factors may lead to fetal asphyxia. Alleviation of stress by the use of anesthetic and analgesic techniques may prevent or alleviate this asphyxia.

Education, psychological and physiologic preparation may be sufficient in some; in others, this maternal preparation may serve as a base, with the addition of some other pain-relieving techniques. Of the available methods, regional anesthesia is probably the best. When properly conducted, side effects are minimal. Maternal consciousness is maintained, allowing cooperation and avoiding the dangers of maternal aspiration. With proper titration, the progress of labor is not impeded. It was thought initially that certain local anesthetics used for epidural anesthesia had adverse effects on early neonatal behavior. More recent studies have shown good neonatal outcome (neurobehavioral scores, umbilical cord blood gases) with all commonly used epidural anesthetic agents, as long as falls in uterine perfusion (e.g., maternal hypotension) and local anesthetic overdoses are avoided.

GENERAL DATA ON USES OF ANALGESIA AND ANESTHESIA

1. There is a wide variation in the amount of analgesia and anesthesia needed. Doses should be carefully titrated so that the smallest effective dose is used.
2. The dose and timing of analgesic and anesthetic medications are

crucial. Given too soon or in excessive amounts, the course of labor may be prolonged. Prescribed at the proper time, pain is relieved and the quality of labor improved.

3. Epidural anesthesia, if started during the accelerating phase of the active stage of labor, will not slow the progress of labor. The dosage can be titrated so that pain is abolished and motor power preserved. This prevents premature paralysis of the perineal muscles and allows flexion and internal rotation of the fetal head to proceed.

4. Unless there is a contraindication, the request of the patient for relief should not be refused.

5. The widespread use of episiotomy has increased the need for anesthesia.

6. Premature infants are exceedingly susceptible to all depressants. Anesthetic techniques which minimize fetal drug exposure, e.g., spinal, epidural, are preferred.

7. Nurses supervising patients in labor must have some familiarity with the anesthetic and analgesic techniques used.

8. The presence of the obstetrician is important in deciding what drugs can be given. Remote control is never as successful as personal management.

9. The availability of a trained anesthetist is essential if complicated techniques are to be employed.

TRAINING FOR CHILDBIRTH

The purpose of training for childbirth is to prepare a woman for labor and delivery so that she approaches the end of her pregnancy with knowledge, understanding, and confidence rather than apprehension and fear. She should be assured that relief will be provided should pain be excessive and that the modern obstetric armamentarium is available to ensure the safety of herself and her unborn child.

One of the first modern advocates of natural childbirth was Grantly Dick-Read. He described the "fear-tension-pain" cycle and hypothesized that fears regarding labor produced tension in the circular muscle fibers of the lower part of the uterus. As a result the longitudinal muscles of the upper part of the uterus have to act against resistance, causing tension and pain. Dick-Read's solution to this problem was to counteract the socially induced expectations regarding labor by providing mothers-to-be with information and assurance to the effect that labor does not have to be painful.

Velvovsky and his followers in the Soviet Union denied that labor was inherently painful. Based on the work of the physiologist Pavlov, they worked out a training procedure designed to inhibit the experience of pain at the cortical level. This is known as the psychoprophylactic method. Lamaze, originator of the Lamaze method, is the best known proponent in the Western world.

Aims of Prenatal Training

1. The apprehension of young women caused by the exaggerated tales of horror told by multiparas is counteracted.
2. The patient is given an opportunity to gain confidence. The facts of childbirth are explained and the methods available to relieve pain are described.
3. Exercises are taught which strengthen certain muscles and relax others.
4. The patient is trained in breath control.
5. The patient is never told that labor and delivery are painless. On the contrary, it is emphasized that analgesia and anesthesia are available should they be needed or desired.
6. It is important that the patient not be placed in competition with other women or with an ideal analgesia-free labor and delivery. Too many women who do need assistance are left with a feeling of failure and remain emotionally disturbed.
7. While patients should be encouraged to take part in the training classes, reluctant women must never be forced to participate.
8. Constant emphasis is placed on the fact that most labors are normal.
9. The program has two parts. The education and exercises are beneficial to all. Whether an individual is desirous of or able to carry on without drugs can be decided only during labor.

Whenever possible the patient should be in a private labor room, with an attendant at all times. This may be her husband, some other relative, a friend, a nurse, or her doctor. Peace and quiet in the labor suite are essential. Nothing that might worry the patient should be said in her hearing. Women in labor read erroneous and worrisome significance into innocent remarks. Unruly and noisy patients should be kept out of earshot, since nothing frightens a woman in labor as much as hearing another's screams.

Achievements of Trained Childbirth

Claims regarding the beneficial effects of trained childbirth include the following:

1. *Psychological effects*: Decreased perception of pain, increased cooperation of the patient during labor, reduced incidence of postpartum depression, and a more positive attitude toward future pregnancy.

2. *Obstetric benefits*: There is a reduction in the need for analgesia and anesthesia, forceps, episiotomy, and cesarean section. The length of labor is reduced and the blood loss is less than in untrained patients.
3. *Benefits to the child*: There is an increase in the oxygenation of fetal blood, quicker initiation of spontaneous respiration, less need for resuscitation, and decrease in the incidence of neonatal morbidity and mortality.

It is unfortunate that opinion regarding training for childbirth has undergone a steady polarization almost since its introduction. On the one hand it has been acclaimed as one of the most significant advances of modern medicine. On the other hand it has been denigrated as primitive and medically unacceptable. Taken as a whole, the reported studies suggest that training for childbirth brings a number of important physical and psychologic benefits to mother and child. The achievements seem impressive. However, critical analysis of these studies reveals that most of them do not meet the most fundamental requirements of the scientific method, including appropriate control groups, double-blind techniques, and statistical tests to rule out chance. As compared with nonusers of the method, followers of natural childbirth were more likely to have the following characteristics: (1) higher social class and income, (2) more advanced levels of education, (3) husband more educated and in an occupation requiring a greater degree of skill.

Leboyer described the ideal birth as one that takes place in a dark and quiet room, the baby is calmed by gentle massage and by placing him in a warm bath, the tying of the umbilical cord is delayed. Leboyer claimed that these infants grow up to be healthier and free of conflict. A recent study did not show that any clear-cut advantages were achieved by the use of this method. The infants were neither more responsive nor less irritable than the control infants during the neonatal period. No differences in temperament or development were seen at 8 months of age. The conclusion was that the Leboyer procedure has no advantage over a gentle, conventional delivery.

Nevertheless, because training programs can do no harm, because the probability is strong that they are helpful, and because patients and spouses enjoy the experience, it is our feeling that prenatal classes should be encouraged.

RELIEF OF PAIN DURING THE FIRST STAGE OF LABOR

During the first stage of labor, the main objective is the relief of pain, while maintaining the mother's cooperation and interfering as little as possible with the progress of labor. To achieve this, each patient must be considered individually. The types and amount of therapy depend on the patient's personality as well as the efficiency of her labor. Multiparas generally need less support than primigravidas.

Because of the more widespread use of regional anasthesia (e.g., epidural), and the better psychological preparation of parturients, the need for systemic narcotics, tranquilizers, and amnestics during the first stage has decreased.

Systemic Medications

These drugs all cross the placenta. Their effect on the fetus depends on the dose, route of administration, proximity to delivery, and degree of fetal well-being.

Narcotics

These agents are used to alleviate pain. If given in excessive quantity during the latent phase, uterine activity and hence rate of cervical dilatation may decrease. If given once labor is well established, the relief of pain and anxiety make the uterine contractions more efficient.

Side effects include respiratory depression, orthostatic hypotension, decreased gastric motility, nausea, and vomiting. All the narcotics are capable of affecting neonatal neurobehavior.

1. *Morphine:* The dose used is approximately 0.1 mg/kg maternal body weight, given every 3 to 4 hours. The peak effect is 1 to 2 hours after intramuscular injection and 20 minutes after an intravenous injection. The duration of action is approximately 4 to 6 hours. The effect on the fetus depends on the time relationship of administration to delivery. If given within 3 hours of delivery, the risk of fetal narcosis is high, especially in premature infants.
2. *Demerol (meperidine, pethidine):* Demerol is a synthetic narcotic, with atropine-like properties. It is given in a dose of 1 mg/kg every 3 to 4 hours. Its peak effect is 40 to 50 minutes after an intramuscular injection and 5 to 10 minutes after an intravenous injection. Duration of action is approximately 3 to 4 hours. Its maternal effect is similar to morphine. The effect on the fetus again depends on dosage and relationship to delivery. The greatest effect on the fetus is reached within 1.5 hours after an intramuscular injection. This is manifested in decreased Apgar scores and impaired neurobehavioral parameters for the first 3 days of life. This prolonged effect may be related to the generation of the metabolite normeperidine, which has a half-life of approximately 23 hours in the neonate.

   Narcotic effects in the newborn are best antagonized with naloxone, 5 to 10 µg/kg.

Amnesics

Scopolamine(hyoscine): Scopolamine is a belladonna alkaloid with amnesic properties. Because of increased popularity of epidural anesthesia for first stage discomfort, its use has markedly decreased in recent years. It is given in a dose of 0.2 to 0.6 mg intramuscularly and usually combined with an analgesic. Its effects on maternal behavior can be very unpredictable. Excitement and delirium can occur, especially in the presence of pain, and close supervision is mandatory. The side effects are related to its antimuscarinic properties. Dry mouth, decreased gastric motility, fetal tachycardia are seen. There are no significant effects on labor.

Sedative Tranquilizers

1. *Barbiturates:* The popularity of these agents in the first stage of labor is declining because of the unpredictable effects on maternal behavior. In large doses, or when combined with narcotics, they may lead to respiratory depression and blunting of upper airway reflexes. In the presence of pain, excitement and disorientation may result. Barbiturates rapidly cross the placenta and the effects on the fetus may be pronounced. Lethargy, somnolence, and decreased feeding may be seen for several days. When used, they should not be given within 12 hours of the anticipated time of delivery. Standard doses of barbiturates have little effect on the progress of labor.

2. *Phenothiazines:* The major tranquilizers in common use today include chlorpromazine (Thorazine), promazine (Sparine) and promethazine (Phenergan). They are anxiolytic and antiemetic and potentiate the effect of narcotics. There is little effect on labor or the fetus, but they should not be used when the baby is premature. Maternal hypotension may be seen, secondary to alpha adrenergic blockade.

3. *Diazepam (Valium):* Diazepam, a benzodiazepine compound, is an excellent tranquilizer and muscle relaxant. It has been used as a sedative and hypnotic during labor and is efficient in the management of preeclampsia and eclampsia. In low doses (less than 30 mg in the 15 hours preceding delivery), there are no adverse fetal or neonatal effects. However, it has been noted that the infants of mothers who were treated with large doses of diazepam during the 24 to 48 hours before delivery manifested symptoms of (1) hypotonia, (2) hypothermia, (3) low Apgar scores, (4) impaired metabolic response to cold, (5) neurologic or respiratory depression, (6) apneic spells, and (7) reluctance to feed. Diazepam and its major active metabolite N-methyl diazepam cross the placenta and accumulate in the fetal tissues. The newborn metabolizes and excretes these compounds very slowly so that significant concentrations may persist for days. Sodium ben-

zoate, one of the preservatives in the intravenous preparation of diazepam, can displace bilirubin from albumin. This is of obvious importance in the newborn with an already elevated level of bilirubin.

Paracervical Block

Paracervical block is an effective, easily performed method of achieving relief of pain during the first stage of labor. Painful impulses from uterine contractions and cervical dilatation pass via sensory and sympathetic pathways to the area of the uterosacral ligaments to the pelvic and hypogastric plexuses, to the lower rami of the tenth, eleventh and twelfth thoracic segments and the first lumbar segment.

The pain of the second stage of labor, produced by distention of the vulva and vagina, is transmitted by sensory fibers of the pudendal nerves to the second, third, and fourth sacral segments. Paracervical block is ineffective in this area, and other methods of pain relief are needed.

Although the technique is easy to master, and the quality of pain relief is good, the high incidence of complications has reduced the popularity of this technique. Some have advocated its abandonment from obstetric practice altogether. Its main advantage, however, is that the block can be performed by the obstetrician, and the attendance of an anesthetist is not required.

Technique

The injection is made transvaginally into the posterolateral fornices, thus blocking the sensory pathways at the junction of the uterosacral ligaments with the cervix. The procedure can be carried out in the patient's bed, but it is done more accurately on the delivery table. The block is instituted during the active phase of labor, with the cervix at least 3 to 4 cm dilated.

The equipment consists of a 20 gauge needle, 13 to 18 cm long, with a sheath or needle guide of such length that about 1.5 cm of the tip of the needle protrudes when it is inserted up to its hub. The needle sheath is guided by the fingers into the vagina and placed in the fornix just lateral to the cervix, at a tangent to the presenting part (Fig. 1). The needle (with attached syringe) is introduced through the guides until the point rests against the mucosa. With quick, slight pressure the needle is pushed through the mucosa to a depth of 6 to 12 mm. Aspiration is performed to guard against direct intravascular injection. If no blood comes back, the desired amount of anesthetic solution is injected. It is advisable to wait a few minutes after the injection of one side. The fetal heart is auscultated. If it is normal the other side is injected. If fetal bradycardia occurs the procedure should be discontinued. Mepivacaine (Carbocaine), lidocaine (Xylocaine), and procaine (Novocain) in 1 percent concentrations are effective. Mepivacaine seems to have a longer lasting effect. Bupivacaine (Marcaine) is no longer recommended in obstetric paracervical block anesthesia because of a high incidence of fetal bradycardia.

The sites of injection vary. Some workers inject the solution at 3 and 9 o'clock. Others give several injections at 3, 4, 8, and 9 o'clock. In any case, 10 ml is given on each side in single or multiple doses.

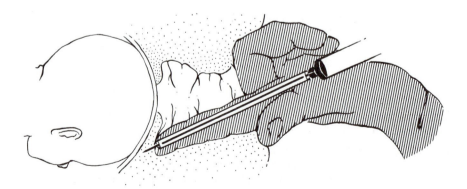

Figure 1. Paracervical block.

Effectiveness

Most patients experience complete or partial relief from pain almost immediately. They remain alert and cooperative. The block gives relief for about 1 hour. In many cases a single block remains effective until the cervix is fully dilated. In others a second block is necessary.

Other forms of anesthesia are required for the actual delivery. Pudendal block or direct infiltration of the perineum are effective and safe.

Effect on Labor

Opinions vary concerning the effect of paracervical block on labor. Some state that labor is shortened, some say it is inhibited, while others feel that the effect varies from one patient to the next and is not predictable. The anesthetized patient may be unaware of strong uterine contractions, and oxytocin augmentation must be used with care, lest the uterus rupture.

Maternal Complications

1. Transient numbness and paresthesias of one or both lower extremities are a common occurence. This is the result of the local anesthetic spreading to the sciatic nerve or part of the lumbosacral plexus.
2. Rapid absorption or intravascular injection causes dizziness, euphoria, anxiety, shaking movements, and, rarely, convulsions.
3. Occasionally there is transient hypotension.
4. A hematoma may form at the site of injection.
5. A rare case of parametritis has been reported.

Fetal Complications

The major limitation of paracervical block is its effect on the fetus. Changes in fetal heart rate occur in approximately 30 percent of cases. Twenty-four percent are bradycardic, 4 percent tachycardic, and 2 percent show a mixed pattern. Five percent have bradycardia sufficient to impair tissue perfusion, with acidosis and neonatal depression the ultimate result.

The etiology of the bradycardia is complex and probably occurs by several pathways:

1. Uterine artery vasoconstriction because of the proximity of injection. This leads to placental hypoperfusion and fetal asphyxia.
2. Direct uterine artery injection.
3. Direct myometrial injection.
4. Diffusion of local anesthetic through the uterine arteries and deposition in the intervillous spaces, with subsequent fetal uptake and direct fetal cardiotoxicity.
5. Direct fetal injection.

Changes in fetal heart rate are seen more often in primigravidas, with prior fetal distress, and in infants of less than 2500 g birth weight. The onset is usually within 2 to 10 minutes of injection and may last 3 to 30 minutes. If bradycardia is prolonged, it may cause fetal acidosis and neonatal depression. This effect is especially prominent if delivery occurs within 30 minutes of injection.

Precautions

1. Paracervical block is unlikely to cause the intrauterine death of a healthy fetus, but it may do so if the fetus is already compromised. Hence this technique should not be used in cases of placental insufficiency, prior fetal distress, and prematurity.
2. Small volumes of a dilute solution of local anesthetic should be used. Vasoconstrictors should be omitted.
3. With rapid cervical dilatation, the chances of aberrant injection are increased and the block should not be performed.
4. The block should not be given if delivery is anticipated within 30 minutes.
5. Because of the high incidence of fetal bradycardia, fetal heart rate should be monitored during and for at least 20 minutes after the block. If bradycardia does occur and is believed to be secondary to the block, it is best to avoid emergency delivery, to allow the fetus time to dispose of the drug.
6. Oxytocin is used with caution. The uterus may become hypertonic; since the patient feels no pain, the excessive contraction is missed by the attendants.
7. Vaginal bleeding and infection are contraindications to the block as is sensitivity to local anesthetic agents.

Lumbar Epidural Block

This block is described later in the chapter.

RELIEF OF PAIN DURING THE SECOND STAGE OF LABOR

Pain relief during the second stage of labor falls into one of four general categories:

1. Inhalational analgesia
2. Inhalational anesthesia
3. Intravenous anesthesia
4. Regional anesthesia which includes lumbar epidural, spinal and caudal anesthesia, pudendal block, and local infiltration.

Of the above techniques, lumbar epidural anesthesia is probably the most satisfactory with regards to quality of analgesia, safety to mother and newborn, and lack of effects on labor. However, it does require the constant availability of a trained anesthetist.

Inhalational Analgesia

The major advantage of using inhalational analgesia is its technical simplicity. It can be instituted with each contraction, and its effects are rapidly eliminated when the agent is withdrawn.

However, there are significant dangers associated with its use. There is a fine line between sufficient analgesia and loss of consciousness at which time the risk of pulmonary aspiration increases and maternal cooperation is lost.

The agents used have dose-related depressant effects on the maternal circulation and on the newborn's level of consciousness.

Inhalational Anesthesia

This technique is generally reserved for situations in which rapid delivery is important, e.g., fetal distress, or when intrauterine manipulation is required.

Because of the attendant risks of maternal aspiration during induction of anesthesia, preventative measures must be undertaken (described later in this chapter).

Nitrous Oxide

Effects on the Mother

1. Because of its relative insolubility in blood, induction and recovery are both rapid.
2. It is rapidly transported to maternal tissues, placenta, and the fetus.
3. Although an effective analgesic during contractions, it is inadequate for delivery, especially if difficult maneuvers such as forceps are planned. A more potent agent (halothane, enflurane) should be added at this time.
4. It is generally nontoxic.
5. It is usually administered as a 50:50 mixture in oxygen. Although this limits its analgesic potency, it decreases the chances of maternal hypoxemia.
6. It can be used as a continuous or intermittent technique.

Effects on the Newborn.   Prolonged use may lead to neonatal depression.

Effects on Labor.   There is little effect on labor.

Halothane, Enflurane, Isoflurane
Halothane is an alkane whereas enflurane and isoflurane are ethers. Their effects are very similar and they will be considered together.

Effects on the Mother

1. There is an initial stage of analgesia. As the dose is increased, anesthesia follows with loss of consciousness and protective airway reflexes.
2. Maternal blood pressure is decreased in a dose-related fashion, secondary to cardiac depression and vasodilatation.
3. Maternal ventilation is also depressed. To avoid maternal and fetal hypoxemia, at least 50 percent oxygen should be administered concurrently.

Effects on the Newborn.   With deep levels of anesthesia, the decreased uterine perfusion may lead to fetal hypoxia, acidosis, and neonatal depression.

Effects on Labor.   There is a dose-related decrease in the intensity of uterine contractions, which may be counteracted with oxytocics. If unchecked, postpartum bleeding may be a result.

Uterine relaxation may be used to advantage when increased uterine tone makes delivery difficult, e.g., delivery of an aftercoming head in a breech presentation.

Intravenous Anesthesia

Agents are administered intravenously for the rapid induction of general anesthesia. They are usually followed by inhalational agents for maintenance of the anesthetic state.

Thiopentone, Ketamine
These intravenous agents are used to induce general anesthesia, followed by the administration of the inhalant agents described above.

When thiopentone is given in a dose of less than 4 mg/kg of maternal body weight, the side effects on mother, neonate, and labor are minimal.

In a dose of less than 1 mg/kg, the same situation applies to ketamine. It may be used as an alternative to inhalational analgesia in a dose of 0.25 mg/kg.

Muscle Relaxants

The currently used muscle relaxants with the exception of gallamine, do not cross the placenta and have no effects on labor or the neonate.

Aspiration of Vomitus During General Anesthesia

The pregnant patient is at high risk for pulmonary aspiration of gastric contents during general anesthesia. The critical factors are volume of gastric juice aspirated and its acidity. A solution of 25 ml with a pH of 2.5 is the threshold quoted most often for the development of symptoms. In pregnancy the gastric pH is low, gastric emptying is impaired, and the lower esophageal sphincter is relaxed, all of which render the parturient especially susceptible.

Maternal aspiration still accounts for a very large percentage of anesthetic-associated morbidity and mortality. One hundred to 400 maternal deaths per year are reported in the United States.

The most important facet of the management of aspiration is taking steps to prevent its occurrence:

1. The use of regional anesthesia allows for maintenance of maternal consciousness, and keeps protective airway reflexes intact.
2. If general anesthesia is to be employed, the airway of each patient should be carefully evaluated. In this way difficult intubations can be anticipated.
3. The gastric volume should be kept at a minimum. Ways of achieving this are minimizing oral intake, and administering drugs such as metaclopramide which enhance gastric emptying. Less popular methods include nasogastric suction and administering emetics such as apomorphine.
4. Reducing the lethality of stomach contents. The goal is to make the stomach contents more alkaline. Antacids can be administered to achieve this. Nonparticulate antacids, such as 30 ml of 0.3 M sodium citrate, may be superior to particulate compounds which may themselves cause pulmonary damage if inhaled. Many delivery rooms now have regimens established for the routine administration of antacids throughout labor and delivery. Ranitidine and cimetidine, histamine antagonists, decrease gastric secretion and acidity. Administration of these drugs can be via the oral or parenteral route and should be 1 to 2 hours before anesthesia to be effective.
5. Preventing regurgitation during the induction of general anesthesia. Induction and paralysis should be done in rapid sequence and followed by manual pressure on the cricoid cartilage (Sellick maneuver). This has the effect of pinching off the esophagus, and prevent-

ing the cephalad migration of stomach contents. Pressure is maintained until the trachea is intubated with a cuffed endotracheal tube. This prevents the entry of any regurgitated materials into the lungs. At the end of anesthesia, the tube is removed. This is done only after the patient has regained consciousness and the protective airway reflexes have returned.

Aspiration of Particulate Matter
Regurgitation and aspiration of particulate matter produces the classic picture of bronchial obstruction and atelectasis. This is an acute and dramatic situation, and, if not treated immediately, may lead to anoxia and death. Treatment includes postural drainage, suction, and, when necessary, bronchoscopy to reestablish patency of the airway.

Mendelson Syndrome
In 1946, Curtis Mendelson, a New York obstetrician, described a syndrome of cyanosis, dyspnea, wheezing, and hypoxia in obstetric patients undergoing general anesthesia. This condition is produced by the aspiration, often silent, of highly acidic gastric fluid, producing a chemical tracheitis and pneumonitis. This leads to destruction of surfactant, capillary damage with intraalveolar hemorrhage, airway closure with alveolar collapse, bronchospasm, and ventilation perfusion mismatching with hypoxemia. At 24 to 36 hours, consolidation occurs and, by 48 hours, hyaline membranes appear. Resolution usually begins at 72 hours. Survivors may have residual scarring.

The diagnosis may be made in several ways:

1. Gastric fluid may be seen entering the trachea at the time of laryngoscopy.
2. Gastric fluid may be suctioned back from the trachea following intubation.
3. Aspiration may be inferred by the unexpected appearance of wheezing and cyanosis, cardiovascular instability, and the radiologic appearance of pulmonary edema.

If aspiration is recognized as it occurs, the patient is intubated with a cuffed endotracheal tube and placed in a lateral decubitus position with the head down. The trachea is suctioned.

Once the syndrome is established, the treatment is that of acute respiratory failure, and is undertaken in an intensive care area. The patient is mechanically ventilated with positive and expiratory pressure in an effort to prevent atelectasis and improve ventilation perfusion matching. The lowest oxygen concentration commensurate with adequate arterial oxygenation is administered. Cardiovascular and fluid management can be exceedingly difficult and is best guided by invasive hemodynamic monitoring.

Bronchodilators are given to counteract wheezing. Steroids are probably of no benefit, and may actually impair long-term healing. Antibiotics are given prophylactically only in the event of a fecal aspiration. Their use is otherwise guided by sputum and blood cultures. The mortality rate depends on the volume and acidity of aspirated material, the presence of large particulate matter, occurrence of infection, prolonged hypoxemia, and general premorbid medical condition. It may be as high as 70 percent. In survivors, the prognosis is generally favorable. Improvement begins at approximately 12 hours and functional clearing in 24 to 48 hours.

Local Anesthesia

The two methods of local anesthesia are (1) direct infiltration of the perineal tissues and (2) pudendal nerve block. Local anesthesia is one of the best choices for obstetrics, but nervous, high-strung women and impatient doctors are not associated with a high degree of success.

Advantages

1. The technique is simple. The obstetrician should administer the drug himself.
2. There are no systemic ill effects as long as dosages of local anesthetic are controlled and drug allergy is not encountered. It is a useful technique in certain forms of cardiopulmonary disease and when other forms of anesthesia are considered unsafe.
3. The baby's vital functions are not affected; it is not narcotized and the respiratory center is not depressed.
4. There is no nausea or vomiting.
5. The cough reflex is not depressed, and there is minimal danger of aspirating.
6. The mother is awake during the delivery.
7. There is no interference with uterine contractions, therefore postpartum bleeding is minimal.
8. Since the baby is not affected, there is no need to hurry and the delivery can be performed gently and carefully.
9. Postpartum nursing care is easy.
10. There is little or no effect on other parts of the body and the vital centers are not depressed. Under proper control complications are minimal.

Disadvantages

1. Not every patient is suitable.
2. The technique does not work in every case. Practice is needed to acquire proficiency.

3. In rare incidences the needle breaks.
4. Care must be taken not to inject into a blood vessel since intravenous injection may cause convulsions, cardiac arrest, or even death.
5. The rare person is allergic to the anesthetic agent and every patient should be asked about history of drug sensitivity.
6. Carelessness in technique may lead to sepsis.
7. A blood vessel may be torn during the procedure leading to formation of a hematoma.
8. Only perineal pain is relieved. The discomfort from the uterine contractions continues.
9. If extensive operative work is necessary, additional anesthesia must be administered.

Direct Infiltration Anesthesia

The main purpose of perineal infiltration is to permit incision and repair of episiotomy, as well as suturing of lacerations (Fig. 2).

Technique

1. Because of its rapid and profound action, we prefer 1 percent Xylocaine (lidocaine hydrochloride). Two percent chloroprocaine or 1 percent mepivacaine can also be used. For the average case 30 to 50 ml of solution is sufficient.
2. Either of two approaches may be used:
   a. The needle is inserted at the posterior fourchette and the injections made laterad.
   b. The needle is inserted at a point halfway between the anus and the ischial tuberosity and the injections made toward the midline.
3. With a small 25 gauge needle a wheal is made by injecting a small amount of the solution into the skin at the point where the needle is to be inserted.
4. The needle is then changed to a No. 20, which is inserted through the wheal. Multiple injections are made into the subcutaneous tissue, muscles, and fascia.
5. During the procedure the plunger of the syringe must be pulled back repeatedly to be sure that the needle is not in a blood vessel.
6. Adequate anesthesia is achieved in about 5 minutes.

Advantages

1. The technique is simple; no special anatomic knowledge is necessary.

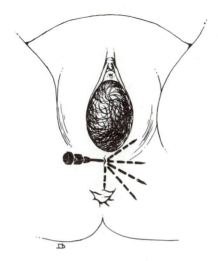

Figure 2. Local anesthesia: direct infiltration.

2. The rate of success is almost 100 percent.
3. The injection can be made at any time, even when the head is on the perineum.

Disadvantages
Complete perineal anesthesia is not achieved. Only the infiltrated areas are affected.

Pudendal Nerve Block

The pudendal nerve originates from S2, S3, and S4. It leaves the pelvis by way of the lower part of the greater sciatic foramen, curves around the ischial spine, crosses the sacrospinous ligament close to its attachment to the ischial spine, and then reenters the pelvis alongside the internal pudendal artery at the lesser sciatic foramen. At this point the pudendal nerve breaks up into the inferior hemorrhoidal (rectal), the perineal, and the dorsal nerve of the clitoris. These nerves are blocked best at the ischial tuberosity. Additional innervation is received from the pudendal branch of the posterior femoral cutaneous nerve, which supplies the posterior labial portion of the perineum. A secondary innervation is provided by the ilioinguinal (L1) and the genitofemoral (L1 and 2) nerves. These nerves must be blocked by supplemental infiltration to achieve thorough anesthesia of the anterior portions of the labia majora and mons pubis.

The time of administration of pudendal anesthesia is important to its success. Once the head or breech is distending the perineum, it is too late. In primigravidas the injection is made when the cervix is fully dilated and the presenting part is at station + 2. In multiparas the anesthetic is given when the cervix is dilated 7 to 8 cm. Pudendal anesthesia is sufficient for spontaneous delivery or low forceps extraction, for breech deliveries, and for episiotomy and repair of lacerations. Many obstetricians combine pudendal block with local infiltration, described above.

Percutaneous Transperineal Approach

The local anesthetic (1 percent Xylocaine, 2 percent chloroprocaine, or 1 percent mepivacaine) is injected around the pudendal nerve through a 5 inch, 20 gauge needle. Effective anesthesia is achieved in about 15 minutes. After an intradermal wheal has been raised, the needle is inserted through the skin midway between the anus and the ischial tuberosity. As the needle is advanced, small amounts of local anesthetic are injected. The index finger of the left hand is inserted into the vagina or rectum and the tuberosity of the ischium is palpated (Fig. 3). The needle is directed toward the ischial spine. The following injections are made: (1) 5 to 10 ml are injected at the anterolateral aspect of the spine, as well as under the tuberosity, to block the inferior pudendal branch of the posterior cutaneous nerve. The syringe is detached from the needle and refilled. (2) The needle is advanced to the medial aspect of the ischial spine, where another 5 to 10 ml of solution are injected to block the branches of the pudendal nerve. Since the pudendal artery and vein run parallel to the nerve, the injection of the anesthetic should be intermittent with aspiration between injections to obviate intravascular injection. If

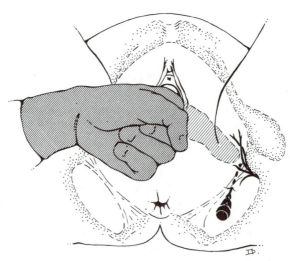

Figure 3. Pudendal nerve block: percutaneous transperineal approach.

blood returns, the needle is withdrawn and repositioned. (3) Another 5 to 10 ml of solution is injected as the needle is advanced 1 inch (2.5 cm) past the ischial tuberosity into the ischial fossa. This blocks the pudendal nerve in Alcock's canal. (4) The point of the needle is advanced posteriorly to the ischial spine. The finger can palpate the sacrospinous ligament, and it guides the needle in this direction until a "popping" sensation indicates that the needle has pierced the ligament. The needle is advanced another 1/4 inch (0.5 cm) and 5 to 10 ml of solution are injected at this point to block the pudendal nerve before it divides. The needle is withdrawn and the other side is blocked.

The final step is to infiltrate the area that lies 5/8 inch (1.5 cm) lateral and parallel to the labium majorum from the middle of the labium to the mons pubis. This blocks the secondary innervation from the iliohypogastric, ilioinguinal, and genitofemoral nerves. This is done bilaterally.

Transvaginal Technique

A 10 or 20 ml syringe is used with a 5 inch, 20 gauge needle. The left puden-dal nerve is blocked first. The index and middle fingers of the left hand are inserted into the vagina, and the ischial spine and the sacrospinous liga-ment are palpated. The syringe is held in the right hand. The needle is placed in the groove formed by the apposition of the index and middle fin-gers, or the tip of the needle may be pressed against the ball of the index finger (Fig. 4). (Some prefer to use the Kobak needle or the Iowa trumpet to prevent the needle from injuring the vagina before it is placed in the correct area.) Protected by the fingers the needle is inserted into the wall of the vagina towards the tip of the ischial spine. The needle is advanced about 5/8 inch (1.5 cm) into the sacrospinous ligament, where 3 ml of solution are in-jected. The needle is then advanced until it "pops" through the sacrospinous ligament, and 5 to 10 ml of the local anesthetic solution (1 percent Xylocaine, procaine, or Metycaine) are injected into this area, with an aspiration test between each 2 to 3 ml. A supplementary infiltration of the area lateral to the labia majora is carried out as described in the section on the transperi-neal technique. The procedure is repeated on the other side.

Continuous Lumbar Epidural Analgesia and Anesthesia

Most of the pain of the first stage of labor is conducted from the uterus by sympathetic pathways to the eleventh and twelfth thoracic segments. These can be effectively blocked, using epidural anesthesia.

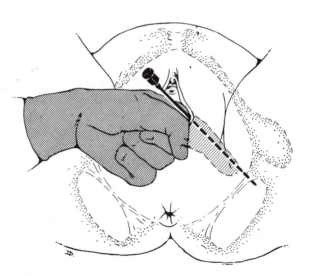

Figure 4. Pudendal nerve block: transvaginal route.

Uterine activity is more dependent on hormonal influences than motor nerve activity. For that reason, labor is usually not interfered with. However, excessive doses of local anesthetic will paralyze the abdominal and pelvic musculature as well as blocking sensory fibers. This interferes with flexion and internal rotation of the baby's head as it passes through the birth canal, and may slow the progress of labor. By proper titration of dosages, pain is abolished and motor activity and maternal cooperation is maintained.

The block may be extended to the sacral segments later in the course of labor, as perineal distention by the presenting part occurs. Sometimes the patient loses the urge to bear down, and must be told when she is having a contraction and instructed to push.

In the adult, the spinal cord extends below the vertebral body of L2 only rarely; more often it ends at L1. The dural sac usually terminates at the level of S1 and S2. Surrounding the dural sac and delineated by the dura mater on one side and the periosteum on the vertebral bodies and ligamentum flavum on the other side, is the epidural space. The latter extends from the foramen magnum superiorly to the sacral hiatus inferiorly.

Technique

While a single shot epidural block is effective for the delivery, the continuous method is better as it provides analgesia for the greater part of labor as well. The needle is inserted into the epidural space; it does not enter the spinal canal.

The patient lies on her side, or sits up. A #17 Tuohy needle (some anesthetists prefer an 18 gauge, thin-walled, short bevelled needle) is inserted into the second or third lumbar interspace with the orifice of the needle pointing toward the head. Epidural puncture is made, using a loss of resistance technique. A vinyl plastic catheter is inserted through the needle which is removed over the catheter. A test dose of 2 to 3 ml of local anesthetic is injected and the patient is observed for signs of systemic toxicity (secondary to intravenous injection) or subarachnoid block (following inadvertent dural puncture). The rest of the anesthetic solution (4 to 6 ml) is then injected. The patient should be kept on her side, or her back with a wedge under the right hip. This prevents aortocaval compression and supine hypotension. Usually subjective relief of pain starts to develop within 3 to 5 minutes and maximum effect is present in 8 to 15 minutes. If there is no evidence of analgesia by 10 minutes, it is likely that the drug was injected outside of the epidural space, or that not enough drug was injected initially. Once the block is established, it can be maintained by a constant infusion of local anesthetic through the catheter or by intermittent injections when discomfort returns. The optimal time to institute this analgesic method is when labor is established in the active phase and the cervix is dilated to 4 to 6 cm in primigravidas and 3 to 4 cm in multiparas.

Satisfactory drugs include bupivacaine (Marcaine) (0.25 to 0.5 percent), lidocaine (0.5 to 1 percent), and mepivacaine (0.5 to 1 percent), and 2 percent chloroprocaine. Adrenalin in a 1:200,000 concentration may be added. The lower strengths are preferable and only when these are ineffective are the stronger concentrations employed. Bupivacaine produces analgesia for 2.5 to 3 hours. To avoid interference with the uterine contractions and to obviate paralysis of the perineal muscles (which would interfere with the mechanism of internal rotation of the fetal head), two approaches are available: One is to use segmental epidural blocks so that the sacral nerves are spared; the other is to employ a low concentration of local anesthetic. This is sufficient to provide relief of pain from uterine contractions without producing significant block of the motor nerves.

As the cervix becomes fully dilated and the head descends, the patient feels pain in the lower pelvis and rectum. The last injection (perineal dose) is given after internal rotation is complete and just prior to delivery. Higher concentrations are used to assure perineal relaxation. In some cases it is advantageous to sit the patient up for 5 minutes or to position her at a 45° angle, to allow the anesthetic solution to descend to the sacral roots. If the block interrupts the afferent sacral nerves, the patient may lose the urge to bear down. However, she will respond to encouragement to bear down when a contraction sets in.

Advantages

1. Almost the entire labor can be made pain free. In a difficult case epidural analgesia brings about a marked change for the better in the patient's general condition and morale. In addition, the relatives are placated.
2. The effect can be maintained as long as necessary.
3. The level of anesthesia is controlled primarily by the volume and concentration of the drug injected, and to a smaller degree by the posture of the patient.
4. The mother is alert and cooperative. She retains the ability to bear down. Delivery may be spontaneous but even if forceps are used the patient can help by pushing down while the operator is exerting traction.
5. The anesthesia is complete and brings about good relaxation; it permits operative deliveries to be performed carefully and without haste.
6. Epidural techniques are valuable in trials of labor. Should cesarean section be necessary, this same anesthetic can be used.
7. There are no postspinal headaches.
8. There is no effect on the fetus, unless marked hypotension occurs.

This may be secondary to intravenous toxicity of the local anesthetic, marked vasodilatation from sympathetic block, or aortocaval compression.

Disadvantages

1. There is danger of masking the strength of the uterine contractions to the point where uterine rupture occurs. The risk is increased by the use of oxytocins.
2. Significant hypotension occurs in approximately 10 percent of women at term if they lie supine for a period of 3 to 7 minutes. With epidural anesthetic a drop of 20 mm Hg systolic or diastolic takes place in close to a third of patients. This hypotension has three main causes:
   a. The sympathetic vasomotor blockade leads to a 15 to 20 percent drop in arteriolar resistance.
   b. The increase in venous capacitance with subsequent venous pooling leads to a decrease in the venous return and cardiac output.
   c. The pregnant uterus may press on the aorta and vena cava and lead to both a decreased placental perfusion and reduced return to the heart.
   Steps to prevent and treat hypotension include (1) Preanesthetic hydration of the patient with 1000 ml of Ringer lactate or saline given intravenously and rapidly through a large bore needle; (2) The use of a wedge under the right hip to displace the uterus to the left and reduce its occlusive pressure on the great vessels; (3) Marked supine hypotension may be a contraindication to the use of the major regional technique; and (4) Ephedrine is the vasopressor of choice if one is needed, because it will help to maintain maternal blood pressure with only little change in uterine blood flow.
3. Accidental intravascular injection or too rapid absorption may cause twitching, convulsions, and maternal hypotension. The cardiotoxicity of bupivacaine may be refractory to resuscitative measures. Because of this, the 0.75 percent preparation, once popular in obstetric anesthesia, is now rarely used.
4. The dura may be punctured. Because of the large needle size, headache often results. Accidental subarachnoid injection may lead to massive motor block with hypotension and respiratory distress.
5. Fetal heart rate (FHR) patterns may be affected. In most cases epidural anesthesia and analgesia have no adverse effects on the fetus. Occasionally late decelerations are noted. These may indicate a

toxic effect of local anesthetic on the fetus but are more likely to represent an effect of hypoxia resulting from decreased maternal-fetal exchange.

6. Rarely, there is infection at the site of injection.
7. A few patients have reported backache.
8. In a few cases, the catheter has broken off and the piece is left in situ. This causes no ill effects.
9. The incidence of neurologic complications secondary to epidural block is widely debated. Obvious problems include epidural hematoma, epidural infection, or injection of the wrong solution. Adhesive arachnoiditis is less convincingly attributed to the block. Peripheral neuropathy is seen after deliveries where epidural anesthesia has not been used. Its incidence secondary to block itself is difficult to determine.
10. Occasionally the uterine contractions become weaker and less frequent, especially when the epidural is initiated before the active phase of labor. An infusion of a dilute solution of oxytocin will improve the labor and bring about the return of good progress.
11. With large doses, the patient loses the desire and ability to bear down. The increased use of midforceps constitutes the most significant complication of the second stage.

Contraindications

1. Allergy to the drug
2. Opposition of the patient or an uncooperative patient
3. Skin infection over the proposed injection site
4. Coagulopathy, because of the risk of forming an epidural hematoma
5. Active, uncontrolled hemorrhage
6. Severe supine hypotension
7. Certain diseases of the central and peripheral nervous systems
8. Certain cardiopulmonary diseases
9. If delivery must be expedient, the time needed to establish a block may be prohibitive.

Safeguards and Precautions

1. The dosage is half that required for surgery.
2. The injection is not made during a uterine contraction because it is forced too high.
3. Full cardiopulmonary resuscitative equipment must be available.
4. Maternal hypotension may occur. Treatment consists of turning the patient on her left side and administering intravenous fluid. When this is not effective, ephedrine, 5 to 10 mg, may be administered intravenously.

5. An intravenous barbiturate must be prepared for treating the patient should convulsions result from accidental intravascular injection.
6. During the delivery, the mother may be given oxygen by mask to increase the level in the blood, and so increase the supply available to the baby.
7. Accidental dural puncture may occur, and with a large needle involved, headache may occur in 75 percent of patients. The treatment is described later in the section on spinal anesthesia.

Caudal Block

The caudal space is the most inferior extension of the epidural space. It is delineated by the periosteum covering the first four fused sacral vertebrae and the sacrococcygeal ligament as it crosses the unfused fifth sacral vertebra. The caudal canal contains the cauda equina in addition to the epidural venous plexus and a loose areolar tissue generally present in the epidural space.

Caudal block is performed by injecting local anesthesia solution through the sacral hiatus into the caudal canal. The extent of anesthesia is largely determined by the volume of the anesthetic injected. In general it is used for procedures below the level of T10. The fetal head may be nearby and care must be taken to avoid accidental injection of the local anesthetic into the scalp. The block should be started only after the active phase of labor has begun because, if given earlier, it may interfere with the uterine contractions. Caudal anesthesia has the potential to paralyze the perineal sling; without perineal resistance, normal internal rotation may not take place.

Because of the large dosage needed, the potential for fecal contamination, and the proximity of the fetal head, epidural block is preferred.

Spinal Anesthesia: Saddle Block

The dural sac extends to the level of S2 and the spinal cord reaches L1 in the great majority, rarely as far as L2. Therefore, a puncture below this level should not encounter the spinal cord and the subarachnoid space may be entered safely through one of the interspaces between L2 and L5.

Saddle block is a low spinal anesthetic confined to the perineal area. In practice, the region of anesthesia is a little more widespread than the saddle area, but this does not interfere with the aims of the technique. With the addition of glucose to the anesthetic agent the solution is made hyperbaric. The subarachnoid injection is made with the patient in the sitting position, so that the heavy solution gravitates downward. Commonly used solutions are 0.5 percent tetracaine (3 mg) and 5 percent lidocaine (35 to 50 mg). The length of time that the patient sits up determines the level of anesthesia. Five minutes is sufficient. In this way complete anesthesia of the perineal region is attained; the perineal muscles are relaxed and there is partial loss of sensation in the abdomen and thighs. The sympathetic fibers that carry the feeling of pain from the uterus are blocked and the pains of labor are relieved or abolished. The injection must not be made during the contraction because the agent may be forced to too high a level.

While uterine contractions do not cease and there is no increase in uterine atony and postpartum hemorrhage, effective progress of labor halts, so this anesthetic is used terminally. The patient is not able to deliver the baby herself and extraction with forceps is necessary. Hence the anesthetic can be given only when labor has reached the point where easy low forceps can be performed. The cervix must be fully dilated.

Advantages
Terminal spinal is an excellent anesthetic especially for difficult deliveries since it provides good anesthesia and excellent relaxation and is easier to administer than epidural anesthesia.

Disadvantages
1. Postdural puncture headache results from the seepage of spinal fluid from the dural tear. The incidence is higher in pregnant women than in others, and is directly proportional to the size of the needle. Spinal fluid pressure falls and pain results from intracranial dural stretching and possibly from tension on intracranial blood vessels. The pain is related closely to posture. It diminishes during recumbency and recurs when the erect posture is resumed. It can be severe and prostrating, with nausea, vomiting, and vertigo. The incidence of this syndrome is lowered when the patient is prehydrated with a liter of Ringer lactate solution, or some other crystalloid solution, infused intravenously. Treatment consists in keeping the patient recumbent and well hydrated. Abdominal binders may decrease the leak of cerebrospinal fluid, as may epidural infusions of Ringer lactate. In severe cases blood patch therapy is used. This consists of the injection of 5 to 10 ml of the patient's own blood into the epidural space to block the opening in the dura and stop the leakage of cerebrospinal fluid. Relief is obtained rapidly.
2. Bladder dysfunction is frequent.
3. Occasionally paresthesias in the lower limbs and abdomen develop, and sometimes there is a temporary loss or diminution of sensation in these areas.
4. It cannot be used in the management of early labor.
5. Nerve palsies occur, but may be secondary to unrelated causes

(nerves entrapped by the stirrups, entrapment of a nerve trunk by the forceps, or by the descending fetal head).
6. A rare complication is nerve damage such as chronic, progressive adhesive arachnoiditis, or transverse myelitis. These lead to paralysis in the lower parts of the body. The mechanism is obscure, and spinal anesthesia has not definitely been implicated.
7. In a few instances, the anesthetic solution has risen in the subarachnoid space high enough to produce difficulty with respiration.
8. The incidence of forceps deliveries has increased.
9. Maternal contraindications are similar to those described for epidural anesthesia.

Epidural and Intrathecal Narcotics

Because of high concentrations of opiate receptors in the spinal cord, narcotics have been injected into the subarachnoid and epidural spaces in an effort to block painful sensation while preserving motor and autonomic function.

Intrathecal narcotics have been found to be useful in the first stage of labor but inadequate in the second. Maternal side effects include nausea and vomiting, pruritis, decrease in respiration, and urinary retention. Fetal outcome has been good. This technique may be used in high-risk maternal cardiac diseases. The effects of epidural narcotics are similar. There have been good neurobehavioral results, and the technique lacks sympathetic block and subsequent hypotension. It may be useful for postcesarean section analgesia.

Transcutaneous Electrical Nerve Stimulation (TENS)

Early experience with this technique of analgesia has been encouraging. Relief is not optimal but narcotic requirements are decreased and there are no major side effects on mother, newborn, or the course of labor.

ANESTHESIA FOR CESAREAN SECTION

There is no single best anesthetic technique for cesarean section. The choice depends on the indication for operation, the prevalence of general maternal problems (e.g., cardiopulmonary disease, coagulopathy), the condition of the fetus, the availability of trained personnel, and the wishes of the patient.

The three main types of anesthesia are local, major conduction (spinal and epidural), and general.

Any anesthetic administered for a cesarean section can affect the fetus:

1. Direct effects of the drug may occur as a result of placental transfer to the fetal circulation.

2. Indirect compromise may take place as the result of reduction of uteroplacental flow of blood secondary to maternal hypotension, or by a direct constrictive effect that some anesthetic drugs have on the uterine blood vessels.

Local Anesthesia

With refinements in general and major conduction anesthesia, the popularity of this technique has declined considerably.

Several agents are available, among them procaine as a 0.5 percent solution, lidocaine, and mepivacaine. Addition of adrenalin to make a dilution of 1:200,000 delays absorption and prolongs the effect of the anesthetic. About 300 ml of solution is used.

Technique

A skin wheal is made just below the umbilicus with a 25 gauge needle. A 20 gauge needle, 4 inches long, is used to inject the solution intradermally and subcutaneously down to the pubic symphysis for a distance of about 3 cm on each side of the midline. After a few minutes have passed the skin and subcutaneous tissue are incised. The tissue must be handled gently and a minimum amount of traction exerted.

The anterior sheath of the rectus muscle is infiltrated in the same way, in the midline and out to the sides to block the nerves at the lateral margins of the recti. A large amount of solution is placed in the suprapubic region, since this is the area of highest sensitivity. The fascia is then incised.

The peritoneum is anesthetized and opened to expose the uterus. About 50 to 60 ml of anesthetic is injected under the bladder flap and spread with the fingers under the bladder and to the sides. The bladder peritoneum is cut and pushed caudad.

The uterus is then opened, the baby extracted, the placenta removed, and the incision closed. The nervous patient may be put to sleep with Pentothal just prior to incision of the uterus.

Advantages

Except for the rare instance of sensitivity to the anesthetic agent or intravascular injection, the method is reasonably safe for the mother and does not depress the fetus. It may be useful in the absence of trained anesthetic personnel.

Disadvantages

1. The patient must be prepared to accept this type of anesthetic. It is not suitable for the nervous or excitable woman.
2. The method is time consuming; it is not good for cases in which rapid operating is necessary.

3. The surgeon must be gentle, patient, and willing to accept slow operating.
4. Because of the large amounts of local anesthetic used, systemic toxicity is a major concern. Full resuscitative facilities must be readily available.
5. Analgesia is often inadequate, and may require some form of supplementation.

General Anesthesia

Although some studies have revealed poorer neonatal outcome with general as compared to other anesthetic techniques, it is accepted to be a good method providing that maternal cardiovascular stability is maintained and excessive fetal depression is avoided. As described earlier, general anesthesia in the parturient is associated with an increased risk of gastric aspiration, and steps to counteract this must be taken.

Technique

1. Prophylaxis against the aspiration of gastric acid can be achieved by giving cimetidine (300 mg intramuscularly 1 to 3 hours before surgery), ranitidine (a longer-acting agent), or sodium citrate (30 ml of a 0.3 M solution by mouth). With elective cesarean section more time is available to tailor the antacid regimen.
2. An intravenous infusion of a balanced salt solution such as Ringer lactate is set up.
3. The patient is given 100 percent oxygen by mask for 2 to 3 minutes.
4. A wedge is placed under the right hip to avoid aortocaval compression.
5. Anesthesia is induced with thiopentone 3 to 4 mg/kg or ketamine 1 mg/kg.
6. Cricoid pressure is applied by a trained assistant.
7. Succinylcholine, 100 mg, is given intravenously as a bolus to promote muscular relaxation.
8. An endotracheal tube is inserted and the cuff inflated.
9. Anesthesia is maintained with nitrous oxide and oxygen in a 50:50 mixture. Small amounts of volatile agent may be safely added to deepen anesthesia and diminish recall. An intravenous infusion of succinylcholine may be used to maintain muscular relaxation.
10. There are differences of opinion as to the ideal interval between the induction of general anesthesia and the delivery of the infant. Some workers feel that this interval should be no longer than 4 minutes, or mild depression may occur. In one study it was found that the number of babies with an Apgar score of under 7 increased progressively as the induction to delivery period was prolonged. The advice

was given that the patient should be prepped and draped before anesthesia is commenced so that there will be no delay once the anesthesia is induced. Other workers have pointed out that, provided there is no maternal hypotension and the anesthetic mixture contains 65 to 70 percent oxygen, prolongation of the induction to delivery interval up to 30 minutes does not alter the acid-base status of the newborn significantly. It is claimed that the crucial factor is the uterine incision to delivery interval. If the latter is less than 1.5 minutes the Apgar scores are excellent. When this period is longer than 3 minutes the incidence of depressed babies and poorer acid-base values is increased. Reasons for this outcome include: (1) Prolonged uterine manipulation may affect adversely uteroplacental and umbilical cord circulation. (2) Pressure on the uterus may cause compression of the aorta or vena cava and lead to interference with placental perfusion. (3) Amniotic fluid may be inhaled when the fetus gasps inside of the uterus. (4) The head may be compressed if there is difficulty and delay in extracting it.

11. Once the infant is delivered, intravenous narcotics can be used to supplement the anesthetic. The patient is extubated at the end of the case when she is fully awake and full muscular strength has returned.

Advantages

1. It is acceptable to the majority of patients.
2. There is usually no hypotension.
3. It is effective in cases such as fetal distress and maternal hemorrhage when rapid delivery is needed.

Disadvantages

1. Aspiration, the largest single cause of maternal mortality in cesarean section is more likely when the patient is rendered unconscious. The prophylactic measures mentioned must be undertaken.
2. The timing must be accurate or fetal depression can occur.
3. The father is generally not permitted in the operating suite during the conduct of a general anesthetic.
4. Maternal/neonatal bonding is delayed.

Lumbar Epidural or Spinal Anesthesia

Technique

This has been described in a previous section.

Advantages

1. The patient remains awake. The risk of gastric aspiration is virtually eliminated.
2. If maternal hypotension is prevented, fetal outcome is excellent.
3. The father is often allowed in the delivery suite.
4. Maternal/fetal bonding is immediate.
5. Uterine incision to delivery time is a less important factor in fetal outcome than with general anesthesia. This may be secondary to vasodilatation of the placental blood vessels secondary to the epidural block.

Disadvantages

1. Maternal hypotension can lead to fetal depression. Prehydration with 1 to 2 liters of a solution, such as Ringer lactate, and avoidance of aortocaval compression are mandatory. Intravenous ephedrine can be used when these measures are inadequate.
2. Systemic local anesthetic toxicity and inadvertent high spinal anesthetic are possible complications.
3. Because it takes 30 to 60 minutes to establish a block, it is unsatisfactory when rapid delivery is needed.

In most situations, properly conducted anesthesia, whether general or regional, is associated with good fetal outcome. Follow-up studies of up to 4 years of age have shown no difference in fetal outcome between the various anesthetic techniques.

PRETERM LABOR

The preterm infant is more susceptible to the depressant effects of sedatives, analgesics, and general anesthetics than is his term counterpart. The preterm infant has less protein to bind drugs and has increased bilirubin to compete for binding so that higher concentrations of free compounds are able to enter the central nervous system, producing greater effects. In addition, there is reduced ability to metabolize and excrete these drugs, and the effects may, therefore, be prolonged. Even small amounts of these agents can depress the respiratory center of the small fetus to the extent of causing severe apnea and asphyxia. Delay in the onset of regular breathing can result in anoxic brain damage.

It is best to avoid prescribing sedatives and analgesics during labor and general anesthesia for the delivery. Continuous lumbar epidural block is the best form of analgesia and anesthesia for preterm labor. Not only is pain relieved, but the incidence of precipitous deliveries, which can cause intracranial bleeding as a result of rapid decompression of the head, is reduced. Oxygen can be given during the delivery to protect the fetus. If epidural block is not used, the delivery can be managed by the use of pudendal block or local infiltration. Cesarean section is carried out best under conduction anesthesia. Note must be made of any drugs used to stop preterm labor. These include beta sympathetic stimulants, methylxanthines, and alcohol. Steroids may have been given in an attempt to induce fetal lung maturation.

MULTIPLE GESTATION

In the presence of twins no special provisions are needed, unless preeclampsia is present. Good perineal relaxation is needed at delivery and this can be achieved with epidural blockade.

With greater numbers of "passengers," problems include:

1. Profound supine hypotension
2. Increased risk of maternal aspiration
3. More marked anemia
4. Premature fetus

Epidural anesthesia has been used successfully for labor, delivery, and cesarean section, but has definite limitations when the above factors are considered. General anesthesia may offer more controlled conditions.

ANTEPARTUM HEMORRHAGE

As a general rule, it may be stated that patients who are bleeding actively, are in hypovolemic shock or have the potential to develop shock, or who need to be delivered rapidly should not be given regional anesthesia. General anesthesia is safer in these instances.

Placenta Previa

The double set-up examination in the operating room should be performed under general anesthesia. If cesarean section is necessary, the anesthesia is maintained.

Abruptio Placentae

An added danger in this condition results from the possible development of consumption coagulopathies resulting in hypofibrinogenemia, thrombocytopenia, and deficiencies of factors V and VIII. Operative deliveries for placental abruption are carried out best under general anesthesia.

MEDICAL COMPLICATIONS OF PREGNANCY

Preeclampsia, Eclampsia

Preeclampsia is defined as hypertension with proteinuria and generalized edema, occurring after the 20th week of gestation. Eclampsia denotes the occurrence of convulsions. The definitive treatment is termination of the pregnancy.

Labor

The management of labor in the mild preeclamptic is best achieved with lumbar epidural analgesia.

Advantages of this technique are:

1. Analgesia is excellent, and the rises in blood pressure with contractions are blunted.
2. Placental perfusion may actually improve.
3. No extra CNS depressants are added to a fetus already at risk.
4. Relaxation is provided if forceps are needed.

Contraindications to this technique are:

1. Coagulopathy
2. Precipitate labor
3. Hypovolemic shock
4. Fetal distress that demands immediate delivery
5. Infection at the site of needle injection
6. Patient refusal

In severe preeclamptics epidural analgesia is still a useful technique, but certain constraints must be adhered to:

1. The above contraindications still apply.
2. Central nervous system hyperexcitability must be controlled. Magnesium sulphate is the drug of choice.
3. The patient's blood pressure and fluid balance must be corrected; the use of invasive hemodynamic monitoring is becoming more prevalent.
4. Epinephrine should not be added to local anesthetic solutions.
5. Fetal monitoring must be used.
6. The mother is given oxygen.
7. A wedge is placed under her right hip.

8. The epidural should not be used merely as a means of lowering blood pressure.

If epidural analgesia is not feasible, low doses of analgesics and tranquilizers may be used. Paracervical block is condemned because of the high incidence of fetal depression.

Vaginal Delivery
Lumbar epidural is best, but in its absence spontaneous delivery may be managed with pudendal block and local infiltration, combined with inhalational analgesia. If pain control is not adequate, or relaxation is needed for operative delivery, general anesthesia may be administered.

Cesarean Section
Both general and epidural anesthesia have their advantages and disadvantages. With general anesthesia intubation may be difficult because of laryngeal edema. Endotracheal intubation may produce an exaggerated hypertensive response, with adverse stress on the central nervous system and the cardiovascular system. Central nervous system depressants are circulated to an already compromised fetus. Epidural anesthesia is effective but is poorly suited to the uncontrolled situation. Maternal cardiovascular status must be controlled beforehand. Hypotension secondary to sympathetic block is managed with oxygen, fluids, left lateral tilt, and the judicious use of intravenous ephedrine.

Diabetes Mellitus

Particular problems in the management of the diabetic patient are preeclampsia, placental insufficiency, neuropathy, nephropathy, and difficulty in estimating insulin requirements.

Labor
Continuous lumbar epidural block provides excellent relief of pain in labor. There is some evidence that this technique reduces maternal endogenous catecholemines during labor, improves the perfusion of the placenta, and reduces fetal acidosis. Small doses of narcotics will provide moderate analgesia when epidural block is not available.

Vaginal Delivery

Spontaneous Delivery. Epidural anesthesia or pudendal block–local infiltration are best for spontaneous births.

Forceps Delivery. Epidural anesthesia is preferred. When it is unavailable and local anesthesia is insufficient, low spinal (saddle block) or general anesthesia may be used.

Cesarean Section

Again both regional and general techniques have their advocates. General anesthesia can be conducted safely, with good neonatal outcome. Epidural anesthesia may result in significant hypotension because of the high sympathetic block, and the possibility of a preexisting autonomic neuropathy. This augments the tendency for diabetic mothers to produce acidotic neonates.If epidural analgesia is used: (1) A separate intravenous line should be used for the maintenance glucose and insulin and the crystalloid used to counteract hypotension. (2) Left lateral tilt and maternal oxygen administration must be used. (3) Maternal hypotension should be aggressively treated. (4) Fetal monitoring is essential.

Cardiac Disease

Cardiac disease has an incidence of 0.5 to 2 percent in childbearing women, and falls into one of two major categories: congenital or acquired.

Congenital heart disease may be further characterized by either a left-to-right shunt (acyanotic) or a right-to-left shunt (cyanotic). In the former, labor and delivery are well tolerated. Antibiotics are given to protect against the development of subacute bacterial endocarditis. In the latter, the fluctuating hemodynamic state of pregnancy, labor, and delivery is poorly tolerated. There is a high degree of fetal wastage and the maternal death rate may reach 50 percent.

The most common form of acquired heart disease in pregnancy is rheumatic mitral stenosis. The ability of the patient to tolerate the added hemodynamic stresses depends on the degree of mitral obstruction. General treatment includes salt restriction, digitalization, diuretics, and antibiotic prophylaxis.

Labor and Delivery

The treatment of acyanotic patients and those with mild mitral stenosis poses no special problems. Epidural anesthesia may be used safely. In the presence of cyanotic heart disease or tight mitral stenosis, management is fraught with danger. Pain must be controlled in order to avoid stressing an already taxed cardiovascular system. Major conduction anesthesia may be contraindicated, especially if the patient is receiving anticoagulants. Relief is obtained with a careful titration of sedatives, analgesics, inhalational agents, paracervical and pudendal blocks. The mother is given oxygen by mask and, depending on the severity of the cardiac disease, invasive hemodynamic monitoring may be indicated. Cesarean section is managed best with general anesthesia.

BIBLIOGRAPHY

Abboud TK, Afrasiabi A, Sarkis F, et al: Continuous infusion epidural analgesia in parturients receiving bupivacaine, chlorprocaine, lidocaine—maternal, fetal, and neonatal effects. Anesth Analg 63:421, 1984

Abboud TK, Kim KC, Noueihed R, et al: Epidural bupivacaine, chlorprocaine, or lidocaine for cesarean section—maternal and neonatal effects. Anesth Analg 62:914, 1983

Abboud TK, Swee SK, Miller F, et al: Maternal, fetal, and neonatal responses after epidural anesthesia with bupivacaine, 2-chlorprocaine, or lidocaine. Anesth Analg 61:638, 1982

Biehl DR: Obstetrical anesthesia update—1984. Canad Anaesth Soc J 31:523 1984

Crawford JS, Davies P: Status of neonates delivered by elective cesarean section. Brit J Anaesth 54:1015, 1982

Datta S, Alper MH: Anesthesia for cesarean section. Anesthesiology 53:142, 1980

Gale R, Zalkinder-Luboshitz I, Slater PE: Increased neonatal risk from the use of general anesthesia in emergency cesarean section—a retrospective analysis. J Reprod Med 27: 715, 1982

Gibbs CP, Spohr L, Schmidt D: The effectiveness of sodium citrate as an antacid. Anesthesiology 57:44, 1982

Hodgkinson R, Glassenberg R, Joyce TH, et al: Comparison of cimetidine with antacid for safety and effectiveness in reducing gastric acidity before elective cesarean section. Anesthesiology 59:86 1983

Kuhnert BR, Harrison MJ, Linn PL, et al: Effect of maternal epidural anesthesia on neonatal behavior. Anesth Analg 64:301, 1984

McCauley DM, Moor J, McCaughey W, et al: Ranitidine as an antacid before elective cesarean section. Anesthesiology 38:108, 1983

Mendelson CL: Aspiration of stomach contents into the lungs during obstetric anesthesia. Am J Obstet Gynecol 52:191, 1946

Nelson NM, Enkin MW, Saigal S, et al: A randomized clinical trial of the Leboyer approach to childbirth. N Engl J Med 302:655, 1980

Ralson DH, Shnider SM: The fetal and neonatal effect of regional anesthesia in obstetrics. Anesthesiology 48:34, 1978

Sellick BA: Cricoid pressure to control regurgitation of stomach contents during induction of anesthesia. Lancet 2:404, 1961

Shnider SM, Wright RG, Levinson G, et al: Uterine blood flow and plasma norepinephrine changes during maternal stress in the pregnant ewe. Anesthesiology 50:529, 1979

Warren TM, Datta S, Ostheimer G: Comparison of the maternal and neonatal effects of halothane, enflurane, and isoflurane for cesarean delivery. Anesth Analg 62:516, 1983

Wright JP: Anesthetic consideration in preeclampsia–eclampsia. Anesth Analg 63:590, 1983

Wynne JW, Modell J: Respiratory aspiration of stomach contents. Ann Int Med 87:466, 1977

Zagorzycki MT: General anesthesia in cesarean section. Effect on mother and neonate. Obstet Gynecol Surg 39:134, 1984

32

Postpartum Hemorrhage

The term postpartum hemorrhage, in its wider meaning, includes all bleeding following the birth of the baby: before, during, and after the delivery of the placenta. By definition, loss of over 500 ml of blood during the first 24 hours constitutes postpartum hemorrhage. After 24 hours it is called late postpartum hemorrhage. The incidence of postpartum hemorrhage is about 10 percent.

At normal delivery an average of 200 ml of blood is lost. Episiotomy raises this figure by 100 ml and sometimes more. Pregnant women have an increased amount of blood and fluid, enabling the healthy patient to lose 500 ml without serious effect. To the anemic patient, however, an even smaller amount of bleeding can be dangerous.

CLINICAL FEATURES

Clinical Picture

The clinical picture is one of continuing bleeding and gradual deterioration. The pulse becomes rapid and weak; the blood pressure falls; the patient turns pale and cold; and there is shortness of breath, air hunger, sweating, and finally coma and death. A treacherous feature of the situation is that because of compensatory vascular mechanisms the pulse and blood pressure may show only moderate change for some time. Then suddenly the compensatory function can no longer be maintained, the pulse rises quickly, the blood pressure drops suddenly, and the patient is in hypovolemic shock. The uterine cavity can fill up with a considerable amount of blood, which is lost to the patient even though the external hemorrhage may not be alarming.

Danger of Postpartum Hemorrhage

The danger of postpartum hemorrhage is twofold. First, the resultant anemia weakens the patient, lowers her resistance, and predisposes to puerperal infection. Second, if the loss of blood is not arrested, death will be the final result.

Studies of Maternal Deaths

Studies of maternal deaths show that women have died from continuous bleeding of amounts which at the times were not alarming. It is not the sudden gush that kills, but the steady trickle. In a large series of cases Beacham found that the average interval between delivery and death was 5 hours 20 minutes. No woman died within 1 hour 30 minutes of giving birth. This suggests that there is adequate time for effective therapy if the patient has been observed carefully, the diagnosis made early, and proper treatment instituted.

ETIOLOGY

The causes of postpartum hemorrhage fall into four main groups.

Uterine Atony

The control of postpartum bleeding is by contraction and retraction of the myometrial fibers. This causes kinking of the blood vessels and so cuts off flow to the placental site. Failure of this mechanism, resulting from disordered myometrial function, is called uterine atony and is the main cause of postpartum hemorrhage. While the occasional case of postpartum uterine atony is completely unexpected, in many instances the presence of predisposing factors alerts the observant physician to the possibility of trouble.

1. *Uterine dysfunction:* Primary uterine atony is an intrinsic dysfunction of the uterus.
2. *Mismanagement of the placental stage:* The most common error is to try to hurry the third stage. Kneading and squeezing the uterus interferes with the physiologic mechanism of placental detachment and may cause partial placental separation with resultant bleeding.
3. *Anesthesia:* Deep and prolonged inhalation anesthesia is a common cause. There is excessive relaxation of the myometrium, failure of contraction and retraction, uterine atony, and postpartum hemorrhage.
4. *Ineffective uterine action:* Ineffective uterine action during the

first two stages of labor is likely to be followed by poor contraction and retraction during the third stage.

5. *Overdistention of the uterus:* The uterus that has been overdistended by conditions such as large baby, multiple pregnancy, and polyhydramnios has a tendency to contract poorly.

6. *Exhaustion from prolonged labor:* Not only is the tired uterus likely to contract weakly after delivery of the baby, but the wornout mother is less able to stand loss of blood.

7. *Multiparity:* The uterus that has borne many children is prone to inefficient action during all stages of labor.

8. *Myomas of the uterus:* By interfering with proper contraction and retraction, uterine myomas predispose to hemorrhage.

9. *Operative deliveries:* This includes operative procedures such as midforceps and version and extraction.

Trauma and Lacerations

Considerable bleeding can take place from tears sustained during normal and operative deliveries. The birth canal should be inspected after each delivery so that the sources of bleeding can be controlled.

Sites of hemorrhage include:

1. Episiotomy. Blood loss may reach 200 ml. When arterioles or large varicose veins are cut or torn the amount of blood lost can be considerably more. Hence bleeding vessels should be clamped immediately to conserve blood.
2. Vulva, vagina, and cervix.
3. Ruptured uterus.
4. Uterine inversion.
5. Puerperal hematomas.

In addition, other factors operate to cause an excessive loss of blood where there is trauma to the birth canal. These include:

1. Prolonged interval between performance of the episiotomy and delivery of the child.
2. Undue delay from birth of the baby to repair of the episiotomy.
3. Failure to secure a bleeding vessel at the apex of the episiotomy.
4. Neglecting to inspect the upper vagina and cervix.
5. Nonappreciation of the possibility of multiple sites of injury.
6. Undue reliance on oxytocic agents accompanied by too long a delay in exploring the uterus.

Retained Placenta

Retention in the uterus of part or all of the placenta interferes with contraction and retraction, keeps the blood sinuses open, and leads to postpartum hemorrhage. Once part of the placenta has separated from the uterine wall, there is bleeding from that area. The part of the placenta that is still attached prevents proper retraction, and bleeding goes on until the rest of the organ has separated and is expelled.

The retention of the whole placenta, part of it, a succenturiate lobe, a single cotyledon, or a fragment of placenta can cause postpartum bleeding. In some cases there is placenta accreta. There is no correlation between the amount of placenta retained and the severity of the hemorrhage. The important consideration is the degree of adherence.

Bleeding Disorders

Any of the hemorrhagic diseases (blood dyscrasias) can affect pregnant women and occasionally are responsible for postpartum hemorrhage.

Afibrinogenemia or hypofibrinogenemia may follow abruptio placentae, prolonged retention in utero of a dead fetus, and amniotic fluid embolism. One etiologic theory postulates that thromboplastic material arising from the degeneration and autolysis of the decidua and placenta may enter the maternal circulation and give rise to intravascular coagulation and loss of circulating fibrinogen. The condition, a failure of the clotting mechanism, causes bleeding that cannot be arrested by the measures usually employed to control hemorrhage.

INVESTIGATION

1. To obtain a reasonable idea of the amount of blood lost, an estimate is made and the figure doubled.
2. The uterine fundus is palpated frequently to make certain it is not filling up with blood.
3. The uterine cavity is explored both for placental remnants and for uterine rupture.
4. The vulva, vagina, and cervix are examined carefully for lacerations.
5. The pulse and blood pressure are measured and recorded.
6. A sample of blood is observed for clotting.

TREATMENT

Prophylaxis

1. Every pregnant woman should know her blood group.
2. Antepartum anemia is treated.

3. Certain patients are susceptible to and certain conditions predispose to postpartum hemorrhage. These include:
   a. Multiparity
   b. History of postpartum hemorrhage or manual removal of the placenta
   c. Abruptio placentae
   d. Placenta previa
   e. Multiple pregnancy
   f. Polyhydramnios
   g. Intrauterine death with prolonged retention of dead fetus
   h. Prolonged labor
   i. Difficult forceps delivery
   j. Version and extraction
   k. Breech extraction
   l. Cesarean section
4. In cases where uterine atony is anticipated, an intravenous infusion is set up before the delivery and oxytocin added to ensure good uterine contractions. This is continued for at least 1 hour post partum.
5. Excessive and prolonged inhalatory anesthesia should be avoided.
6. As long as the child is in good condition and there is no need for rapid extraction, the body is delivered slowly. This facilitates placental separation and permits the uterus to retract sufficiently to control bleeding from the placental site.
7. Once the placenta has separated it should be expelled.
8. Squeezing or kneading the uterus before the placenta has separated is traumatic and harmful.
9. Careful postpartum observation of the patient is made, and the uterine fundus is palpated to prevent its filling with blood. The patient remains in the delivery room for at least 1 hour postpartum.
10. Fibrinogen studies are done in cases of placental abruption and retained dead fetus.
11. When hemorrhage is anticipated adequate amounts of blood should be cross-matched and available.

Supportive Measures

1. The key to successful treatment is the transfusion of blood. The amount must be adequate to replace at least the amount lost. Usually a minimum of 1 liter is needed, and it is given quickly. When response to blood replacement is not satisfactory the following conditions must be considered:

    a. Continued unappreciated ooze
    b. Bleeding into an atonic uterus
    c. Silent filling of the vagina
    d. Bleeding behind and into a uterine pack
    e. Hematoma formation
    f. Intraperitoneal bleeding as with ruptured uterus
    g. Afibrinogenemia or hypofibrinogenemia
2. Until blood is available plasma expanders are used.
3. If the blood pressure is falling, the foot of the table is elevated.
4. General anesthesia should be discontinued and oxygen given by face mask.
5. Warmth is provided by blankets.
6. Morphine is given by hypodermic injection.
7. If bleeding continues, the coagulation factors of the blood must be measured and deficiencies corrected.

Placental Bleeding

In the presence of excessive bleeding associated with the third stage, no time should be wasted. Manual removal of the placenta is carried out immediately and oxytocics given. The uterus should not be manhandled in efforts to squeeze out the placenta.

Uterine Atony

Uterine Massage. The uterine fundus is massaged through the abdomen.

Ergometrine. Ergometrine 0.125 or 0.25 mg is given intravenously and/ or 0.5 mg intramuscularly.

Oxytocin. Oxytocin can be given intramuscularly, but the best method is by an intravenous drip containing 20 units of oxytocin in a liter of fluid. This is run at a speed sufficient to keep the uterus contracted.

Uterine Exploration. Manual exploration of the uterus is carried out, and blood clots and fragments of placenta and membrane are removed.

Lacerations. The cervix, vagina, and vulva are examined for lacerations.

Uterine Compression. Bimanual compression of the uterus (Fig. 1) is a valuable method of controlling uterine atonic bleeding. One hand is placed in the vagina against the anterior wall of the uterus. Pressure is exerted against the posterior aspect of the uterus by the other hand through the abdomen. With a rotatory motion the uterus is compressed and massaged between the two hands. This provides twice the amount of uterine stimulation that can be achieved by abdominal massage alone. In addition, compression of the venous sinuses can be effected and the flow of blood reduced. As part of this procedure, the atonic uterus is elevated, anteverted, and anteflexed.

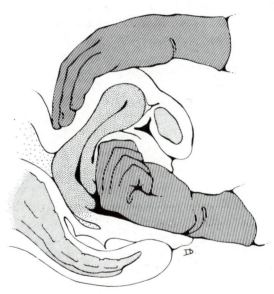

Figure 1. Bimanual compression of the uterus.

Uterine Packing. Packing the uterine cavity is a controversial subject (Fig. 2). Most authorities condemn its use in that the procedure is unphysiologic. Up to this point attempts had been made to empty the uterus; now it is to be filled. It is unlikely that a uterus that does not respond to powerful oxytocic drugs will be stimulated to contract by the gauze pack. It is impossible to pack an atonic uterus so tightly that the blood sinuses are closed off. The uterus simply balloons and fills up with more blood. Thus the packing not only does no good but is dangerous in that it leads to a false sense of security by obscuring the flow of blood. Ten yards of 3-inch packing gauze absorbs 1000 ml of blood. Furthermore, packing favors infection.

Despite these antipacking arguments, many obstetricians believe that it is worth trying to control bleeding by this method before more radical measures are employed. The patient must be observed carefully. Deterioration of the vital signs, ballooning of the uterus, or continuation of the bleeding are signs that the pack is ineffective and must be removed. Packing must be done properly. One or two 5- or 10-yard rolls of gauze are needed. With one hand on the abdomen the operator steadies the uterine fundus, while the pack is pushed through the cervix and into the cavity of the uterus with the fingers of the other hand. The gauze is placed first into one corner of the uterus and then the other, so coming down the cavity from side to side. The uterus must be packed tightly. Then the vagina is packed. A large, firm pad is placed on the abdomen above the uterus, and a tight abdominal and perineal binder is applied. The gauze packing is removed in 12 hours.

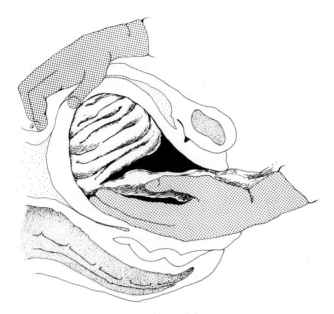

Figure 2. Packing of the uterus.

Compression of Aorta. In thin women compression of the aorta against the spine may slow down the bleeding.

Prostaglandin. Prostaglandins appear to be involved in postpartum hemostasis by means of their versatile biologic properties, including the function of platelets, vasoactive effects, and, especially, myometrial stimulation. These drugs have a powerful ecbolic effect. Postpartum hemorrhage resulting from uterine atony has been treated by vaginal suppositories containing 20 mg of PGE_2, intramuscular injections of $PGF_{2\alpha}$ and direct intramyometrial injection of $PGF_{2\alpha}$. The latter technique is the most effective. The dose is 1 mg administered transabdominally into the myometrium. (A transvaginal approach has been used also.) A sustained uterine contraction develops rapidly and bleeding is reduced within 2 to 3 minutes. Side effects include nausea and hypertension, both of which are controlled easily. Care must be taken to avoid direct intravenous injection. In patients who have asthma or hypertension a test dose of 0.25 mg should be tried before giving the full amount (Fig. 3).

Embolization of Pelvic Arteries. This technique can be used instead of, or after failure of, hysterectomy or ligation of the internal iliac artery for the treatment of pelvic hemorrhage. Under radiologic angiographic control, a polyethylene catheter is introduced into the aorta via the right femoral artery. Each internal iliac artery is catheterized and occluded with small (2 to 3 mm) fragments of Gelfoam. In situations of pelvic hemorrhage other than that caused by uterine atony the specific bleeding vessel can be identified and selectively embolized. The procedure can be carried out in less than 2 hours, and imposes little additional morbidity and no mortality. An advantage over internal iliac ligation is that the distal blood vessels are occluded, so that bleeding from reconstituted distal vessels is rare. In addition, the uterus is retained and further childbearing is possible.

Hysterectomy. If the bleeding continues, the abdomen must be opened and hysterectomy performed. Deaths following and during hysterectomy have been reported; these resulted from delaying the operation until the patient was nearly moribund. Performed in time, hysterectomy is effective and lifesaving.

Ligation of Uterine Arteries. Since most of the uterine blood is supplied by the uterine arteries, their ligation can control postpartum hemorrhage. The collateral supply is sufficient to maintain the viability of the organ. The abdomen is opened, the uterus is elevated by the surgeon's hand, and the area of the uterine vessels is exposed. Using a large nee-

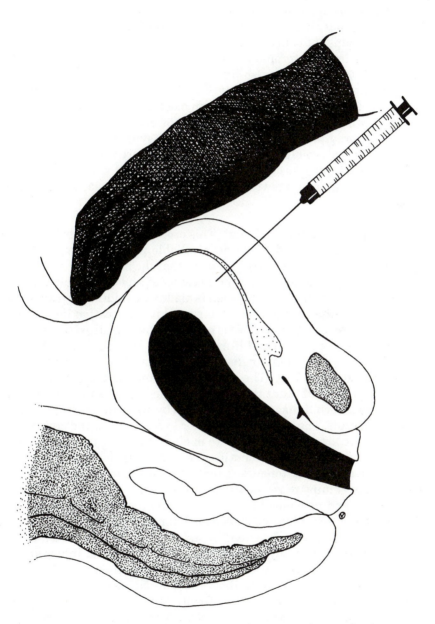

Figure 3. Transabdominal intramyometrial injection of prostaglandin.

dle and No. 1 chromic catgut, the suture is placed through the myometrium of the lower segment of the uterus, 2 to 3 cm medial to the vessels. It is brought out through the avascular area of the broad ligament. A substantial amount of myometrium is included in the suture to occlude some of the inferior coronary branches of the uterine artery. In most cases the uterine vein is also ligated, but the hypertrophied ovarian veins drain the uterus adequately. The vessels are ligated, but not divided. Recanalization will take place in most cases. The uterus becomes blanched with a pink hue, and bleeding subsides. Subsequent menstruation and pregnancy are unaffected. Transvaginal ligation of the uterine arteries is a blind and hazardous procedure which is not recommended. Subsequent pregnancy has been successful without the occurrence of intrauterine growth retardation, preeclampsia, or any other problems.

Ligation of Internal Iliac Arteries.   This procedure may be performed in any situation associated with uncontrollable pelvic bleeding (Fig. 4). The collateral circulation is so extensive that the pelvic arterial system is never deprived of blood, and no necrosis of any of the pelvic tissue takes place. Entry into the abdomen is made by a midline or transverse incision. First the common iliac artery and its bifurcation into the external and internal iliac arteries is palpated and visualized through the posterior peritoneum. The bifurcation feels like the letter Y. The branch coming off at right angles is the internal iliac artery; it courses medially and posteriorly. The continuing branch is the external iliac artery. It is essential that these two branches be identified positively. Should the external iliac artery be ligated by accident, loss of the lower limb may result. The ureter lies anterior to the vessels, and crosses the common iliac artery from lateral to medial at a point just proximal to the bifurcation. It must be identified to prevent its being damaged.

The posterior peritoneum is tented and incised in a longitudinal direction, beginning proximal to the bifurcation of the common iliac artery and extending caudad for 4 to 6 cm. The incision is lateral to the ureter. The ureter is located on the medial peritoneal flap and usually remains attached to it. The external and internal iliac arteries must be reidentified to avoid any error. Care is taken to avoid injury to the veins. The internal iliac artery is elevated from the vein gently and with care to avoid damage to the vein. Two No. 2–0 silk sutures are placed beneath the artery and tied firmly, but gently. The artery is not transected. The peritoneum is closed with interrupted 3–0 catgut. A continuous suture might kink the ureter. The procedure is repeated on the other side.

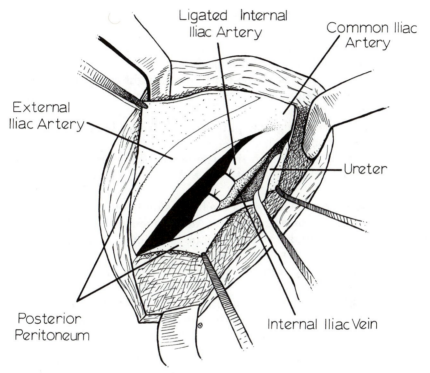

Figure 4. Ligation of internal iliac artery.

Umbrella Pack Following Total Hysterectomy

Described by Logothetopulos in 1925, the umbrella pack (Fig. 5) is of value in desperate situations where, after hysterectomy, pelvic bleeding is uncontrollable even by such drastic measures as ligation of the internal iliac arteries.

Technique

1. The outside of the pack is a 24-inch square piece of nonadhesive nylon (or cotton).
2. Into the center of this cloth is placed 15 to 20 yards of firm, noncompressible 2-inch gauze packing.
3. The four corners of the cloth are brought together to form a funnel-shaped sling, similar to a parachute, with the gauze packing inside.
4. The end of the gauze packing put in last is left protruding through the funnel.
5. The pack is placed in the true pelvis (the uterus having been removed previously) with the tail coming out through the vagina.
6. Traction on the tail pulls the bolus snugly into the pelvis, compressing the bleeding points. An intravenous bottle containing 1000 ml of fluid is attached to the tail to provide traction. Sometimes two bottles are needed.
7. Traction is maintained for 24 hours. The pack is left in for 36 hours.
8. The pack is removed by pulling on the end of the gauze which is outside the vagina. Once the gauze is removed the nylon cloth container collapses and comes out easily.

Insertion of the pack is accomplished in one of two ways. Using the abdominal technique (Fig. 5A), the pack is formed outside of the patient and is inserted via the abdominal incision. A dressing forceps is passed up through the vagina, the tail of the pack is grasped, and it is pulled down and out. For the vaginal application (Fig. 5B),the nylon square is held in front of the vagina, and the center is pushed up gradually through the vagina and into the pelvis by packing the gauze into the cloth with a ring forceps (Fig. 5C).

Complications

1. Tangling of the gauze within the cloth makes its removal difficult.
2. The cloth may stick to the raw surfaces of the pelvis. Hence nonadherent nylon is best.

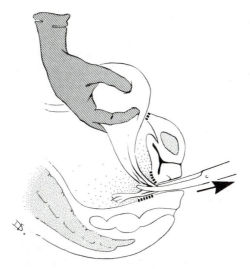

Figure 5A. Umbrella pack. Insertion through the abdominal incision during laparotomy. The tail of the pack is pulled down through the vagina.

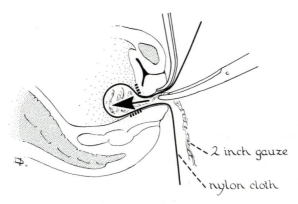

Figure 5B. Umbrella pack. Insertion through the vagina. The gauze is packed inside the nylon cloth.

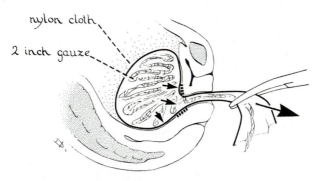

Figure 5C. Umbrella pack in place. Traction on the tail of the pack compresses the bleeding points.

3. In rare cases the flow of urine is obstructed.
4. Serious infection has not been encountered; but where life-threatening hemorrhage is present, infection is a secondary consideration.

Lacerations

1. Rupture of the uterus necessitates laparotomy with either repair of the tear or hysterectomy.
2. Lacerations of the cervix, vagina, and vulva are repaired and the bleeding controlled with figure-8 sutures.
3. In some cases the bleeding from the vaginal tears cannot be controlled with sutures. Where there are large varicosities each passage of the needle through the tissue seems to provoke fresh bleeding. In such cases the vagina should be packed firmly with gauze that is left in for 24 hours.
4. Rarely, bleeding from a small superficial laceration in the lower uterine segment can be controlled by packing.

PITUITARY INSUFFICIENCY

Insufficiency of the anterior lobe of the pituitary gland was described by Simmonds in 1914. In 1937 Sheehan described the syndrome in women of childbearing age. Symptoms include:

1. Mammary involution and failure to lactate.
2. Weakness and lethargy.
3. Hypersensitivity to cold.
4. Diminished sweating.
5. Excessive involution of the uterus.
6. Atrophy of the external genitalia.
7. Amenorrhea or oligomenorrhea.
8. Loss of body hair, including the pubic area.
9. Absence of menopausal symptoms.
10. Later signs of failure of the thyroid and adrenal glands may appear.

The condition is initiated by severe shock, the result of massive hemorrhage. The pituitary gland undergoes ischemia followed by necrosis. From 5 to 99 percent of the anterior lobe may be affected. As long as 10 percent of the gland is left in a functioning state, the patient will be in a reasonably normal condition. In severe cases death may occur. In less acute situations the patient can live for years in a subnormal state, a prey to infection.

The exact nature of the vascular disturbance is not known. Possible conditions include:

1. Arterial spasm
2. Interruption of the portal circulation of the pituitary
3. Coagulation in the capillaries
4. Venous thrombosis
5. Disseminated intravascular coagulation.

LATE POSTPARTUM HEMORRHAGE

Late postpartum hemorrhage is the loss of 500 ml of blood after the first 24 hours and within 6 weeks. While most of these episodes occur by the 2lst day, the majority take place between the 4th and 9th postpartum days. The incidence is around 1 percent.

Nonuterine Bleeding

In a few cases the origin is the cervix, vagina, or vulva. Local infection leads to sloughing of sutures and dissolution of thrombi, with hemorrhage at the site of the episiotomy or lacerations. The amount of blood lost depends on the size of the vessels. Treatment includes cleaning out infected debris, suturing bleeding points, and if necessary, pressure packing the vagina. Blood transfusion is given as needed.

Uterine Bleeding

Etiology

1. Retained fragments of placenta.
2. Intrauterine infection.
3. Subinvolution of the uterus and the placental site.
4. Uterine myoma, especially when submucous.
5. Occasionally the use of estrogens to inhibit lactation results in profuse bleeding at the first postpartum menstrual period.

Mechanism of Bleeding

The exact sequence of events is not known, but some type of subinvolution is present. Three probable factors are: (1) late detachment of thrombi at the placental site, with reopening of the vascular sinuses; (2) abnormalities in the separation of the decidua vera; and (3) intrauterine infection, leading to dissolution of the thromboses in the vessels. The basic mechanism is similar, regardless of whether placental tissue has been retained.

Clinical Picture

The amount of bleeding varies. Most of these patients require hospital-ization and many need blood transfusion. A few go into shock.

Treatment

1. Oxytocics are given.
2. If bleeding continues, curettage is performed carefully, so as not to perforate the soft uterus. In many cases no placental tissue is found, the histologic examination showing organized blood clot, decidual tissue, or fragments of muscle. The results of curettage are satisfactory regardless of whether placenta was present. Re-moval of the inflamed tissue with its superficial bleeding ves-sels permits the uterus to contract around the deeper, healthier vessels, thus producing more effective hemostasis.
3. Blood is replaced by transfusion.
4. Antibiotics are given to control infection.
5. Repeat curettage may be necessary.
6. If all other treatment fails, hysterectomy is performed.

ETIOLOGY OF SHOCK IN OBSTETRICS

Direct Obstetric Causes

Placental Site

1. Abortion
2. Placenta previa
3. Abruptio placentae
4. Retained placenta
5. Postpartum uterine atony

Trauma

1. Lacerations of vagina and vulva
2. Uterine rupture
3. Uterine inversion

Extraperitoneal

1. Broad ligament hematoma
2. Paravertebral hematoma

Intraperitoneal

1. Ectopic pregnancy

Related Obstetric Conditions

1. Embolism
   a. Thrombotic
   b. Amniotic
   c. Air
2. Eclampsia
3. Sepsis
4. Neurogenic
5. Anesthetic complications
   a. Aspiration of gastric fluid (Mendelson syndrome)
   b. Extended spinal or regional block
6. Drug reactions

Nonobstetric Conditions

1. Cardiac, e.g., myocardial infarct
2. Respiratory, e.g., spontaneous pneumothorax
3. Cerebrovascular accidents
4. Abdominal causes
   a. Ruptured spleen
   b. Torsion or rupture of ovarian cyst
   c. Perforated peptic ulcer
   d. Acute pancreatitis

BIBLIOGRAPHY

Brown B, Heaston DK, Poulson AM, et al: Uncontrollable postpartum bleeding: A new approach to hemostasis through angiographic arterial embolization. Obstet Gynecol 54:361, 1979

Hertz RH, Sokol RJ, Dierker LJ: Treatment of postpartum uterine atony with prostaglandin E_2 vaginal suppositories. Obstet Gynecol 56:129, 1980

Hester JD: Postpartum hemorrhage and re-evaluation of uterine packing. Obstet Gynecol 45:501, 1975

Hibbard BM: Postoperative complications. Clin Obstet Gynecol 7:639, 1980

Jacobs MM, Arias F: Intramyometrial prostaglandin $F_{2\alpha}$ in the treatment of severe postpartum hemorrhage. Obstet Gynecol 55:665, 1980

O'Leary JL, O'Leary JA: Uterine artery ligation for control of post cesarean section hemorrhage. Obstet Gynecol 43:849, 1974

Pais SO, Glickman M, Schwartz P, et al: Embolization of pelvic arteries for control of postpartum hemorrhage. Obstet Gynecol 55:754, 1980

Toppozada M, El-Bossaty M, El-Rahman HA, et al: Control of intractable atonic postpartum hemorrhage by 15-methyl prostaglandin $F_{2\alpha}$. Obstet Gynecol 58:327, 1981

Antepartum Hemorrhage

33

Hemorrhage in the latter part of pregnancy poses a serious threat to the health and life of both mother and child. Placenta previa and abruptio placentae make up the vast majority of these cases.

CLASSIFICATION

1. Placenta previa
2. Abruptio placentae (premature separation)
3. Vasa previa
4. Rupture of marginal sinus
5. Local lesions
6. Idiopathic: no discoverable cause

PLACENTA PREVIA

In this condition the placenta is implanted in the lower uterine segment and lies over or near the internal os of the cervix. It is in front of the presenting part of the fetus. The incidence is 1:200 pregnancies.

Etiology

The etiology is unknown, but placenta previa is more common in multiparas and when the placenta is large and thin. It is thought that when the endometrium and decidua of the upper segment of the uterus are deficient, the placenta spreads over more of the wall of the uterus in an effort to obtain an adequate supply of blood.

Classification

Placenta Previa

1. *Total or central:* The entire internal os of the cervix is covered by placenta (Fig. 1A).
2. *Partial:* Part of the internal os of the cervix is covered by placenta (Fig. 1B).
3. *Marginal:* The placenta extends to the edge of the cervix, but does not lie over the os (Fig. 1C). When the cervix effaces and dilates in late pregnancy, a marginal placenta previa may be converted into the partial variety.

Low-lying Placenta

The placenta is in the lower uterine segment, but does not encroach on the internal os of the cervix (Fig. 1D).

Clinical Manifestations

The main or only symptom is painless vaginal bleeding. In most cases the bleeding is unprovoked, but it may be preceded by trauma or coitus. The first hemorrhage is almost never catastrophic. It may stop and start again later. Sometimes there is a continuing trickle of blood so that the patient becomes anemic. A feature of placenta previa is that the degree of anemia or shock is equivalent to the amount of blood lost.

Source of the Bleeding

As the lower segment of the uterus develops and the cervix effaces and dilates, there is a degree of separation of the placenta from the wall of the uterus. This is associated with rupture of the underlying blood vessels. If these are large the bleeding will be profuse.

Associated Conditions

1. Failure of engagement.
2. Abnormal presentations, such as breech and transverse lie, are more common, probably because the placenta occupies the lower part of the uterus.
3. Congenital fetal anomalies.
4. Placenta accreta. The incidence is higher than when the placenta is implanted in the upper segment of the uterus.
5. Postpartum hemorrhage is seen more often.

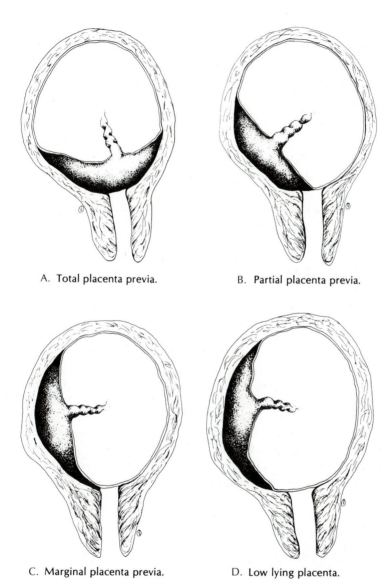

A. Total placenta previa.   B. Partial placenta previa.

C. Marginal placenta previa.   D. Low lying placenta.

Figure 1. Placenta previa.

Physical Findings

1. The patient feels no pain, unless labor has begun.
2. The uterus is soft and not tender.
3. The presenting part is high.
4. The fetal heart is usually present.
5. Shock is rare.

Placental Localization

1. Ultrasonic examination is the safest and most accurate, and is the procedure of choice.
2. Radioactive isotope. This method is accurate and safe for the fetus.
3. Soft tissue x-ray may locate the placenta but is not as reliable as the above techniques.

ABRUPTIO PLACENTAE

This condition, known also as premature separation of the placenta, involves the detachment of the placenta from the wall of the uterus. Abruptio placentae is initiated by hemorrhage into the decidua basalis which divides, leading to separation of the part of the placenta adjacent to the split. A hematoma forms between the placenta and the uterus.

In most cases the bleeding progresses to the edge of the placenta. At this point it may break through the membranes and enter the amniotic cavity or, more often, the blood tracks down between the chorion and the decidua vera until it reaches the cervix, and then comes out of the vagina. Occasionally there is extensive extravasation of blood into the myometrium, a condition described as uteroplacental apoplexy, or Couvelaire uterus. The incidence of abruptio placentae is around 1:200 pregnancies.

Etiology

The cause of placental abruption is not known. The condition is associated with the following:

1. Hypertensive disorders of pregnancy
2. Overdistention of the uterus, including multiple pregnancy and polyhydramnios
3. Trauma
4. Short umbilical cord

Classification

Degree of Separation of the Placenta

1. *Total:* Fetal death is inevitable.
2. *Partial:* The fetus has a chance. Separation of more than 50 percent of the placenta is incompatible with fetal survival.

Location of the Bleeding

1. *External or apparent* (Fig. 2A): The blood may be bright red or dark and clotted. The pain is mild unless the patient is in labor. The degree of anemia and shock is equivalent to the apparent blood loss.
2. *Internal or concealed* (Fig. 2B): There is little vaginal bleeding. The blood is trapped in the uterus. The pain is severe and the uterus is hard and tender. The fetal heart is absent. The degree of shock is greater than expected for the amount of visible bleeding.
3. *Mixed or combined:* All varieties of the above groups are seen.

Clinical Picture

This depends upon the location of the blood (apparent or concealed) and the amount of blood lost. The latter may be relatively small or large

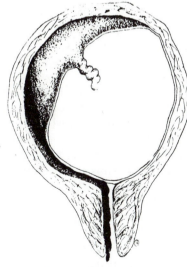 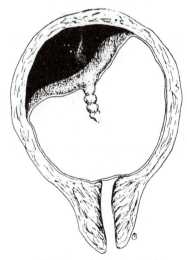

A. External or apparent.   B. Internal or concealed.

Figure 2. Abruptio placentae.

enough to lead to hypovolemic shock and even maternal death. The clinical picture includes vaginal bleeding, abdominal pain, and uterine tenderness with high tonicity. The uterus may exhibit a board-like rigidity, and may enlarge as blood accumulates in the cavity. Often the patient is in labor.

Fetal distress is common and the fetal heart tones are absent in many cases. The perinatal mortality ranges from 25 to 50 percent.

The diagnosis of abruptio placentae is made on clinical grounds; ultrasonography is essential to rule out placenta previa. The diagnosis may be confirmed at delivery when inspection of the placenta reveals an adherent retroplacental clot with disruption of the underlying tissue.

Complications

1. Hemorrhagic shock is due to blood loss, apparent or concealed.
2. Disseminated intravascular coagulation. Thromboplastin from the decidua and amniotic fluid enters the circulation and leads to hypofibrinogenemia.
3. Postpartum hemorrhage is caused both by the failure of the uterus to contract properly and by the coagulopathy.
4. Renal lesions. Ischemic necrosis of the kidneys, acute tubular necrosis, and/or bilateral cortical necrosis leads to renal shutdown.
5. Sheehan syndrome results from ischemic necrosis of the anterior lobe of the pituitary gland as a consequence of shock.

Painless Abruption

Several cases have been reported of separation of a posteriorly implanted placenta, severe enough to cause fetal death, but differing from the usual clinical presentation in that the only symptoms are vaginal bleeding and backache. The uterus is not tender, relaxes between contractions if the patient is in labor, and allows for easy palpation and auscultation of the fetus. The diagnosis depends on the demonstration, by ultrasound, of a posterior, upper segment, placental implantation.

VASA PREVIA

Vasa previa refers to a condition in which the umbilical vessels, unsupported by either the umbilical cord or placental tissue, traverse the fetal membranes of the lower uterine segment, and lie over the internal os of the cervix, in front of the presenting part. Often the placenta is low-lying. A velamentous insertion of the cord is a prerequisite. In the latter the umbilical cord inserts into the membranes, and the branching vessels run between the amnion and the chorion before joining the placenta. Unprotected by Wharton jelly, the blood vessels are vulnerable. If they are compressed the fetus becomes asphyxiated. If they are ruptured the fetus exsanguinates rapidly. In either case fetal death is frequent. Rupture of the blood vessels can occur even when they do not cross the os. The velamentous vessels may rupture before labor, at the onset of labor, during labor, or not at all. They may rupture at the time of rupture of the membranes or afterward. The exact incidence of vasa previa is unknown, but it is rare. However, in association with velamentous insertion of the cord the incidence of vasa previa is 1 in 50. The incidence of velamentous insertion of the cord is from 0.24 to 1.8 percent.

Clinical Picture

The two symptoms are (1) fetal bradycardia when the vessels are compressed and (2) vaginal hemorrhage when the vessels are torn.

Antepartum diagnosis is uncommon and here lies the main problem. When labor has started and the cervix opens, leaving the membranes unsupported, rupture of the vasa previa is almost inevitable. Once hemorrhage has occurred there is little hope for the fetus unless the origin of the blood is suspected and rapid treatment instituted. The fetus is at maximum risk, the mother not at all. The fetal prognosis remains poor.

Diagnosis

1. *Fetal heart rate:* Vasa previa may be suspected when each episode of vaginal bleeding is followed by irregularities of the fetal heart.
2. *Vaginal examination:* The vessels may be felt by the fingers. The condition may be confused with presentation of the umbilical cord.
3. *Amnioscopy:* The blood vessels may be seen.
4. *Kleihauer test:* This procedure demonstrates the presence of fetal red blood cells and establishes that the bleeding is of fetal origin.
5. *Cesarean section:* Severe fetal bradycardia may lead to emergency cesarean section without the diagnosis being made until after the operation.

RUPTURE OF MARGINAL SINUS

The marginal sinus rims the circumference of the placenta and is one of the channels by which blood from the intervillous spaces is returned to the maternal circulation. Normally it is torn during the third stage of labor as the placenta separates from the wall of the uterus.

Occasionally the marginal sinus ruptures in the third trimester of pregnancy. The etiology is unknown. The clinical picture is that of mild, painless bleeding, unaccompanied by uterine rigidity or changes in the fetal heart.

LOCAL LESIONS

1. Neoplasms
   a. Cervical polyp
   b. Cervical cancer
2. Infection
   a. Vaginitis
   b. Cervicitis

IDIOPATHIC

In this case no cause or reason for the bleeding is ever found. Probably it results from a slight separation of the membranes from the uterine wall. The bleeding is usually small in quantity and there is no effect on the mother, fetus, or pregnancy. Sometimes an excessive amount of bloody show is a sign of impending labor.

Treatment involves the ruling out of serious conditions, followed by expectant management. Most patients go to term.

GENERAL MANAGEMENT OF THIRD TRIMESTER BLEEDING

Preliminary Evaluation

1. The patient is admitted to hospital.
2. Blood loss is estimated.
3. Vital signs are determined.
4. The degree of shock is evaluated.
5. The hemoglobin and hematocrit are measured.
6. Clotting factors, including fibrinogen, are assayed.

Obstetric Evaluation

1. The period of gestation is calculated.
2. The abdomen is palpated for consistency and tenderness of the uterus.
3. Fetal position is determined.
4. The fetal heart is auscultated.
5. The placenta is localized by ultrasound or radioactive isotopes.

Preliminary Management

1. An intravenous infusion with a transfusion unit and a large bore needle or intracath is set up.
2. Blood is cross-matched, at least two units.
3. The patient is kept in bed.
4. No vaginal or rectal examinations are performed at this time.

Treatment

1. If the bleeding stops and there is no recurrence for several days, and if placenta previa is not present, a speculum examination is performed to rule out local lesions. If all findings are negative, discharge of the patient from hospital is considered.
2. If the bleeding goes on, treatment of the specific condition is carried out.

DIFFERENTIAL DIAGNOSIS

	Placenta Previa	Abruptio Placentae
Onset	Quiet and sneaky	Sudden and stormy
Bleeding	External	External and concealed
Color of blood	Bright red	Dark venous
Anemia	= Blood loss	> Apparent blood loss
Shock	= Blood loss	> Apparent blood loss
Toxemia	Absent	May be present
Pain	Only labor	Severe and steady
Uterine tenderness	Absent	Present
Uterine tone	Soft and relaxed	Firm to stony hard
Uterine contour	Normal	May enlarge and change shape
Fetal heart tones	Usually present	Present or absent
Engagement	Absent	May be present
Presentation	May be abnormal	No relationship

MANAGEMENT OF PLACENTA PREVIA

Expectant Treatment

Because the first episode of bleeding is rarely catastrophic and because the fetus may be too premature to survive outside of the uterus, an attempt is made to prolong the pregnancy in the interests of the infant. A reasonable goal is 37 to 38 weeks.

1. Hospitalization. The time and amount of the next episode of bleeding are unpredictable. Therefore the patient must remain in hospital.
2. Transfusion. At least two units of blood should be available.
3. Anemia. Blood transfusion and supplements of iron are given if anemia is present.
4. Pulmonary maturity. The lecithin/sphingomyelin (L/S) ratio of the amniotic fluid helps determine the optimum time for delivery.

Termination of the Pregnancy

Indications

1. Excessive bleeding. Fetal maturity is ignored.
2. The pregnancy has reached 38 weeks, and fetal pulmonary maturity is assured. Nothing is gained by waiting longer. There is the danger that a sudden hemorrhage may jeopardize the infant if one waits for the pregnancy to go to term.

Cesarean Section

This is performed for the following indications:

1. Profuse bleeding
2. Total or partial placenta previa; certain diagnosis by ultrasound
3. Fetal distress
4. Abnormal presentation (e.g., breech, transverse lie)

Double Set-up Examination

This procedure is carried out when the diagnosis is uncertain. The patient is taken to the operating room, where all preparations have been made for immediate cesarean section. Under anesthesia, abdominal and vaginal examinations are performed to ascertain the fetal presentation, the condition of the cervix, and the location of the placenta.

Treatment is based on these findings. However, vaginal examination may provoke heavy bleeding, and a double set-up procedure is not employed when the diagnosis of placenta previa is certain. It is reserved for those patients whose placenta previa is only suspected, or whose vaginal bleeding is of unclear etiology.

Cesarean Section. This is performed when the diagnosis is made of complete or partial placenta previa, when profuse bleeding is provoked by the examination, when there is fetal distress, or when the presentation is abnormal. Many obstetricians prefer the lower segment vertical uterine incision in this situation because it provides easier access to bleeding sinuses if suture is necessary and because, if the placenta is anterior, it is easier to find a path around it to extract the baby than when the incision is transverse. Some physicians perform the transverse lower segment procedure, while a few believe that the classic incision is best for placenta previa.

Induction of Labor. The membranes are ruptured and an oxytocin infusion is instituted. The descent of the head, by causing pressure on the placenta, will control the bleeding from the uterine sinuses. This procedure is carried out when:

1. The bleeding is minimal.
2. The placenta covers no more than 10 percent of the internal os.
3. The cervix is effaced and at least 3 cm dilated.
4. The fetal head is in the pelvis.

Await Onset of Labor. Patient is returned to the ward when:

1. No placenta previa is found.
2. No indication for induction is present.

Prognosis

Mother. Good as long as shock and severe anemia are prevented.

Fetus. The mortality rate is around 15 percent. Factors that worsen the chances for fetal survival include:

1. Uncontrollable maternal hemorrhage and shock
2. A marked degree of placental separation
3. Excessive anesthesia
4. Delivery of premature infant

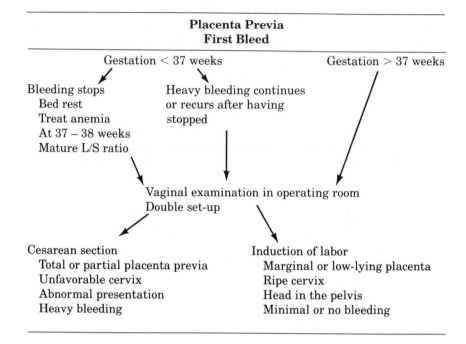

Placenta Previa
First Bleed

Gestation < 37 weeks   Gestation > 37 weeks

Bleeding stops   Heavy bleeding continues
  Bed rest   or recurs after having
  Treat anemia   stopped
  At 37 – 38 weeks
  Mature L/S ratio

Vaginal examination in operating room
Double set-up

Cesarean section   Induction of labor
  Total or partial placenta previa   Marginal or low-lying placenta
  Unfavorable cervix   Ripe cervix
  Abnormal presentation   Head in the pelvis
  Heavy bleeding   Minimal or no bleeding

MANAGEMENT OF ABRUPTIO PLACENTAE

Initial Evaluation and Stabilization

1. History and physical examination
2. Blood for hemoglobin, hematocrit, platelets, prothrombin time, and fibrinogen
3. Intravenous line with 18-gauge needle
4. Cross-match four units of blood
5. Tranfuse as necessary

Time of Delivery

Except for mild cases, when bleeding is minimal, the aim is to effect delivery as soon as possible and for the following reasons:

1. A number of intrauterine fetal deaths occur after the mother has been admitted to hospital and is awaiting delivery.
2. The neonatal mortality rises as the interval between abruption and birth is lengthened.
3. Early delivery and consequent reduction of the period of fetal hypoxia reduces both fetal and neonatal mortality.

4. In these cases the fetuses do not tolerate the process of labor too readily.
5. Final control of the bleeding cannot be achieved until the uterus has been emptied.

Vaginal Delivery

The vaginal route is preferred, especially if the mother is in good condition and rapid delivery is anticipated by the cervix being dilated to 4 or 5 cm and the presenting part lying well into the pelvis.

Spontaneous labor will have begun in the majority of patients. If not, labor is induced. In either case amniotomy is performed. The release of amniotic fluid reduces the intraamniotic pressure, may retard the abruptive process, lessens the extravasation of blood into the uterine wall, decreases the entry of amniotic fluid into the circulation and, hence, the incidence of amniotic fluid embolism and disseminated intravascular coagulation. Amniotomy will also accelerate labor. Occasionally an infusion of oxytocin is necessary to augment labor.

Cesarean Section

1. If the fetus is viable, the fetal heart tones are present, the presenting part is not in the pelvis, and the cervix is closed, suggesting that rapid labor and delivery will not occur, cesarean section is indicated in the interests of both mother and child.
2. In the situation where the fetus is dead, cesarean section is performed in the interest of the mother only when bleeding is so profuse that maternal life is threatened.

Treatment of Bleeding

1. Adequate transfusion.
2. Disseminated intravascular coagulation. Delivery within 8 hours prevents this complication in most cases. If it occurs, cryoprecipitate, fibrinogen, or fresh plasma may be given once the delivery is under way.
3. Hysterectomy may be necessary if bleeding from a noncontracting uterus cannot be controlled.

Prognosis

Maternal
The maternal prognosis depends on (1) the extent of placental separation; (2) the blood loss; (3) whether the hemorrhage is apparent or con-

cealed (the latter is more grave); (4) the extent of uteroplacental apoplexy; (5) the degree of interference with the clotting mechanism; and (6) the interval between the placental abruption and the institution of treatment. With proper management the mortality is less than 1 percent.

Fetal

Perinatal mortality ranges between 30 and 50 percent. The outlook for the fetus is influenced by (1) the extent of placental separation, (2) the interval between the accident and delivery, and (3) prematurity.

MANAGEMENT OF VASA PREVIA

1. In the presence of fetal bleeding immediate delivery is essential, vaginally or by cesarean section.
2. If there is no bleeding, cesarean section may be necessary, but if vaginal delivery is imminent the membranes can be ruptured away from the vessels and the baby extracted.
3. In the presence of a dead fetus, vaginal delivery is awaited.
4. Postpartum the baby's blood picture must be studied, and if necessary, immediate transfusion carried out.

BIBLIOGRAPHY

Cotton DB, Read JA, Paul RH, et al: The conservative aggressive management of placenta previa. Am J Obstet Gynecol 137:687, 1980

Hurd WM, Miodovnik M, Hertzberg V, Lavin JP: Selective management of abruptio placentae: A prospective study. Obstet Gynecol 61:467, 1983

Knab DR: Abruptio placentae, an assessment of the time and method of delivery. Obstet Gynecol 52:625, 1978

Kouyoumdjian A: Velamentous insertion of the umbilical cord. Obstet Gynecol 56:737, 1980

Pallewela CS: Antepartum diagnosis of vasa previa—report of a case causing sudden fetal death. Postgrad Med J 50:723, 1974

Quek SP, Tan KL: Vasa previa. Aust NZ J Obstet Gynaecol 12:206, 1972

Weiser EB, Cefalo RC: Managing second trimester placenta previa. Contemp OB/GYN 15:187, 1980

34

Episiotomy, Lacerations, Uterine Rupture, Inversion

EPISIOTOMY

An episiotomy (perineotomy) is an incision into the perineum to enlarge the space at the outlet, thereby facilitating the birth of the child.

Maternal Benefits

1. A straight incision is simpler to repair and heals better than a jagged, uncontrolled laceration.
2. By making the episiotomy before the muscles and fascia are stretched excessively, the strength of the pelvic floor can be preserved and the incidence of uterine prolapse, cystocele, and rectocele reduced.
3. The structures in front are protected as well as those in the rear. By increasing the room available posteriorly, there is less stretching of and less damage to the anterior vaginal wall, bladder, urethra, and periclitoral tissues.
4. Tears into the rectum can be avoided.
5. The second stage of labor is shortened.

Fetal Benefits

It is also advantageous to the child. A well-timed episiotomy not only makes the birth easier but lessens the pounding of the head on the perineum and so helps avert brain damage. This is true for any baby but is especially important for those who have a low resistance to trauma, such as premature infants, babies born to diabetic mothers, and those with erythroblastosis.

Indications

1. Prophylactic: To preserve the integrity of the pelvic floor
2. Arrest of progress by a resistant perineum
   a. Thick and heavily muscled tissue
   b. Operative scars
   c. Previous well-repaired episiotomy
3. To obviate uncontrolled tears, including extension into the rectum
   a. When the perineum is short, there being little room between the back of the vagina and the front of the rectum
   b. Where large lacerations seem inevitable
4. Fetal reasons
   a. Premature and infirm babies
   b. Large infants
   c. Abnormal positions such as occipitoposteriors, face presentations, and breeches
   d. Fetal distress, where there is need for rapid delivery of the baby and dilatation of the perineum cannot be awaited

Timing of Episiotomy

There is a proper time to make the episiotomy. Made too late, the procedure fails to prevent lacerations and to protect the pelvic floor. Made too soon, the incision leads to needless loss of blood. The episiotomy is made when the perineum is bulging, when a 3 to 4 cm diameter of fetal scalp is visible during a contraction, and when the presenting part will be delivered with the next three or four contractions. In this way lacerations are avoided, overstretching of the pelvic floor is prevented, and excessive bleeding is obviated.

There are three types of episiotomy: (1) midline; (2) mediolateral, left or right; and (3) lateral episiotomy, which is no longer used (Fig. 1A).

Midline Episiotomy

Technique
In making the incision two fingers are placed in the vagina between the fetal head and the perineum. Outward pressure is made on the perineum, away from the fetus, to avoid injury to the baby. The scissors (some prefer a scalpel) are placed so that one blade lies against the vaginal mucosa and the other on the skin. The incision is made in the midline from the fourchette almost to but not through the external fibers of the anal sphincter (Fig. 1B). The cut is in the central tendinous portion

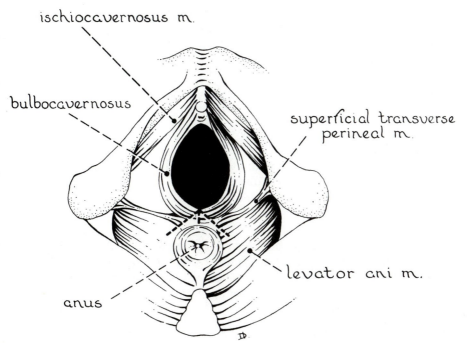

ischiocavernosus m.

bulbocavernosus

superficial transverse perineal m.

levator ani m.

anus

A. Muscles of the pelvic floor and perineum. The sites of median and mediolateral episiotomy are shown.

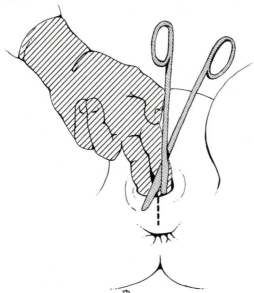

B. Incision of the midline episiotomy.

Figure 1. Midline episiotomy.

of the perineal body to which are attached the bulbocavernosus muscle in front, the superficial transverse perineal and part of the levator ani muscles at the sides, and the anal sphincter behind (Fig. 1B). This is an excellent anatomic incision.

Advantages

1. The muscle belly is not cut.
2. It is easy to make and easy to repair.
3. The structural results are excellent.
4. Bleeding is less than with other incisions.
5. Postoperative pain is minimal.
6. Healing is superior and dehiscence is rare.

Disadvantages

The one drawback is that should there be extension of the incision as the head is being born, the anal sphincter is torn and the rectum entered. Although most bowel injuries heal well if repaired properly, this accident should be avoided. Median episiotomies are not ideal in the following situations:

1. Short perineum
2. Large baby
3. Abnormal positions and presentations
4. Difficult operative deliveries

Repair

Since in most cases the third stage is completed soon after the birth of the child, the repair of the episiotomy is performed after the placenta is delivered, the uterus contracted, and the cervix and vagina found to be uninjured. Not only are intrauterine procedures, such as manual removal of the placenta, and intravaginal procedures more difficult to perform after the episiotomy has been closed, but the repair may be broken down.

Except for the subcuticular layer, a medium, round needle is employed. In the deep tissues a cutting edge needle may lacerate a blood vessel and cause a hematoma. Our preference is for 000 chromic catgut.

First the vaginal mucosa is sewn together (Fig. 2A). The procedure is begun at the top of the incision, the first bite being taken a little above the apex to include any retracted blood vessel. The suture is tied leaving one end long. The edges of the wound are then approximated but not strangulated, using a simple continuous or a lock stitch to assure hemostasis. Each bite includes the mucous membrane of the vagina and the tissue between the vagina and rectum. This reduces bleeding, eliminates dead space, and makes for better healing. The repair is carried past the hymenal ring to the skin edges. The last two bites include the subcutaneous tissue at the base of the episiotomy but do not come through the skin. This end of the continuous suture may be tied, or it may be left untied and held with a hemostat.

The second stitch near the base of the wound is the crown suture (Fig. 2B). The needle passes under the skin deeply enough to catch and

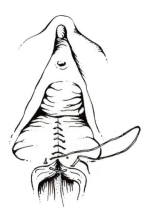

A. Closure of the vaginal mucosa by a continuous suture.

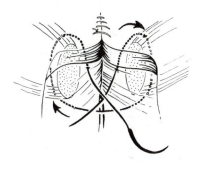

B. The crown suture, reuniting the divided bulbocavernous muscle.

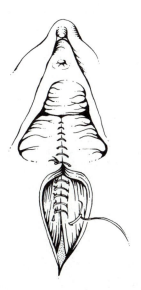

C. Drawing together the perineal muscles and fascia with interrupted sutures.

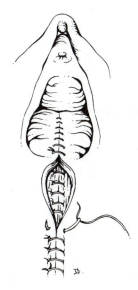

D. Approximation of the skin edges with interrupted sutures.

Figure 2. Repair of the midline episiotomy.

bring together the separated and retracted ends of the bulbocavernosus muscle and fascia. The crown suture is important: If these tissues are approximated too tightly coitus is painful, and if too loose, the introitus gapes.

Next the transverse perineal and levator ani muscles and fascia are approximated in the midline anterior to the rectum with three or four interrupted sutures (Fig. 2C). One layer is enough in most cases.

Finally the incision is closed by one of several methods:

1. The skin edges are united by interrupted, or mattress, sutures which pass through the skin and subcutaneous tissue. These are tied loosely to prevent strangulation as postpartum swelling takes place (Fig. 2D).

2. The skin edges are approximated using a continuous subcuticular stitch on a small cutting needle, starting at the lower end of the incision. The first bite is taken in the subcuticular tissue just under but not through the skin, going from side to side until the base (upper end) of the wound is reached. Here it is tied separately, or if the suture used to repair the vaginal mucosa has been left untied, this suture and the subcuticular one are tied together. This completes the repair (Fig. 3D).

Aftercare

Aftercare of the episiotomy is essentially a matter of cleanliness. The perineum is cleaned with a mildly antiseptic solution after each urination and bowel evacuation. Heat, as from an electric bulb, may be used to dry the area and to reduce the swelling. Daily showers and washing with mild soap and water are excellent ways of keeping the perineum clean and free from irritating discharges.

Mediolateral Episiotomy

When a large episiotomy is needed, or when there is danger of rectal involvement, the mediolateral variety is advised. Included here are patients with short perineums, contracted outlets, large babies, face to pubis deliveries, attitudes of extension, breech births, and midforceps operations.

Technique

The incision is made from the midline of the posterior fourchette toward the ischial tuberosity, far enough laterally to avoid the anal sphincter. The average episiotomy is about 4 cm long and may reach the fatty tissues of the ischiorectal fossa. Whether it is placed on the left or right side is unimportant.

The following structures are cut:

1. Skin and subcutaneous tissue.
2. Bulbocavernosus muscle and fascia.
3. Transverse perineal muscle.
4. Levator ani muscle and fascia. The extent to which this structure is involved is determined by the length and depth of the incision.

Repair

The technique is essentially the same as for the median perineotomy. The vaginal mucosa is repaired starting at the apex, and brings together the mucous membrane and the underlying supporting tissue (Fig. 3A). The crown suture is placed carefully (Fig. 3B).

The muscles and fascia which were cut are approximated with interrupted sutures (Fig. 3C). The tissues on the medial side tend to retract, and care must be taken not to enter the rectum. Some operators prefer to place these sutures, leaving them untied, before the vaginal mucosa is repaired. In many patients a single layer of four or five stitches is sufficient. When the wound is deep or when there is much bleeding two layers may be necessary, one in the muscles, and one to bring together the overlying fascia. The skin edges are joined by a subcuticular stitch beginning at the apex (Fig. 3D), or by interrupted sutures through skin and subcutaneous tissue.

Disruption of Episiotomy: Infection

Etiology

Like incisions in other parts of the body, an episiotomy may dehisce. Predisposing factors include:

1. Poor healing powers:
   a. Nutritional deficiencies
   b. Anemia
   c. Exhaustion after a long and difficult labor
   d. Avascular scarred tissue
2. Failure of technique:
   a. Careless approximation of the wound
   b. Incomplete hemostasis leading to hematoma formation
   c. Failure to obliterate dead space
3. Devitalization of tissue:
   a. Use of crushing instruments
   b. Strangulation of tissue by tying sutures too tightly
   c. Employment of too heavy catgut
4. Infection:
   a. Infected lochia in puerperal sepsis
   b. Poor technique and neglect of aseptic standards
   c. Proximity of the rectum
   d. Extension of the incision into or passage of the needle through the bowel
   e. Sepsis in a hematoma
   f. Improper postpartum cleanliness

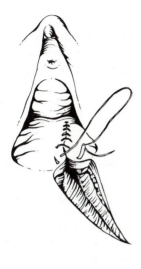

A. Closure of the vaginal mucosa by a continuous suture.

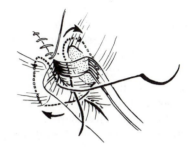

B. The crown suture.

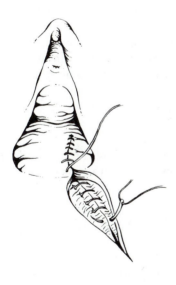

C. Drawing together the perineal muscles and fascia with interrupted sutures.

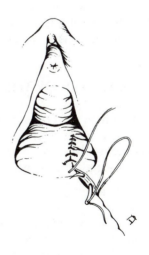

D. Approximation of the skin edges with a continuous subcuticular suture.

Figure 3. Repair of left mediolateral episiotomy.

Clinical Course

The episiotomy becomes extremely painful, tender, swollen, red, and indurated. The patient may or may not have fever. Sometimes there is a discharge from the incision. By the fourth or fifth day the edges of the wound separate.

Management of Disruption

Supportive Management. The area is kept clean and free from irritating discharge and debris by warm sitz baths twice daily for 20 minutes. Following this the perineum is lamped for 30 minutes. The wound granulates in and heals from the deep layers up. The patient may go home at the usual time and continue the treatment there. Unless there has been damage to the rectum, this management has always been successful in our experience. The wound heals well, no aftereffects are noted, and prolonged hospitalization is avoided.

Secondary Repair. Supportive treatment is carried on until the area is clean. This takes 5 to 6 days. Then the patient is anesthetized, the devitalized tissue debrided, and the episiotomy repaired.

In our experience supportive therapy alone has given the best results and is the simplest to carry out.

A late complication of an infected episiotomy is a rectovaginal fistula. This results from an unrecognized tear of the rectum or from a suture being passed through the rectal wall and left there.

LACERATIONS OF THE PERINEUM

Many women suffer tears of the perineum at birth of the first child. In about half the cases these tears are extensive. Lacerations must be repaired carefully.

Maternal causes include:

1. Precipitate, uncontrolled, or unattended delivery (the most frequent cause)
2. The patient's inability to stop bearing down
3. Hastening the delivery by excessive fundal pressure
4. Edema and friability of the perineum
5. Vulvar varicosities weakening the tissue
6. Narrow pubic arch with outlet contraction, forcing the head posteriorly
7. Extension of episiotomy

Fetal factors are:

1. Large baby
2. Abnormal positions of the head—e.g., occipitoposterior and face presentations
3. Breech deliveries
4. Difficult forceps extractions
5. Shoulder dystocia
6. Congenital anomalies, such as hydrocephaly

Classification of Perineal Lacerations

First Degree Tear
First degree tear involves the vaginal mucosa, the fourchette, and the skin of the perineum just below it.

Repair. These tears are small and are repaired as simply as possible. The aim is reapproximation of the divided tissue and hemostasis. In the average case a few interrupted sutures through the vaginal mucosa, the fourchette, and the skin of the perineum are enough. If bleeding is profuse, figure-8 stitches may be used. Interrupted sutures, loosely tied, are best for the skin because they cause less tension and less discomfort to the patient.

Second Degree Tear

Second degree lacerations are deeper. They are mainly in the midline and extend through the perineal body. Often the transverse perineal muscle is torn, and the rent may go down to but not through the rectal sphincter. Usually the tear extends upward along the vaginal mucosa and the submucosal tissue. This gives the laceration a doubly triangular appearance with the base at the fourchette, one apex in the vagina, and the other near the rectum.

Repair.   Repair of second degree lacerations is in layers:

1. Interrupted, continuous, or lock stitches are used to approximate the edges of the vaginal mucosa and submucosa (Fig. 4A).
2. The deep muscles of the perineal body are sewn together with interrupted sutures (Fig. 4B).
3. A running subcuticular suture or interrupted sutures, loosely tied, bring together the skin edges (Fig. 4C).

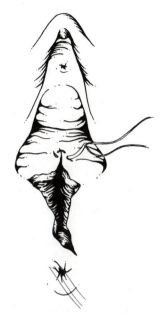

A. Closure of the rent in the vaginal mucosa with a continuous suture.

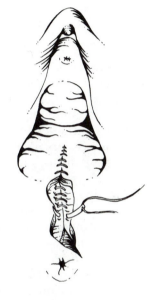

B. Drawing together the perineal muscles and fascia with interrupted sutures.

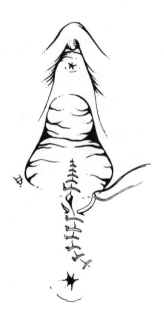

C. Closure of the skin edges with interrupted sutures tied loosely.

Figure 4. Repair of a second degree perineal laceration.

Third Degree Tear

Third degree tears extend through the perineal body, the transverse perineal muscle, and the rectal sphincter. In partial third degree tears only the rectal sphincter is torn; in complete tears the rectal sphincter is severed, and the laceration extends up the anterior rectal wall for a variable distance. Some authors refer to this as a fourth degree tear.

Repair of Complete Tear. Complete third degree tear (Fig. 5A) is repaired in layers:

1. The anterior wall of the rectum is repaired with fine 000 or 0000 chromic catgut on a fused needle. Starting at the apex, interrupted sutures are placed submucosally so that the serosa, muscularis, and submucosa of the rectum are apposed (Fig. 5B). Some authors advise that the knot be tied in the lumen of the bowel. Others approximate the edges of the rectum with a continuous suture going through all layers. This part of the repair must be performed meticulously.
2. The line of repair is oversewn by bringing together the perirectal fascia and the fascia of the rectovaginal septum. Interrupted or continuous sutures are used.
3. The torn ends of the rectal sphincter (which have retracted) are identified, grasped with Allis forceps, and approximated with interrupted sutures or two figure-8 sutures (Figs. 5C and D).
4. The vaginal mucosa is then repaired as in a midline episiotomy, with continuous or interrupted sutures.
5. The perineal muscles are sewn together with interrupted stitches.
6. The skin edges are sewn together with a continuous subcuticular suture or loosely tied interrupted sutures.

Repair of Partial Tear. Repair of partial third degree tear is similar to that of the complete variety, except that the rectal wall is intact and the repair starts with reapproximation of the torn ends of the rectal sphincter.

Aftercare. Aftercare of third degree tears includes:

1. General perineal asepsis.
2. Low-residue diet.
3. Encouragement of soft bowel movements with mild laxatives.
4. A suppository or carefully given enema is prescribed on the fifth or sixth day if the bowels have not moved.

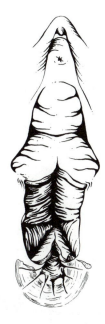

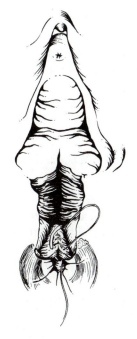

A. Torn and retracted ends of the rectal sphincter, laceration of the anterior wall of the rectum, and the torn vagina and perineum.

B. Closing the tear in the anterior wall of the rectum with interrupted sutures tied in the lumen.

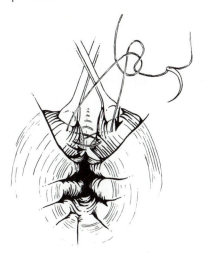

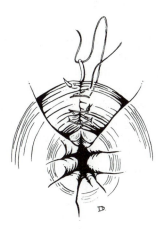

C. Retracted ends of the rectal sphincter are grasped with Allis forceps, and the first figure-eight suture is being placed.

D. Reunion of torn rectal sphincter completed with two figure-eight sutures.

Figure 5. Repair of a third degree laceration (complete tear).

527

LACERATIONS OF ANTERIOR VULVA AND LOWER ANTERIOR VAGINAL WALL

Various areas may be involved. Superficial tears are not serious, but with deep tears the bleeding may be profuse.

Locations of Lacerations

1. Tissue on either side of the urethra.
2. Labia minora.
3. Lateral walls of the vagina.
4. Area of the clitoris: With deep tears the corpora cavernosa may be torn. Because of the general vascularity of this structure, as well as the presence of the deep and dorsal blood vessels of the clitoris, these lacerations are accompanied by severe bleeding.
5. Urethra, under the pubic arch.
6. Bladder: The bladder is close to the anterior vaginal wall and may be damaged. Vesicovaginal fistula can occur. The main causes of fistula are prolonged labor with pressure necrosis of the wall of the bladder and instrumental damage during difficult deliveries.

Repair of Lacerations

Superficial small lacerations do not need repair in many cases. When the legs are brought together the torn edges are approximated and heal spontaneously. Larger tears should have the edges brought together with interrupted sutures to promote healing.

Deep lacerations must be repaired. Profuse bleeding is controlled best by figure-8 sutures placed to include and shut off the torn and bleeding vessels. Unfortunately in many cases the lacerated area is the site of varicosities, and passage of the needle through the tissue provokes fresh bleeding. If sutures do not stop the bleeding, a firm pack should be applied against the bleeding site and the hemorrhage controlled by tamponade.

Often the area of bleeding is *near the urethra*, and when the periclitoral region is involved the hemorrhage can be excessive. Repair is difficult because of the proximity of the urethra. To prevent damaging the urethra a catheter should be inserted to guide the needle away from it (Fig. 6).

Tears of the *urethra and bladder* are repaired in three layers to approximate the bladder mucosa, bladder wall, and anterior wall of the vagina. An indwelling catheter should be inserted into the bladder for drainage.

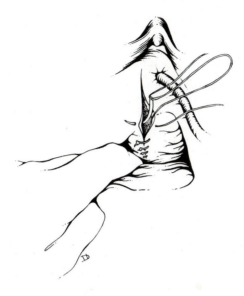

Figure 6. Anterior paraurethral laceration: placing of fine interrupted sutures. A catheter is in the urethra.

LACERATIONS OF UPPER VAGINA

These lacerations may take place during spontaneous delivery but are more common with operative deliveries and are associated with a variety of conditions. Predisposing factors include congenital anomalies of the vagina, a small or infantile vagina, loss of tissue elasticity in elderly primigravidas, scar tissue following the use of caustic substances in attempting to induce abortions, and unhealthy tissues, which tear like wet blotting paper.

Forceps rotation and extractions following deep transverse arrest, persistent occipitoposteriors, or face presentations often cause vaginal tears. The fact that these malpositions are frequently associated with small or male type pelves aggravates the situation and increases the incidence and extent of the lacerations. During rotation the edge of the blades may shear off the vaginal mucosa. Improper traction tends to overstretch the tissues and may result in a large tear. A large infant increases the danger of extensive lacerations.

The majority of vaginal tears are longitudinal and extend in the sulci along the columns of the vagina. In many cases the lacerations are bilateral.

Technique of Repair

Lacerations of the upper vagina bleed profusely; the bleeding must be controlled as soon as possible. As the tear is often high and out of sight, good exposure, good light, and good assistance are essential. Bleeding from the uterus may obscure the field. The placenta should be removed and oxytocics given before the repair is begun. The operator must be certain that the apex of the tear is included in the suture, or hemorrhage may take place from a vessel that has retracted. If the apex cannot be reached, several sutures are placed below it, and traction on these then expose the apex of the laceration (Fig. 7). Figure-8 sutures are preferable if bleeding is profuse, or a continuous lock stitch may be employed.

In some instances the sutures do not control the bleeding adequately. The vagina should be packed tightly with a 5-yard gauze. This reduces the oozing and helps prevent the formation of hematomas. The pack is removed in 24 hours.

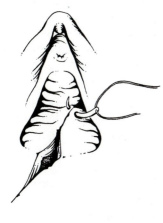

A. Introduction of first suture at highest point visible.

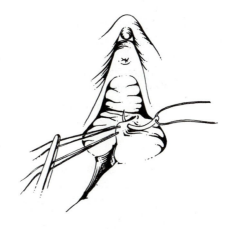

B. Traction on first suture exposes apex of the laceration and enables top suture to be placed. The remainder of the vaginal laceration is closed with continuous or interrupted sutures.

Figure 7. Right mediolateral episiotomy with high left vaginal sulcus tear.

VESICOVAGINAL FISTULA

A fistula is an abnormal communication between two or more organs. One variety is formed between the vagina and the urinary tract—the urethra, bladder, or ureter. Urine passes into the vagina, and there is an uncontrollable vaginal discharge.

Fistulas occur: (1) at childbirth, (2) during surgery, or (3) as a complication of cancer and radiation therapy. Although, because of improved obstetrics, most fistulas are associated with surgery, they do occur in association with parturition in the following ways:

1. During prolonged and obstructed labor the bladder is trapped between the fetal head and the maternal pubic symphysis. The resulting ischemic necrosis and slough results in fistulas of varying sizes. The proximal urethra, vesical neck, and trigone are involved.
2. Direct injury can occur during a difficult forceps delivery. Usually the trigone and urethra are damaged.
3. At cesarean section the bladder and ureter may be cut or torn.

Management

If the injury is recognized, an immediate two- or three-layer repair should be performed, followed by continuous bladder drainage for 10 days. When the damage is not recognized or if repair is not possible, continuous bladder drainage is instituted. Sometimes spontaneous closure of the fistula takes place. Should the fistula persist, active treatment is delayed for 2 to 3 months to allow the edema to subside, the slough to separate, and a new circulation to be established. Repair of the fistula is then carried out. However, the loss of urine from the vagina causes considerable distress to these women, and it is difficult for them to carry on. With the use of new techniques for repair and antibiotics to control infection, early correction of the problem has been carried out with success.

RECTOVAGINAL FISTULA

This is an opening between the rectum and the vagina. The patient notices the passage of air from the vagina and an irritating vaginal discharge.

Most of these occur as the result of an unsuccessful repair of a third degree laceration. The sphincter, or part of it, heals, while the area above the sphincter breaks down. A low rectovaginal fistula is the result. Occasionally a stitch in the apex of the episiotomy enters the rectum. Most of these cause no trouble. Once in a while healing does not take place and a fistula develops.

Treatment is by surgical repair.

HEMATOMAS

Vulva and Vagina

Puerperal Hematoma

1. *Vulvar:* The bleeding is limited to the vulvar tissue and is readily apparent.
2. *Vulvovaginal:* The hematoma involves the paravaginal tissue and the vulva, perineum, or ischiorectal fossa. The extent of the bleeding is only partially revealed on inspection of the vulva.
3. *Vaginal or concealed:* The hematoma is confined to the paravaginal tissue and is not visible externally.
4. *Supravaginal or subperitoneal:* The bleeding occurs above the pelvic fascia and is retroperitoneal or intraligamentous.

These result from rupture of the blood vessels, especially veins, under the skin of the external genitals and beneath the vaginal mucosa. The causal trauma occurs during delivery or repair. In rare cases the accident takes place during pregnancy or very early labor, in which case a large hematoma can obstruct progress. Damage to a blood vessel may lead to its necrosis, and the hematoma may not become manifest for several days.

Most hematomas are small and are located just beneath the skin of the perineum. While they cause pain and skin discoloration, they are not important. Since the blood is absorbed spontaneously no treatment is required beyond ordinary perineal care.

Rupture of the vessels under the vaginal mucosa is serious, since large amounts of blood can collect in the loose submucosal tissues. Many vaginal hematomas contain over half a liter of blood by the time the diagnosis is made. The mass may be so large that it occludes the lumen of the vagina, and pressure on the rectum is intense. When bleeding occurs at the base of the ligament the blood may extend in the retroperitoneal space even as far as the kidneys.

Many hematomas occur after easy spontaneous deliveries as well as in association with traumatic deliveries. The hematoma often is located on the side opposite the episiotomy. Stretching of the deep tissues can result in rupture of a deep vessel without visible external bleeding.

Varicosities play a predisposing role. The possibility of a coagulation defect must be considered. Failure to achieve perfect hemostasis is an important etiologic factor.

Diagnosis

The diagnosis is made within 12 hours of delivery. Classically, the patient's complaints of pain are dismissed as being part of the usual postpartum perineal discomfort. After a time it is realized that the pain is out of proportion to that associated with the ordinary trauma of delivery. Sedatives and analgesics do not alleviate the pain. Careful examination of the vulva and vagina reveals the swelling, discoloration, extreme tenderness, rectal pressure, and large fluctuant mass palpable per rectum or vaginam. Where large amounts of blood have been lost from the general circulation there is pallor, tachycardia, hypotension, and even shock. If the hematoma is high and ruptures into the peritoneal cavity, sudden extreme shock may occur and the patient may die.

Treatment

Active treatment is not needed for small hematomas and those which are not getting larger. The area should be kept clean; and since tissue necrosis may be followed by infection, antimicrobial agents are prescribed.

Big hematomas and those which are enlarging require surgical therapy. The wound is opened, the blood clots are evacuated, and if bleeding points can be found these are ligated. The area is packed with sterile gauze and a counter pack is placed in the vagina. This is left in situ for 24 to 48 hours. Antibiotics are given, blood transfusion is used as needed, and the patient is observed carefully for fresh bleeding. An indwelling catheter should be placed.

Since there is a tendency for the bleeding to recur and the hematoma to re-form, careful observation is necessary. Most cases do well, but several weeks pass before the wound heals and the perineum looks normal.

Broad Ligament

The danger of broad ligament hematomas is that they can rupture into the general peritoneal cavity and cause sudden and extreme shock.

Diagnosis

Diagnosis is made by vaginal examination. Rupture of the lower uterine segment must be ruled out. If the hematoma is large the uterus is pushed to the opposite side.

Treatment

Treatment depends on the degree of bleeding. Conservative therapy consists of bed rest, antibiotics, blood transfusion, and observation. Serial blood counts are done.

In the event of continued bleeding or progressive anemia, surgical intervention is carried out. The abdomen is opened, and the blood clots are evacuated. Where possible the bleeding points are tied off, care being taken to avoid the ureter. An extraperitoneal drain may be inserted. In older women hysterectomy is considered, and this operation may be necessary in young women to control the situation.

LACERATIONS OF THE CERVIX

As a result of its dilatation, superficial lacerations of the cervix occur during almost every confinement. They are partly responsible for the bloody show. These small tears heal spontaneously and require no treatment.

Deep lacerations, on the other hand, can cause severe hemorrhage and shock to the extent of endangering the life of the patient. This is particularly so when the laceration extends into the lower uterine segment where the large uterine vessels may be involved. The lacerations may be unilateral or bilateral. The most common sites are at the sides of the cervix, at 3 or 9 o'clock.

Etiology

The etiology of deep lacerations includes precipitate labor, a rigid or scarred cervix, the forceful delivery of the child through an undilated cervix, breech extraction, and a large baby.

Diagnosis

Diagnosis is made by careful inspection. We believe that the cervix and vagina should be inspected after every delivery. Some obstetricians do not agree. There is no question, however, that this examination must be made after all difficult confinements and whenever bleeding is excessive. Ring forceps are used to grasp the lips of the cervix so that the whole circumference can be visualized.

Repair

Repair of cervical tears is important. The cervix is exposed with a vaginal speculum or with retractors. An assistant is invaluable. Ring forceps are placed on each side of the laceration. Interrupted or figure-8 sutures are placed starting at the apex and are tied just tightly enough to control the bleeding and to approximate the tissues. Care must be taken not to include the ring of the forceps in the stitch. It is important that the first stitch be placed a little above the apex (Fig. 8) to catch any vessel that may have retracted. If the tear is high there is danger of injury to the ureter. When the tear has extended into the lower uterine segment or into the broad ligament, repair from below may be impossible and laparotomy necessary.

Careful repair of the torn cervix is important, not only to control bleeding but as prophylaxis against scarring, erosions, and chronic ascending infections. Lacerations more than a centimeter in length warrant treatment.

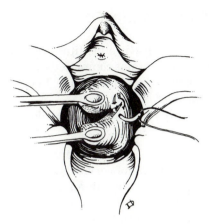

Figure 8. Laceration of cervix on the left side. Uppermost suture is placed just above the apex of the tear. The laceration is being closed with interrupted sutures. Figure-8 sutures may be used.

DÜHRSSEN CERVICAL INCISIONS

Incisions of the cervix are used to facilitate immediate delivery when the cervix is fully effaced but not completely dilated. This procedure is used rarely today, the incidence being under 1 percent and being needed more often in primigravidas.

Reasons why this procedure is used so seldom today include the following:

1. The employment of the intravenous oxytocin drip has reduced the incidence of failure of cervical dilatation.
2. The increased safety of cesarean section has steered obstetricians away from incising the cervix.
3. It is realized that nondilatation of the cervix may be an indication of disproportion.
4. In the presence of fetal distress cervical incisions and midforceps may be more than the baby can stand.

Indications

This operation may be employed in the presence of fetal distress or arrest of progress when it is considered that vaginal delivery would be relatively easy if the cervix were fully dilated. The obstetrician must beware of diagnosing cervical dystocia when fetopelvic disproportion is the real problem.

Prerequisites

1. There must be no cephalopelvic disproportion.
2. The cervix must be completely effaced.
3. The cervix must be at least half dilated.
4. The station of the fetal skull is at +1 or +2.
5. The patient must have been in good labor for 6 to 8 hours with ruptured membranes.

Technique

The cervix is grasped with ring forceps, and the incisions are made between them at 2, 6, and 10 o'clock (Fig. 9). These are extended to the junction of the cervix and vaginal wall. When the three incisions have been made, the diameter of the cervix is equivalent to full dilatation.

Because the bladder is pulled upward as effacement takes place, its dissection from the anterior vaginal wall is not required.

Appropriate measures for delivery of the child are then carried out. The incisions are repaired with continuous, interrupted, or figure-8 sutures. While there is rarely much bleeding, preparations to treat hemorrhage should be at hand. Most cervices heal well, and future pregnancies deliver normally.

ANNULAR DETACHMENT OF THE CERVIX

The anterior lip of the cervix may be compressed between the fetal head and the pubic symphysis. If this situation continues for a long time, edema, local anemia, anoxia, and even necrosis may develop. Rarely, an entire ring of cervix undergoes anoxic necrosis, and a section of the vaginal part of the cervix comes away. This is known as annular detachment of the cervix. Because the prolonged pressure has caused the blood vessels to thrombose, excessive bleeding from the cervix is unusual.

Etiology

1. Seventy-five percent of cases occur in primigravidas.
2. Prolonged labor is almost always the rule.
3. There is often a history of early rupture of the membranes.
4. The fetal head is low in the pelvis.

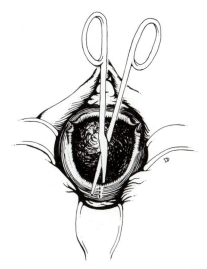

Figure 9. Dührssen cervical incisions at 2, 6, and 10 o'clock.

5. The cervix is well effaced and often quite thin. It is the external os that does not dilate. Several observers have reported that the cervix feels rigid to palpation during the first stage of labor.
6. The uterine contractions are strong and efficient.

Mechanism

The myometrial contractions press the presenting part against the thinned out, rigid external os; in addition, the retracting upper segment of the uterus pulls the cervix upward. This double action leads to poor circulation in the cervix, anoxia, and necrosis. A tear starts at the cervicovaginal junction, and a line of cleavage develops and continues until the separation is complete. The characteristic doughnut-shaped ring of tissue becomes detached when the cervix is about 3 to 5 cm dilated. Gross histologic examinations have revealed these cervices to be no different from the normal term organ.

Clinical Picture

The clinical picture is one of good labor obstructed by an unyielding external os. In almost every case the fetus is delivered without difficulty once the cervical obstruction is overcome. Annular detachment is the result of true cervical dystocia.

Treatment

Because the vessels are thrombosed, serious bleeding from the stump is rare. No active treatment is needed. The rare maternal death occurs either from sepsis or from uterine bleeding associated with prolonged labor and postpartum uterine atony. Any hemorrhage that originates in the cervix must be controlled by figure-8 sutures.

Prevention

Prevention is achieved by recognizing the situation before the actual detachment takes place. When the cervix is effaced and thin, cervical incisions are indicated; delivery usually follows. If the situation is not right for the cervical incisions, cesarean section must be done.

Prognosis

Many women avoid future pregnancy. Stenosis and hematometra have been recorded. Several subsequent gestations have been delivered vaginally with no difficulty and there has been one elective cesarean section and one abortion from an incompetent os reported.

RUPTURE OF THE UTERUS

Rupture of the uterus is a dangerous complication of pregnancy. It is responsible for 5 percent of maternal deaths in the United States and Canada, and is an even greater hazard in the underdeveloped countries.

Incidence

The reported incidence varies from 1:93 confinements to 1:8741, depending on the source of the material. The average incidence is around 1:2000. Recent publications suggest that the number of uterine ruptures is increasing and blame this fact on (1) more frequent use of cesarean section, leaving a scarred uterus for the next pregnancy, (2) careless administration of oxytocic drugs, (3) inadequate professional care during labor, and (4) lackadaisical and poor management of labor and delivery, i.e., nonrecognition of an obstructed labor.

Types of Rupture

1. *The rupture is complete* when all the layers of the uterus are involved and there is a direct communication between the uterine and abdominal cavities. This is the common variety.
2. *The incomplete rupture* includes the whole myometrium; the peritoneum covering the uterus remains intact.
3. A *third variety* may occur. In this instance the serosa and part of the external myometrium are torn, but the laceration does not extend into the cavity. A severe intraperitoneal hemorrhage may take place without the condition being diagnosed. This situation should be suspected when there are signs of an intraabdominal catastrophe during or after labor, but no uterine defect is detectable on manual exploration of the uterine cavity.

Site and Time of Rupture

Tears that take place during pregnancy are more often in the upper segment of the uterus, at the site of previous operation or injury. During labor the rupture is usually in the lower segment. The longer the labor, the more thinned out the lower segment, and the greater the danger of rupture. The tear may extend into the uterine vessels and cause profuse hemorrhage. Tears in the anterior or posterior walls of the uterus usually extend transversely or obliquely. In the region of the broad ligament the laceration runs longitudinally up the sides of the uterus.

It may occur during pregnancy, normal labor, or difficult labor, or it may follow labor. Most ruptures take place at or near term. Those happening before the onset of labor are usually dehiscences of cesarean section scars.

Classification

Spontaneous Rupture of the Normal Uterus
These accidents occur during labor, are more common in the lower segment of the uterus, and are the result of mismanagement and neglect. Etiologic factors include:

1. Multiparity
2. Disproportion
3. Abnormal presentation (brow, breech, transverse lie)
4. Improper use of oxytocin

Traumatic Rupture
This is caused by ill-advised and poorly executed operative vaginal deliveries. The incidence is decreasing. Etiologic factors include:

1. Version and extraction
2. Difficult forceps operations
3. Forceful breech extraction
4. Craniotomy
5. Excessive manual pressure on the fundus of the uterus
6. Manual dilatation of the cervix

Postcesarean Rupture
This is the most common variety seen today. It may occur before or during labor. Upper segment scars rupture more often than lower segment incisions. While hysterograms done 3 months after operation may give an indication as to whether good healing has taken place, there is no accurate way of predicting the behavior of a uterine scar. All cesarean section scars present a hazard.

Rupture Following Trauma Other Than Cesarean
The danger is that often the damage is not recognized, and the accident comes as a surprise. Included in this group are:

1. Previous myomectomy
2. Too vigorous curettage
3. Perforation during curettage
4. Cervical laceration
5. Manual removal of an adherent placenta
6. Placenta percreta
7. Endometritis and myometritis
8. Hydatidiform mole
9. Cornual resection for ectopic pregnancy

10. Hysterotomy
11. Amniocentesis during the pregnancy may lead to a weakened area in the myometrium.

Silent Bloodless Dehiscence of a Previous Cesarean Scar

This is a complication of lower segment cesarean sections. Part or all of the incision may be involved. Usually the peritoneum over the scar is intact. Many of these windows are areas not of current rupture but of failure of the original incision to heal. This complication is in no way as serious as true uterine rupture. Features of this complication include:

1. Usually diagnosed during repeat cesarean section, being unsuspected before operation
2. No hemorrhage at site of dehiscence
3. No shock
4. Hysterectomy not necessary
5. No fetal death
6. No maternal mortality

Clinical Picture

The clinical picture of uterine rupture is variable in that it depends on many factors:

1. Time of occurrence (pregnancy, early or late labor)
2. Cause of the rupture
3. Degree of the rupture (complete or incomplete)
4. Position of the rupture
5. Extent of the rupture
6. Amount of intraperitoneal spill
7. Size of the blood vessels involved and the amount of bleeding
8. Complete or partial extrusion of the fetus and placenta from the uterus
9. Degree of retraction of the myometrium
10. General condition of the patient

On a clinical basis rupture of the uterus may be divided into four groups.

1. *Silent or quiet rupture:* The accident occurs without (initially) the usual signs and symptoms. Diagnosis is difficult and often delayed. Nothing dramatic happens, but the observant attendant notices a rising pulse rate, pallor, and perhaps slight vaginal

bleeding. The patient complains of some pain. The contractions may go on, but the cervix fails to dilate. This type is usually associated with the scar of a previous cesarean section.

2. *Usual variety:* The picture develops over a period of a few hours. The signs and symptoms include abdominal pain, vomiting, faintness, vaginal bleeding, rapid pulse rate, pallor, tenderness on palpation, and absence of the fetal heart. These features may have arisen during pregnancy or labor. If the diagnosis is not made, hypotension and shock supervene.

3. *Violent rupture:* It is apparent almost immediately that a serious accident has taken place. Usually a hard uterine contraction is followed by the sensation of something having given way and a sharp pain in the lower abdomen. Often the contractions cease, there is a change in the character of the pain, and the patient becomes anxious. The fetus can be palpated easily and feels close to the examining fingers. The presenting part is no longer at the pelvic brim and can be moved freely. Sometimes the uterus and fetus can be palpated in different parts of the abdomen. Fetal movements cease, and the fetal heart is not heard. The symptoms and signs of shock appear soon, and complete collapse may occur.

4. *Rupture with delayed diagnosis:* Here the condition is not diagnosed until the patient is in a process of gradual deterioration. Unexplained anemia leads to careful investigation, a palpable hematoma develops in the broad ligament, signs of peritoneal irritation appear, or the patient goes into shock (either gradually or suddenly as when a hematoma in the broad ligament ruptures). Sometimes the diagnosis is made only at autopsy.

Diagnosis

The diagnosis is made easily when the classic picture is present or when the rupture is catastrophic. In atypical cases the diagnosis may be difficult. A high index of suspicion is important. If routine exploration of the uterus is not carried out after every birth, then at least following all difficult deliveries whenever there is unexplained shock or postpartum bleeding the interior of the cavity should be explored manually and the lower segment searched for tears.

Palpatory findings, as described in the previous section, may be pathognomonic. The fetal heart beat is absent in most cases. An x-ray of the abdomen may demonstrate the fetus lying in the peritoneal cavity surrounded by the intestines, with the shadow of the uterus to one side.

Treatment

Treatment must be prompt and in keeping with the patient's condition. Laparotomy is performed, and the bleeding is controlled as quickly as possible. Aortic compression (by the hand or by using a special instrument) is useful in reducing the bleeding until the situation can be evaluated. Most patients are critically ill and are unable to stand prolonged surgery.

In most cases total hysterectomy is the procedure of choice. If the patient is in poor condition rapid subtotal hysterectomy may be performed. If, however, the tear has extended into the cervix, the bleeding will not be controlled by subtotal hysterectomy. In such cases, if it cannot be removed, the cervix must be sutured carefully to tie off all bleeding points.

In young women and in those who desire more children, treatment may be limited to repair of the tear. This should be done only when the uterine musculature can be so reconstituted as to assure a reasonable degree of success and safety for a future pregnancy. In repairing the laceration, the edges of the wound are freshened and the tissues approximated carefully in two or three layers. As supportive treatment blood must be replaced rapidly. Subsequent fertility is impaired, and the reported rate of recurrent rupture is between 4 and 19 percent.

Maternal Mortality

The reported maternal death rate ranges from 3 to 40 percent. Spontaneous rupture of the uterus is responsible for the largest number of deaths, followed by the traumatic variety. The amount of hemorrhage is greatest in these types. The lowest death rate is associated with postcesarean ruptures, probably because these patients are observed so carefully during labor.

The main causes of death are shock and blood loss (usually over 1000 ml). Sepsis and paralytic ileus are contributory factors.

The prognosis for the mother depends on (1) prompt diagnosis and treatment, the interval between rupture and surgery being important; (2) the amount of hemorrhage and the availability of blood; (3) whether infection sets in; and (4) the type and site of the rupture.

The mortality rate is lower today because of:

1. Early diagnosis
2. Immediate laparotomy
3. Blood transfusion
4. Antibiotics

5. Reduction or elimination of traumatic vaginal operative deliveries
6. Better management of prolonged or obstructed labor

Fetal Mortality

Fetal mortality is high, ranging from 30 to 85 percent. Most fetuses die from separation of the placenta. There is a reduction of blood supply available to the fetus after the uterus has ruptured. Probably the prolonged labor before rupture plays a part in causing fetal hypoxia. Many of these babies are premature. The highest mortality is associated with fundal rupture where the fetus has been extruded into the abdominal cavity.

Pregnancy After Rupture of the Uterus

Ritchie reported 28 patients who had 36 pregnancies following repair of a ruptured uterus. Repeat rupture occurred in 13 percent with two maternal deaths. The risk of repeat rupture is:

1. Least when the scar is confined to the lower segment
2. Greater if the scar extends into the upper segment
3. Greatest in women whose original rupture occurred following classic cesarean section

Management
Cesarean section should be performed before the scar is subjected to stress.

1. Scar in lower segment: cesarean section at 38 weeks
2. Scar in upper segment: cesarean section at 36 weeks

INVERSION OF THE UTERUS

Uterine inversion is a turning inside out of the uterus. In the extreme case the doctor may see the purplish endometrium, with the placenta often still attached. In the severe situation the patient may be bleeding profusely, hypotensive, and sometimes pulseless. The reported incidence ranges from 1:100,000 to 1:5000 deliveries. It occurs rarely in the nongravid uterus in association with a pedunculated submucous myoma. The rate of maternal mortality varies between 0 and 18 percent, depending on diagnosis and management.

Hippocrates (460-370 BC) recognized uterine inversion and Avicenna (980-1037 AD) described uterine inversion and prolapse, but it is chiefly since the time of Ambroise Paré in the sixteenth century that a true understanding of uterine inversion exists.

Etiology

The disorder's mechanism is not understood completely. It is believed to be related to an abnormality of the myometrium. Some inversions are spontaneous and tend to recur at subsequent deliveries; however, it occurs more often in primigravidas.

Many are caused by improper obstetric manipulations, but they may take place after normal or abnormal labor. Most often inversion is a catastrophe of the third stage of labor.

Predisposing Factors

1. Abnormalities of the uterus and its contents
   a. Adherent placenta
   b. Short umbilical cord
   c. Congenital anomalies
   d. Weakness of uterine wall at the placental site
   e. Fundal implantation of the placenta
   f. Neoplasm of the uterus
2. Functional conditions of the uterus
   a. Relaxation of the myometrium
   b. Disturbance of the contractile mechanism

Exciting Causes

1. Manual removal of the placenta
2. Increase in abdominal pressure
   a. Coughing
   b. Sneezing
3. Mismanagement of third stage of labor
   a. Improper fundal pressure
   b. Traction on the cord
   c. Injudicious use of oxytocics

Classification

Classification on the basis of stage is as follows:

1. *Acute,* occurring immediately after birth of the baby or placenta, before there is contraction of the cervical ring
2. *Subacute,* beginning when contraction of the cervix becomes established

3. *Chronic,* present for more than 4 weeks

Classification on the basis of degree includes three types:

1. *Incomplete,* when the fundus is not beyond the internal os of the cervix
2. *Complete,* when the fundus protrudes through the external os of the cervix
3. *Prolapse,* in which the fundus protrudes through the vulva

Pathology

The following sequence of events may take place, especially if the diagnosis is not made:

1. Acute inversion
2. Contraction of the cervical ring and lower segment of the uterus around the encircled portion of the uterus
3. Edema
4. Reduction of blood supply
5. Gangrene and necrosis
6. Sloughing

Clinical Picture

Sometimes the symptoms are minor so the diagnosis is not made, or the condition is recognized but treatment is not carried out at the time. These are the chronic inversions. Those that cause shock and require immediate therapy are the acute ones.

In the typical case, after the birth of the infant, traction on the cord, in an effort to deliver the placenta, leads to its advancement, but, if the patient is awake there is a good deal of pain. Finally, with continued traction on the cord, the placenta is delivered, but it is attached to a bluish-gray mass that fills the vaginal outlet. This is the interior of the uterine fundus. If the diagnosis is made and replacement accomplished quickly, the patient will remain in good condition and bleeding will not be excessive.

In a different situation the placenta is delivered with some difficulty by fundal pressure and traction on the umbilical cord. As the episiotomy is being repaired the physician notes that bleeding is profuse. The uterus cannot be felt by the nurse as she tries to massage it. On vaginal examination the cervix cannot be located. Instead, a grayish mass, oozing blood, fills the vagina. Rapid diagnosis and deinversion of the uterus will avoid blood loss, trauma, and shock. The latter will take place if the diagnosis is not made.

When the inversion is complete the diagnosis is easy. Partial inversions may fool the observer. Classically, shock is greater than expected for the amount of bleeding. The extreme shock is probably caused by tension on the nerves of the broad ligament, which are drawn through the cervical ring, and by irritation of the peritoneum. In any situation where shock is out of proportion to hemorrhage the accoucheur should think of uterine inversion. The placenta may have separated or may remain attached. The hemorrhage may be excessive or minimal.

Diagnosis

1. High index of suspicion
2. Absence of uterine fundus on abdominal examination
3. Vaginal examination
4. Uterine rupture must be excluded

Prophylaxis

1. No attempt should be made to deliver the placenta until it has separated.
2. To deliver the placenta, the Brandt maneuver is safer than the Credé method of expression by fundal pressure, or by traction on the cord.
3. Routine exploration of the postpartum uterus will detect a uterine inversion in its incomplete stage, before it has descended through the vaginal introitus.

Treatment of Acute Inversion

The aim of treatment is to replace the uterus as soon as possible. The patient should be cross-matched and blood given as necessary. Replacement of the uterus must not be delayed until shock has been treated, since the latter may not be overcome as long as the uterus remains inverted.

In most cases the placenta will have been delivered. If it is still attached, it can be removed manually or replaced with the fundus, whichever is easier. On the one hand, attempts to remove the placenta prior to the uterine replacement may lead to profuse bleeding. On the other hand, if the placenta has been removed, correction of the inversion will be easier because the mass that has to be replaced is smaller.

Technique of Replacement

The patient is anesthetized. In the first step of the procedure the uterus is grasped so that the inverted fundus lies in the palm of the hand with the fingers placed near the uterocervical junction (Fig. 10A.). As pressure is exerted on the uterus it gradually returns into the vagina. In the second step (Fig. 10B.) the uterus is lifted out of the pelvis and held in the abdominal cavity above the level of the umbilicus. This stretches and tautens the uterine ligaments. As the uterine ligaments are placed under tension, the resultant pressure widens the cervical ring and then pulls the fundus through it. In this way the uterus is replaced to its normal position. Success may not be immediate and it may take 3 to 5 minutes until the uterine fundus recedes from the palm of the hand.

Treatment of Subacute Inversion

Once the cervix has contracted, immediate replacement of the uterus is no longer feasible.

1. The vagina is packed with 2-inch gauze, without replacing the uterus, pushing the cervix into the abdominal cavity. A Foley catheter is inserted into the bladder.
2. The patient is treated for shock, and blood transfusion is given in the amount lost.
3. Antibiotics may be used.
4. During the next 48 hours fluids and electrolytes are infused in an attempt at restoring the patient to a condition suitable for surgery. At the same time it is hoped that some uterine involution will take place.
5. Laparotomy is carried out and the inversion corrected by a combined abdominovaginal operation, as for chronic inversion.

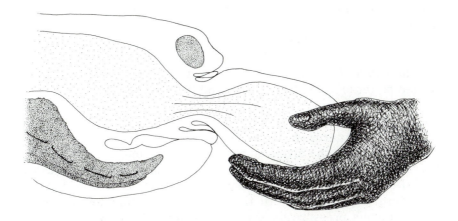

Figure 10A. Replacement of the inverted uterus: Step 1.

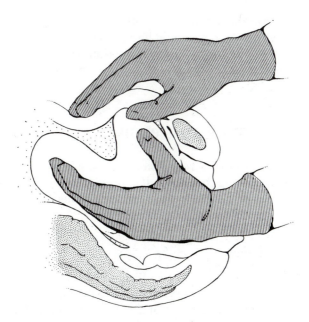

Figure 10B. Replacement of the inverted uterus: Step 2.

Treatment of Chronic Inversion

Spinelli Procedure. Using the vaginal approach, the contracted cervical ring is incised anteriorly, so that the fundus of the uterus can be pushed back into place.

Haultain Procedure. Laparotomy is performed. The cervical ring is incised posteriorly and the uterine fundus is drawn up.

Huntington Procedure. The approach is per abdominal incision. The surface of the uterus inside the crater is grasped with Allis forceps about 2 cm below the inversion cup on each side and upward traction exerted. As the uterus comes up through the ring additional forceps are placed below the original ones and further traction is exerted. This procedure is continued until the inversion is completely reversed. Simultaneous pressure on the fundus through the vagina by an assistant may make the procedure easier.

Prognosis

The reported rate of recurrence is over 40 percent. Some authorities believe that further pregnancy should be avoided. It is probable that subsequent delivery should be by cesarean section. However, this does not obviate the problem entirely as inversion can occur even at cesarean section.

SEPARATION OF SYMPHYSIS PUBIS

During pregnancy there is relaxation and weakening of the pelvic joints. This begins during the first half of pregnancy and reaches a maximum in the seventh month. Return to normal begins after delivery and is complete by the sixth month.

Incidence and Etiology

This varies from 1:250 to 1:30,000 confinements. Minor degrees of separation take place, but since the symptoms are minimal the diagnosis is not made and spontaneous correction follows. This accident may occur during labor or in the second half of pregnancy.

Rupture of the pubic symphysis occurs in patients with excessive relaxation of the pelvic joints. Precipitating factors include:

1. Tumultuous labor
2. Difficult forceps extractions

3. Cephalopelvic disproportion
4. Excessive abduction of the thighs at delivery
5. Any condition that might place sudden and excessive pressure on the pubic symphysis

Many cases occur following spontaneous delivery.

Pathology

There is an actual tear of the ligaments connecting the pubic bones. The rupture is usually incomplete, and a fibrocartilagenous bridge remains. Hemorrhage and edema are present. Arthritis or osteomyelitis are possible complications.

Clinical Picture and Diagnosis

The onset of symptoms is usually sudden but may not be noted until the patient tries to walk. At the time of rupture the patient may experience a bursting feeling, or a cracking noise may be heard.

Motion of the symphysis (as by moving the legs) causes great pain. If the patient can walk, she does so with a waddling gait.

There is a marked tenderness of the pubic symphysis. Edema and ecchymosis are present frequently. A gaping defect in the joint is often palpable. Walking or pressure causes motion of the loose joint.

Diagnosis is made by the symptoms and signs. X-ray helps, but the degree of separation seen on radiologic study may not be proportional to the clinical manifestations. To be considered pathologic the separation seen on x-ray should be greater than 1 cm.

Management of symptomatic separation must be directed at relieving the patient's discomfort and compensating for her disability. Treatment is governed by the severity of the condition. Analgesia is essential.

Some patients require prolonged bed rest, with a tight corset or peritrochanteric belt to keep the separated bones as nearly apposed as possible. The local injection of Novocain may help. While in hospital the patient should sleep with a bed board under the mattress; she should also use a trapeze to pull herself to a sitting position so as not to strain the pelvis.

When the rupture is minor early ambulation is permissible. When the problem is more severe crutches should be used. Support is needed for 6 weeks. The patient must limit her use of stairs.

Surgical intervention is indicated rarely. When necessary, fusions may be carried out, often supplemented by bone grafts, bolts, and crossed wires.

BIBLIOGRAPHY

Harris BA: Acute puerperal inversion of the uterus. Clin Obstet Gynecol 27:134, 1984

Lee WK, Baggish MS, Lashgari M: Acute inversion of the uterus. Obstet Gynecol 51:144, 1978

Ritchie EA: Pregnancy after rupture of the pregnant uterus. J Obstet Gynecol Brit Commonw 78:642, 1971

Schrinsky DC, Benson RC: Rupture of the pregnant uterus: A review. Obstet Gynecol Surv 33:217, 1978

Spaulding LB, Gallup DG: Current concepts of management of rupture of the gravid uterus. Obstet Gynecol 54:437, 1979

Thacker SB, Banta HD: Benefits and risks of episiotomy: An interpretive view of the English language literature, 1860–1980. Obstet Gynecol Survey 38:322, 1983

Watson O, Besch N, Bowes WA: Management of acute and subacute puerperal inversion of the uterus. Obstet Gynecol 55:12, 1980

35

The Placenta, Retained Placenta, Placenta Accreta

THE PLACENTA

Normal Placenta

Size and Shape. The placenta is a round or oval disk, 20 x 15 cm in size and 1.5 to 2.0 cm thick. The weight, usually 20 percent of that of the fetus, is between 425 and 550 g.

Organization. On the uterine side there are eight or more maternal cotyledons separated by fissures. The term fetal cotyledon refers to that part of the placenta that is supplied by a main stem villus and its branches. The maternal surface is covered by a layer of decidua and fibrin, which comes away with the placenta at delivery. The fetal side is covered by membranes.

Location. Normally the placenta is implanted in the upper part of the uterus. Occasionally it is placed in the lower segment, and sometimes it lies over the cervix. The latter condition is termed placenta previa and is a cause of bleeding in the third trimester. Ultrasonic examinations in early pregnancy have demonstrated the placenta to be in the lower segment, suggesting placenta previa. At reexamination late in pregnancy the placenta is found in the upper segment. Probably the normal growth of the placenta is away from the cervix. In addition, the uterus enlarges faster than the placenta and, as pregnancy progresses, a proportionately smaller area of the wall of the uterus is occupied by placenta. No cases of downward migration of the placenta have been reported.

Abnormalities of the Placenta

Succenturiate Lobe. This is an accessory lobe that is placed at some distance from the main placenta. The blood vessels that supply this lobe run over the intervening membranes and may be torn when the latter rupture or during delivery. A succenturiate lobe may be retained after birth and cause postpartum hemorrhage.

Circumvallate Placenta. The membranes are folded back on the fetal surface and insert inward on themselves. The placenta is situated outside of the chorion.

Amnion Nodosum. This is a yellow nodule, 3 to 4 cm in diameter, situated on the fetal surface of the amnion. It contains vernix, fibrin, desquamated cells, and lanugo hairs. It may form a cyst. This condition is associated with oligohydramnios.

Infarcts. Localized infarcts are common. The clinical significance is not known, although if the condition is excessive, the functional capacity of the placenta may be reduced.

Discoloration. Red staining is associated with hemorrhage. Green color is caused by meconium and may be an indication of fetal hypoxia.

Twin Placenta. In monochorionic twins the placenta forms one mass, whereas in dichorionic twins the placentas may be fused or separate.

Weight. Placentas weighing over 600 g or under 400 g are usually associated with abnormal pregnancy.

The Placenta in Various Conditions

Prematurity. The placenta is small and often pale.

Postmaturity. The size and weight are usually normal. There may be meconium staining. If there is excessive fibrosis or infarction, the placental function may be reduced.

Intrauterine Growth Retardation. The placenta tends to be small, the decrease in weight being proportional to the weight of the infant.

Diabetes Mellitus. The placenta is usually larger than normal, but in severe cases, when the mother's circulation is affected, the placenta may be small.

Toxemia of Pregnancy. No specific changes are seen. Often the placenta appears normal.

Erythroblastosis. The placenta is boggy, is pale pink to yellow in color, and may weigh as much as 2000 g.

Congenital Syphilis. The placenta is large, thick, and pale.

Amnionitis. The membranes are opaque and have yellow discoloration. The placenta may be foul smelling.

RETAINED PLACENTA

Retention of the placenta in utero falls into four groups:

1. *Separated but retained*: Here there is failure of the forces that normally expel the placenta.
2. *Separated but incarcerated*: An hourglass constriction of the uterus, or cervical spasm, traps the placenta in the upper segment.
3. *Adherent but separable*: In this situation the placenta fails to separate from the uterine wall. The causes include failure of the normal contraction and retraction of the third stage, an anatomic defect in the uterus, and an abnormality of the decidua which prevents formation of the normal decidual plane of cleavage.
4. *Adherent and inseparable*: Here are the varying degrees of placenta accreta. The normal decidua is absent, and the chorionic villi are attached directly to and through the myometrium.

Technique of Manual Removal

Manual removal of the retained placenta is not considered to be as dangerous as it once was. Many of the bad outcomes of this procedure were the result of too long a delay in treatment until hemorrhage had put the patient in a precarious state. When bleeding is present the placenta must be removed immediately. If there is no associated hemorrhage and the patient is in good condition, a delay of 30 minutes is permissible.

If the patient has been bleeding actively, an intravenous infusion is set up and blood is made available. Anesthesia is necessary. The procedure is carried out under aseptic conditions.

The uterus is steadied by one hand holding the fundus through the maternal abdomen (Fig. 1). The other hand is inserted into the vagina and through the cervix into the uterine cavity. The placenta is reached by following the umbilical cord. If the placenta has separated it is grasped and removed. The uterus is then explored to be sure that nothing has been left.

If the placenta is still adherent to the uterine wall it must be separated. First some part of the margin of attachment is identified and the fingers inserted between the placenta and the wall of the uterus. The back of the hand is kept in contact with the uterine wall. The fingers are forced gently between the placenta and uterus, and as progress is made they are spread apart. In this way the line of cleavage is extended, the placenta is separated from the uterine wall, and it is then extracted. Oxytocics are given to ensure good uterine contraction and retraction.

PLACENTA ACCRETA

Placenta accreta is defined as the abnormal adherence, either in whole or in part, of the afterbirth to the underlying uterine wall. The placental villi adhere to, invade into, or penetrate through the myometrium.

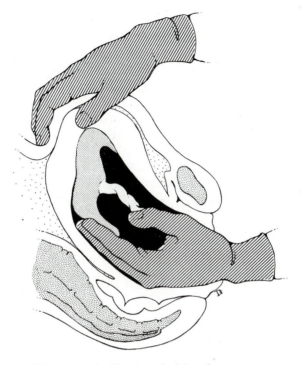

Figure 1. Manual removal of the placenta.

Pathology

Normally the decidua basalis lies between the myometrium and the placenta (Fig. 2A). The plane of cleavage for placental separation is in the spongy layer of the decidua basalis. In placenta accreta the decidua basalis is partially or completely absent (Fig. 2B), so that the placenta is attached directly to the myometrium. The villi may remain superficial to the uterine muscle or may penetrate it deeply. This condition is caused by a defect in the decidua rather than by any abnormal invasive properties of the trophoblast.

In the superficial area of the myometrium a large number of venous channels develop just beneath the placenta. Rupture of these sinuses by forceful extraction of the placenta is the source of the profuse hemorrhage that occurs.

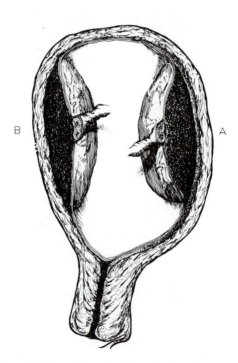

Figure 2. Uteroplacental relationships. A. Normal: decidua separates placenta from myometrium. B. Placenta accreta: absence of decidua.

Classification

1. By extent
   a. Complete: The whole placenta is adherent to the myometrium.
   b. Partial: One or more cotyledons or part of a cotyledon is adherent.
2. By depth
   a. Accreta: The placenta is adherent to the myometrium. There is no line of cleavage.
   b. Increta: The villi penetrate the uterine muscle but not its full thickness (Fig. 2C).
   c. Percreta: The villi penetrate the wall of the uterus and perforate the serosa (Fig 2D). Intraperitoneal bleeding occurs frequently. Occasionally the uterus is ruptured. The villi may grow into the cavity of the bladder and cause gross hematuria.

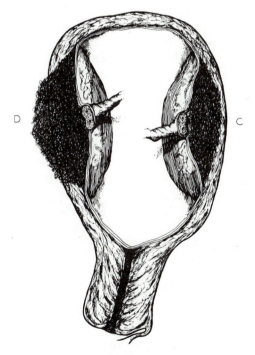

Figure 2. (cont.) Uteroplacental relationships. C. Placenta increta: villi penetrate the myometrium. D. Placenta percreta: villi extend through the uterine wall.

Incidence

The true incidence is impossible to determine. The reported range varies from 1:540 to 1:93,000 deliveries.

Etiology

1. Maternal factors:
   a. Older gravidas.
   b. Multiparity. Placenta accreta is rare in primigravidas.
2. Uterine factors:
   a. Previous cesarean section. Often the placenta is implanted over the uterine scar.
   b. Previous uterine surgery.
   c. Previous uterine curettage, mainly following a pregnancy or abortion.
   d. Previous manual removal of placenta.
   e. Previous endometritis.
3. Placental factors:
   a. Placenta previa.
   b. Cornual implantation.

The significance of most of the etiologic factors is uncertain. The two most frequent predisposing factors are placenta previa and previous cesarean section.

The underlying condition that appears to be common to all causal conditions is a deficiency of the endometrium and the decidua:

1. The decidua overlying the scar of a previous cesarean section is often deficient.
2. In women who have placenta previa the decidua of the lower uterine segment is relatively poorly developed.
3. The decidua of the uterine cornu is usually hypoplastic.
4. With increasing age and parity there is, in many women, a progressive inadequacy of decidua.
5. Previous curettage or manual removal of placenta is probably not an etiologic factor but an indication that an abnormal adherence of the placenta was the reason for the procedure's being necessary.

Clinical Picture

Pregnancy

1. Most patients have a normal pregnancy.
2. The incidence of antepartum bleeding is increased, but this is usually associated with placenta previa.

3. Premature labor occurs, but only when precipitated by bleeding.
4. Rarely, rupture of the uterus takes place.

Labor: First and Second Stages
These are normal in almost all cases.

Third Stage of Labor

1. *Retained placenta.* This is the main and presenting feature.
2. *Postpartum hemorrhage.* The amount of bleeding depends on the degree of placental attachment. In complete placenta accreta there is no bleeding. In the partial variety bleeding takes place from the uterine vessels underlying the detached area, while the adherent portion prevents the uterus from retracting properly. Often the bleeding is precipitated by the obstetrician as he attempts manual removal of the placenta. In a recent report of 22 cases the average loss of blood was 3826 ml, and the mean amount of blood transfused was 8 units.
3. *Uterine inversion.* A rare, but serious complication, is uterine inversion. This may occur spontaneously, but is more often the result of attempts to remove the placenta.
4. *Rupture of the uterus.* This may occur during too vigorous attempts to extract the afterbirth.

Diagnosis

The gross diagnosis is provisional and is made in two ways. (1) Direct intrauterine palpation. No line of cleavage can be found between the placenta and uterus. The examining fingers slide over the fetal side of the placenta. (2) Study of the uterus and placenta following hysterectomy.

Microscopic examination establishes the diagnosis by demonstrating chorionic villi in the myometrium.

The differential diagnosis includes:

1. Retained incarcerated placenta
2. Adherent placenta, where there is a line of cleavage
3. Retained placental fragments
4. Subinvolution of the placental site
5. Choriocarcinoma

Management

The safest treatment is hysterectomy. Since this puts an end to childbearing, a conservative method of therapy has evolved based on the

availability of blood and antibiotics. When placenta accreta is suspected, the following plan of management is useful.

Diagnosis and Preliminary Treatment

1. An intravenous infusion is started with a wide-bore needle.
2. Blood is cross-matched.
3. Expert anesthesia should be available.
4. The operating room must be ready for an emergency.
5. Intrauterine exploration is performed to see whether placenta
   accreta is present, and if so whether it is complete or partial.
6. In making the diagnosis an attempt is made to remove the placenta. In most instances placenta accreta is not present. Overzealous attempts to extract the placenta must be avoided since
   the uterus can be ruptured.

Indications for Hysterectomy

1. Further pregnancy is not desired
2. Uncontrollable hemorrhage
3. Failure of conservative management
4. Intrauterine suppuration
5. Placenta previa accreta

Conservative Management: Total Placenta Accreta

1. There is no bleeding unless attempts are made to remove the
   placenta.
2. The cord is cut short and the blood drained from the placenta.
3. The placenta is left in the uterus.
4. Broad-spectrum antibiotics are given.
5. The placenta becomes organized and partially absorbed, and the
   superficial portion sloughs off.
6. In some cases suppuration takes place and generalized infection
   may set in.

Conservative Management: Partial Placenta Accreta

1. All separated placenta is removed manually. The part of the placenta that is abnormally attached is left.
2. An intravenous oxytocin infusion is maintained for 48 hours.
3. The patient is observed carefully and constantly.
4. Broad-spectrum antibiotics are given.
5. If there is no bleeding after 48 hours, the first stage of conservative management has been successful.

Placenta Previa Accreta

Because the decidua of the lower segment is less abundant than that in the fundus, a placenta implanted near the cervix may be abnormally adherent. The treatment is total hysterectomy.

Maternal Mortality

Maternal mortality has decreased greatly from the rate of 37 percent reported before 1934. Fox's review summarized maternal mortality rates from 1945 to 1955 as 10.1 percent and from 1955 to 1969 as 9.5 percent. Three recent reports of a total of 4 deaths in 129 cases gives a maternal mortality rate of only 3.1 percent. The danger of death has decreased because of (1) a greater awareness of the problem, (2) the availability and use of adequate replacement of blood, (3) the effectiveness of antibiotics in combatting infection, and (4) the performance of hysterectomy before the patient is moribund.

Fetal Results

An incidence of intrauterine fetal death of 9.6 percent indicates that a risk to the fetus exists. Fetal death is associated with antepartum bleeding, uterine rupture, and no discernible cause in equal proportions.

BIBLIOGRAPHY

Breen JL, Gregori CA, Franklin JE: Placenta accreta, increta, and percreta. Obstet Gynecol 49:43, 1977

Cario GM, Adler AD, Morris N: Placenta percreta presenting as intraabdominal antepartum hemorrhage. Brit J Obstet Gynaecol 90:491, 1983

Fox H: Placenta accreta 1945–1969. Obstet Gynecol Survey 27:475, 1972

Read JA, Cotton DB, Miller FC: Placenta accreta: Changing clinical aspects and outcome. Obstet Gynecol 56:31, 1980

36

The Amniotic Fluid

In normal pregnancy the volume of amniotic fluid increases gradually to around 1000 ml (600 to 1500) at 36 weeks. Thereafter it decreases, and in postterm pregnancy there may be only a couple of hundred ml.

The major source of amniotic fluid is assumed to be the amniotic epithelium, but there are other mechanisms. During the first half of pregnancy the volume of amniotic fluid correlates with fetal weight, its composition resembles that of the fetal extracellular fluid, and it is believed that there is some diffusion of fluid across the fetal skin. In the second half of gestation, rapid diffusion across fetal skin is impaired by its cornification. Other sources of fluid, such as filtrate of maternal plasma and fetal urine play an increasingly important part in the maintenance of the volume of amniotic fluid. The turnover is rapid; some 500 ml enter and leave the amniotic sac each hour.

The normal fetus swallows around 500 ml of amniotic fluid per day, and this is one way by which the fluid is removed. In many, but not all, cases where there is obstruction between the fetal mouth and the intestinal tract an excessive amount of amniotic fluid is present.

Fetal micturition is an important source of amniotic fluid. An 18-week fetus voids approximately 7 to 17 ml per 24 hours. By term this increases to 40 to 45 ml per hour. Fetal abnormalities that cause anuria are nearly always associated with oligohydramnios, a reduction in the amount of amniotic liquor.

Secretions from the fetal respiratory tract do enter the amniotic cavity, but it is not known whether this is a major source of amniotic fluid.

POLYHYDRAMNIOS

Polyhydramnios (hydramnios) is a pathologic condition characterized by an excessive amount of amniotic fluid; by definition over 2000 ml. In severe cases as much as 15 liters of fluid have been reported. The amniotic fluid in polyhydramnios has the same composition as in normal pregnancy.

Minor degrees of polyhydramnios (2 to 3 liters) are common, the reported incidence being 1:150 to 1:280 pregnancies. Polyhydramnios sufficient to cause clinical symptoms (over 3 to 4 liters) occurs less than once in every 3000 deliveries.

Etiology

1. Idiopathic. In 35 percent of cases no cause can be found.
2. Diabetes mellitus is the underlying factor in about 25 percent. How diabetes causes polyhydramnios is not known.
3. Congenital anomalies are implicated in some 20 percent. Those found most often include anencephaly, microcephaly, hydrocephaly, spina bifida with meningocele or meningomyelocele, and intestinal abnormalities, such as esophageal atresia and tracheoesophageal fistula. The latter conditions interfere with fetal swallowing. Suspected reasons for the association of polyhydramnios and anencephaly include: a decrease in fetal swallowing, increased production of fluid by transudation from the exposed meninges, and the lack of production of antidiuretic hormone which leads to fetal polyuria.
4. Erythroblastosis accounts for about 10 percent of cases of polyhydramnios.
5. Multiple gestation is seen in around 10 percent.

Symptoms

The maternal symptoms depend on the stage of the gestation, the amount of amniotic fluid, and the rapidity of accumulation.

Mild symptoms include abdominal discomfort and slight dyspnea.

In severe cases (over 4000 ml of fluid) there is abdominal pain, dyspnea and orthopnea, edema of the abdomen, vulva, and legs, and nausea and vomiting.

Types of Polyhydramnios

Acute Polyhydramnios

Less than 2 percent of cases of polyhydramnios are in the acute group. This variety occurs in the second trimester of pregnancy, before the fetus is viable. The accumulation of fluid is rapid, over a short period of time. Preterm labor, before 28 weeks, is frequent. The fetal prognosis is guarded, mainly because of prematurity.

Chronic Polyhydramnios
This occurs later in pregnancy, usually between 32 and 40 weeks. The fluid accumulates gradually, and the maternal symptoms are less marked than in the acute group. The prognosis depends on the underlying cause. In the idiopathic group the prognosis is good. When there is erythroblastosis or diabetes the prognosis is guarded. With congenital anomalies the outcome depends on the type of abnormality and whether it is treatable.

Diagnosis

Abdominal Examination
1. The uterus is larger than expected.
2. The fetal parts are difficult to outline.
3. The fetus may be ballotable.
4. The fetal heart cannot be heard clearly.

Sonography
1. There is a large, echo-free space between the fetus and the uterine wall.
2. Sometimes an abnormality can be detected, such as anencephaly or spina bifida with meningocele or myelomeningocele.

X-ray of Abdomen
1. A large radiolucent area with a typical ground glass appearance is seen surrounding the fetal skeleton.
2. Fetal abnormalities can be identified, especially anencephaly.

Amniography
X-ray, following the injection of a contrast medium injected into the amniotic cavity, helps identify:
1. Excessive amount of fluid
2. Fetal abnormalities
3. Fetal swallowing

Work-Up
This includes:
1. Blood sugar studies

2. Maternal antibodies to rule out erythroblastosis
3. Search for fetal anomalies

Management

Mild Symptoms

1. Diet: high protein, low sodium.
2. Bed rest as required.
3. Mild sedation.
4. Diuretics may relieve the maternal edema, but they have no effect on the volume of amniotic fluid, and are not recommended.

Severe Symptoms

1. Diet: high protein, low sodium
2. Bed rest, hospitalization in many cases
3. Mild sedation
4. Diuretics may relieve the maternal edema
5. Mature fetus: induction of labor
6. Immature fetus:
   a. Normal fetus: amniocentesis and removal of fluid
   b. Abnormal fetus: induce labor

Amniocentesis

The main purpose is to relieve the mother's symptoms.

1. Ultrasonography is utilized to:
   a. Locate the fetus.
   b. Establish position of the placenta.
   c. Determine the depth to which penetration of the needle is required.
2. An 18-gauge needle that is covered tightly by a plastic catheter is inserted into the amniotic cavity and the needle is withdrawn, leaving the catheter in place. This reduces the chance of injury to the fetus.
3. The fluid is removed by either dependent drainage or gentle suction at the rate of 500 ml per hour.
4. Enough fluid is removed to bring relief to the patient. In most cases the amount is between 1000 and 1500 ml.
5. The procedure has to be repeated every 2 to 3 days, as the reaccumulation of fluid is rapid.
6. A beta-mimetic drug (isoxsuprine, ritodrine) may be given to reduce uterine contractions.
7. When the L/S ratio becomes mature, labor is induced.

Complications of Polyhydramnios

1. Abnormal presentations are common.
2. Premature rupture of the membranes causes several problems:
   a. Preterm labor.
   b. Sudden decompression of the uterus may lead to:
      i. Abruption of the placenta.
      ii. Prolapse of the umbilical cord.
3. Artificial rupture of the membranes can cause the same problems as when the membranes rupture spontaneously. Hence, the procedure must be carried out on a delivery table, the fluid should be removed as slowly as possible through a needle puncture, and care taken to prevent prolapse of the umbilical cord.
4. The overstretched myometrium leads to a high incidence of:
   a. Inefficient contractions and prolonged labor.
   b. Postpartum atony and hemorrhage.

Prognosis

Fetal

1. Serious malformations occur in 20 percent.
2. Incidence of prematurity is more than twice the general rate.
3. Erythroblastosis may be lethal.
4. Diabetes complicates the situation.
5. Prolapse of the cord may occur when the membranes rupture.
6. Placental abruption when the membranes rupture and the uterus decreases in size adds to the rate of fetal mortality.

Maternal
Maternal prognosis is good.

OLIGOHYDRAMNIOS

In rare instances the amount of amniotic fluid is reduced far below the normal. It may be as little as a few ml of dark, thick fluid.

Etiology

The cause is unknown. Oligohydramnios is seen in association with the following conditions:

1. Anuria, the result of renal agenesis or an obstruction to the fetal urinary tract

2. Pregnancies that are prolonged several weeks beyond term
3. Intrauterine growth retardation

Early Pregnancy

When oligohydramnios occurs in early pregnancy the fetus may be damaged.

1. Amniotic adhesions or bands may cause deformities, amputation of fetal limbs, or constriction and obstruction of the umbilical cord.
2. Pressure deformities, such as club feet.
3. Pulmonary hypoplasia has been reported.
4. The skin becomes dry, leathery, and wrinkled.

Later Pregnancy

The markedly reduced volume of amniotic fluid can cause several problems.

1. It is a sign of fetal distress.
2. Close adaptation between the fetus and the uterine wall can lead to pressure on the umbilical cord and obstruction to the flow of blood to and from the fetus. Fetal hypoxia may result.
3. Meconium passed into an amniotic sac in which there is a paucity of fluid will not be diluted. Aspiration of this thick meconium by the fetus will lead to bronchiolar obstruction.

Diagnosis

In the past most diagnoses were made at delivery. Use of the real-time ultrasonic scanner has enabled the diagnosis to be made in the later stages of gestation. On this basis patients have been divided into four groups.

1. Oligohydramnios. No pocket of amniotic fluid greater than 1 cm in its greatest diameter is revealed on real-time scanning. There is a distinct impression of fetal crowding in utero. In some cases the fetus is seen as being closely adapted to the uterine wall without intervening fluid.
2. Pockets of amniotic fluid are seen greater than 1 cm in their greatest diameter.
3. Adequate amniotic fluid. Fluid is seen everywhere between the fetus and the uterine wall.
4. Polyhydramnios. There is a large echo-free space between the

uterine wall and the fetus. In some cases the latter seems to be floating freely in a large amount of fluid.

Treatment

There is no treatment for oligohydramnios.

In some cases termination of the pregnancy is carried out to forestall severe fetal hypoxia or fetal death in utero.

AMNIOTIC FLUID EMBOLISM

Amniotic fluid embolism is a syndrome in which, following the infusion of a large amount of amniotic fluid into the maternal circulation, there is the sudden development of acute respiratory distress and shock. Twenty-five percent of these women die within 1 hour. The condition is rare. Probably many cases are unrecognized, the diagnosis being obstetric shock, postpartum hemorrhage, or acute pulmonary edema.

Amniotic fluid embolism was discovered by Meyer in 1926 at postmortem examination. In 1947 the clinical syndrome was described by Steiner and Lusbaugh. They showed that the sudden infusion of amniotic fluid of sufficient quantity into the maternal circulation is fatal.

Etiology

Predisposing factors:

1. Multiparity
2. Age over 30
3. Large fetus
4. Intrauterine fetal death
5. Meconium in the amniotic fluid
6. Strong uterine contractions
7. High incidence of operative delivery

Diagnosis

Definitive diagnosis requires the demonstration of the components of amniotic fluid in the maternal circulation. On histologic preparations of the lungs, edema, alveolar hemorrhages, and emboli consisting of fetal squamous cells, fat, mucin, bile, and lanugo hair are seen. More recent techniques include the detection of squamous cells and lanugo hair on cytologic examination of blood aspirated through a Swan-Ganz catheter.

Clinical Picture

Steiner and Lusbaugh wrote:

> Profound shock coming on suddenly and unexpectedly in a woman
> who is in unusually severe labor or has just finished such a labor, es-
> pecially if she is an elderly multipara with an excessively large, per-
> haps dead, fetus, and with meconium in the amniotic fluid, should
> lead to a suspicion of this possibility [amniotic fluid embolism]. If also
> the shock is introduced by a chill, which is followed by dyspnea, cya-
> nosis, vomiting, restlessness and the like, and accompanied by a pro-
> found fall in blood pressure and a rapid weak pulse, the picture is
> more complete. If pulmonary edema now develops quickly in the
> known absence of previously existing heart disease, the diagnosis is
> reasonably certain.

Nothing has been added to this description except the recognition
that there may be an associated failure of coagulation of the patient's
blood, and hemorrhage from the placental site.

The picture includes the following:

1. Respiratory distress.
2. Cyanosis.
3. Cardiovascular collapse.
4. Failure of coagulation and hemorrhage.
5. Coma.
6. Death.
7. In nonfatal cases scan of the lungs using macroaggregated I^{131}
   albumin may reveal the embolization and establish the diagnosis.

Differential Diagnosis

1. Thrombotic pulmonary embolism
2. Air embolism
3. Fat embolism
4. Aspiration of vomitus
5. Eclampsia
6. Anesthetic drug reaction
7. Cerebrovascular accident
8. Congestive heart failure
9. Hemorrhagic shock
10. Ruptured uterus
11. Inverted uterus

Clinicopathologic Findings

Mode of Infusion

For the passage of amniotic fluid into the maternal circulation to take place, there must be a tear in the fetal membranes and an opening into the maternal vasculature. The two major sites of entry into the maternal blood stream are the endocervical veins (which may be torn even in normal labor) and the uteroplacental area. Rupture of the uterus increases the chance of amniotic fluid embolism taking place. Abruption of the placenta is a common occurrence, this accident preceding or coinciding with the embolic episode.

Pathogenesis

The exact mechanism is unknown. Two theories have been advanced: (1) There is an overwhelming mechanical blockade of the pulmonary vessels by emboli of the particulate material in the amniotic fluid, especially meconium. (2) An anaphylactoid reaction to the particulate matter occurs.

The three major aspects of the syndrome are produced probably by a combination of mechanical and spastic processes.

1. The sudden reduction of the amount of blood returning to the left heart and the decreased left ventricular output lead to peripheral vascular collapse.
2. The acute pulmonary hypertension, cor pulmonale, and failure of the right heart produce peripheral edema.
3. The uneven capillary blood flow with derangement of the ventilation/perfusion ratio leads to anoxemia and tissue hypoxia. This can explain the cyanosis, restlessness, convulsions, and coma.

Lungs

The significant findings are:

1. Edema
2. Alveolar hemorrhage
3. Emboli composed of the particulate material of amniotic fluid (squames, amorphous debris, mucin, vernix, and lanugo)
4. Dilated pulmonary vessels at the area of embolization

Heart

The right side is often dilated. Blood aspirated from the right side reveals amniotic fluid elements.

Coagulation Defects

The hemorrhage that ensues is the result of a failure of blood coagulation and diminished tonus of the uterus. The probable cause of the failed coagulation process is the release of thromboplastin into the circulation leading to disseminated intravascular coagulation and followed by hypofibrinogenemia and fibrin degradation products. Uterine atony is common, but the exact reason is not known.

Management

While in severe cases nothing does any good, the aims of treatment include reduction of pulmonary hypertension, increased tissue perfusion, relief of bronchospasm, control of hemorrhage, and general supportive measures.

1. Oxygen is given under pressure, either by positive pressure breathing or artificial ventilation.
2. Antispasmodics and vasodilators such as papaverine, aminophylline, and trinitroglycerine may help. Isoproterenol increases pulmonary ventilation and reduces bronchospasm. One way of administering aminophylline is to infuse 250 to 500 mg in 50 ml of 5 percent dextrose in water, given over 20 minutes.
3. Coagulation defects must be corrected using heparin, fibrinogen, or cryoprecipitate.
4. Fresh blood is given to combat deficits, care being taken not to overload the circulation.
5. Digitalis is used to prevent or treat cardiac failure. Digoxin 0.5 mg is given intravenously, followed by 0.125 mg IV every 2 hours for 6 doses.
6. Manual exploration of the uterus is performed to rule out uterine rupture and retained placenta.
7. Hydrocortisone is prescribed both to help combat the overwhelming stress and for its ionotropic action. The dose is 1.0 g intravenously, then 250 mg every 4 hours.
8. Morphine 5 to 15 mg intramuscularly is useful to reduce anxiety and pain.
9. A Swan-Ganz catheter, placed into the pulmonary artery, is helpful in monitoring the patient's condition.

Mortality

Maternal

While maternal mortality is high, amniotic fluid embolism is not fatal in every instance. Sublethal cases do occur. About 75 percent of the deaths are a direct result of the effects of embolism. The rest perish from hemorrhage.

Fetal

Fetal mortality is high. Fifty percent of the deaths occur in utero.

BIBLIOGRAPHY

Flowers WK: Hydramnios and gastrointestinal atresias: A review. Obstet Gynecol Survey 38:685, 1983

Hill LM, Breckle R, Wolfgram KR, O'Brien PC: Oligohydramnios: Ultrasonically detected incidence and subsequent fetal outcome. Am J Obstet Gynecol 147:407, 1983

Masson RG, Ruggieri J, Siddiqui MM: Amniotic fluid embolism: Definitive diagnosis in a survivor. Am Rev Respir Dis 120:187, 1979

Queenan JT, Kubarych SF: Detecting and managing polyhydramnios. Contemp OB/GYN 16:113, 1980

Quinlap RW, Cruz AC, Martin M: Hydramnios: Ultrasound diagnosis and its impact on perinatal management and pregnancy outcome. Am J Obstet Gynecol 145:306, 1983

37

Assessment of the Fetus in Utero

Denis K.L. Dudley

INDICATIONS FOR FETAL ASSESSMENT

There are numerous situations where it is important to ascertain both the maturity and the health of the fetus while it is still in utero. Among these are the following:

A. During pregnancy
  1. Patients at risk for uteroplacental insufficiency
    a. Diabetes mellitus
    b. Hypertension and preeclampsia
    c. Renal disease
    d. Previous stillbirth
    e. Intrauterine growth retardation, suspected
    f. Postterm pregnancy, over 42 weeks
    g. Rhesus sensitization
    h. Premature rupture of membranes
    i. Multiple gestation
  2. Obstetric reasons
    a. Previous cesarean section
    b. When induction of labor is necessary
      i. In the interests of the mother
      ii. In the interests of the fetus
B. During labor
  1. Obstetric reasons
    a. Clinically detected abnormalities of the fetal heart rate (FHR)
    b. Passage of meconium
    c. Oxytocin stimulation of labor

    d. Preterm labor

    e. Slow progress in labor

    f. Abnormal presentation

  2. Patients at risk for uteroplacental insufficiency

There is a group of infants for whom the intrauterine environment is unfavorable, who fare better outside of the uterus than in it, and whose chances of survival are improved by effecting delivery, even in the preterm period. The obstetrician must decide which babies should be delivered early, and he has to select the best time for the delivery. The risk of delay has to be measured against the danger of prematurity.

DETERMINATION OF FETAL MATURITY

Clinical Methods

Clinical history and examination are useful. One cannot rely upon a single finding, but by assembling a number of symptoms and signs a reasonably accurate assessment of fetal maturity can be made. Such symptoms and signs include the following:

1. Date of the onset of the last menstrual period. In most cases this is a valid and important parameter. Sources of error include uncertainty of the last menses, bleeding in the early part of pregnancy mistaken for a period, oligomenorrhea, and delay of ovulation after discontinuance of the contraceptive pill.
2. One of the most accurate and important pieces of evidence in establishing the duration of pregnancy is pelvic examination in the first 6 to 8 weeks of pregnancy to evaluate the size of the uterus and to correlate it with the menstrual history. This should be done carefully at the first visit in every pregnancy.
3. Onset of the symptoms of pregnancy.
4. Well-documented evidence of when conception took place, such as an isolated act of coitus or the induction of ovulation in infertile women.
5. Correlation of date of positive pregnancy test and menstrual history.
6. First fetal movement is noticed at 18 to 20 weeks.
7. The fetal heart is heard at 18 to 20 weeks using a fetal stethoscope.
8. Abdominal palpation. In the hands of experienced observers the accuracy is within 1 pound in 80 percent of cases and within 8 ounces in 55 percent. However, the rate of unacceptable esti-

mates is high at the extremes of 2300 and 4300 g. There is a tendency to overestimate in the lower and underestimate in the higher ranges of birth weight.

9. Measurement of the height of the uterine fundus (Fig. 1) and the abdominal girth is helpful. In the second part of pregnancy the distance from the symphysis pubis to the top of the fundus of the uterus, measured in centimeters, equals the weeks of gestation. These measurements are rough approximations and, while aberrations from the normal will arouse suspicion, they cannot be relied upon in making important decisions.

Radiologic Techniques

Flat Plate of Abdomen

A search is made for the epiphyses at the ends of the long bones of the lower limb. The distal (inferior) femoral epiphyseal ossification center is present in 80 percent of fetuses from the 36th week of gestation onward. The proximal (superior) tibial epiphyseal center appears at week

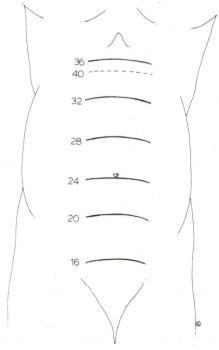

Figure 1. Uterine fundal height at various weeks of pregnancy.

38. Sometimes these centers do not ossify until term. The demonstration of the distal femoral center indicates that the fetus is mature in 90 percent of cases. Unfortunately neither the size nor the age of the fetus can be determined accurately by radiography. Identification of the epiphyses is often technically difficult. Therefore abdominal radiographs are used no longer to assess fetal age and maturity except in areas where better methods, such as ultrasonography and amniocentesis, are unavailable.

Amniocentesis

Examination of a sample of amniotic fluid is of great value in determining both the maturity and the state of health of the fetus. The constituents of amniotic fluid change all through pregnancy. The fetus swallows amniotic fluid and contributes to it by urination. Fetal pulmonary secretions pass into the amniotic fluid, and cells from the fetal skin are exfoliated into it.

Technique of Amniocentesis

A careful abdominal examination is made first and the fetal position assessed. Ultrasonic scanning performed immediately prior to, and during, amniocentesis provides information as to the fetal position, the location of the placenta, and the area where amniotic fluid is most accessible (sometimes there are only pockets of fluid). In this way both the site and the depth of the tap can be determined accurately, thus increasing the safety of the procedure.

There are two commonly used sites for amniocentesis (Fig. 2): (1) In advanced pregnancy when the head is in the pelvis, the fetal position can be palpated, and the placenta is posterior, the favored site of puncture is in the upper segment of the uterus, in the area of the fetal small parts (Fig. 2A). (2) When the placenta is anterior and in the upper segment of the uterus, and the fetal head can be elevated away from the pelvis, the needle can be inserted easily between the pubic symphysis and the presenting part (Fig. 2B).

The selected area is cleaned with an antiseptic solution and draped. The site of puncture is infiltrated with a local anesthetic. A stylet-containing 18- to 22-gauge needle is used. Entry into the amniotic cavity produces an abrupt loss of resistance.

The return of blood through the needle indicates that the needle is either in the wall of the uterus or in the placenta. If the placenta has been localized by ultrasound one may assume that the needle is in the myometrium and it should be advanced into the amnion. If the placental site is unknown and the depth of the puncture is judged to be adequate, the needle should be removed and another site selected.

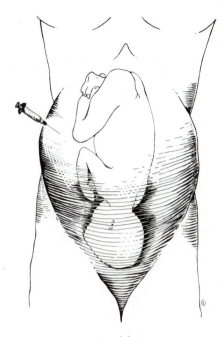

A. Fundal site.

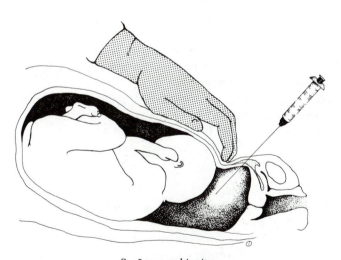

B. Supra pubic site.

Figure 2. Amniocentesis.

Ten milliliters of amniotic fluid are aspirated and sent to the laboratory for testing. Occasionally no fluid is obtained. This is more common in term or postterm pregnancy in which the volume of amniotic fluid is reduced. In such cases an attempt is made in a different area. However, the procedure may have to be abandoned.

Postamniocentesis care consists of a 20- to 30-minute period of observation with frequent auscultation of the fetal heart. Acceleration of the FHR is the normal response to amniocentesis and is in the order of 20 to 60 beats per minute, lasting for 2 to 3 minutes. The absence of this tachycardia may indicate that the fetus is not in good condition.

Complications of Amniocentesis
Diagnostic amniocentesis is an important procedure. The rate of complications is less than 1 percent. However, they do occur and, as with any invasive technique, amniocentesis should be used only when necessary.

Maternal Complications

1. Infection, chorioamnionitis.
2. Puncture of uterine vessels leading to hemorrhage, hemoperitoneum, and formation of hematoma.
3. Vaginal bleeding.
4. Premature rupture of membranes. Leakage of fluid from the site of puncture may track down through the cervix and vagina. This is an occasional and benign event. Rarely, the membranes actually rupture.
5. Preterm labor. It is common for patients to experience a few contractions following amniocentesis, but actual labor is rare.
6. Supine hypotension may occur.
7. A rare case of uterine rupture during labor in a woman who had had an amniocentesis has been reported, but a direct etiologic relationship has not been established.

Fetal Complications

1. Fetal death is rare.
2. Abortion occurs in less than 1 percent of cases.
3. Infection is rare.
4. Hemorrhage can occur as the result of direct puncture of fetal vessels on the placenta, the cord, or the fetus itself.
5. Fetal injury. In most cases needle trauma is in noncritical areas and no permanent damage results. Occasionally serious injury does take place. The danger is greater in postterm pregnancy, when the volume of fluid is small.

6. Feto-placental-maternal bleeding and potential isoimmunization. This occurrence is especially serious when the mother is Rh negative and the fetus Rh positive. This complication can be reduced by ultrasonic localization of the placenta preceding amniocentesis. In any case, Rh immunoglobulin should be administered to Rh negative women following amniocentesis.

Phospholipids in Amniotic Fluid: Pulmonary Maturity

Since the survival of a newborn infant depends, to a large extent, upon its ability to breathe efficiently and to effect proper exchange of gases in the lungs, the determination of the state of "pulmonary maturity" of the fetus is of inestimable value. For the pulmonary alveoli to attain stability so that they do not collapse after each expiration, and for normal respiration to take place, pulmonary surfactant must be present. Surfactant phospholipids, which originate principally from the lungs of the fetus, appear in the amniotic fluid by 24 to 26 weeks, and can be measured. As the fetus approaches maturity the amounts of phospholipids in the amniotic fluid increase. When they reach a certain level, the lungs have attained a degree of development so that the occurrence of the respiratory distress syndrome (RDS) is unlikely.

Lecithin (phosphatidylcholine) makes up almost 80 percent of the surfactant phospholipids, and is the most important one. Phosphatidylglycerol (PG) comprises 10 percent of surfactant in the adult. Other phospholipids include phosphatidylinositol (PI), phosphatidylethanolamine (PE), phosphatidylserine (PS), and sphingomyelin (S).

Lecithin/Sphingomyelin (L/S) Ratio

From 20 to 30 weeks of pregnancy the amount of sphingomyelin in amniotic fluid is higher than that of lecithin. By 30 weeks the concentrations are equal. From this point on the amount of lecithin rises gradually above that of sphingomyelin, until between 32 and 35 weeks it increases sharply. The levels of sphingomyelin cease rising at week 32, and then decline progressively until at term they are at a low level. A ratio of lecithin to sphingomyelin (L/S) of 2 or more indicates that the fetal lungs are able to sustain the respiratory needs of extrauterine life, and that RDS will not develop. In normal pregnancy this takes place between 33 and 37 weeks, the mean being about 35 weeks.

Contamination of amniotic fluid by blood or meconium may alter the L/S ratio and render it unreliable. Their presence in amniotic fluid tends to lower high ratios and to elevate low ones. The L/S ratio of both maternal and fetal blood is between 1.31 and 1.46. The effect of meconium is to lower the L/S ratio of amniotic fluid. The L/S ratio of amniotic fluid obtained from the vagina following rupture of the membranes is contaminated by constituents of the vagina, and is unreliable as a predictor of fetal outcome.

In most situations the L/S ratio is an excellent forecaster of the likelihood of the occurrence of RDS. However there appears to be a false-positive rate of around 2 percent, i.e., the baby develops RDS even when the L/S ratio is 2.0 or more. About half of these cases occur in diabetics. The false-negative rate (absence of RDS despite an "immature" L/S ratio) is substantial, in that RDS does not develop in over 25 percent of infants when the L/S ratio is less than 1.5, and in 60 percent of babies with ratios between 1.5 and 2.0. Thus, while a mature L/S ratio predicts, with a certainty of 98 percent, that RDS will not occur, an immature L/S ratio does not ensure that RDS will develop.

Other Phospholipids

Because the L/S ratio was found to be less than 100 percent reliable in certain situations, other phospholipids in the amniotic fluid were measured. Phosphatidylglycerol (PG) appears in the amniotic fluid after 35 weeks, and the levels continue to rise for the duration of the pregnancy, thus correlating with gestational age. In normal pregnancy the levels of phosphatidylinositol (PI) rise after 30 weeks, peak at 36 to 37 weeks, and then fall gradually.

Phosphatidylglycerol

PG occurs in no body fluids other than amniotic fluid, pulmonary effluent, and semen. Hence, in contrast to the L/S ratio, the contamination of amniotic fluid, obtained by abdominal amniocentesis, by blood or meconium (neither of which contain PG) has no effect upon the accurate determination of the presence or absence of PG. The presence of PG can be noted reliably in the amniotic fluid in the vagina when the membranes are ruptured. In these cases, i.e., when PG is present in the vaginal pool after the membranes have ruptured, the development of RDS in the newborn infant is rare.

It was found that in those cases where RDS occurred even when the L/S ratio indicated pulmonary maturity, there was an absence of PG. On the other hand, RDS did not develop when PG was present. In pregnancies under stress (e.g., diabetes, Rh-immunization) and in situations where the amniotic fluid is contaminated by blood or meconium, an absolute diagnosis of pulmonary maturity should not be made without measuring the level of PG in the amniotic fluid. The study of both the L/S ratio and the level of PG increases the accuracy of prediction of the development of RDS in the newborn.

Correlations: PG and L/S Ratio

The following correlations appear to be valid in both normal and stressed pregnancies:

1. PG present, L/S ratio 2 or more: It is virtually certain that the lungs are mature and that RDS will not develop.
2. PG present, L/S ratio less than 2: The risk of RDS is almost zero, less than 3 percent.
3. PG absent, L/S ratio 2 or more: The incidence of RDS is almost zero. However, in diabetics these babies may be at risk for RDS and immediate delivery is not advised unless the indications to do so are strong.
4. PG absent, L/S ratio less than 2: There is a substantial risk of the development of RDS. Delivery is postponed if possible. Administration of corticosteroids to accelerate the development of pulmonary maturity should be considered when gestational age is less than 31 weeks. The use of steroids to enhance pulmonary maturity remains controversial. There is evidence, however, that steroids are beneficial in improving pulmonary maturity when the gestational age is less than 31 weeks

The L/S Ratio in Diabetic Pregnancy
Despite some reports to the contrary, it has been our experience, as well as that of others that, as long as the diabetes is well controlled, there is no delay in fetal pulmonary maturation and the L/S ratio is reliable. Further, we have found that in well-controlled diabetic patients, whose expected date of confinement is based on an accurate menstrual history and early ultrasonography and who are being delivered at a gestational age of 37 weeks or more, amniocentesis to determine pulmonary maturity may be unnecessary. However, in diabetic pregnancy associated with poor control, preterm delivery, or uncertain dates, amniocentesis should be carried out before delivery and both the L/S ratio and the presence of phosphatidylglycerol determined.

Declining Use of the L/S Ratio
Recent reports suggest that, while the L/S ratio is an excellent predictor of fetal pulmonary maturity in most pregnancies, its value and use are declining for the following reasons:

1. Improvement in neonatal care, especially in ventilatory support of babies with respiratory distress, has led obstetricians to regard RDS with less fear than was once the case, and they are less likely to order an invasive test that predicts this condition.
2. In many situations such as fulminating preeclampsia, severe abruption of the placenta, or acute fetal distress, the pregnancy must be terminated whatever the L/S ratio may be.
3. Many women have an ultrasonic scan in the early part of pregnancy. If the duration of gestation can be set reliably as being

past 36 weeks, there is little to be gained by determining the L/S ratio.

4. Accuracy of the L/S ratio is less than perfect in predicting the maturity of the fetal lungs in poorly controlled diabetic pregnancies. In this area the presence of phosphatidylglycerol in amniotic fluid is a more reliable indicator.

5. When the amniotic fluid is collected from the vagina, the demonstration of the presence of phosphatidylglycerol is a more accurate indicator of fetal pulmonary maturity than the L/S ratio.

Other Parameters in Amniotic Fluid

In the assessment of fetal maturity and especially the prediction of development of RDS, the levels of creatinine, bilirubin, and "fat cells" are of low sensitivity, and are used rarely today.

Creatinine. A level of 180 mmol/L or higher per 100 ml of amniotic fluid indicates that the gestation is over 35 weeks.

Fat Cells. A drop of amniotic fluid is stained with Nile blue. When over 20 percent of the cells are mature, orange-stained fat cells, the gestational age is at least 36 weeks.

Bilirubin. As pregnancy progresses there is a gradual fall in the concentration of bilirubin in the amniotic fluid. The spectrophotometric reading of bilirubin at 450 mμ should be zero at 36 weeks. A reading over 0.01 suggests a gestational age of less than 35 weeks.

ULTRASONOGRAPHY

Ultrasonography has many uses and a variety of structures can be visualized. The technique is discussed in this section only in the field of determining fetal maturity and size.

Crown Rump Length

The most accurate method of determining gestational age is by the measurement of the crown rump length, from the top of the head to the bottom of the buttocks, in the first trimester of pregnancy. Excluding the fetal limbs it is the longest fetal diameter. Calculation of the gestational age is made from standard tables. If these are not available, a good approximation can be made by adding 6.5 to the crown rump length in centimeters. The result equals the menstrual age in weeks. Between 9 and 13 weeks of pregnancy, estimates of gestational age by the crown rump length are accurate to less than 5 days at the 95 percent confidence level.

Fetal Cephalometry

Biparietal Diameter (BPD)
Between 14 and 28 weeks of pregnancy a single measurement of the BPD is accurate to within ± 10 to 11 days in calculating gestational age. Paired scans done in the same period 8 to 10 weeks apart increase the accuracy to ± 1 week. After 28 weeks the accuracy is only to within 3 weeks. However, a BPD greater than 8.5 cm denotes a gestation of at least 35 weeks in 90 percent of cases. Recent studies have shown that a BPD greater than 9.2 cm indicates fetal pulmonary maturity, both clinically and as shown by the L/S ratio. It may be that when the BPD is greater than 9.2 cm amniocentesis to determine the L/S ratio is unnecessary. Certainly, in the presence of a BPD greater than 9.2 cm and a grade 3 placenta, the determination of the L/S is not needed.

Circumference of the Head
An approximation of the cephalic circumference can be calculated from the formula:

$$\text{BPD} + \text{Occipitofrontal diameter} \times \frac{3.14}{2}$$

Abdominal Circumference

The anteroposterior and transverse diameters of the fetal abdomen are measured at the reference plane when the umbilical vein is perpendicular to the spine. The abdominal circumference (AC) is then calculated using the formula:

$$\text{Anteroposterior diameter} + \text{transverse diameter} \times \frac{3.14}{2}$$

The abdominal circumference, however, is not always of uniform shape, and may vary with fetal respiration. Hence, AC measurements are less accurate than the BPD in predicting gestational age except after 36 weeks. It is used primarily in combination with the BPD to estimate fetal weight.

Femoral Length

The length of the fetal femur is the measurement of only the central diathesis of the shaft. The neck of the femur is excluded. Femoral length increases in almost linear fashion with gestational age at a rate of slightly less than 2 mm/week. Femoral length is no more accurate than the BPD in determining gestational age, but it is a useful alternative when the BPD cannot be measured.

Assessment of femoral length is useful in distinguishing symmetrical from asymmetrical fetal growth retardation. In the asymmetrical variety, growth of the brain and the skeleton remains within the normal range until the very late stages. On the other hand, the growth of the abdominal circumference and the fetal weight is retarded.

Measurement of femoral length can diagnose a variety of skeletal dysplasias.

Placental Maturation

Based upon changes (demonstrated by ultrasonography) that occur in three separate zones of the placenta (chorionic plate, placental substance, and basal layer), four relatively distinct phases of placental maturation have been identified and graded from zero (immature) to III (most mature). Preliminary studies have found a high correlation (100 percent in some reports) between grade III placentas and mature L/S ratios. A limiting feature is that the grade III placenta is present in only 15 percent of pregnancies at term. When it is present amniocentesis to determine pulmonary maturity may be unnecessary.

Estimation of Gestational Age: Summary

First Trimester.   Crown rump length is the most accurate.

Second Trimester.   Biparietal diameter is the most useful.

Third Trimester: Multiple Fetal Growth Parameters.   An improvement in the accuracy of calculation of the gestational age over a single parameter may be obtained by using several fetal measurements. Prior to 36 weeks the optimal combination is biparietal diameter, abdominal circumference, and femoral length. After 36 weeks the calculations are based on head circumference, abdominal circumference, and femoral length. Each parameter is used separately to determine gestational age from standard reference tables. The average is then taken for the final result.

DETERMINATION OF FETAL HEALTH: ANTEPARTUM

The reduction of perinatal mortality has been achieved largely by the decrease in the rate of neonatal death. As a result, antepartum fetal deaths, which used to account for less than 50 percent of perinatal deaths, now constitute approximately two-thirds of perinatal mortality. The prevention of fetal death represents a major therapeutic goal, and is the reason for antepartum fetal surveillance.

Biochemical assessment of the fetus has largely been replaced by biophysical and biometric evaluation. Fetal biophysical activities are initiated, modulated, and regulated by mechanisms of the central nervous system (CNS). The fetus compromised by hypoxia demonstrates one or both of the following changes:

1. A decrease or cessation of biophysical activity.
2. A significant reduction in the volume of amniotic fluid which becomes evident as oligohydramnios on sonography.

The fetal CNS is exquisitely sensitive to changes in PO_2. Hypoxia and its resultant metabolic acidosis produce pathologic CNS depression with changes in biophysical activity. Any biophysical response, however, has its own inherent periodicity and circadian (diurnal) rhythm. Hence the absence of a given biophysical event may reflect physiologic periodicity, and a normal "sleep state" in the fetus must be differentiated from the comatose state of hypoxic CNS depression.

The important principle in antepartum testing, regardless of the method used, is that a normal test is reliable in indicating present fetal well-being, and is an accurate predictor of a good outcome. However, the diagnosis of fetal jeopardy based on a single absent or abnormal biophysical event is frequently inaccurate. Hence, in any scheme of antepartum testing our goal must be to reduce and, if possible, eliminate the incidence of falsely positive results. This is achieved by increasing the period of observation for any single biophysical event and/or utilizing multiple observations. The demonstration of several biophysical activities showing a normal pattern collectively negates a single abnormal result.

Fetal Movement

Fetal movement, first perceived by the mother at 16 to 20 weeks' gestation, may be recorded subjectively or objectively using active or passive techniques. Using B-mode and real-time ultrasonography (an active technique) the fetal movements may be classified into various patterns:

Types of Movement

1. *Movements lasting longer than 3 seconds*: These are complex or rolling movements of the trunk and fetal limbs, usually perceived by the mother, and often seen by an observer because they distort the maternal abdominal wall.
2. *Movements of duration 1 to 3 seconds*: These movements appear to be single gross trunk or limb movements or both. There is no clear distinction between simple and rolling fetal movements except for their duration.
3. *Movements of duration less than 1 second*: These are seen as either isolated or repetitive events. They are characteristically of short duration and include abrupt fetal chest and abdominal wall movements resembling neonatal startles or hiccups. Episodes of hiccups lasting 1 to 23 minutes appear to be a common event in normal pregnancy.

Fetal movements are not random phenomena. They are regulated and modulated by complex CNS mechanisms and reflexes. They occur in cyclic periods or in epochs associated and integrated with respiratory, cardiac, behavioral, and "sleep" cycles. The acceleration of the fetal heart rate which occurs after certain fetal movements provides the basis of the nonstress test (NST). Movements lasting more than 3 seconds elicit fetal heart rate accelerations 99.8 percent of the time. Movements of lesser duration rarely do so.

Counting Methods

1. The "count to 10" method: In this simple method the patient counts fetal movements starting at 9 AM in the morning. After ten movements are perceived, the counting comes to an end. This routine is carried on daily and the patient is asked to alert her physician if (1) less than ten movements occur after 12 hours on 2 successive days or (2) no movements are perceived after 12 hours in a single day. In such a situation a nonstress test should be performed. In most pregnancies ten movements are perceived within 1 hour of counting.
2. In the periodic method the number of fetal movements is counted during three periods of observation lasting 30 to 60 minutes each. The number of daily movements is extrapolated from these data. In one study a normal variation of from 4 to 1440 movements per day was reported. A frequency of fetal movement less than four per 12 hours is abnormal, and calls for further investigation.

Fetal activity may be decreased in late pregnancy but in the normal fetus this is not great. The possible reasons for the reduction in fetal movement at this time include decreasing amounts of amniotic fluid and the larger fetus having less room to move in the uterus. It could also be related to sleep states, which are thought to occur for longer periods in the mature fetus. Finally, sedatives and drugs that produce autonomic blockade reduce fetal activity.

Most studies report that, of those pregnant women who carry on a protocol of formal counting of fetal movement, only a small number report diminished activity. Therefore, the procedure does not lead to an unmanageable situation. A random study of 2250 patients has shown that a group of women who carried out a formal protocol of counting fetal movements had no fetal deaths compared to 8 deaths in the control group. It appears that reduced fetal activity may be a good predictor of fetal compromise.

Ultrasonography

Measurement of Fetal Growth
Fetal growth retardation may be defined as occurring when the estimated weight of the fetus is below the 10th percentile for gestational age. On the one hand, half of the fetuses diagnosed as having intrauterine growth retardation show no evidence of fetal malnutrition when they are born.

On the other hand, some fetuses who are growth retarded are missed because their weights have been estimated as being above the 10th percentile for gestational age.

Growth retardation may be divided into two categories although differentiation of the varieties is not always possible by clinical examination and ultrasonography.

1. *Early onset or symmetrical fetal growth retardation.* This is caused by an insult occurring in early pregnancy, usually due to a chromosomal aberration, congenital anomaly, viral infection, or severe protein calorie maternal malnutrition. The fetus retains the relative proportions of head size to length, and overall weight but all are reduced for gestational age. Hence, measurements of BPD, abdominal circumference, femur length, and overall weight are less than the 10th percentile for gestational age. However, the head:abdomen ratio is within the mean for gestational age and shows the normal reversal—after 35 weeks the abdominal circumference is larger than that of the head. In making a diagnosis the possibility of an error in gestational dates must be considered. Often it is difficult to distinguish a fetus that is growth retarded from a normal one who is simply destined to be small.
2. *Late onset or asymmetrical fetal growth retardation.* This occurs

as a result of placental insufficiency and usually becomes manifest in the late second or third trimester. The decreased transfer of oxygen and metabolic substrate results in decreased soft tissue and muscle mass, and in decreased deposition of glycogen in the fetal liver. Hence, initially, the growth of abdominal circumference decreases but as blood flow to the brain is maintained, fetal head size remains normal with normal increases in the biparietal diameter. This results in an asymmetrical profile which may be demonstrated on sonography:

a. There is a decrease in the abdominal circumference while the BPD remains normal. This results in an increase in the head:abdomen ratio to a value greater than the 95th percentile for gestational age. Subsequent scans will show a further increase in this ratio in contrast to the normal fetus, in whom the abdomen gradually becomes larger than the fetal head, giving a head:abdomen ratio which is usually less than 1 after 35 weeks' gestation.

b. The biparietal diameter may remain within the normal range in the initial stages of this disorder. A normal rate of growth (1.6 to 2.0 mm/week) in the third trimester can occur until the very late stages because the brain-sparing effect makes the BPD the last ultrasonic parameter to be affected. Hence estimates of BPD alone cannot be used to diagnose fetal growth retardation.

c. The femur length, like the BPD, remains relatively normal until the insult is prolonged or severe. The femur length is proportional to crown heel length and is an indirect measure of the length of the fetus. Hence the femur length to abdominal circumference ratio increases as the severity of the growth retardation progresses.

Oligohydramnios

This is a common finding in both varieties of fetal growth retardation (FGR). The presence of a normal volume of amniotic fluid casts serious doubt on a diagnosis of FGR. It may be more consistent with an error in dates or a normal fetus, genetically determined to be small. This condition is also significant in two other ways: (1) It may be associated with an underlying congenital anomaly. (2) It introduces a further risk factor as the absence of the protective fluid cushion may lead to cord compression after fetal movements and uterine contractions, and eventual hypoxia.

Disproportion

In cases where disproportion is suspected, measurement of the BPD and abdominal circumference may be useful. In large-for-gestational age fetuses weighing more than 4 kg, or in macrosomic infants associated with maternal diabetes, the head:abdomen ratio provides valuable information. A head:abdomen ratio of less than 0.90 in this situation indicates significant head-to-body disproportion with a significant risk of shoulder dystocia during vaginal delivery. In such cases delivery by elective cesarean section would seem preferable.

Fetal Breathing

Ultrasonic studies have shown that by 30 to 31 weeks the healthy fetus makes respiratory movements 30 percent of the time. Fetal breathing decreases after consumption of alcohol, smoking of cigarettes, and during active labor. It increases postprandially and during maternal sleep. Preliminary data indicate that ultrasonic demonstration of fetal breathing may be a useful guide in selecting which patients in preterm labor are suitable candidates for tocolysis. It seems that absent fetal breathing over a 45-minute period of observation correlates with a tocolytic success rate of less than 5 percent in contrast to better than 90 percent efficacy when fetal breathing is observed. The explanation could be that prostaglandin E_2 is known to be a potent inhibitor of respiratory centers in the fetal medulla. Absent breathing probably indicates high levels of placental prostaglandin E_2 which reduces the likelihood of tocolytic success. Furthermore the absence of fetal breathing may indicate a compromised and hypoxic fetus requiring delivery instead of tocolysis to postpone birth.

Hypoxemia produces a dramatic decrease of fetal breathing movements and severe acidosis produces apnea and cessation of gross body movements. This is seen in cases of fetal growth retardation, intrapartum fetal distress, and neonatal depression. The presence of fetal breathing movements is a reliable index of an intact and functioning CNS. Patrick and associates have shown that prolonged episodes of absent fetal breathing movements and diminished fetal movement and heart rate nonreactivity of up to 108 minutes do occur in normal fetuses. Subsequently these fetuses exhibited the presence of normal activity. Hence the absence of fetal breathing in a single period of observation may indicate normal periodicity, and assessment of other biophysical activities is required to substantiate a diagnosis of fetal hypoxia and acidosis.

Maternal Levels of Estriol

There is a relationship between the amount of estriol in the maternal serum and urine and the condition of the fetus. The measurement of maternal estriol used to be a popular method of trying to ascertain the condition of the fetus in utero. This test has a number of drawbacks. Single determinations are unreliable and serial studies have to be performed. The assay is subject to wide fluctuation, making interpretation ambiguous. The obtaining of results from the laboratory may take 1 to 2 days. The test is expensive. In addition the levels of estriol do not correlate well with fetal outcome.

At one time measurement of maternal estriol was the only test available to assess fetal well-being. Today the nonstress test, the contraction stress test, and the biophysical profile have proven to be so much more accurate, quicker, and less expensive, that the measurement of the levels of maternal estriol as a test of the fetal condition has fallen into almost complete disuse.

Human Placental Lactogen (HPL)

This hormone is synthesized by the placenta and transferred into the maternal circulation. It is related immunologically to growth hormone and has the biologic activity of growth hormone and prolactin. Its function is not known.

HPL can be detected in the maternal blood by the fifth week of pregnancy using radioimmune assay. It rises progressively until the last month of pregnancy, increasing to 500 to 1000 times the levels of early pregnancy.

Because HPL is of solely trophoblastic origin, it was hoped that it would be an index of placental function. Normal values have not been standardized, the results are controversial, and at present it is believed that HPL levels are of no clinical importance in managing complicated pregnancies.

Meconium

Meconium, or fetal stool, is thick, viscous, and green. It consists of bile pigment, bile salts, fetal hair, squamous cells, mucopolysaccharides, and cholesterol. The incidence of meconium staining of the placenta and/or fetal body is between 5 and 10 percent. Once meconium has been passed it takes 4 to 6 hours for the placenta and the fetus to become discolored.

Suggested explanations for the passage of meconium include two extremes: On the one hand it may be a normal physiologic function, no more than a sign of increasing fetal maturity. On the other hand the sequence of events may be that fetal hypoxia leads to hyperperistalsis, sphincteric relaxation, and expulsion of intestinal contents.

Meconium is not prominent in acute emergencies such as prolapse of the umbilical cord, placenta previa, or abruptio placentae. Rather, it is seen in chronic stresses including toxemia of pregnancy, prolonged gestation, intrauterine growth retardation, and chorioamnionitis.

The presence of meconium-stained amniotic fluid is not an absolute sign of severe hypoxia, acidosis, or acute fetal distress. It probably indicates a previous episode of intrauterine hypoxia or a state of compensated fetal distress. It is possible that repeated or prolonged episodes of stress could produce intrauterine or neonatal death.

The exact seriousness of this symptom is not known. Marked fetal distress occurs frequently in the absence of meconium, and meconium is often present in the amniotic fluid with no evidence of fetal distress or asphyxia. Yet, studies of large series of cases have shown that the neonatal mortality rate is higher, and the 1- and 5-minute Apgar scores are lower in infants that have passed meconium during labor than in controls. In most cases the fetal heart rate (FHR) patterns in infants who passed meconium are not markedly different from those who did not. However, the combination of late passage of meconium and abnormalities of the FHR has been shown to be accurately predictive of fetal distress and low Apgar scores. Certainly, the passage of meconium does enhance the potential for aspiration.

While the passage of meconium is not a reason for panic, it alerts the physician. These patients should be monitored closely so that any further signs of trouble can be noted immediately.

Fetoscopy

Fetoscopy may be described as the introduction of an instrument transabdominally into the amniotic cavity. The instrument used most frequently is the Dionics needlescope. The procedure is best performed between the 17th and 20th week of pregnancy under strictly aseptic conditions. It is difficult and special training is required to perform it properly. A preliminary ultrasonic examination is necessary to: (1) confirm fetal viability; (2) diagnose multiple pregnancy; (3) confirm gestational age by measurement of the fetal biparietal diameter; (4) to localize the placenta, especially the site of insertion of the umbilical cord; (5) establish the fetal position. Concurrent real-time ultrasonography during fetoscopy is a useful adjunctive technique. Fetoscopy was most useful in obtaining fetal blood samples to diagnose hemaglobinopathies and perform enzyme studies in the diagnosis of certain inborn errors of metabolism. Recently, newer techniques of gene mapping and DNA analysis of cells taken from amniotic fluid are being used to diagnose these conditions. Consequently, amniocentesis provides almost all the answers, and fetoscopy has a small or no role in clinical practice at the present time.

Nonstress Test (NST)

This test is performed on the patient who is not in labor. It utilizes the observation that the occurrence of accelerations of the fetal heart rate in response to fetal movement or a uterine contraction is a reliable indicator of immediate fetal well-being.

Advantages

1. There are no contraindications and no complications.
2. The test is simple, inexpensive, and takes less time than a contraction stress test or a biophysical profile.
3. It can be used in an office setting and provides an immediate answer.
4. Performance of the test requires no special expertise.

Indications

1. Patients at risk for uteroplacental insufficiency. (See first page of this chapter.)
2. The absence of normal fetal movements.

Instrumentation and Technique

1. A fetal heart rate tracing is obtained using external ultrasound in preference to phonocardiography or abdominal electrocardiography.
2. The recording is obtained with the patient in the lateral recumbent position or with a lateral tilt so as to avoid supine hypotension.

Frequency of Testing

1. Weekly testing is indicated and adequate in most conditions.
2. The test must be repeated immediately if any change in the clinical condition of mother or fetus occurs.
3. Certain conditions require twice weekly testing:
   a. Maternal diabetes
   b. Postterm pregnancy
   c. Fetal growth retardation with oligohydramnios
   d. Maternal hypertension when the mother is taking medication, such as methyldopa or propanolol.

Timing of Testing

In most patients testing is instituted at 32 to 34 weeks of gestation. In selected cases, such as poor past obstetric performance or specific high-risk condition in the current pregnancy, testing may begin at 26 to 28 weeks. At this time many fetuses may show nonreactive patterns because of immaturity and the significance of the test is questionable. However, the finding of a normal reactive pattern in early gestation has a reassuring value.

Classification
1. Reactive pattern: Normal NST
   a. The presence of two or more accelerations of the fetal heart rate in a 10- to 20-minute period of observation (Fig. 3A).
   b. Each acceleration with fetal movement (AFM) must be of amplitude greater than 15 beats per minute (BPM) and of duration more than 15 seconds.
   c. The baseline fetal heart rate
      i. Is within the normal rage of 120 to 160 beats per minute.
      ii. There is normal fetal heart rate variability of 5 to 15 beats per minute.
      iii. There are no periodic decelerations.
         However, since fetal heart rate variability may be artificially increased in external ultrasonic recordings, this parameter is of lesser significance. Interpretation of the test rests on the presence or absence of accelerations of the FHR.
2. Nonreactive pattern: Abnormal NST
   a. Less than two accelerations meeting the stated criteria have occurred. Usually there are no accelerations in a 20- to 40-minute period of observation. If accelerations do occur their amplitude and duration are less than the stated criteria.
   b. The occurrence of persistent late decelerations in a nonreactive NST is usually an ominous sign of severe fetal compromise in which uteroplacental insufficiency is present even during basal or Braxton-Hicks uterine activity.

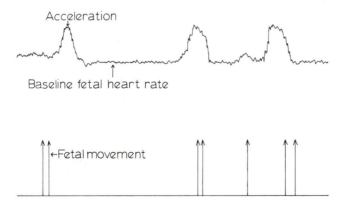

Figure 3A. Reactive nonstress test. Showing accelerations of FHR with fetal movement. Amplitude more than 15 beats per minute, duration longer than 15 seconds.

Isolated variable decelerations may occur in conjunction with either reactive or nonreactive patterns. This would indicate transient cord compression occurring with fetal movement or uterine contractions. Repeated and persistent variable decelerations may indicate the presence of oligohydramnios, and ultrasonography should be performed. In the absence of oligohydramnios the occurrence of intermittent variable decelerations during a NST is often associated with the umbilical cord's being wound around the neck of the fetus.

The time in which two accelerations should occur is arbitrarily taken as 10 or 20 minutes. The presence of accelerations is perhaps more important than the time base over which they occur. Using 10 minutes instead of 20 minutes makes a 1 percent difference in the overall reactive rate. That is, with a 10-minute time base approximately 92 percent of tests are reactive compared to 93 percent for a 20-minute time base.

Significance of the Nonstress Test

Normal Reactive Nonstress Test
The normal reactive NST is a reliable indicator of present fetal health. The risk of fetal death within 1 week of a reactive pattern is only 3.2 per 1000. Hence, the test is highly sensitive, with a falsely negative rate (normal test, abnormal fetus) of less than 0.5 percent.

Abnormal Nonreactive Nonstress Test
A nonreactive pattern may be caused by the following:

1. Hypoxia
2. Effects of drugs
   a. Sedative or tranquilizing agents
   b. Parasympatholytic drugs (e.g., atropine)
   c. Sympatholytic drugs (beta-blockers)
3. Fetal immaturity
4. Fetal sleep cycle

In contrast to the reliability of the reactive pattern of the NST, the falsely positive (abnormal test, normal fetus) rate is high, approximately 75 percent. This is almost certainly a reflection of the normal periodicity of the function of the fetal central nervous system. Hence, a nonreactive NST, defined as absent accelerations over a 40-minute period must be interpreted with caution. Either prolonged observation or repeated testing is indicated. A NST that remains nonreactive for longer than 80 minutes is virtually always associated with a significantly compromised fetus. A prolonged period of nonreactivity appears to be the most ominous finding in a NST and, therefore, extending the period of observation or repeating the test will improve its validity.

Under usual circumstances a nonreactive pattern after 40 minutes requires one of the following:

1. Performance of an alternate test (biophysical profile or contraction stress test).
2. A repeat nonstress test within 24 hours.
3. Extending the test to an 80-minute NST.

Contraction Stress Test (Oxytocin Challenge Test) (CST)

This test is based on the principle that, in late pregnancy, the response of the fetal heart rate to oxytocin-induced uterine contractions is a useful method of evaluating the status of the fetoplacental unit, and of predicting the capacity of the fetus to withstand the stress of labor. The CST has been largely replaced as a primary method of fetal surveillance by the NST. However, some workers still claim that the CST is more reliable than the NST, and use it as a first line of testing.

Technique

1. The patient is placed in the semi-recumbent or lateral tilt position.
2. Fetal heart rate and uterine contractions are recorded for a suitable observation period (10 to 30 minutes).
3. Maternal blood pressure is recorded every 10 minutes.
4. If uterine contractions are occurring at a frequency of three per 10 minutes or greater, or with a duration of more than 40 seconds, no stimulation is necessary as this constitutes a spontaneous CST.
5. In the absence of spontaneous uterine contractions, oxytocin is given intravenously by pump, starting with a dose of 0.5 milliunits per minute. The dose is increased incrementally every 15 minutes until at least three uterine contractions, each lasting 60 seconds, occur per 10 minutes. To avoid uterine hypertonus the maximum safe dose is 20 milliunits per minute. If no contractions occur by the end of 30 minutes the procedure is discontinued.
6. Nipple stimulation has been proposed recently as a less expensive and less time-consuming alternative to intravenous oxytocin. In the 60 percent of cases in which it is effective, the results are comparable. First, a warm moist cloth is placed on each breast for 5 minutes. Then the patient massages and/or rolls the nipple on one breast for 10 minutes. If this does not produce the desired uterine contractions, both breasts are stimulated in the same way for 10 minutes. Once the contractions begin, the nipples are massaged intermittently, enough to maintain the con-

tractions at the desired frequency. If no contractions result, the oxytocin-stimulated test is used.

Indications

1. Patients at risk for fetoplacental insufficiency
2. Nonreactive NST
3. Abnormal biophysical profile

Contraindications

Absolute

1. Previous classical cesarean section
2. Known placenta previa
3. Active antepartum hemorrhage

Relative

Patients at high risk for preterm labor:

1. Ruptured membranes
2. Multiple gestation
3. Incompetent cervix
4. Uterine malformations
5. Previous preterm labor

Recent studies do not demonstrate that a CST induced by oxytocin leads to an increased incidence of preterm labor. However the test is usually not performed in patients with any of the relative contraindications shown above. In these patients nonstress testing is utilized as the routine surveillance method and a biophysical profile is performed if a secondary method of testing is required.

When to Begin Testing

A CST is usually performed following a nonreactive NST. When utilized as a primary method of surveillance, testing is begun at 32 to 34 weeks in most patients. However, in women with insulin-dependent diabetes, severe hypertension, intrauterine growth retardation (IUGR), or whose NST is nonreactive, testing may be started as early as 26 to 28 weeks.

Frequency of Testing

1. Once weekly is usually sufficient for most patients.
2. Testing is sometimes performed at 3- to 5-day intervals in diabetes, postterm pregnancies, severe IUGR with oligohydramnios,

and when antihypertensive drugs are introduced in the treatment of hypertension.
3. Any change in the clinical condition of the fetus or mother should be an indication for immediate repetition of the CST.

Interpretation of CST

1. *Negative CST (normal)*. This pattern is defined as the absence of late decelerations with a contraction frequency of three per 10 minutes.
2. *Positive CST (abnormal)*. Repetitive late decelerations occur with the majority of contractions.
3. *Equivocal CST*. This is defined as an isolated or intermittent late deceleration where the majority of contractions show no evidence of late decelerations. Some authorities interpret an equivocal test as negative if a 10-minute negative window in which no late decelerations have occurred can be found.
4. *Unsatisfactory CST*. A poor quality tracing or a contraction frequency of less than three in 10 minutes is deemed unsatisfactory. This test requires repeating. However if a contraction frequency of less than three in 10 minutes is associated with persistent late decelerations then the test is interpreted as being positive. In this situation the fetus is probably severely compromised.

Variable decelerations are often noted on a contraction stress test and one must consider the possibility of oligohydramnios. Since oligohydramnios may be a manifestation of severe placental insufficiency, the presence of persistent variable decelerations or mixed late/variable deceleration patterns should be interpreted in the clinical context.

Significance of the Contraction Stress Test

A weekly negative CST is a sensitive indicator of immediate fetal condition. It allows the physician to avoid intervention with a low risk of antepartum fetal death, recently determined to be 0.4 per 1000 (corrected). Critics of the test point to the high false-positive rate of 8 to 50 percent reported in the literature. A false-positive test is defined as one in which an abnormal test result is subsequently associated with a normal fetal heart rate pattern (no late decelerations) in labor and eventually normal fetal outcome. The true false-positive rate for all CSTs is probably around 15 percent. However better specificity and improved reliability can be obtained by categorization of CST results into four groups. This is based on the presence or absence of FHR accelerations in association with fetal movements or uterine contractions during the CST:

1. *Reactive-negative CST.* This pattern is obtained in just over 85 percent of all CSTs. It is indicative of a normal healthy fetus with good placental reserve (Fig 3B).
2. *Nonreactive-negative CST.* This pattern is rarely observed (approximately 0.4 percent of tests) and should be interpreted with extreme caution (Fig. 3C). Three possibilities must be considered:
   a. Subtle late decelerations are being missed in a severely compromised fetus with a nonreactive pattern. The fetus is so acidotic that it is no longer able to accelerate or decelerate its heart rate.
   b. The fetus has a congenital CNS or cardiac anomaly.
   c. Maternal therapy with a CNS depressant or autonomic blocking agent.

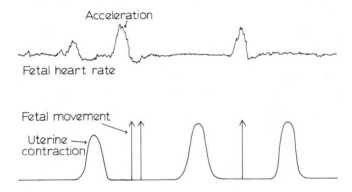

Figure 3B. Reactive-negative contraction stress test. Normal accelerations of FHR (more than 15 BPM) with fetal movement. No late decelerations.

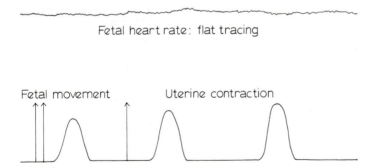

Figure 3C. Nonreactive-negative CST. Absence of accelerations of FHR. No late decelerations.

3. *Reactive-positive CST.* This pattern accounts for virtually all the false-positive test results obtained with CSTs (Fig. 3D). The false-positive rate in this group of patients is over 50 percent. However a minority of these patients will eventually demonstrate fetal distress in labor or other evidence of morbidity. It must be emphasized that a reactive-positive CST, with its high false-positive rate, must not be taken as an indication for intervention.

4. *Nonreactive-positive CST.* Several studies show that a nonreactive-positive pattern is an accurate indicator of fetal growth retardation, intrapartum fetal distress, and fetal morbidity. The false-positive rate is virtually zero and is certainly less than 5 percent (Fig. 3E).

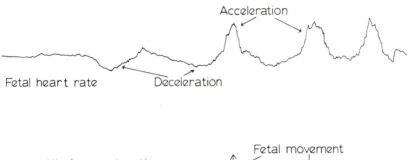

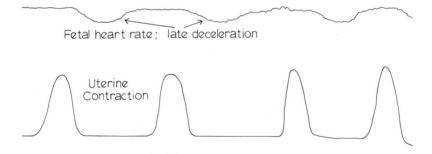

Figure 3D. Reactive-positive CST. Normal accelerations of FHR despite the presence of late decelerations with some uterine contractions.

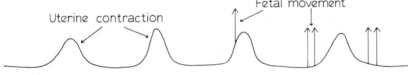

Figure 3E. Nonreactive-positive CST. Absence of accelerations of FHR. Persistent late decelerations with each uterine contraction.

Fetal Biophysical Profile

A different approach to the assessment of fetal status is the biophysical profile. The basic concept is that a multiple variable assessment of fetal biophysical activities is a more sensitive and reliable test of fetal well-being than the examination of a single parameter.

The biophysical profile is made up of five components (Table 1). One is the standard nonstress test. The other four fetal parameters are observed by using real-time ultrasonography, and include fetal breathing movements, gross fetal body movements, fetal tone, and the volume of amniotic fluid. A normal fetal response in these areas indicates that the part of the central nervous system that controls that activity is functioning normally. Any factor that leads to depression of the fetal CNS will reduce or abolish the biophysical actions of the fetus.

Two points are assigned for each normal and zero for each abnormal finding. Recent reports indicate that a biophysical score of 8 to 10 correlates well with a normal outcome of pregnancy. Scores of 0 to 2 were associated with a high incidence of perinatal morbidity. Scores of 0 to 2 have never been shown to improve, and have a low falsely positive rate. However, improvement has taken place when the scores are 4 or 6, especially if there is betterment in the condition of the mother. It appears that a score of 4 or 6 is the equivalent of a reactive positive contraction stress test, and is not to be taken as an indication for active intervention; except when oligohydramnios is present.

The biophysical profile is a reliable indicator of a healthy fetus, comparable with the NST and CST. Each is associated with a falsely negative (normal test, depressed fetus) of less than 0.5 percent. The rate of falsely positive results (abnormal test, score 0 to 4, and a normal fetus) has recently been reported to be in the order of 43.5 percent. This is lower than that of an NST, but greater than the false-positive rate for CST.

At present an abnormal biophysical profile score is defined as less than or equal to 4. The falsely positive score in this group is 43.5 percent. However, a score of 0 or 2 has an extremely low falsely positive rate. Hence, it may be that the scores should be reclassified:

Normal:	8 or 10
Equivocal:	4 or 6
Abnormal:	0 or 2

The biophysical profile is less time consuming than a contraction stress test, and should replace the CST as the next step following a nonreactive nonstress test.

TABLE 1. FETAL BIOPHYSICAL PROFILE

Biophysical Parameter	Normal: Score = 2	Abnormal: Score = 0
Nonstress test	Reactive pattern: At least 2 FHR accelerations of ≥15 BPM and ≥15 seconds' duration, associated with fetal movement in a 20-min period.	Nonreactive pattern: <2 FHR accelerations of ≥15 BPM and 15 seconds' duration associated with fetal movement in 40 min.
Fetal breathing movements	Present: Presence of at least 1 episode of fetal breathing of ≥ 60 seconds' duration within a 30-min period of observation.	Absent: Absence of fetal breathing movements or the absence of an episode of fetal breathing movements of ≥ 60 seconds' duration during a 30-min period of observation.
Gross fetal body movement	Present: Presence of at least 3 discrete episodes of fetal movement within a 30-min period. Simultaneous limb and trunk movements are counted as a single movement.	Decreased: Two or fewer discrete fetal movements in a 30-min period of observation.
Fetal tone	Upper and lower extremities in full flexion. Trunk in position of flexion and head flexed on chest. At least 1 episode of extension of limbs with return to position of flexion and/or extension of spine with return to flexion.	Decreased: Limbs in position of extension or partial flexion. Spine in extension. Fetal movement not followed by return to flexion. Fetal hand open.
Volume of amniotic fluid	Fluid evident throughout the uterine cavity. Largest pocket of fluid greater than 1 cm in vertical diameter.	Decreased: Fluid absent in most areas of uterine cavity. Largest pocket of fluid measure 1 cm or less in vertical axis. Crowding of fetal small parts.

An Integrated Approach to Antepartum Testing

A protocol outlining an approach to antepartum testing, which utilizes the three methods, is presented in Figure 4. Our primary method of fetal surveillance is the nonstress test.

Nonstress Test

1. *Reactive pattern*. The test is repeated once or twice a week as the clinical condition requires.
2. *Nonreactive pattern*. A nonreactive result that persists for 40 minutes is managed as follows:
   a. The testing time is increased to 80 minutes, OR
   b. The test is repeated within 24 hours, OR
   c. A biophysical profile is performed, OR
   d. A contraction stress test is carried out

A biophysical profile is a more practical procedure than a CST, but is not always available. Either a reactive-negative CST or a biophysical profile score of 8 or more would negate the nonreactive NST, and the latter would be repeated at the appropriate interval.

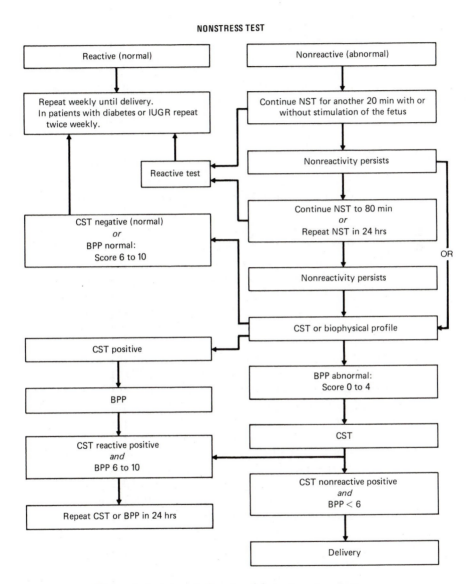

Figure 4. An integrated protocol for antepartum testing.

Contraction Stress Test

1. *Nonreactive-positive CST.* The presence of this pattern indicates that the fetus is compromised severely, and is a sufficient reason to terminate the pregnancy (Fig. 3E). However, it is advisable to confirm the abnormal result by means of a biophysical profile.

   Preliminary data suggest that a nonreactive-positive CST is always associated with a biophysical score of 0 or 2, with one exception. This is in the fetus of less than 30 weeks' gestation, when accelerations of the FHR may be absent because of immaturity.

   If the biophysical score is 6 or 8, especially when fetal breathing is normal and the amount of amniotic fluid is adequate, it appears that delivery may be postponed safely for 1 day at a time in the immature fetus. Daily reevaluations are mandatory.

   If a nonreactive-positive CST, confirmed by a biophysical score of 0 or 2 is obtained, then delivery by cesarean section is warranted. Preliminary evidence indicates that the correlation of a nonreactive 80-minute NST with a nonreactive-positive CST and a biophysical profile score of 0 or 2 is 100 percent. Hence all of these test results would seem to be equivalent in their predictive value as far as low false-positive rates are concerned.

2. *Reactive-positive CST.* This pattern is no longer accepted as an indication for immediate intervention (Fig. 3D). It is associated with a high false-positive rate, but a minority of fetuses demonstrating such a pattern do exhibit intrapartum distress and eventual morbidity. Although the majority are normal fetuses, the presence of late decelerations could indicate that some fetuses are in a state of marginal compromise or early uteroplacental insufficiency. The presence of FHR accelerations is reassuring and would indicate the absence of significant hypoxia or acidosis, thereby allowing normal biophysical activity such as accelerations, fetal breathing, and gross body movements. A reactive-positive tracing should be managed in the following way:

   a. A biophysical profile could be performed immediately. A normal score of 8 or 10 would negate the CST result and allow continued observation.

   b. If a biophysical score is not available then the CST should be repeated on the next day. It is also prudent to keep such a patient at bed rest in hospital and perform daily NSTs.

   c. A reactive-positive tracing in a patient at term with a ripe cervix is managed by induction of labor. In such a case moni-

toring of the FHR by means of a scalp electrode should be instituted as soon as the membranes are ruptured.

d. A reactive-positive CST in combination with a biophysical
score of 0 or 2 does not occur often. The management in this
situation is individualized, depending on fetal maturity:

   i. If the fetus is at term then induction of labor with fetal
scalp electrode monitoring is advisable.

   ii. If a reactive-positive tracing is obtained in a preterm fetus
with a biophysical score of 4 or greater, delivery can be
postponed on a day-by-day basis with continued observation. If the biophysical score is 0 or 2 then immediate delivery must be considered. In this situation the demonstration of a mature L/S ratio and pulmonary maturity
would be helpful.

Biophysical Profile Score

If the second testing method employed after a nonreactive NST is biophysical scoring, management is based on the test score obtained:

1. A score of 0 or 2 is usually an indication of fetal compromise and
provides sufficient basis for delivery based on this test result
alone. However it is also prudent to confirm the abnormal test
result when possible by an 80-minute NST or CST.

2. Test scores of 4 or 6 after a nonreactive NST should be evaluated
by repeat testing or the performance of a CST.

3. A score of 8 after a nonreactive NST is an indication of a healthy
fetus in whom the NST may then be repeated at the appropriate
interval.

Summary

The basic principles underlying the interpretation of antepartum tests
are as follows:.

1. A single normal test result, based on the observation of a single
biophysical activity, is a reliable sign of immediate fetal well-
being. Hence there would be little justification for the performance of a CST or biophysical profile if the NST is normal under
most circumstances.

2. An abnormal NST should be evaluated further by either a CST
or a biophysical profile score. A normal result from either of
these tests would then negate the significance of the nonreactive
NST. If the second testing method also gives an abnormal result,
confirmation should be sought by performing the remaining
test. Abnormal results from three tests virtually rule out the
chance of a falsely abnormal situation, and indicate the need for
urgent delivery.

It must be emphasized that, although antepartum tests can be misinterpreted so that a healthy fetus appears compromised, it is difficult to make a hypoxic infant appear well.

DETERMINATION OF FETAL HEALTH: INTRAPARTUM

Intermittent Auscultation of Fetal Heart

Instruments

1. Conventional fetal stethoscope
2. Handheld Doppler ultrasonic fetal stethoscope.

Intermittent auscultation of the fetal heart beat is a satisfactory method in many cases. When the fetal heart cannot be heard by the conventional fetal stethoscope, it can be located, if it is present, by Doppler ultrasound.

In the first stage of labor the fetal heart is auscultated every 15 minutes for at least 30 seconds, immediately following a uterine contraction. In the second stage of labor, auscultation is performed every 5 minutes.

Disadvantages of Periodic Auscultation

1. It is not continuous and variable or prolonged decelerations may be missed.
2. The proper categorization of a deceleration in relationship to uterine contractions cannot often be made.
3. Studies show that intermittent auscultation is of no value in diagnosing early fetal distress.
4. Fetal heart rate variability, which is the most important component of the fetal heart rate record in the assessment of fetal status, cannot be evaluated.
5. There is no permanent record to allow for the progressive analysis or retrospective evaluation. This may be of medicolegal importance.

Uterine Activity Recording

Technique

External. An external tocodynamometer or pressure transducer is placed on the abdominal wall. Semiquantitative recordings are obtained which do not actually reflect intrauterine pressure. However, they do indicate when the contractions begin and end. The advantage of this method is that it is noninvasive.

Internal. A transcervical intrauterine catheter connected to a strain gauge transducer is used to obtain direct pressure measurements which are recorded on the second channel of the apparatus.

Insertion of the intrauterine pressure catheter has been attended by an occasional complication. The reported incidence of uterine perforation ranges from 1 per 1400 to 1 per 376 monitored cases.

Indications

1. Patients with a previous cesarean section undergoing a trial of labor. Sudden loss of uterine pressure will be the first sign of uterine rupture in these cases.
2. In obstructed labor the assessment of the strength of uterine contractions may be helpful in ruling out uterine inertia. It is also useful to monitor oxytocin stimulation in these cases.

Continuous Electronic Fetal Heart Rate Recording

The fetal heart rate (FHR) is modulated by reflex neurogenic mechanisms. Normal rate and variability of the FHR indicate an intact fetal CNS with normal cardiac responsiveness. Changes in the fetal P_{O_2} produce alterations in the CNS. Biochemical changes (metabolic acidosis) through their effect on the CNS ultimately produce hemodynamic alterations. The clinical use of continuous electronic FHR monitoring is based on the assumption that there is metabolic evidence of asphyxia and hemodynamic change before permanent neurologic damage occurs.

All conventional FHR monitors provide a continuous record of the rate derived from serial calculations of instantaneous or beat-to-beat heart rate. A counter processes each consecutive pair of cardiac signals and measures the elapsed time between each beat. The reciprocal of this beat-to-beat interval is used to calculate the instantaneous heart rate required to produce that time interval. This is then printed out on the FHR record in beats per minute. As the interval of each cardiac cycle changes with varying neurogenic input, the instantaneous heart rate as recorded by the monitor changes constantly. This allows evaluation of intrinsic variability within the heart rate signal as well as the baseline rate.

Methods of Recording

1. Internal or direct. By this technique an electrode is applied to the fetal scalp or buttocks by means of which a fetal electrocardiogram signal is obtained.

   a. *Advantages*:
     i. It is noninvasive.
     ii. Suitable in patient with intact membranes or closed cervix.
     iii. Allows for antepartum monitoring.
   b. *Disadvantages*:
     i. High level of artifact.
     ii. May artificially increase the variation in instantaneous heart rate and give an erroneous interpretation of FHR variability.
     iii. Abscess of the scalp is a rare and usually benign complication. The lesions are single and localized in most cases. They are more common after prolonged labor and an extended period of monitoring of the fetal heart. In most instances spontaneous evacuation takes place following local treatment. Occasionally incision and drainage is needed. Rarely parenteral antibiotics are given.

2. External or indirect. A fetal heart tracing is obtained by using a Doppler ultrasonic technique. The transducer is applied to the mother's abdomen.

   In Doppler ultrasound detection of fetal cardiac motion a transducer of ultrasound crystals directs a broad ultrasound beam toward the fetal heart. Continuous or repetitive bursts of ultrasound energy are emitted from the crystal which serves both as a transmitter and a receiver for ultrasound energy. Moving cardiac structures produce a Doppler shift in reflected frequencies. The fastest moving objects, usually the cardiac valves, produce the greatest Doppler shift and the greatest increase in frequency. These changes in frequency are detected by the ultrasound crystal and converted to an electronic signal. This signal is measured by the cardiotachometer which calculates an instantaneous heart rate from measuring the time interval between two heart beats.

   a. *Advantages*:
     i. It is noninvasive.
     ii. Suitable in patient with intact membranes or closed cervix.
     iii. Allows for antepartum monitoring.
   b. *Disadvantages*:
     i. High level of artifact.
     ii. May artificially increase the variation in instantaneous heart rate and give an erroneous interpretation of FHR variability.

Components of the Fetal Heart Rate Tracing

1. Baseline heart rate
2. Baseline variability
3. Periodic changes:
   a. Accelerations
   b. Decelerations

Baseline Fetal Heart Rate

The baseline fetal heart rate is the average rate observed when the patient is not in labor or between uterine contractions.

Definitions

1. Normal range: 110 to 160 beats per minute
2. Tachycardia
   a. Mild: 161 to 180 beats per minute
   b. Severe: greater than 180 beats per minute
3. Baseline bradycardia
   a. Mild: 90 to 109 beats per minute
   b. Moderate: 70 to 89 beats per minute
   c. Severe: less than 70 beats per minute

The baseline FHR decreases with advancing gestational age, reflecting increased parasympathetic control. The baseline FHR is the least sensitive indicator of the degree of fetal oxygenation, and a compromised fetus could have a normal baseline rate. On the other hand, changes in the baseline rate should be considered as indicating asphyxia until it has been ruled out by other evidence. In cases of asphyxia, changes in the baseline rate are usually accompanied by late or variable decelerations and decreased beat-to-beat variability. By definition, to be accepted as a baseline change, the alteration in the FHR must be sustained for more than 10 to 15 minutes.

Tachycardia

Tachycardia is defined as a rate over 160 beats per minute. It reflects increased adrenergic tone with decreased vagal input. Tachycardia is usually accompanied by some decrease in heart rate variability.

Causes of Tachycardia

1. Fetal hypoxia
2. Fetal anemia
3. Fetal cardiac failure

4. Fetal tachyarrhythmia
5. Prematurity
6. Maternal fever (and therefore elevated fetal temperature)
7. Maternal anxiety
8. Maternal or fetal hyperthyroidism
9. Chorioamnionitis
10. Parasympatholitic drugs (atropine, Atarax, phenothiazines)
11. Betamimetic drugs (ritodrine, salbutamol, isoxsuprine)

Outcome

1. The outcome is good if decelerations are absent and fetal heart rate variability is normal.
2. The outcome is poor if decelerations, with or without a decrease in fetal heart rate variability, are present.

Tachycardia alone is not a good indicator of fetal infection or asphyxia. It may however be an early sign of hypoxia and indicates fetal distress when accompanied by periodic changes and absent variability. There is some evidence that in postterm fetuses fetal distress is manifest as a tachycardia with loss of variability. These changes may precede fetal death without the appearance of late or variable decelerations.

Bradycardia

A fetal heart rate less than 120 beats per minute is defined as bradycardia. Clinically this definition would seem stringent as many normal fetuses have a baseline rate of 100 to 120 beats per minute. Any bradycardia in the presence of good heart rate variability is usually benign. Bradycardias must be distinguished from prolonged decelerations (periodic bradycardia) as the significance and subsequent management are different in the two situations.

Causes of Bradycardia

1. Asphyxia (usually a late sign)
2. Physiologic
3. Arrhythmia
4. Drug effect

A baseline fetal heart rate of less than 70 beats per minute may represent a congenital heart block which is often associated with congenital heart disease and in rare cases maternal systemic lupus erythematosis.

Outcome

Fetal bradycardia is a late sign of fetal distress when:

1. Variability and accelerations are absent.
2. There are periodic decelerations. However, in a severely compromised fetus, late decelerations may be absent because the fetus is so acidotic that it can neither accelerate or decelerate its heart rate.

Baseline Variability of the Fetal Heart Rate

In the normal FHR there is a beat-to-beat variation of 5 to 15 beats per minute. A minor baseline irregularity is normal and indicates that the CNS is functioning normally and is capable of controlling the FHR (Fig. 5A).

In predicting the immediate status of the fetus, variability of the baseline FHR is a most significant parameter. Loss of variability indicates that the fetus may be suffering from anoxia and acidosis, and correlates well with the measurement of the pH of blood obtained from the fetal scalp antepartum and the cord blood postpartum.

Fetal heart variability may be divided into two types:

1. Short-term variability (STV): This represents the normal variance in intervals between successive cardiac cycles. It is difficult to identify and assess, and is of less clinical value than long-term variability.
2. Long-term variability (LTV): This represents the cumulative changes in the FHR occurring over a time base of 5 to 30 seconds. It is responsible for the waviness of the FHR tracing. The usual frequency is 3 to 5 cycles per second, with an amplitude of at least 5 beats per minute and duration of at least 5 seconds. Because LTV may be increased artificially by external monitoring, the assessment of heart rate variability is made best from a scalp electrode recording whenever possible.

Changes in Long-term Variability

1. Increased long-term variability. In this situation the amplitude of the cycle exceeds 30 beats per minute. There are several possible explanations:
   a. Mild fetal hypoxia. Increased long-term variability is one of the early FHR signs of a decrease in fetal oxygenation.
   b. Fetal hemorrhage. In this case there is usually an accompanying tachycardia. A Kleihauer test on maternal blood will reveal fetal red blood cells. Assessment of the hematocrit from a scalp sample will show anemia.
   c. Vulnerable cord syndrome. This results from the compression of an umbilical cord made vulnerable by shortening or oligohydramnios.

2. Decreased long-term variability. This is a common pattern and is caused by several factors:.
   a. Fetal hypoxia. This is the most serious situation.
   b. Physiologic sleep cycle. In labor this lasts 20 to 40 minutes.
   c. Central nervous system depressing drugs.
   d. Parasympatholytic drugs cause decreased variability and tachycardia.
   e. Sympatholytic drugs lead to decreased variability and brady-cardia.

Interpretation. When decreased variability is the result of hypoxia there are, in most cases, periodic changes in the FHR with or without a change in the baseline rate. Decreased variability occurs during fetal sleep, and if the tracing is normal in other respects, no action need be taken. Normal variability will return either spontaneously or following stimulation of the fetus.

A difficult pattern to evaluate is one where the baseline rate is persistently flat although the FHR is within the normal range and there are no abnormal periodic changes. Possible causes include (1) congenital anomalies of the heart or CNS; (2) prematurity; (3) previous hypoxia; (4) some cases are idiopathic and no etiologic factor is identifiable. Estimation of fetal pH from a sample of scalp blood should be performed before active treatment is instituted.

Poor or absent variability may not show up on tracings from an external monitor. Therefore, in problem cases a scalp electrode should be applied so that a more accurate assessment can be made. However, absence of variability demonstrated by the external monitor is significant because the true variability is never more than that displayed on the external monitor.

Periodic Changes in the Fetal Heart Rate

Accelerations
These occur most commonly in the antepartum period, in early labor, and along with variable decelerations. There are two possible physiologic mechanisms:

1. They represent an intact CNS in a state of arousal indicating a healthy fetus.
2. Partial cord occlusion results in compression of the umbilical vein while the umbilical artery remains patent. This causes decreased fetal cardiac output and fetal hypotension. Hypotension elicits a baroreceptor response resulting in a FHR acceleration. Hence these accelerations are often seen just at the start of a uterine contraction and often precede a variable deceleration.

Decelerations
Four types are identified according to their shape and temporal relationship to uterine contractions.

Classification

1. Uniform: When the pattern of the FHR relates to the curve of the uterine contraction
   a. Early deceleration (Fig. 5B)
   b. Late deceleration (Fig. 5C)
2. Variable: When there is no relationship between the uterine contraction and the FHR
   a. Variable (Fig. 5D)
   b. Prolonged

Significant Features
In interpreting the FHR patterns (Fig. 5), the following features are significant:

1. The baseline FHR
2. The increase or decrease of the FHR in response to a uterine contraction
3. Whether the curve of the FHR is uniform or variable
4. The time relationship between the onset of the contraction and the start of the deceleration of the FHR
5. The lag time, i.e., the interval between the peak of the intrauterine pressure curve and the lowest level of the FHR
6. The recovery time, i.e., the interval from the nadir of the FHR until its return to the baseline

Early Deceleration of FHR

Characteristics. All the following must apply (Fig. 5B):

1. The shape of the curve is uniform and appears the same from one contraction to the next.
2. The pattern of the FHR mirrors that of the contraction.
3. Onset of the deceleration is early in the contraction cycle.
4. Nadir of the deceleration occurs at the peak of the contraction.
5. The FHR returns to the baseline before the contraction is over.
6. The lowest amplitude is proportional to the strength of the contraction.
7. Baseline FHR rarely falls below 100 beats per minute.
8. The amplitude of deceleration is usually less than 30 beats per minute.
9. The pattern is repetitive in most cases.
10. Baseline beat-to-beat variation is maintained.

Proposed Mechanism. Early deceleration is believed to be the result of fetal head compression resulting in altered cerebral blood flow which initiates a vagal reflex and cardiac slowing. This deceleration may be abolished by atropine.

Interpretation. This is a benign FHR pattern. It is not usually associated with baseline changes or loss of beat-to-beat variability. It is not associated with fetal hypoxia, acidosis, or low Apgar scores. It may represent a physiologic mechanism by which the fetus conserves energy in labor. During a uterine contraction the fall in placental perfusion results in decreased transfer of oxygen. Slowing of the fetal heart at this time would conserve cardiac glycogen at a time when the energy yield is lowest.

Management. No treatment is indicated.

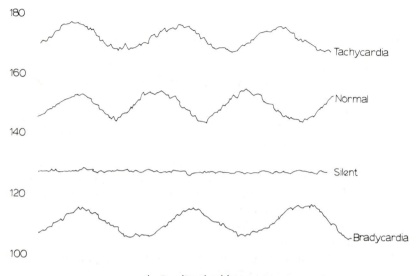

A. Baseline fetal heart rate.

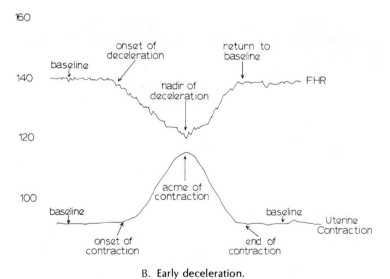

B. Early deceleration.

Figure 5. Fetal heart rate patterns.

Late Deceleration of FHR

Characteristics.   All the following must apply (Fig 5C):

1. The shape of the curve is uniform; one is similar to the next.
2. The onset of the deceleration occurs late in the uterine contraction cycle, 20 to 30 seconds after the start of the contraction.
3. The FHR does not return to baseline until after the end of the uterine contraction. The deceleration may persist for 30 to 60 seconds after the contraction.
4. The lag time (interval between the peak of the uterine contraction and the lowest level of the FHR) is greater than 20 seconds.
5. The duration of the deceleration of the FHR is proportional to the uterine contraction.
6. The amplitude of the deceleration is proportional to the strength of the contraction.
7. The deceleration is usually 20 to 30 beats per minute. Rarely does it exceed 40 beats per minute.
8. The pattern is usually repetitive.

Proposed Mechanism

1. Decreased uterine blood flow (uteroplacental insufficiency)
2. Reduction of Po_2 below a critical level during the peak of contraction
3. Initially mediated by hypoxic depression of CNS
4. Severe hypoxia also leads to direct depression of fetal myocardium

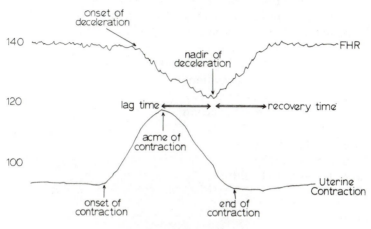

C. **Late deceleration.**

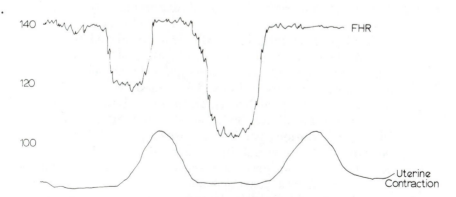

D. **Variable deceleration.**

Figure 5. (cont.) Fetal heart rate patterns.

Interpretation. Late decelerations are potentially ominous and a repetitive pattern may lead to fetal acidosis. Management of this pattern is often based on whether the cause of the uteroplacental insufficiency is considered to be potentially reversible or is known to be irreversible.

1. Potentially reversible causes
   a. Hyperstimulation with oxytocic agents
   b. Maternal hypotension
      i. Supine position
      ii. Associated with epidural anesthesia
      iii. Maternal hypovolemia
2. Usually irreversible causes
   a. Fetal growth retardation
   b. Diabetes
   c. Hypertension
   d. Postmaturity
   e. Placental abruption

Management

1. Corrective measures:
   a. Relief of maternal hypotension by turning the patient on her side.
   b. Reduction of uterine overactivity by discontinuing the administration of oxytocin.
   c. Administration of high concentrations of oxygen to the mother by tight-fitting face mask.
2. If the pattern persists for over 15 minutes, preparation should be made for early delivery.
3. The presence of good FHR variability would indicate the absence of fetal acidosis. In this situation if delivery is anticipated within 1 hour, a fetal scalp pH should be performed. If the pH is normal then vaginal delivery may be awaited.
4. Persistent late decelerations accompanied by baseline changes (bradycardia or tachycardia) and decreased FHR variability indicate significant fetal distress and acidosis. Delivery should be carried out immediately, by cesarean section if necessary.
5. In certain situations, persistent late decelerations in the face of normal heart rate variability or normal scalp pH, delivery by cesarean section may still be carried out. An example would be late decelerations appearing in a patient known to have an irreversible cause for placental insufficiency in early labor. In this situation although the presence of normal variability or the demonstration of a normal scalp pH would indicate absence of

fetal acidosis at that time, it is obvious that the fetus would eventually become compromised during the course of many hours of labor.

Variable Deceleration of FHR

Characteristics

1. Variable shape and wave form. It may be U, V, or W shaped, etc. It differs from one deceleration to the next (Fig. 5D).
2. Variable onset.
3. Variable lag time.
4. Variable amplitude and duration.
5. Need not be repetitive. For any single contraction a variable deceleration can mimic an early or late deceleration.
6. It is frequently preceded or followed by accelerations ("shoulders").

Proposed Mechanism

1. Cord compression initially produces obstruction of umbilical vein blood flow while the umbilical artery remains patent. This produces a fall in fetal cardiac output, hypotension, and a baroreceptor response. The baroreceptor response initiates a period of FHR acceleration.
2. As umbilical cord compression proceeds, the flow through the umbilical artery is finally impaired. This isolates the fetal cardiovascular system from the low pressure placental unit. The increased peripheral vascular resistance in the fetus increases fetal blood pressure. This always provokes a reflex vagal slowing of the FHR. If cord compression is sustained and persistent this may eventually lead to hypoxia and metabolic acidosis. Hence a variable deceleration has two components: (1) A neurogenic or reflex vagal deceleration usually accompanied by a reversible respiratory acidosis due to the accumulation of carbon dioxide and increased P_{CO_2} in the fetus. (2) A late component due to hypoxic depression of the CNS after sustained or persistent cord compression. When this occurs metabolic acidosis will supervene.

Interpretation. Variable decelerations are the most common periodic change observed in labor. There is a higher incidence in association with a nuchal, short, or prolapsed cord, and when oligohydramnios is present. The potential for cord compression exists each time there is fetal movement or a uterine contraction.

Variable decelerations are also noted with occipitoposterior positions. In this situation the deceleration does not result from compression of the umbilical cord, but from other mechanisms. The distinguishing feature is the absence of the "shoulders" (accelerations of the FHR) that usually accompany variable decelerations caused by compression of the cord. Variable decelerations are not, under usual circumstances, associated with low Apgar scores or fetal acidosis.

Criteria which suggest that the variable deceleration is benign and does not require operative intervention are as follows:

1. The FHR deceleration lasts no more than 45 seconds on a repetitive basis.
2. The return of the FHR to the baseline is abrupt. There is no late component manifested by a slow return or a late deceleration after the return to baseline.
3. The baseline rate is not increasing.
4. Baseline variability is not decreasing.

Management. When any of these criteria are exceeded it may mean that the fetus is becoming hypoxic and acidotic. Treatment varies and is based upon the clinical situation.

1. A patient in early labor having variable decelerations of a severity exceeding the above criteria is treated best by delivery by cesarean section. It is unreasonable to expect any improvement as labor progresses since variable deceleration tends to worsen as descent of the fetus increases traction on the umbilical cord.
2. On the other hand, a patient in the second stage of labor having variable decelerations that exceed the stated criteria may be managed expectantly. As long as FHR variability is present and there is no progressive rise in the FHR, it is unlikely that fetal acidosis is present. Variable decelerations that occur repetitively during the second stage and last more than a minute are seen frequently. Difficult forceps deliveries are best avoided as long as heart rate variability is maintained. Fetal scalp sampling is of limited use and may be misleading in patients with variable deceleration. Any interpretation of a scalp sample performed in association with variable decelerations must take account of the profound but reversible respiratory acidosis which may occur during and just after the deceleration.

The presence of beat-to-beat variability in this situation is a good guide to the absence of significant acidosis. Careful correlation of persistent severe variable decelerations with variability and other baseline changes will obviate unnecessary intervention. It may be stated that variable decelerations are responsible for most unnecessary cesarean sections when inexperienced personnel overreact to their significance.

Prolonged Deceleration of FHR

Characteristics

1. Abrupt in onset and variable in nature
2. High amplitude deceleration of at least 30 beats per minute
3. Duration longer than 2.5 minutes
4. The pattern varies considerably in:
   a. Rapidity of onset
   b. Relationship to uterine contraction
   c. Speed of recovery
   d. Patterns during and after recovery
   e. Duration and amplitude
5. Must be distinguished from baseline bradycardia
6. Also denoted as periodic bradycardia

Proposed Mechanism

1. This is uncertain.
2. It is probably reflex and vagal in origin.
3. The potential for fetal hypoxia is present if the deceleration is prolonged.

Causes

1. Tetanic contraction (spontaneous or oxytocin induced)
2. Severe placental abruption
3. Vaginal examination
4. Application of an internal fetal scalp electrode
5. Fetal scalp blood sampling
6. Prolapsed umbilical cord
7. Maternal convulsion
8. Paracervical block
9. Epidural anesthesia
10. Supine hypotension
11. CNS anomalies
12. Prolonged umbilical cord compression often associated with rapid descent of the fetus during expulsion
13. Maternal respiratory arrest due to a high spinal or intravenous narcotic agent
14. Following epidural top-up injections

Interpretation and Management. If the deceleration is related to an identifiable event it is best to correct the problem and to allow labor to continue. In the absence of a known cause the patient should be prepared for operative delivery in case the deceleration recurs. If significant hypoxia occurred during the deceleration, the latter is usually followed by rebound tachycardia. The usual corrective measures of lateral recumbency, discontinuation of oxytocin, and administration of oxygen should be instituted as soon as the deceleration is noted.

Prolonged decelerations often follow repetitive severe variable decelerations, and in this case are indicative of significant fetal hypoxia and acidosis. Immediate cesarean section is the treatment of choice.

Summary

1. A normal FHR tracing with normal heart rate variability indicates a healthy fetus and is associated with normal Apgar scores virtually 100 percent of the time.
2. FHR changes represent a hemodynamic response to a fetal *stress* and should not be interpreted to mean the presence of fetal *distress*.
3. Late or persistent variable decelerations occurring over a 30- to 60-minute period may lead to fetal acidosis.
4. The presence or absence of beat-to-beat variability determines the degree of hypoxia and is an accurate guide to fetal pH.

The Role of Continuous FHR Monitoring

Continuous bioelectronic FHR monitoring was developed to improve the predictive accuracy of intermittent auscultation. At present bioelectronic fetal monitoring during labor is a widely used and clinically accepted technique. As with most fetal assessment methods, the incidence of false-negative results is extremely low. Great care in the interpretation of abnormal tracings must be exercised, however, in order to reduce the incidence of false-positive results. Failure to do this will lead to an increased incidence of interference and unnecessary cesarean sections. A proper understanding of the physiologic and pathologic basis of FHR changes allows the knowledgeable physician to make effective use of electronic monitoring. Some institutions utilize adjunctive fetal scalp pH estimations in an attempt to reduce the errors of the fetal monitoring. As better understanding of the significance of changes in the FHR develops, the need for fetal scalp blood sampling is reduced. Careful attention to the entire FHR record, and the assessment of the degree of FHR variability, allows for accurate and reliable assessment of immediate fetal status.

Indications for Continuous FHR Monitoring

1. Obstetric reasons:
   a. Clinically detected abnormalities of the FHR
   b. Meconium in the amniotic fluid
   c. Oxytocin stimulation of labor
   d. Premature labor
   e. Slow progress in labor
   f. Abnormal presentation
2. Patients at risk for uteroplacental insufficiency. (See first page of this chapter.)

The Role of Periodic Auscultation of the FHR

Periodic auscultation of the FHR, immediately following a uterine contraction, for at least 30 seconds in the first stage of labor, and every 5 minutes during the second stage of labor, is an acceptable method of assessing the fetal condition in women at low risk for intrapartum fetal distress. Interpretation of auscultated FHR data must be done on the basis of an understanding of the relationship between changes in the FHR and the uterine contractions. To achieve excellence with this method an almost one-to-one relationship is necessary between the patient and an experienced nurse. Auscultation of the FHR every 1 to 2 hours, seen not infrequently on a busy obstetric service, is inadequate observation of the laboring patient.

Proper use of both intermittent auscultation and continuous electronic fetal monitoring in both high- and low-risk patients should include an explanation to the patient of the purpose of these examinations, and a discussion with her about her concerns and wishes. Ideally, this should take place during the prenatal visits and again upon her admittance to the labor suite.

Psychologic Response to Fetal Monitoring

Valuable as the fetal monitor is, it transforms the labor room into an intensive care environment, and some patients manifest strong reactions.

Positive Response. Many women find that their state of anxiety is relieved, the machine providing valuable information that is otherwise unavailable. The clicking of the monitor confirms that the baby is alive. Both patient and husband can tell when the next contraction is coming and are able to prepare for it. Women who have had a fetal loss in a previous pregnancy are strongly in favor of fetal monitoring.

Negative Response. The patients complain about the discomfort from the abdominal transducers and from the wires of the intravaginal electrode, which hangs between their thighs. They are unhappy with their enforced immobility, the loss of privacy, and their loss of control of the labor. Some are concerned that the electrode may damage the baby or that fetal monitoring is carried on only in dangerous situations and become anxious by variations in the FHR. A few resent the doctor and the husband paying more attention to the equipment than to the patient and feel that they are being used as guinea pigs.

The solution to these problems lies in educating the patient in the antepartum period. A description and demonstration of the apparatus, correction of erroneous impressions as to the purposes of and indications for fetal monitoring, reference to the scalp electrode as a small clip attached to the skin, and reassurance that the procedure is not part of a research project will make electronic monitoring more acceptable.

During labor the working and purposes of the monitor should be explained, the patient should be allowed as much mobility as possible, her comfort must be a paramount consideration, and her privacy maintained.

Biochemical Analysis of Fetal Capillary Blood

When significant fetal hypoxia occurs metabolic acidosis develops. As anaerobic metabolism proceeds, increasing amounts of lactic acid progressively lower the pH of fetal blood. Saling developed a method of testing fetal blood for acidosis before birth. A blood sample is obtained from the presenting part. Microanalysis is performed mainly to measure the pH, P_{CO_2}, and bicarbonate levels, but glucose, electrolytes, blood type, and antibodies can be determined.

It must be emphasized that a proper interpretation of fetal scalp pH requires a complete analysis of fetal blood gases. Also to minimize errors a measurement of maternal pH should be taken at the same time.

Indications

1. When a confusing FHR pattern is present with some elements that suggest fetal hypoxia
2. When there is a sustained baseline heart rate without variability but showing no ominous periodic changes
3. When uncorrectable late decelerations in the presence of good variability occur in a patient where vaginal delivery may be anticipated within 60 minutes

Technique
To be successful fetal capillary blood sampling requires an organized routine, availability of equipment for immediate analysis, and operators with expertise. The membranes must be ruptured, the presenting part fixed in the pelvis, the position known, the cervix dilated more than 3 cm, and good lighting available. Under aseptic conditions, and with the patient lying preferably in the left lateral position, an amnioscope is introduced into the posterior fornix of the vagina. Slow withdrawal of the scope at an angle allows the end to slip through the cervix and, with light pressure, to come against the fetal scalp (or rarely, the buttocks). The site for sampling is wiped clean of maternal blood and amniotic fluid, and a thin layer of silicone gel is applied to induce beading of blood to aid in its collection. The commercially available scalpels are preset so that the depth of incision is 3 mm. A cruciate incision is made, and a brief, moderate flow of blood follows. Approximately 150 μL is collected into two capillary tubes. The samples must be analyzed immediately. Excessive or prolonged bleeding is rare; it is easily controlled by pressure. In less than 1 percent of cases a mild localized infection occurs.

Correlation Between FHR Patterns, Fetal pH, and Outcome
The normal fetus has a pH of 7.25 to 7.35 prior to the start of labor. During labor there is a gradual shift in pH towards 7.25. If fetal hypoxia produces metabolic acidosis, fetal pH falls through preacidosis (7.20 to 7.25) to frank acidosis (less than 7.20).

Certain correlations between fetal pH and neonatal condition have been observed:

1. pH over 7.25: More than 90 percent of these neonates will be healthy, nondepressed, with high Apgar scores, and would have shown normal FHR patterns during labor.
2. pH between 7.20 and 7.25: This level indicates mild preacidosis. It is often associated with a prolonged second stage of labor and mild hypoxemia. FHR patterns often demonstrate late or variable decelerations, but beat-to-beat variability is normal. Most of these neonates will have high Apgar scores. Operative intervention is not indicated, but the sampling should be repeated in 30 minutes.
3. pH less than 7.20: This is usually indicative of significant fetal acidosis. In 80 percent of neonates the Apgar score will be under 6. FHR patterns often show persistent late or persistent severe variable decelerations with loss of heart variability.

4. pH less than 7.10: This indicates profound asphyxia. Significant neonatal depression is present in 90 percent of cases.

The correlation between fetal scalp pH measurements and neonatal Apgar score increases as the sample is taken closer to the time of birth. If taken within 5 minutes of delivery Hon and associates have shown a high correlation between low pH and low Apgar scores. However there appears to be a poor correlation between fetal pH and Apgar scores between 7 and 10. This could be accounted for partially by local factors that may make the fetal pH low at the scalp when the central fetal circulation is normal, especially at the time of delivery when caput formation is greatest.

A low fetal pH should not be interpreted in isolation. A full review of the entire blood gas picture must be carried out. An assessment of the P_{CO_2}, bicarbonate, and base deficit values are required to substantiate a diagnosis of metabolic acidosis. Respiratory acidosis, unassociated with hypoxia, may follow cord compression. Hence if a scalp sample is obtained during or just after a variable deceleration, an extremely low fetal pH due to respiratory acidosis may be obtained. Interpreted in isolation of other acid-base parameters, this would lead to erroneous diagnosis of severe fetal distress and result in unnecessary intervention.

False Results

False normal results (pH over 7.20, low Apgar score) occur in association with sedative drugs, anesthesia, obstruction of the airway, congenital anomalies, prematurity, hypoxia subsequent to the sampling, trauma of delivery, or a previous episode of asphyxia (the acid-base balance returns to normal, but the central nervous system does not).

False abnormal results (pH under 7.20, good Apgar score) may occur in the presence of maternal acidosis. Hence, it is important to measure the maternal pH when low values are obtained in the fetus before definitive action is taken.

Management During Labor

1. An abnormal FHR is an indication for analysis of the fetal blood.
2. If the pH is over 7.25, labor is allowed to go on and the analysis is repeated only if the FHR remains abnormal.
3. When the pH is 7.20 to 7.25, another sampling is performed in 30 minutes.
4. With the pH under 7.20, another sample is collected and preparations are made for operative delivery. If the second analysis confirms the first one, delivery is carried out immediately.

BIBLIOGRAPHY

Brame RG, MacKenna J: Vaginal pool phospholipids in the management of premature rupture of the membranes. Am J Obstet Gynecol 145:992, 1983

Brown, R, Patrick JE: The nonstress test: How long is enough. Am J Obstet Gynecol 141:646, 1981

Collea JV, Holls WH: The contraction stress test. Clin Obstet Gynecol 25:707, 1982

Cordero L, Anderson CW, Zuspan FP: Scalp abscess: A benign and infrequent complication of fetal monitoring. Am J Obstet Gynecol 146:126, 1983

Cruickshank DP: Amniocentesis for determination of fetal maturity. Clin Obstet Gynecol 25:773, 1982

Elias S: Fetoscopy in prenatal diagnosis. Clin Perinatol 10:357, 1983

Freeman RK, Garite TJ: Incidence of premature delivery following the oxytocin challenge test. Am J Obstet Gynecol 141:5, 1981

Freeman RK, Garite TJ: Fetal Heart Rate Monitoring. Baltimore/London: Williams and Wilkins, 1981, pp 84–112

Grannum T, Berkowitz RL, Hobbins JC: The ultrasonic changes in the maturing placenta and their relation to fetal pulmonary maturity. Am J Obstet Gynecol 133:915, 1979

James DK, Tindall VR, Richardson T: Is the lecithin/sphingomyelin ratio outdated? Brit J Obstet Gynaecol 90:955, 1983

Holer CW: Ultrasound estimation of gestational age. Clin Obstet Gynecol 27:314, 1984

Kochenour NK: Estrogen assay during pregnancy. Clin Obstet Gynecol 25:659, 1982

Leveno KJ, William ML, DePalma RT, Whalley PJ: Perinatal outcome in the absence of antepartum fetal heart acceleration. Obstet Gynecol 61:347, 1983

Lin CC, Moawad AH, River P, Pishotta FT: An OCT-reactivity classification to predict fetal outcome. Obstet Gynecol 56:17, 1980

Madanes AE, David D, Cetrulo C: Major complications associated with intrauterine pressure monitoring. Obstet Gynecol 59:389, 1982

Manning FA, Lange IR, Morrison I, Harman CR: Determination of fetal health: Methods for antepartum and intrapartum fetal assessment. Curr Prob Obstet Gynecol Vol 7, No. 4, 1983

Miller RC: Meconium staining of the amniotic fluid. Clin Obstet Gynecol 6:359, 1979

Molfese V, Sunshine P, Bennett A: Reactions of women to intrapartum fetal monitoring. Obstet Gynecol 59:705, 1982

Patrick J, Campbell K, Carmichael L, et al: Patterns of human fetal breathing during the last 10 weeks of pregnancy. Obstet Gynecol 56:24, 1980

Patrick J: Fetal breathing movements. Clin Obstet Gynecol 25:787, 1982

Petrucha RA, Golde SH, Platt LD: The use of ultrasound in the prediction of fetal pulmonary maturity. Am J Obstet Gynecol 144:931, 1982

Plauché WC, Faro S, Letellier R: Phosphatidyl-glycerol and fetal lung maturity. Am J Obstet Gynecol 144:167, 1982

Sadovsky E, Polishuk WZ: Fetal movements in utero: Nature, assessment prognostic value, timing of delivery. Obstet Gynecol 50:49, 1977

Sorokiny Y, Dierker LJ: Fetal movement. Clin Obstet Gynecol 25:719, 1982

Timor-Tritsch IE, Dierker LJ, Hertz RH, Rosen MG: Fetal movement: A brief review. Clin Obstet Gynecol 22:583, 1979

Tulchinsky D: Use of biochemical indices in the management of high risk obstetric patients. Clin Perinatal 7:413, 1980

Yeh SY, Read JA: Plasma unconjugated estriol as an indicator of fetal dysmaturity in postterm pregnancy. Obstet Gynecol 62:22, 1983

Young DC, Gray JH, Luther ER, et al: Fetal scalp blood pH sampling: Its value in an active obstetric unit. Am J Obstet Gynecol 136:276, 1980

38

Ultrasonography and Radiography

Henry F. Muggah

ULTRASONOGRAPHY

In the diagnosis of obstetric and fetal conditions ultrasound is a valuable and frequently used tool. Because no clinically significant adverse effects have been reported in humans, ultrasound is believed to be safe at the intensities currently employed for diagnoses, i.e., at the low MHz frequency range below 100 mW/cm^2.

Since 1880, it has been known that when a mechanical force such as sound is applied to a piezoelectric crystal an electric current is generated. Conversely, when an electric current is passed across the surface of such a crystal, a high frequency vibrational sound wave is produced. In most of the equipment used in the medical field, a pulsed ultrasonic system is used by which a single transducer both transmits ultrasonic vibrations and receives the sound echoes when they return. The pulsed system sends out signals less than $1/10$ of 1 percent of the time, and receives their returning echoes the rest of the time. In some bedside fetal monitoring units and handheld apparatuses, continuous ultrasound is employed.

As ultrasound is transmitted poorly through air, the face of the transducer is coupled to the body by a fluid medium, such as water or mineral oil, enabling the sound waves to penetrate the skin surface–air interface. When the high frequency waves cross a tissue interface, an echo is reflected and this is picked up by the transducer. The latter changes the returning vibrations into electric energy, amplifies them, and either converts this signal into an audible sound or records it on an oscilloscope screen as a two-dimensional image. As objects of different densities vary in the amount of reflected energy, the pictures produced by different tissues are characteristic, thus enabling diagnoses to be made.

Types of Ultrasonography

Doppler Effect

Doppler ultrasound employs a two-crystal transducer that emits and receives sound waves continually. Echoes returning from moving structures are recorded as audio signals or peaks on an oscilloscope. In obstetrics, Doppler ultrasound is used mainly for the monitoring of the fetal heart rate. An exciting new area is in the measurement of uterine, placental, and fetal blood flow. This may lead to more accurate diagnoses and better management of those conditions where reduced blood flow has significant fetal implications. Problems, such as pregnancy-induced hypertension and fetal growth retardation, may be more successfully monitored by these techniques.

A-Scan

The use of A or amplitude mode scanning is of historic interest in obstetrics and gynecology. The A-mode gives a unidimensional view, measuring the space between two interfaces. It can determine the biparietal diameter of the head and the midline cerebral falx shifts that occur with intracranial hemorrhage or neoplasms.

B-Scan

This sonar system utilizes pulsed ultrasonic waves, which produce cross-sectional pictures of internal organs and structures, enabling size and position to be determined. The B-scan shows what would be seen if the subject were cut tangentially along a plane defined by the beam and the cut surface surveyed. It can outline the fetal skull, thorax, extremities, and the placenta. The machine measures the time interval between the two echoes, and converts this to distance on the basis of assumed speed of transmission through the tissues. In clinical use, repeated scans are performed in both longitudinal and transverse planes to obtain a composite display.

Real-time Imaging

Real-time imaging displays moving structures. It is particularly valuable for viewing fetal movement, breathing, and cardiac activity. The method uses either a linear or a sector transducer.

Linear Technique. This employs a single handheld probe which has multiple transducers that fire in sequence. The images produced are similar to those seen in a motion picture.

Sector Scanner. This uses a revolving or rapidly firing transducer to produce a pie shaped image of increased resolution.

Safety of Ultrasonography

At the present time, enough data are not available to permit the conclusion that the use of diagnostic ultrasound is without biologically adverse effects. The American Institute of Ultrasound in Medicine Bioeffects Committee has noted: "In the low megahertz frequency range, 0.5–10 megahertz, there have been no independently confirmed significant biological effects in mammalian tissue exposed to intensities below one hundred mW/cm^2." Despite these findings, ultrasound is recommended for diagnostic use only when medically indicated. The Society of Obstetricians and Gynecologists of Canada and the American Institute of Ultrasound in Medicine have published lists of recommended indications for the use of diagnostic ultrasound, noting that the *routine* use of ultrasound in pregnancy has not been supported on the basis of favorable cost benefit studies or the known absence of adverse side effects.

Indications for the Use of Diagnostic Ultrasound

1. To determine the expected date of confinement: To avoid unnecessary and unrewarding examinations during the third trimester for gestational dating, the physician should remember that the best estimate of fetal age from a single scan is obtained between the 15th and 18th weeks. Therefore in any of the following indications an ultrasound scan should be performed early in pregnancy, i.e., before the 20th week:
    a. Uncertain gestational age
    b. Discrepancy between duration of amenorrhea and uterine size
    c. A repeat cesarean section is planned
2. Suspicion of fetal and/or placental abnormalities:
    a. Potential or actual growth retardation: as soon as suspected
    b. Amniocentesis for genetic indications: during the procedure
    c. Suspicion of fetal death
    d. Bleeding during pregnancy
    e. Suspicion of ectopic or molar pregnancy
    f. High-risk pregnancy: Rhesus isoimmunization, diabetes, hypertension
    g. As part of an approved investigative protocol
3. Postpartum, postabortion:
    a. Retained products of conception
    b. Hematoma
    c. Pelvic abscess

4. In gynecologic practice:
   a. Pelvic mass: to confirm the diagnosis and, possibly, to define the type
   b. To locate an intrauterine contraceptive device

Uses of Ultrasonography in Obstetrics

Early Pregnancy

Diagnosis of Pregnancy

In the first trimester, the patient's bladder should be full to act as a sonic "window," allowing sound waves to pass through the bladder and reach the pelvic uterus. The amniotic sac can be seen by 6 weeks. Fetal echoes are obtained from the 7th week onward. If a sac is not visible by 6 weeks from the last menstrual period, and the date of conception is known, it is doubtful that a normal pregnancy exists.

Abortion

Ultrasonic examination can differentiate a normally developing pregnancy, a blighted ovum, and a missed abortion. This may require serial scans 1 week apart to demonstrate the presence or absence of the amniotic sac or fetal growth. Signs of early failure of pregnancy include:

1. A poorly formed gestational sac or a fragmenting sac
2. An empty sac, perhaps with a low uterine implantation site
3. Absence of fetal heart action
4. A gestational sac whose size is over 2 weeks behind the dates with no growth in the next week

Ectopic Pregnancy

The diagnosis of ectopic pregnancy may be difficult. The presence of an intrauterine sac with a fetal echo rules out ectopic pregnancy, except in that rare instance when there is both an intrauterine and ectopic gestation (1/30,000). In some cases, an adnexal mass can be seen, and, more rarely, the presence of a fetal heart outside the uterine cavity confirms the diagnosis. In clinical practice, serial ultrasonic scans are required, combined with the use of beta-human chorionic gonadotropin (hCG) assays to properly evaluate cases of suspect ectopic pregnancy. The presence of free fluid (blood) in the pelvic cul-de-sac is supporting evidence for this diagnosis.

Hydatidiform Mole

The appearance of a hydatidiform mole is that of a diffuse intrauterine "snowstorm" pattern, representing multiple vesicles and areas of hemorrhage. Theca lutean cysts may be detected in the adnexal areas. Following evacuation of the mole, regression in the size of these cysts and absence of intrauterine vesicles may be observed by serial ultrasonic scans.

Fetal Condition

Fetal Heart Activity
The fetal heart beat has been detected as early as 45 days of gestation. It is accurate after 7 weeks, and by the use of real-time imaging, fetal movement can be detected at 6 to 7 weeks. The application of adult echocardiographic techniques to the fetal situation is currently undergoing evaluation, and has allowed the diagnosis of fetal cardiac abnormalities such as hypoplasia and valvular defects.

Multiple Pregnancy
This can be diagnosed as early as the 8th week and should be confirmed by serial scans. Not infrequently, one of the pregnancies fails to develop and the patient ultimately delivers a single child. It is important with serial scans to note the development of each fetus so as to detect growth discrepancies that may indicate fetal/fetal transfusion or growth retardation.

Fetal Presentation
The lie of the fetus and whether the head or breech is presenting can be determined easily.

Fetal Anomalies
The ability to identify both large and small fetal parts has improved with developments in instrumentation. Many fetal anomalies can be detected early in pregnancy, although some of the diagnoses are difficult to make and require specialized techniques and experience.

1. *Anomalies incompatible with life*: In this group (e.g., anencephaly) elective termination of pregnancy can be carried out.
2. *Anomalies amenable to surgical correction*: Conditions in this group include hydrocephalus, spina bifida, cardiac malformations, intrathoracic cysts, gastrointestinal abnormalities, urologic anomalies, diaphragmatic hernia, skeletal dysplasias, and fetal neoplasms. Diagnosis of these conditions before birth permit preparations to be made so that surgical treatment can be carried out immediately after birth before postnatal deterioration sets in.
3. *Anomalies amenable to intrauterine therapy*: This work is still experimental and results to this date are disappointing. In-

cluded here are shunting procedures for hydrocephalus and out-
flow obstructions to the urinary bladder. Diagnostic ultrasound
has been utilized in the management of erythroblastosis fetalis
secondary to Rh and atypical antibody sensitization. It has permitted more accurate placements of fetal intraperitoneal cathe-
ters for blood transfusions.

Fetal Death

In most cases this will be diagnosed when a fetal heart is unobtainable
by Doppler techniques, and is confirmed with the use of linear or sector
ultrasound machines. The absence of fetal cardiac activity when scanning the thorax is unmistakable evidence of fetal demise. Other signs of
fetal death include loss of fetal tone with extension of the spine, collapse
of the fetal skull, and oligohydramnios.

Fetal Size and Growth

Crown Rump Length

The determination of crown rump length is the most accurate method of
determining the gestational age of the fetus and the probable date of
confinement. Measurements between the 7th and 13th weeks of gestation permit dating to within ±5 days.

Cephalometry

The fetal head may be visible as early as 11 weeks of pregnancy. The
biparietal diameter (BPD) correlates most accurately with the gestational age between the 14th and 25th week of pregnancy. At this time
the correlation may be ±10 days. The best estimate of fetal age from a
single measurement of the BPD is obtained between the 15th and 18th
week. After 25 weeks the BPD is accurate to only ±3 weeks. Therefore,
a single determination of the BPD at, for example, 38 weeks to establish
fetal maturity can be misleading. In addition, when the head is deep in
the pelvis or the fetus is presenting as a breech, it may be difficult to
view the head properly and to determine the BPD accurately.

Length of Femur

The determination of fetal femoral length is obtained easily from 15
weeks of gestation onwards. Femoral length is linear in a fashion similar to BPD and may be helpful in confirming growth impressions derived from BPD estimations or in those cases where BPDs are difficult
to obtain.

Intrauterine Growth Retardation

One of the most common indications for diagnostic ultrasound is uterine size less than expected for the gestational age. Serial ultrasonic

scans are required to make this diagnosis. They are performed at an interval of 2 to 3 weeks so that a meaningful growth curve can be obtained.

The BPD alone is not always conclusive and the ratio between body and head size must be calculated to obtain significant evidence. Up to 34 to 36 weeks, the circumference of the head is generally greater than that of the body. At 34 to 36 weeks the measurements are the same, while after 36 weeks the circumference of the body increases at a greater rate than that of the head. In many cases of intrauterine growth retardation, this reversal of the head:abdominal circumference ratio does not take place and is a point in favor of the diagnosis.

Puerperal or Postabortal Uterus
This organ may be scanned when retained products of conception are suspected. Blood clot may confuse the picture.

Amniotic Fluid

Polyhydramnios
In about 20 percent of cases of excessive amounts of amniotic fluid (greater than 2000 ml) there are congenital fetal anomalies. In the presence of central nervous system (CNS) abnormalities, polyhydramnios may result from impaired fetal swallowing, from the transudation of fluid through the meninges, or from a deficiency of antidiuretic hormone leading to polyuria. In gastrointestinal abnormalities, polyhydramnios may be caused by diminished fetal swallowing.

Ultrasonography shows an excessive amount of amniotic fluid and displacement of the fetus posteriorly and away from the anterior wall of the uterus. Normally, in the third trimester, the fetus is in contact with both the anterior and posterior walls of the uterus.

Once the diagnosis of polyhydramnios is made, a search for fetal abnormalities must be carried out. The head should be examined for anencephaly, encephalocele, hydrocephaly, and hydroencephalocele. A meningocele or cystic hygroma, such as one might find in Turner syndrome (XO), should be sought. Cystic structures within the fetal abdomen may represent dilated fluid-filled bowel, where there is gastrointestinal obstruction (double bubble sign in duodenal atresia), or a large hydronephrotic kidney.

Oligohydramnios
Occasionally the amount of amniotic fluid is reduced far below the normal. Both moderate and severe oligohydramnios are detectable by ultrasonography. The reduced amount of fluid gives the impression of fetal crowding in utero. A diagnosis of severe oligohydramnios can be made when there is no pocket of fluid greater than 1 cm in diameter.

This finding may indicate significant intrauterine growth retardation or occasionally a fetal genetic abnormality.

Placentography

Ultrasonography provides the most reliable method of locating the site of the placenta and determining its texture, quality, thickness, and margins. In the first part of pregnancy, sonograms may show placentas that are low lying and even over the cervix in up to 25 percent of cases. Later in pregnancy the placenta will be found to be more properly located in all but 1 to 2 percent of such cases. As pregnancy advances, the normal growth of the placenta is away from the cervix and, as the uterus enlarges faster than the placenta, a proportionately smaller area of the uterus will be covered by it. The finding of a low-lying placenta in early pregnancy is an indication for reexamination later— nothing more. No cases have been reported of a placenta moving downward once it has located itself in the upper segment.

Placenta Previa

The value of ultrasonography in the diagnosis of placenta previa is both positive and negative. The observation that the placenta is lying over the cervical os confirms the diagnosis. Finding the placenta to be in the fundus of the uterus rules out placenta previa.

Abruptio Placentae

The diagnosis of placental abruption (separation from the wall of the uterus) may be made by excluding placenta previa. Sometimes a retroplacental blood clot can be identified and its volume measured. Occasionally serial scans may demonstrate an enlarging retroplacental hematoma; this finding suggests that concealed bleeding is occurring.

Placental Maturity

The placenta is a dynamic organ which grows and matures throughout pregnancy. There appears to be some correlation between ultrasonically defined placental maturity and fetal pulmonary development, with the suggestion that advanced placental maturity may be accurate in predicting the ability of the fetal lungs to sustain effective postnatal respiration. One study reported 100 percent correlation between grade III placentas and mature L/S ratios, and 88 percent correlation between grade II placentas and mature L/S ratios. While these findings are preliminary and more evidence is needed, the presence of a grade III placenta can be considered presumptive evidence of advanced pulmonary maturity. It does not rule out, however, the development of respiratory distress syndrome in a small percentage of cases.

Based on changes in the placenta that are demonstrable by ultrasonography, four phases of maturation can be recognized.

Grade 0. This phase is seen in the first and second trimesters of pregnancy. The chorionic plate is a smooth, straight, dense, and unbroken line. The placental substance and the basal layer are homogenous and contain no marked echogenic areas.

Grade I. This grade is seen as early as 30 to 32 weeks, and may persist to term. The chorionic plate appears as a well-defined unbroken line with undulations. The placental substance contains a number of scattered echogenic areas so that the state of homogenity is lost. There are no identifiable changes in the basal layer.

Grade II. The chorionic plate indentations become more marked and deeper. The placental substance undergoes two changes: (1) It appears divided by echogenic densities that are contiguous with the indentations of the chorionic plate; these do not reach the basal layer. (2) The echogenic areas are more numerous and larger than those in grade I. The basal layer contains linear echoes that lie parallel to it. These are larger and more dense than those in the placental substance.

Grade III. This is the phase of placental maturity. The indentations of the chorionic plate extend to the basal layer, and probably represent the septa between the cotyledons. In the center of these compartments echo-free areas are seen. Dense, irregular, echogenic areas up to 2 cm in size appear close to the chorionic plate. The echogenic areas near the basal layer are larger than those in the placental substance, more dense, confluent, and may cast acoustic shadows.

Ultrasonic Multiple Variable Assessment: Fetal Biophysical Profile

A method of biophysical profile scoring using diagnostic ultrasound has evolved recently, and is of help in managing high-risk pregnancy, including intrauterine growth retardation. The parameters that make up the biophysical profile include (1) the nonstress test, (2) fetal breathing movements, (3) gross fetal body movements, (4) fetal tone, and (5) the volume of amniotic fluid. (For details of the examination see Chapter 37.)

The use of several variables improves the predictive value of the examination. Two points are assigned for each normal and zero for each abnormal finding. A score of 8 to 10 correlates well with a normal outcome of pregnancy. A score of 6 or less should be viewed with caution; the test is repeated in 1 to 2 days. A score of 0 to 2 is associated with significant fetal morbidity and mortality.

Routine Screening of All Pregnant Women

In many cases the need to assess gestational age or to determine whether there is a deviation in fetal growth does not arise until late in pregnancy. The most accurate ultrasonic evidence of gestational age, however, is obtainable in the early part of the pregnancy (crown rump length 8 to 14 weeks; biparietal diameter 15 to 22 weeks). Where intrauterine growth retardation is suspected, the degree of growth can be evaluated much more accurately if there is an early sonographic reading that can be used as a baseline. A routine scan at 17 weeks will detect certain congenital abnormalities that might require early neonatal care (e.g., gastrointestinal abnormalities), or suggest therapeutic termination of pregnancy (e.g., anencephaly).

The value of routine ultrasonography lies in the following groups: (1) accurate determination of gestational age, (2) fetal growth abnormalities, (3) detection of fetal malformations, (4) diagnosis of multiple pregnancy, and (5) cases of unsuspected placenta previa. For these reasons, it has been suggested that all pregnant women should have ultrasonography at 17 and again at 33 weeks' gestation.

There appears to be no doubt that the examination of all pregnant women by ultrasonography has real benefits. How great these advantages are, in how many women the management of pregnancy would be changed, and whether this routine is cost effective, have not been proven. It is believed that ultrasound does not pose a danger to the mother or the fetus. The same conviction, however, was once held about x-ray pelvimetry. Ultrasonography has been in wide use for too short a time to be certain as to its safety.

Neonatal Head Scanning

There have been recent marked improvements in the management of very low-birth-weight infants resulting in a decline in neonatal mortality rates. Intraventricular hemorrhage and its sequelae continue to be an important contributor to neonatal illness. Postmortem studies have revealed intraventricular hemorrhage in approximately 50 to 70 percent of nonsurviving premature infants. Real-time ultrasound scanning offers a number of advantages over radiologic studies using computerized axial tomography (CAT). It may be performed without moving the infant from his incubator in the neonatal intensive care unit, handling of the infant is minimized, and there are no known harmful effects of ultrasound. Some investigators suggest that real-time scanning should be used as a screening procedure in all very low-birth-weight infants (less than 1500 g), and where there is suspicion of intracranial pathology in large infants. With good visualization of the ventricular and paraventricular areas, ultrasound allows the accurate diagnosis of hydrocephaly and even small intraventricular hemorrhages to be made.

RADIOGRAPHY

As a diagnostic aid, x-ray has a limited range of uses in modern obstetics. Because the exact effects of the gamma rays on the maternal ovaries and on the fetus are not known, radiography should be employed in pregnancy only when there is a clear and definite indication. The first trimester is considered to be the most dangerous time. The use of diagnostic ultrasound has almost eliminated the need for x-ray examination of the developing fetus. In the absence of ultrasound, however, and where management of labor is concerned, certain areas of benefit may be described.

Fetus

Multiple Pregnancy
The presence of multiple pregnancy can be proved, and the positions of the babies in utero shown.

Fetal Maturity
Sometimes fetal maturity can be determined. From 36 weeks onward, well-developed bony structure is seen in all major parts of the skeleton. The distal (lower) femoral epiphyseal ossification center is present in over 80 percent of infants from week 36 onward. The proximal (upper) tibial epiphyseal ossification center appears at about week 38. It is ill defined at this time, but becomes clearly visible at 40 weeks. Between weeks 40 and 43 the proximal tibial epiphyseal ossification center becomes as large as the distal femoral center. The demonstration by films of the maternal abdomen of the distal femoral center indicates that the fetus is mature in 96 percent of cases. However, negative findings, i.e., the absence of these epiphyses, is inconclusive, because in a small number of cases ossification does not occur until term or even later.

Presentation, Position, Station
When abdominal and vaginal examinations are inconclusive, x-ray can be used to establish the lie, presentation, position, and attitude of the fetus. Engagement and descent of the presenting part can also be demonstrated.

Fetal Abnormalities

Abnormalities such as hydrocephaly, microcephaly, anencephaly, and spina bifida may be demonstrable.

Intrauterine Death

Loss of Fetal Tone. When the fetus dies the muscles become flaccid and there is loss of flexion. The uterus becomes reduced in size as it tends to become more spheric. This loss of height is accentuated by resorption of amniotic fluid. The fetus appears rolled up and the term "ball sign" has been used. This sign takes several days to become apparent, but it is fully established by 1 week after death.

Spalding Sign (1922). The overlapping and angulation of the cranial bones is consequent to the shrinkage of the brain and the collapse of the skull. In late pregnancy, before the onset of labor or rupture of the membranes, disalignment of more than 4 mm is indicative of fetal death. Spalding sign may be present as early as 7 days after death, and can be identified without difficulty by 10 days.

Halo Sign (Devel, 1947). The fetal skull is covered by the scalp. The fat-containing subcutaneous layer has a lower density than the other soft tissue and appears on the x-ray of the fetus in utero as a dark line. When there is edema of the scalp, the fluid elevates the fat-containing layer from the skull. On x-ray the fat layer is seen as a dark line apart from the skull and more or less parallel to it. This sign appears no sooner than 3 days after fetal death. Severe erythroblastosis with hydrops fetalis is the only condition in which the halo sign is seen in a live fetus.

Mother

The following conditions of the mother can be determined by radiography:

1. Abdominal pregnancy. The fetus may be seen to lie outside of the uterus.
2. Congenital anomalies of the pelvis.
3. Bony injury to the pelvis, e.g., after an accident.
4. Pelvimetry: investigation of fetopelvic disproportion.

Amniography

Amniography is primarily of historic interest. Amniocentesis is performed and some 30 ml of amniotic fluid removed. An equal amount of radiopaque fluid is injected into the amniotic cavity. The opaque fluid disperses quickly through the amniotic fluid. For the identification of external fetal abnormalities the x-ray films are taken within 15 minutes of the injection of the dye. The fetus swallows the dye-containing amniotic fluid, which can be identified in the intestines by 3 hours. The highest density is reached in 12 to 24 hours after injection. The fluid is excreted via the kidneys. Modern applications of this technique are confined to the evaluation of fetal congenital abnormalities, such as small spina bifidas and gastrointestinal or genitourinary obstructions.

X-ray Pelvimetry

X-ray pelvimetry is a valuable aid to mensuration of the pelvis, but should be used only in conjunction with clinical examination and judgment. Information is obtained concerning (1) the shape and inclination of the pelvis, (2) the length of its diameters, and (3) the relationship and fit of the fetus to the pelvis.

X-ray pelvimetry not only provides greater precision of mensuration, but makes possible the measurement of important diameters that cannot be obtained manually, e.g., the transverse diameter of the inlet and the distance between the ischial spines. Moreover, it affords a better understanding of the configuration of the pelvis. This has enabled the female pelvis to be classified according to shape, permitting a more accurate clinical prognosis to be made of the outcome of labor.

Three x-ray views are taken to obtain maximal information when performing x-ray pelvimetry.

Abdominal View

An anteroposterior view is taken of the abdomen with the patient positioned on her back. This view gives a good picture of the entire fetus.

Information Obtained

1. Attitude of the fetus
2. Lie, presentation, and position
3. Rough estimate of the size of the baby
4. Presence of more than one fetus
5. Ossification centers that may provide an estimate of maturity
6. Fetal abnormalities or death

Standing Lateral View

A lateral view of the pelvis is taken with the patient erect. A metal ruler with notches or perforations 1 cm apart is placed in the gluteal folds between the buttocks. The ruler has the same degree of distortion as the pelvis and the desired diameters can be measured.

Information Obtained

1. Inclination, curve, and length of the sacrum
2. Depth of the pelvis
3. Relationship of the promontory of the sacrum to the inlet
4. Sacrosciatic notch—whether it is wide or narrow
5. Anteroposterior diameters of the inlet, the obstetric conjugate; midpelvis, the plane of least dimensions; and the outlet
6. Posterior sagittal diameter of the midpelvis and the outlet
7. Size and shape of the ischial spines. Are they small or large? Are they prominent and posterior? Do they shorten the posterior sagittal diameter and narrow the sacrosciatic notch?
8. Length and inclination of the symphysis
9. Station of the fetal presenting part
10. In cephalic presentations, the presence of synclitism or asynclitism
11. Attitude of the fetus: flexion or extension
12. Relationship or fit of the head to the pelvis

Anteroposterior View

The anteroposterior film is taken with the patient positioned in a semirecumbent position so that the x-ray tube is aimed at the inlet, looking into the midpelvis. A special grid is used for making measurements.

Information Obtained

1. Shape of the inlet, the posterior and anterior segments. Is the posterior segment well rounded or heart shaped? Is the anterior segment round or wedge shaped?
2. Widest transverse diameter of the inlet.
3. Distance between the ischial spines, the transverse diameter of the plane of least dimensions.
4. Anterior and posterior sagittal diameters of the inlet.
5. Size and shape of the ischial spines.
6. Slope of the sidewalls. Are they straight, convergent, or divergent?
7. Classification of the pelvis.

Indications for X-ray Pelvimetry

1. Nonpregnant state
   a. Grossly abnormal pelvis, e.g., fracture
2. During pregnancy, before labor
   a. Breech presentation when a trial of labor is contemplated

3. During active labor
   a. Breech undiagnosed antepartum
   b. Cephalic presentation; arrest in first or second stage when the station, attitude, or position are unclear. Decision to be made: further trial of labor, forceps application, or cesarean section

Once an important tool in the diagnosis and management of obstetric problems, x-ray pelvimetry plays a reduced role today. Clearer understanding of uterine dysfunction, the realization that most disproportion is relative and its seriousness can be assessed properly only by a trial of labor, acceptance of the use of oxytocin stimulation in trials of labor, elimination of the fear of doing a cesarean section after the patient has been in labor for some time, and the knowledge that radiation may be harmful have all helped narrow the indications for pelvimetry.

X-ray pelvimetry is needed rarely in modern times because:

1. In most cases the decision can be made on clinical examination and a trial of labor.
2. Often the reason for failure of progress is not demonstrated by x-ray.
3. In cases of disproportion the cause is a large baby more often than a contracted pelvis.
4. Inefficient labor is a frequent factor when progress ceases, and this is not shown by x-ray.
5. Most cesarean sections are performed in women with normal pelves.

Dangers of Radiation

About 1 percent of women have abdominal x-rays in the first trimester of pregnancy. In later pregnancy the amount of radiation to which the fetus is exposed during x-ray pelvimetry is approximately 1.1 rads. The degree of risk to the fetus in utero engendered by radiologic examination of the mother is not known accurately and may prove to be minimal. Doses below 10 rads have not been shown to cause congenital malformations or intrauterine growth retardation. Until the final truth is established, however, diagnostic x-ray should be used only when there is a clear and necessary indication and should be avoided whenever possible.

Type of Effect

1. *Developmental effects:* A disturbance of growth during organogenesis may result in hypoplasia, absence, or gross distortion of

part or all of an organ. If the effect is of major proportions death and abortion will occur.

2. *Mutation:* This refers to an unusual and permanent change in the structure of the genetic material or the chromosome. In such cases the infant may appear normal at birth, the abnormalities appearing only later in life.

3. *Effects on the central nervous system:* The CNS is unique in being susceptible to radiation-induced damage through the entire period of gestation.

4. *Late effects:* There may be a higher incidence of neoplasia (especially leukemia) in children who were exposed to radiation in utero.

Stage of Pregnancy

1. *Preimplantation period* (1st week postconception): The embryo is in danger of succumbing to the lethal effects of radiation, but the probability of teratogenic or growth-retarding consequences are low if the embryo survives and implantation and continued development take place.

2. *Period of major organogenesis* (3 to 8 weeks postconception): The embryo is extremely sensitive to the teratogenic, growth-retarding, lethal, and postnatal neoplastic effects of radiation.

3. *Fetal period* (9 weeks or more postconception): There is decreased sensitivity to the teratogenic effects of radiation, but growth retardation, functional abnormalities (especially of the CNS), and postnatal neoplasia may occur.

BIBLIOGRAPHY

Alexander ES, Spitz HB, Clark RA: Sonography of polyhydramnios. Am J Roentgenol 138:343, 1982

Barton JJ, Garbaciak JA, Ryan GM.: The efficacy of X-ray pelvimetry. Am J Obstet Gynecol 143:304, 1982

Fine EA, Bracken M, Berkowitz RL: An evaluation of of the usefulness of X-ray pelvimetry: Comparison of the Thoms and Modified Ball methods with manual pelvimetry. Am J Obstet Gynecol 137:15, 1980

Grannum PAT, Berkowitz RL, Hobbins JC: The ultrasonic changes in the maturing placenta and their relation to fetal pulmonary maturity. Am J Obstet Gynecol 133:915, 1979

Mossman KL, Hill LT: Radiation risks in pregnancy. Obstet Gynecol 60:237, 1982

Persson PH, Kullander S: Long-term experience of general ultrasound screening in pregnancy. Am J Obstet Gynecol 146:942, 1983

Sarda P, Bard H, Teasdale F, Grignon A: The importance of an antenatal ultrasonographic diagnosis of correctable fetal malformations. Am J Obstet Gynecol 147:443, 1983

Varner MW, Cruickshank DP, Laube DW: X-ray pelvimetry in clinical practice. Obstet Gynecol 56:296, 1980

39

Normal and Abnormal Uterine Action

DEFINITIONS

CONTRACTION Contraction is the shortening of a muscle in response to stimulus, with return to its original length after the contraction has worn off.

RETRACTION The muscle shortens in response to a stimulus but does not return to its original length when the contraction has passed. The muscle becomes fixed at a relatively shorter length, but the tension remains the same. In this way the slack is taken up and the walls of the uterus maintain contact with the contents. Retraction is responsible for descent. Without this property the fetus would move down with the contraction, only to return to the original level once the contraction had ceased. With retraction, on the other hand, the fetus remains at a slightly lower level each time. During contraction it is as though three steps are taken forward and then three backward. With retraction, three steps are taken forward and then two backward. In this way a little ground is gained each time. In the control of postpartum bleeding retraction is essential. Without it many patients might bleed to death.

PHYSIOLOGIC RETRACTION RING As labor and retraction proceed, the upper part of the uterus becomes progressively shorter and thicker, while the lower portion gets longer and thinner. The boundary between the two segments is the physiologic retraction ring (Fig. 1).

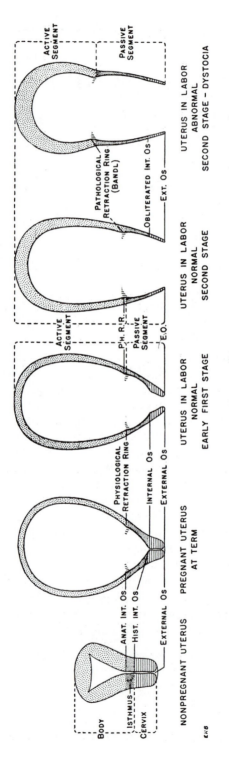

Figure 1. Progressive development of the segments and rings of the uterus at term. Note comparison between the nonpregnant uterus, uterus at term, and uterus in labor. The passive segment is derived from the lower uterine segment (isthmus) and cervix; the physiologic retraction ring form the anatomic internal os. The pathologic ring which forms under abnormal conditions develops from the physiologic ring. (*From Pritchard, MacDonald and Gant. Williams Obstetrics, 17th ed., 1985. Courtesy of Appleton-Century-Crofts.*)

PATHOLOGIC RETRACTION RING   In cases of obstructed labor the physiologic ring becomes extreme and is known as the pathologic retraction (Bandl) ring.

CONSTRICTION RING   This is a localized segment of myometrial spasm which grips the fetus tightly and prevents descent.

TONUS   Tonus is the lowest intrauterine (intraamniotic) pressure between contractions. It is expressed in millimeters of mercury (mm Hg). The normal resting tension is 8 to 12 mm Hg.

INTENSITY   Intensity or amplitude is the rise in intrauterine pressure brought about by each contraction. It is measured from the baseline, resting pressure (tonus) rather than from zero. The normal is 30 to 50 mm Hg.

FREQUENCY   Caldeyro-Barcia defined this as the number of contractions per 10 minutes. For the patient to be in good labor the frequency must be at least two per 10 minutes.

UTERINE ACTIVITY   The Montevideo unit (MU) was introduced by Caldeyro-Barcia and represents the average intensity of the uterine contractions multiplied by the number of contractions observed during a 10-minute period of monitoring (intensity × frequency). To incorporate the third variation, duration of the contraction, the Alexandria unit (AU) was evolved. It represents the product of the average intensity of the contractions in millimeters of mercury, the frequency of contractions per 10 minutes, and the average duration of the contractions in minutes (intensity × frequency × duration).

POLARITY OF THE UTERUS   When the upper segment contracts, the lower segment relaxes. Actually the lower part does contract, but much less than the upper part. The effect is as though the lower portion did relax.

PAIN OF LABOR

Pain during labor is related to contractions of the uterus. In normal labor the pain is intermittent. It starts as the uterus contracts, becomes more severe as the contraction reaches its peak, and disappears when the uterus relaxes. The degree of pain varies in different patients, in the same patient during succeeding labors, and at different stages in the same labor. In some cases the contractions are painless.

Causes

1. Distention of the lower pole of the uterus.
2. Stretching of the ligaments adjacent to the uterus.

3. Pressure on or stretching of the nerve ganglia around the uterus.
4. Contractions of the muscle while it is in a relatively ischemic state (similar to angina pectoris). This occurs especially when the uterine tonus is too high or when the contractions are too frequent and last too long. Adequate amounts of blood do not get to the muscles and they become hypoxic.

Pain in Lower Abdomen

Pain in the lower abdomen seems to be related to activity in the upper uterine segment and is present during efficient labor.

Pain in Back

Pain in the back is related to tension in the lower uterus segment and the cervix. In normal labor back pain is prominent only at the start of a contraction and in the early stages of cervical dilatation. When the cervix is abnormally resistant the backache is severe. Backache is prominent also in posterior positions. In general, the less the backache the more efficient the uterus.

Pain in the Incoordinate Uterus

1. An excessive amount of pain is felt in the back.
2. Because of persistent high tonus or spasm in some parts of the uterus the pain seems to be present even in the intervals between contractions.
3. The patient complains of pain before the uterus is felt to harden, and the pain persists even after the uterus relaxes and softens.

NORMAL UTERINE CONTRACTIONS

Uterine contractions occur spontaneously in patterns that are characteristic of individuals and of various stages of gestation. The frequency, duration, and strength of the myometrial contractions can be estimated by feeling them with a hand placed on the mother's abdomen or by electronic techniques. The latter employ either a noninvasive external tocodynamometer that consists of a pressure sensor held in place on the abdomen over a prominent part of the uterus, or by an invasive internal method using an open-ended, fluid-filled catheter placed through the cervix into the uterine cavity. The last is the most accurate technique of monitoring uterine contractions.

The recorded curve of a normal uterine contraction is bell shaped. The steep crescentic slope leading to the apex of the curve represents the actual power of the contraction and comprises only one-third of the total contraction. The period of relaxation makes up two-thirds of the process and is shown by a curve that is, initially, a steep decrescentic slope that becomes more horizontal in the last third, reflecting the gradualness of the final stage of relaxation.

Caldeyro-Barcia has published a logical and understandable description of the normal uterine contraction wave.

Triple Descending Gradient (TDG) of Caldeyro-Barcia

Each contraction wave has three components:

1. *The propagation* of the wave is from above downward. It starts at the pacemaker and works its way to the lower part of the uterus.
2. *The duration* of the contraction diminishes progressively as the wave moves away from the pacemaker. During any contraction the upper portion of the uterus is in action for a longer period of time than the lower.
3. *The intensity* of the contraction diminishes from top to bottom of the uterus. The upper segment of the uterus contracts more strongly than the lower.

In order that normal labor may take place all parts of the triple descending gradient must perform properly. The activity of the upper part dominates and is greater than that of the lower part. All parts of the uterus contract, but the upper segment does so more strongly than the lower segment; in turn, the latter's contractions are stronger than those of the cervix. Were this not so there would be no progress. This is the modern interpretation of uterine polarity.

The normal contractions are regular and intermittent. There is contraction (systole) and relaxation (diastole). The most efficient uterus is one showing moderately low tonus and strong contractions.

Pacemakers

Normally there are two, one situated at each uterine end of the fallopian tube. Since one pacemaker is responsible for initiation of a contraction, their activities must be coordinated. In the abnormal uterus new pacemakers may spring up anywhere in the organ, resulting in incoordinate uterine action.

Propagation

The wave begins at the pacemaker and proceeds downward to the rest of the uterus. A small wave goes up to the fundal portion of the uterus above the level of the pacemaker.

Coordination

Coordination is such that, while the wave begins earlier in some areas than in others, the contraction attains its maximum in the different parts of the uterus at the same time. The places where the contraction starts later achieve their acme more rapidly. Thus at the peak of the contraction the entire uterus is acting as a unit. Relaxation, on the other hand, starts simultaneously in all parts of the uterus. For normal uterine action there must be good coordination between the two halves of the uterus as well as between the upper and lower segments.

Dilatation of the Cervix

Dilatation of the cervix is caused by two mechanisms:

1. The pressure on the cervix by the presenting part: When this part of the fetus is regular and well fitting—e.g., the flexed head—it favors effective uterine action and smooth cervical dilatation. The bag of waters does not play an important role in helping promote good contractions and rapid cervical opening.
2. The longitudinal traction on the cervix by the upper part of the uterus as it contracts and retracts: After each contraction the upper segment becomes shorter and thicker; the lower uterine segment becomes longer, thinner, and more distended; and the cervix becomes more and more dilated.

Cervical dilatation is the result of a gradient of diminishing activity from the fundus through the lower uterine segment.

Round Ligament Contraction

These ligaments contain muscle and they contract at the same time as the upper segment of the uterus. This anchors the uterus, prevents its ascending in the abdomen, and so helps force the presenting part down.

Uterine Contractions During Pregnancy

Some uterine activity goes on throughout pregnancy. During the first 30 weeks the frequency and strength of the contractions are low, less than 20 Montevideo units.

After 30 weeks and especially after 35 weeks the contractions become more frequent and may be noticed by the patient. Sometimes they are painful and are called false labor pains. Prelabor, as evidenced in the increasing activity of the uterus during the later weeks of pregnancy, is an integral part of the process of evacuating the human uterus. The contractions of this period are associated with steadily increasing uterine activity, cervical ripening, and general readiness for true labor (Braxton-Hicks contractions). Prelabor merges into clinically recognizable labor by such small degrees that the exact point at which so-called true labor begins is difficult to determine.

CLASSIFICATION OF UTERINE ACTION

Clinical Conditions with Normal Contractile Waves

Normal Labor
The intensity or amplitude of the contractions varies from 30 to 50 mm Hg, and frequency is two to five contractions per 10 minutes.

True Inertia
When the intensity of the contractions is less than 25 and the frequency is under two per 10 minutes, progress is slow and labor prolonged. If the intensity is less than 15, labor does not begin, or if it has started it ceases.

The uterine tonus is normal, the pattern of activity is coordinated, and the relaxation of the lower segment is adequate. The uterus, however, is inactive, and the expulsive efforts are weak, infrequent, or both. There is progress neither in descent of the presenting part nor in dilatation of the cervix. It is often difficult to be sure that the patient is in labor. Pain is mild or even absent entirely.

The force exerted on the fetus is small and no caput succedaneum is formed. No damage is done to either mother or child.

Precipitate Labor
Precipitate labor lasts less than 3 hours. In some cases an amplitude over 50 is responsible for the rapid labor. In most instances, however, the chief factor enabling the baby to pass easily through the pelvis is the lack of resistance of the maternal tissues.

Conditions that predispose to or contribute to the etiology of precipitate labor include:

1. Multiparity
2. Large pelvis
3. Lax and unresistant soft tissues
4. Strong uterine contractions
5. Small baby in good position
6. Induction of labor by rupture of membranes and oxytocin infusion
7. Previous precipitate labor

The distinction must be made between precipitate labor and precipitate delivery. The latter, being sudden and unexpected, carries with it the dangers of an unattended birth.

While many authors have warned of the dangers of rapid labor, such as maternal lacerations, cerebral hemorrhage, brain damage in the fetus, and asphyxia from interference with the placental circulation, some recent studies suggest that the risk to mother and child is not greater than the average labor.

Cervical Dystocia

Cervical dystocia includes two main groups:

1. Primary dystocia
   a. Achalasia of the cervix: The failure or inability of the structurally normal cervix to relax and open
   b. Rigid cervix: An anatomic abnormality of the cervical tissue
   c. Conglutination of the external os: The sticking together of the lips of the cervix
2. Secondary dystocia
   a. Postdelivery
   b. Postoperative scarring
   c. Cancer

If the condition is not treated the cervix may rupture or annular detachment may take place. The constant and prolonged pressure on the cervix leads to anoxia and devitalization of the tissue, which eventually separates and comes away as a ring. Usually there is thrombosis in the vessels at the site of separation, so bleeding is rarely a problem.

In some cases the cervix becomes well effaced and the external os very thin, but dilatation does not take place. In this situation incision of the rim of cervix is followed by easy delivery.

Obstructed Labor

Etiologic factors range from fetopelvic disproportion through malpresentations to neoplasms blocking the birth canal. As labor proceeds and the uterus tries to overcome the obstruction, the contractions become more frequent and stronger, and the tonus rises. There is progressive retraction of the upper segment with stretching and thinning of the lower part of the uterus. The physiologic retraction ring becomes the pathologic (Bandl) ring. The round ligaments are tense and may be palpable through the abdomen. The pain is severe.

If the obstruction is not relieved and the contractions go on, rupture of the lower segment is the final outcome. In some cases the myometrium becomes exhausted and inertia sets in before rupture occurs.

While the uterus itself does not impede the descent and birth of the baby, the strong, frequent contractions and high tonus may cut off the placental circulation and kill the baby.

Rapid Overdistention of the Uterus
Acute polyhydramnios is an example. The rapidly accumulating amniotic fluid leads to a rise in tonus and a fall in the intensity of the contractions.

Slow Distention of the Uterus
Slow distention of the uterus is seen in multiple pregnancy or in chronic polyhydramnios. The increase in the intrauterine volume is slow and gradual, so there is time for compensatory hypertrophy and hyperplasia of the uterine muscles. For this reason the tonus and intensity of the contractions are normal.

Contractile Waves with Inverted Gradient

Caldeyro-Barcia described the normal contraction wave as having three properties:

1. The propagation of the wave is from above downward.
2. The duration of the contraction diminishes progressively as the wave moves away from the pacemaker.
3. The intensity of the contraction decreases from the top of the uterus to the lower part.

One of the varieties of inefficient uterine action takes place when the gradients of the normal contraction are inverted. The inversion may be total or partial.

1. Total: All three gradients are affected. The uterine contractions are completely ineffective. There is no progress—neither dilatation of the cervix nor descent of the fetus.
2. Partial: One or two of the gradients are involved. Some cervical dilatation may take place, but it is very slow.

Inversion of the propagation gradient means that the contraction begins in the lower segment and moves upward. Normally it goes the other way. Inversion of the duration gradient means that the contraction lasts longer in the lower than in the upper segment. This is the opposite of the normal wave. When there is inversion of the intensity gradient, the lower segment contractions are stronger than those of the upper segment. Normally the opposite is true.

When these conditions are present the polarity of the uterus is reversed. The contractions are of no value in furthering progress as they produce no effacement or dilatation of the cervix. They are the type of contraction seen often in false labor and prelabor.

Clinically, as compared with true inertia, these patients do have pain and it may be severe. Backache is often the main complaint. Typically, the fetus remains high, and the cervix stays thick, uneffaced, and poorly applied to the presenting part.

Incoordination of the Uterus: Localized Contraction Waves

Asymmetrical Uterine Action

The pacemakers do not work in rhythm, and each half of the uterus acts independently. Small contractions alternate with large ones. The minor contractions are entirely ineffective. The major ones do bring about some cervical dilatation but much less effectively than normal waves. Progress is painfully slow.

Uterine Fibrillation: The Colicky Uterus

In this condition new pacemakers appear all over the uterus. The myometrium contracts spasmodically, frequently, irregularly, and purposelessly. The tonus is elevated slightly, but the action is not effectively expulsive. The fetus is not pushed down, and the cervix does not dilate well.

Pain is present all the time—before, during, and after contractions. The pain is out of proportion to the intensity of the contractions.

Constriction Ring

A constriction ring is a localized phenomenon. A ring of myometrium goes into tetanic contraction. The most common site is 7 to 8 cm above the external os of the cervix. A constriction ring can develop rapidly. Causes include:

1. Intrauterine manipulations
2. Failed forceps
3. The use of oxytocin when the uterus is hypertonic
4. Spontaneous constriction ring, which usually occurs in a colicky uterus

The constriction ring grips the fetus tightly and prevents its descent. It is the cause of the obstruction. In the pathologic contraction ring of Bandl, on the other hand, the obstruction to the passage of the fetus comes first and it is the cause of the ring.

The area of spasm is thick, but the lower segment is neither stretched nor thinned out. Constriction rings never lead to uterine rupture. The patient experiences severe pain, and the tenderness of the uterus makes her resist palpation of the abdomen.

While deep surgical anesthesia is needed to relax the major rings, lesser degrees of anesthesia, sedation, or Adrenalin Chloride may be effective in the milder forms.

Diagnosis is made by abdominal, vaginal, and intrauterine examinations:

1. The ring may be felt on abdominal examination.
2. There is no change in the station of the presenting part during a contraction.
3. The fetal head is loose in the pelvic cavity both during and between uterine contraction.
4. The portion of the uterus between the external os and the ring is lax during the contraction.
5. The cervix is floppy and is not well applied to the presenting part.
6. Because of the laxity of the cervix a hand can be passed into the uterine cavity and the ring palpated.
7. By placing a finger between the cervix and the head, the impact on the finger during a strong contraction is found to be quite weak

The differential diagnosis may be made by studying Table 1.

TABLE 1. DIFFERENTIAL DIAGNOSIS OF CONSTRICTION RING AND THE PATHOLOGIC RETRACTION RING

Constriction Ring	Pathologic Retraction Ring
Localized ring of spastic myometrium.	Formed by excessive retraction of upper segment.
May occur in any part of the uterus.	Always at junction of upper and lower segments.
Muscle at the ring is thicker than above or below it.	Myometrium is much thicker above than below the ring.
Uterus below the ring is neither thin nor distended.	Wall below is thin and overdistended.
Uterus never ruptures.	If uncorrected, uterus may rupture.
Uterus above ring is relaxed and not tender.	Uterus above ring is hard.
Round ligaments are not tense.	Rounded ligaments are tense and stand out.
May occur in any stage of labor.	Usually occurs late in the second stage.
Position of the ring does not change.	The ring gradually rises in the abdomen.
Presenting part is not driven down.	Presenting part is jammed into the pelvis.
Fetus may be wholly or mainly above the ring.	Part of the child must be below the ring.
Patient's general condition is good.	Patient's general condition is poor.
Uterine action is inefficient.	Uterine action is efficient or overefficient.
Abnormal polarity.	Normal polarity.
Results in obstructed labor.	Caused by an obstruction.

Spasm of the Internal or External Cervical Os

The cervix does not relax and does not dilate. The contractions of the cervix are stronger than those of the lower uterine segment, and no progress is made.

Abnormal Uterine Action: Third Stage of Labor

Separation and expulsion of the placenta and the control of hemorrhage are dependent on normal uterine action. Abnormal uterine contractility can lead to the following complications:

1. Uterine inertia may cause delayed separation of the placenta and postpartum hemorrhage.
2. The colicky uterus interferes with normal separation.
3. A constriction ring prevents normal expulsion.
4. Cervical spasm may trap the placenta in the uterus.
5. Incoordinate uterine action may lead to inversion of the uterus.

INCOORDINATE UTERINE ACTION

Etiology

The quoted incidence varies from 1 to 7 percent, but it is doubtful that the real syndrome occurs in more than 2 percent of labors. Mild disproportion and malpresentations predispose to abnormal uterine action.

Age and Parity

This is mainly a condition of primigravidas. About 95 percent of severe cases occur in first labors, and the uterus is almost always more efficient during the next pregnancy. The incidence in elderly primigravidas is only a little higher than in young women.

Constitutional Factors

Especially prone to incoordinate uterine action is the thickset, obese, masculine, relatively infertile woman. There appears to be a familial tendency. It is not associated with general debility or malnutrition.

Nervous and Emotional Conditions

We do not know how nervous and emotional problems act in causing or aggravating incoordination of the uterus in labor. It has been claimed that fear increases the tension of the lower uterine segment. However, there are placid women who have difficult labors, and highly emotional ones who have easy deliveries. Most grave disorders of the central nervous system do not affect labor adversely.

Errors of the Uterus

While some workers believe that overdistention, fibroids, and scars of the uterus predispose to poor uterine contractions, others deny it. Certainly the congenitally abnormal, incompletely fused, or bicornuate uterus does not behave well in labor.

Rupture of the Membranes

Rupture of the membranes under proper conditions stimulates the uterus to better contractions and speeds progress. However, rupture of the bag of waters when the cervix is unripe—i.e., uneffaced, hard, thick, and closed—does lead to a prolonged and inefficient type of labor.

Mechanical Errors in the Relation of Fetus to Birth Canal

A close and even application of the presenting part to the cervix and lower uterine segment during the first stage of labor and to the vagina and perineum in the second stage results in good reflex stimulation of the myometrium. Anything that prevents this good relationship causes the reflex to fail, and poor contractions may be the result.

The relationship of posterior positions, extended attitudes, and transverse arrest to faulty uterine action is well known. The malposition precedes the uterine disturbance, and if it can be corrected good contractions often return.

Late engagement and incomplete formation of the lower uterine segment may be an early sign of an incoordinate uterus. Mild degrees of cephalopelvic disproportion predispose to incoordinate uterine action.

Irritation of Uterus

Improper stimulation of the uterus by drugs or intrauterine manipulations may bring about incoordination.

Clinical Picture

Labor

The clinical picture is of prolonged labor in the absence of fetopelvic disproportion. There is hypertonus, increased tension, and spasm in some areas of the uterine muscle which persist even between the contractions. The resting intrauterine pressure is increased. The contractions may be frequent and are usually irregular in strength and periodicity. Despite uterine contractions that are often strong and always painful, progress is slow or absent. The cervix dilates slowly, and the presenting part advances little or not at all. This condition occurs in all degrees, from mild to most severe.

Labor may be normal at first or it may be incoordinate from the beginning. Premature rupture of the membranes while the cervix is closed and uneffaced is seen frequently. The patient complains bitterly of pain, and when examination shows no progress the assumption is made that she is making more fuss than the condition warrants. The experienced obstetrician, however, recognizes the condition and orders sedation. After a rest the contractions may resume in a normal pattern, or they may still be incoordinate. As time passes the colicky nature of the pain increases. The patient holds her hands over the sensitive uterus to protect it. Eventually more sedation is needed.

Labor is long, especially the first stage, because with incoordinate uterine action the cervix fails to dilate normally. After a long period: (1) the cervix may dilate fully, and the baby may be born spontaneously or by forceps; (2) some method of promoting cervical dilatation may have to be used before the baby can be extracted; or (3) vaginal delivery may be abandoned and cesarean section performed.

It is characteristic of this condition that the patient complains of the pain before the uterus is felt to harden, and the pain persists after the uterus softens. Sometimes there is continual pain, especially severe in the back. The patient realizes that she is not making progress, and her anxiety and loss of morale aggravate the situation. Eventually she becomes exhausted and dehydrated, and the pulse and temperature rise.

The cervix may be thick or thin, it may be applied tightly to the presenting part or hang loosely in the vagina. It dilates very slowly and may never reach full dilatation. In most cases dilatation stops at 6 to 7 cm. Sometimes a thick, edematous anterior lip is caught between the pubis and the fetal head.

The patient often experiences the acute desire to bear down before the cervix is fully dilated. The attendant must stop the patient from doing this, for it exhausts her without furthering progress. There is a tendency to urinary retention. Vomiting is common and adds to the dehydration.

Diagnosis

Diagnosis is based on the following:

1. The patient's subjective impression of the strength and duration of the pains
2. The physician's objective impression of the duration of the contractions, and his partly objective opinion of their strength (Table 2)
3. Observation of the effectiveness of the contractions in promoting progress, especially cervical dilatation
4. The use of electronic equipment to monitor the uterine contractions and the fetal heart rate

TABLE 2. MANUAL EVALUATION OF UTERINE CONTRACTIONS

	Frequency	Duration	Indentibility of Uterus
Good	q 2–3 min	45–60 sec	None
Fair	q 4–5 min	30–45 sec	Slight
Poor	q 6+ min	<30 sec	Easy

Maternal Dangers

1. Exhaustion
2. Hemorrhage and shock
3. Infection
4. Lacerations of the vagina during difficult deliveries
5. Annular detachment or lacerations of the cervix

Fetal Dangers

1. Asphyxia from prolonged labor
2. Injury during traumatic delivery
3. Pulmonary complications from aspiration of infected amniotic fluid

The fetal mortality is under 15 percent. The prognosis used to be bad, especially because of traumatic forceps deliveries performed often before the cervix was fully dilated and with the head not engaged. The improvements in the results are due to:

1. Early diagnosis of ineffective uterine action
2. More timely forceps extractions
3. Increased use of cesarean section
4. Better anesthesia
5. Early diagnosis of fetal hypoxia by electronic monitoring of the fetal heart rate

False Labor

False labor is attended by irregular contractions. There is no progress, no dilatation of the cervix, and no descent of the presenting part. No damage is done to the fetus. The contractions may be painful and prevent the patient from resting. Sometimes they do have an effect in effacing the cervix and are called prelabor contractions. Treatment is sedation and rest.

Secondary Uterine Inertia

Secondary uterine inertia is a condition of myometrial and general fatigue. It is often associated with prolonged obstructed labor. The contractions become feeble, infrequent, and irregular and may stop altogether. Progress ceases. Treatment is hydration and rest.

Management of Incoordinate Uterine Action

Investigation and Diagnosis

1. The patient is observed as to her general condition, the amount of pain, and the degree of progress.
2. The uterus is palpated to determine the type and severity of the contractions.
3. Vaginal examination shows the position, station, size of the caput, condition of the cervix, presence of a constriction ring, and any disproportion.
4. In cases of doubt, x-rays are taken to rule out fetopelvic disproportion or abnormal position.
5. Questions to be answered include:
   Is there disproportion?
   Is the fetus placed badly?
   Is the woman in true labor?
   Is the uterus hypertonic or hypotonic?
   Is the uterine action incoordinate?
   Is the basic problem at the cervix?

Prevention

1. Fear is counteracted by good prenatal care.
2. Analgesia is used when necessary to prevent loss of control.
3. Heavy sedation is prescribed for false labor, so that the patient is not exhausted when she goes into true labor.

General Measures

1. The morale of the patient should be maintained.
2. An intravenous infusion of crystalloid solution (e.g., Ringer) will maintain hydration and prevent acidosis.
3. The bladder should be emptied when necessary.

Sedation and Analgesia

While an excessive amount of sedation can inhibit uterine contractions, properly used it does not interfere with true labor. The patient needs sedation to relieve her anxiety and analgesia to make the pain less severe. Often sedation and rest change poor labor into a better variety. Continuous lumbar epidural analgesia is frequently effective in improving uterine coordination.

Uterine Stimulation

The uterus should be stimulated only in hypotonic conditions. If the uterus is hypertonic, stimulation makes the situation worse. Methods include.

1. Keeping the patient walking around to maintain the presenting part against the cervix
2. Oxytocin, given best as a dilute intravenous infusion
3. Artificial rupture of the membranes

Operative Measures

1. When the head is low and the cervix thin, the cervix may be dilated manually or an anterior rim pushed over the fetal head.
2. Forceps rotation and extraction can be performed when the cervix is fully dilated. The operation should not be delayed until the mother and fetus are in poor condition.
3. Cesarean section is used more often today. It is safer for mother and child than a traumatic vaginal delivery.

Constriction Ring

Relaxing drugs and deep anesthesia can be tried. If these succeed in releasing the constriction, the fetus is extracted with forceps. Cesarean section, however, is probably the method of choice.

Bandl Pathologic Retraction Ring

Since the basic problem here is cephalopelvic disproportion, cesarean section is the proper therapy.

Cervical Dystocia

1. Cesarean section is the procedure of choice when the cervix does not dilate.
2. Manual dilatation or incisions of the cervix are used rarely.

BIBLIOGRAPHY

Friedman EA: The labor curve. Clin Perinatol 8:15, 1981

40

Uterotonic Agents: Oxytocin, Ergot, Prostaglandin

OXYTOCIN, PITUITRIN, PITOCIN, AND PITRESSIN

Posterior pituitary extract has been used for many years to stimulate uterine contractions. In the beginning whole posterior pituitary extract (pituitrin) was employed. It contains mainly an oxytocic agent and an antidiuretic-hypertensive factor. To eliminate the undesirable side effects of the latter, the extract has been divided into its two main components: an almost pure oxytocic factor (pitocin) and a hypertensive agent (pitressin).

During the early 1950s DuVigneaud and his colleagues succeeded in the purification, chemical identification, and synthesis of oxytocin and vasopressin. The natural and synthetic products are equally efficient in regard to their action on the myometrium. Synthetic oxytocin is a chemically pure substance and is free from the danger of reaction to animal protein. At the present time all commercial preparations of oxytocin used in obstetrics are synthetic.

Oxytocin, an octopeptide, is produced in the supraoptic and paraventricular nuclei of the hypothalamus. The hormone migrates down the supraoptic-neurohypophyseal nerve pathways and is stored in the posterior pituitary gland. Oxytocin-releasing stimuli include (1) cervical dilatation, (2) coitus, (3) emotional reactions, (4) suckling, and (5) drugs such as acetylcholine, nicotine, and certain anesthetics.

Maternal levels of oxytocin increase throughout gestation; secretion seems to occur in a pulsatile fashion. Fetal blood contains much more oxytocin at the end of the second stage of labor than does maternal blood. The blood in the umbilical cord of anencephalic infants, however, has no oxytocin. It is possible that the fetus may be an important source of oxytocin during parturition.

In experimental animals the establishment of neurohypophyseal deficiency leads to difficulty in parturition. The same is not true in humans. Pregnant patients who have had an hypophysectomy or have idiopathic diabetes insipidus experience no difficulty in labor.

The exact role of oxytocin in human labor is not known. It may be that oxytocin has only a facilitating role in the physiology of uterine activity during pregnancy, and not a primary role in the initiation and maintenance of labor.

Effects of Oxytocin

Uterus

In causing the uterus to contract, oxytocin is believed to act on the myometrial cell membrane. It increases the normal excitability of the muscle but adds no new properties. The myometrial sensitivity to oxytocin rises as pregnancy progresses.

Cardiovascular System

Oxytocin has numerous effects on the cardiovascular system.

1. Heart rate: a small to moderate increase.
2. Systemic arterial blood pressure: a decrease results mainly from a lowering of peripheral resistance.
3. Cardiac output: given as a single dose oxytocin causes a rise in cardiac output, followed by a fall; continuous infusion results in an increased cardiac output.
4. Renal blood flow: no significant change.
5. Skin: the blood vessels are sensitive to the vasodilatory action of oxytocin, and flushing of the face, neck, and hands may occur.
6. Uterine flow: the decrease is caused mainly by the extravascular resistance around the uterine blood vessels as the result of the increased uterine contractions.

Kidneys

Oxytocin can induce antidiuresis. The human kidney is not damaged, the excretion of electrolytes is not changed, and renal blood flow is not reduced. The antidiuretic action probably occurs by resorption of water from the distal convoluted tubules and the collecting ducts.

Breast

Oxytocin stimulates the myoepithelial cells of the breast and causes the passage of the milk from the alveoli to the mammary ducts.

Administration

Routes of administration include intramuscular or repeated subcutaneous injections of small or large doses and the placing of a cotton pledget soaked in 5 or 10 units of oxytocin in the nostril, whence the drug is absorbed. However, the intravenous infusion of a dilute solution of oxytocin is so superior to other methods that it is the procedure of choice, to the virtual exclusion of the others.

Advantages of the Intravenous Route

1. The amount of oxytocin entering the bloodstream can be regulated. With other techniques the amount given to the patient is known, but there is no control over the rate of absorption. It can be fast or slow, regular or intermittent, and it may accumulate in the tissues to be released later in a large amount and high concentration.
2. Minute amounts are effective.
3. The blood level and the activity of oxytocin are constant as long as the rate of the drip is maintained. It can be speeded up or slowed down with instant changes in effect.
4. The plasma of pregnant women near term contains an enzyme, pitocinase, in such high concentration that half of an intravenously given dosage of pitocin is destroyed in 2 to 3 minutes. Thus, within 3 to 4 minutes of shutting off an intravenous infusion, the oxytocic activity has ceased.
5. The contractions brought on by this technique seem to be mainly of the normal triple descending gradient type.

Technique of Intravenous Administration

The two methods of intravenous infusion are by the use of a constant infusion pump or by a Murphy drip. Whichever system is employed it is advisable to start the drip at a rate of 1.0 mU per minute to test for untoward reactions. If none occur the speed of the infusion is increased until the desired effect is achieved. The maximum safe dose is 20 mU per minute. In most cases doses of less than 10 mU per minute are adequate.

In high-risk cases, when extreme accuracy and control are essential, the constant rate infusion pump should be used. Changes in the patient's position or movement will not affect the speed at which the solution is being infused.

In many cases the drip technique is satisfactory. The popular strengths of the solutions are 5 or 10 units of oxytocin in a liter of crystalloid (e.g, normal saline or Ringer lactate). In many instances a concentration of 2 U of oxytocin per liter will be effective. The advantages of a dilute solution are that the dose is physiologic rather than pharmacologic, the control is easier, and the danger of excessive uterine contraction is reduced. The disadvantage is that too much fluid may be given. When used for induction or augmentation of labor, it is advisable to maintain the infusion for 1 hour postpartum to obviate uterine atony. To avoid water intoxication, the amount of oxytocin and fluid must be controlled: less than 45 mU per minute of the former and 1 liter per 24 hours of the latter.

When the drip method is used, the two-bottle system is advised. One bottle contains a liter of crystalloid solution. The other contains a liter of crystalloid to which the oxytocin has been added; this must be labeled clearly. The two tubes leading from the bottles are connected by a Y adapter, which connects to the needle in the vein. The Y adapter should be close to the needle so that a change from one solution to the other will be immediate.

The drip is started with the crystalloid solution. When it is running at 10 to 15 drops a minute the switch is made to the oxytocin solution. Careful observation is made as to the type, strength, and duration of the contractions and to their effect on the fetal heart. If no untoward reactions are noted, the drip is continued. If excessive uterine contractions occur, or if there is fetal bradycardia (under 100), tachycardia (over 160), or irregularity of the heart, the oxytocin is stopped and plain crystalloid is infused. Oxytocin is a potent drug. It may vary a hundredfold in its actions on different people. The dosage is regulated by the effect on the individual receiving it. The speed of the drip is determined by and correlated to the frequency, intensity, and duration of the resulting contractions, rather than by any arbitrary number of drops per minute. The aim is to bring about strong uterine contractions lasting 40 to 50 seconds, and recurring every 2 to 3 minutes. Care must be exercised to avoid tumultuous contractions so frequent and prolonged that there is no interval between them. This carries the danger of uterine rupture, placental separation, and fetal asphyxia.

Indications for Use of Oxytocin

Management of Abortions
Oxytocin is used during abortions to stimulate the uterus to pass retained tissue and to control bleeding.

Inevitable Abortion.   The symptoms are bleeding and cramps. The cervix is partly open, but the products of conception have not been passed. Oxytocin stimulates the uterus to contract and expel its contents after the cervix has been opened widely. Curettage is easier through an open cervix. The oxytocin keeps the uterus firm, makes it easier to avoid perforation of the uterine fundus, and helps control hemorrhage.

Incomplete Abortion. The fetus has been passed, but part or all of the placenta is in situ. Oxytocin helps expel what is left, makes curettage easier, and controls hemorrhage.

Complete Abortion. Oxytocin is used to reduce postabortal bleeding.

Missed Abortion. While most missed abortions terminate spontaneously, in some instances (e.g., danger of hypo- or afibrinogenemia) one can wait only so long and then steps must be taken to empty the uterus. Oxytocin is valuable to soften the cervix, to open it sufficiently so that dilatation and curettage can be performed safely, and to keep the uterine tone high so that bleeding is controlled.

Induction of Labor

Elective Induction of Labor. Elective induction of labor is performed for a variety of reasons including the following:

1. Convenience to the mother and doctor
2. Patients with a history of precipitate labors
3. Patients who live a long distance from the hospital

As long as the cervix is ripe (soft, less than 1.3 cm [0.5 in] long, effaced, open to admit at least one finger, and easily dilatable) and the head is well in the pelvis, induction of labor is feasible. Artificial rupture of the membranes increases the efficiency of inducing labor with oxytocin.

Spontaneous Rupture of the Membranes. If the membranes rupture prematurely, much before term, an attempt is made to prolong the pregnancy until the baby is mature enough to survive. On the other hand, most patients who rupture the membranes near or at term go into spontaneous labor. If this does not take place within 24 hours induction of labor is indicated.

Fetal Salvage. In certain instances where the pregnancy has gone past the date of expected confinement by 2 weeks or more, induction is indicated. Rupture of the membranes and an oxytocin drip are the methods of choice, providing the cervix is ripe and the head engaged. In diabetic mothers and in those who are sensitized to the Rhesus factor, induction of labor before term may be necessary. If conditions are right this can be done with oxytocin and rupture of the membranes. If the cervix is not ripe and the presenting part is high, cesarean section may be safer.

Maternal Indications. In conditions such as preeclampsia, premature separation of the placenta, and fetal death in utero, the time comes when medical management or watchful expectancy is no longer indicated and the pregnancy must be terminated artificially in the interests of the mother. This is especially true if her condition is deteriorating.

Ripening of the Cervix. As a general rule, induction of labor by artificial rupture of the bag of waters is not attempted unless the cervix is ripe and the head is in the pelvis. Should induction be essential in the presence of an unripe cervix, an attempt is made to ripen it. The patient is given an oxytocin drip several hours daily for a few days. In most instances, this does not institute true labor, but the oxytocin-induced contractions often bring the head down into the pelvis and ripen the cervix so that the membranes can be ruptured and good labor instituted.

To Improve Efficiency of Uterine Contractions

Prolonged Labor Due to Hypotonic Uterine Inertia. In prolonged labor due to hypotonic uterine inertia oxytocin is most valuable. The effect is to increase the type of contraction already present. In true hypotonic inertia the pattern is normal, but the contractions of the upper segment are weak and progress is not made. Before using oxytocin in these conditions one must be sure that there is no disproportion or malpresentation, since these abnormalities signal poor uterine action.

In hypotonic uterine action an oxytocin drip may result in an immediate improvement of the labor, with steady progress to successful delivery of the child. The proper use of pitocin in these cases has resulted in:

1. Successful termination of the labor
2. Reduction in the incidence of midforceps, cervical lacerations, cesarean section, Dührssen incisions, and traumatic deliveries
3. Shortening of prolonged labor

Treatment of Postpartum Hemorrhage. In postpartum hemorrhage caused by uterine atony an oxytocin drip is a good method of treatment. Other causes of the bleeding must, of course, be ruled out. The drip is effective in improving the tone of the uterus, and it can be kept running as long as necessary.

Prevention of Postpartum Hemorrhage. Such conditions as uterine inertia, twin pregnancy, polyhydramnios, difficult delivery, and excessive anesthesia predispose to uterine atony and postpartum hemorrhage. The complication should be anticipated and guarded against by starting an oxytocin drip before the hemorrhage takes place.

Normal Management of the Third Stage. To hasten delivery of the placenta and to reduce the bleeding of the placental stage, oxytocin may be given before or after delivery of the placenta.

Prerequisites for the Use of Oxytocin

1. The presenting part should be well engaged.
2. The cervix must be ripe, effaced, soft, and partially dilated.
3. There must be a normal obstetric history and the absence of an abnormal one.
4. There must be no fetopelvic disproportion.
5. The fetus should be in normal position.
6. The fetus should be in good condition with normal fetal heart.
7. Adequate personnel must be available to watch the patient.
8. The patient must be examined carefully before the oxytocin is started.
9. The doctor in charge of the case should:
   a. Examine the patient himself before the drip is set up.
   b. Be present when the infusion is started.
   c. Observe the patient and the fetal heart for the first few contractions. He should then regulate the speed.
   d. Not order the drip by telephone.
   e. Be in hospital and available while the drip is running.
10. The response of the human uterus to intravenous oxytocin increases with the length of pregnancy, reaching a peak during the 36th week. After this the reactiveness changes little. Induction is as successful during weeks 36 to 39 as later. However, in the earlier period the induction takes longer, and more oxytocin is needed.

Contraindications to the Use of Oxytocin

1. Absence of proper indication.
2. Absence of the prerequisites.
3. Disproportion, generally contracted pelvis, and obstruction by tumors.
4. Grand multiparity: There is too great a chance of uterine rupture.
5. Previous cesarean section.

6. Hypertonic or incoordinate uterus. The hypertonic or incoordinate uterus is made worse by oxytocin and may lead to a constriction ring.
7. Maternal exhaustion. This condition should be treated by rest and fluids, not by oxytocin stimulation.
8. Fetal distress. Not only should oxytocin not be given, but the appearance of an irregular or slow heart while the drip is running demands that the drip be stopped.
9. Abnormal presentation and position of all types.
10. Unengaged head.
11. Congenital anomalies of the uterus.
12. Placenta previa.
13. Previous extensive myomectomy.

Dangers of Oxytocin

Maternal Dangers

1. Uterine rupture. If the patient is oversensitive to the drug she may get hard and even tetanic contractions, enough to rupture the uterus, whereas normal contractions would do no harm.
2. Cervical and vaginal lacerations can be caused by too rapid passage of the baby through the pelvis.
3. Uterine atony and postpartum hemorrhage may develop when the oxytocin is discontinued.
4. Abruptio placentae has been reported.
5. Water intoxication is induced by retention in the body of large amounts of water in excess of electrolytes.

Water Intoxication

Oxytocin has an antidiuretic effect that begins when the rate of infusion is 15 mU per minute and is maximal at 45 mU per minute. Single doses have no effect; the antidiuretic activity seems to depend on the maintenance of a constant and critical level. The action is on the distal convoluted tubules and collecting ducts of the kidneys, causing increased resorption of water from the glomerular filtrate. The combination of oxytocin and large amounts of electrolyte-free glucose in water leads to retention of fluid, low serum levels of sodium chloride, and often progressive oliguria.

The symptoms range from headache, nausea, vomiting, mental confusion, and seizures to coma and death. These have been attributed to edema and swelling of the brain.

Management of Water Intoxication

1. Prevention. Patients receiving an infusion of oxytocin should not receive more than 1 liter of electrolyte-free fluid in 24 hours.
2. Mild cases. Discontinue the oxytocin and withhold all fluids.
3. Severe cases require, in addition, the infusion of hypertonic (3.0 percent) sodium chloride intravenously. This will withdraw fluid from the tissues and bring about a diuresis. The rate of infusion must be slow and should be discontinued when the diuretic phase ends to avoid overcorrection, lest the cerebral effects of hypernatremia be imposed upon those of water intoxication.

Fetal Dangers From Oxytocin

1. Anoxia caused by contractions that are too hard, too frequent, and last too long. The uterus never relaxes enough to maintain adequate circulation. In some cases separation of the placenta has taken place.
2. Damage to the baby from too rapid propulsion through the pelvis.
3. Forcing the fetus through a pelvis too small for it.

In a large series it was shown that the signs of fetal distress are more common in patients receiving an oxytocin drip than in those without stimulation of labor. In almost all instances slowing or stopping the oxytocin infusion resulted in the rapid return to normal of the fetal heart. The incidence of emergency obstetric intervention was no higher, and the final fetal results were comparable.

ERGOT DERIVATIVES

The first pure ergot alkaloid, ergotamine, was isolated in 1920. Later another active alkaloid was discovered and named ergometrine (ergonovine). Only the latter is used in obstetrics. It has no adrenergic blocking action and the emetic and cardiovascular effects are less than those of ergotamine. These are powerful ecbolic agents, exciting a tonic contraction of the myometrium. The maximum effect is during labor and the puerperium. They are never used during the first and second stages of labor.

Undesirable effects include (1) hypertension, (2) tachycardia, (3) headache, and (4) nausea and vomiting. The vasomotor effects are worse in patients delivered under regional anesthesia. The ergot alkaloids should not be used in hypertensive patients, in women with cardiac disease, or in those being delivered under spinal or epidural anesthesia.

PROSTAGLANDIN

Prostaglandins are 20-carbon carboxylic acids that are formed enzymatically from polyunsaturated essential fatty acids. Most organs are capable of synthesizing prostaglandins, as well as metabolizing them to less active compounds.

On the basis of their structure prostaglandins are divided into four groups, namely E, F, A, and B. Three of the E group and three of the F group are primary compounds. The other eight are metabolites of the parent six. Thirteen of the 14 known prostaglandins occur in man.

First isolated from the seminal fluid, these substances are distributed widely in all mammalian tissues. Their exact mode of action is not known, but prostaglandins are thought to be part of the mechanism that controls transmission in the sympathetic nervous system. Two generalized activities are apparent: (1) alteration of smooth muscle contractility and (2) modulation of hormonal activity. How an organ will respond depends upon (1) the specific prostaglandin, (2) the dose, (3) the route of administration, and (4) the hormonal or drug environment. Prostaglandins are metabolized rapidly and their systemic effects are of short duration.

Prostaglandins produce a wide variety of physiologic responses. Both E and F have profoundly stimulating effects on the myometrium. In adequate dosage they can initiate labor at any stage of pregnancy. Prostaglandins can be given intravenously, intramuscularly, intravaginally, and directly into the myometrium. The latter technique will control postpartum hemorrhage when other methods fail. In cases where induction of labor is indicated in the presence of an unripe cervix, the use of vaginal suppositories containing prostaglandin is effective in softening, effacing, and dilating the cervix. Sometimes true labor will be induced.

Adverse Reactions and Contraindications

1. Gastrointestinal symptoms, including nausea, vomiting, and diarrhea, occur in half the patients. In most cases these effects are short in duration and not severe.
2. A syndrome of bronchial constriction (asthma attack) with tachycardia, vasovagal effects, and alterations in blood pressure may take place. Should this occur the drug is discontinued and

supportive therapy instituted. The vital signs return to normal within a few minutes, probably because the drug is metabolized rapidly.

3. Hyperpyrexia occurs occasionally.
4. Convulsive seizures have been reported, and patients with epilepsy should not be given prostaglandin.
5. Contraindications include asthma, cardiovascular disease, and hypertension.

BIBLIOGRAPHY

Dawood MY, Ylikorkala O, Trivedi D, Fuchs F: Oxytocin in maternal circulation and amniotic fluid during pregnancy. J Clin Endocrinol Metab 49:429, 1979

Sogolow SR: An historical review of the use of oxytocin prior to delivery. Obstet Gynecol Surv 21:155, 1968

41

Induction of Labor

Induced labor is labor started by artificial methods.

INDICATIONS FOR THE INDUCTION OF LABOR

Maternal Indications

SPONTANEOUS RUPTURE OF MEMBRANES   If the pregnancy is within 2 weeks of term and labor does not begin after 24 hours, induction with oxytocin should be considered.

TOXEMIA OF PREGNANCY   When medical therapy is unable to control toxemia the pregnancy must be terminated.

POLYHYDRAMNIOS   Polyhydramnios is the accumulation of an excessive amount of amniotic fluid. Pressure symptoms and dyspnea may be so severe that the patient is unable to carry on.

ANTEPARTUM BLEEDING   Included here are cases of low-lying placenta and mild placental separation, in which the bleeding is not controllable by bed rest, or when the baby is dead.

INTRAUTERINE FETAL DEATH   In selected cases labor is induced to relieve the mother of the strain of carrying a dead child and to prevent the development of afibrinogenemia.

CANCER   Termination of the pregnancy is for the purpose of permitting surgical, radiation, or chemical treatment of the lesion, or simply to remove a drain on the patient's resources and powers of resistance.

HISTORY OF RAPID LABORS   The aim is to avoid birth of the baby at home or en route to hospital.

PATIENTS LIVING FAR FROM HOSPITAL

ELECTIVE   Here the procedure is being carried out for the convenience of the patient, the doctor, or both. Because there is no pressing medical reason for the induction, great care must be taken in selecting the patient and no risks should be taken. The labor must be supervised constantly. If there is the least doubt about the procedure it should not be instituted.

Fetal Indications

MATERNAL DIABETES   There is a risk of fetal death in utero during the later weeks of pregnancy. If tests of fetal well-being indicate that the baby is in jeopardy the pregnancy must be terminated before 40 weeks.

RHESUS INCOMPATIBILITY   When the fetus is being sensitized or when there has been fetal death in utero during previous pregnancies, premature induction of labor is sometimes indicated.

RECURRENT INTRAUTERINE DEATH   Intrauterine death near term in past pregnancies is a rational reason for premature induction of labor.

EXCESSIVE SIZE OF THE FETUS

POSTTERM PREGNANCY   There is some evidence that there is a progressive decrease in placental function and in the oxygen content of fetal blood as pregnancy proceeds past term. Occasionally there is fetal death in utero, or the baby is born in poor condition. If tests show that the condition of the baby is deteriorating, induction of labor must be considered.

Advantages

1. The patient is admitted to hospital the previous night and a hypnotic is prescribed to assure her of sleep.
2. No food is given by mouth; the empty stomach decreases the anesthetic risk.
3. The rush to hospital is avoided.
4. It is a daytime procedure when full staff is available.
5. The doctor chooses a day when he has no other duties and can remain in hospital with the patient.
6. The length of labor is shortened.

PREREQUISITES AND CONDITIONS

PRESENTATION   The presentation should be cephalic. Labor is never induced in the presence of attitudes of extension, transverse lies, or compound presentations, and almost never when the breech presents.

STAGE OF THE PREGNANCY   The closer the gestation is to term the easier is the induction.

STATION   The head must be engaged: the lower the head, the easier and safer the procedure.

CERVICAL RIPENESS   The cervix must be effaced, less than 1.3 cm (0.5 inch) in length, soft, dilatable, and open to admit at least one finger and preferably two. The firm ring of the internal os should not be present. It is advantageous for the cervix to be in the center of the birth canal or anterior. When the cervix is posterior conditions for induction are less favorable.

PARITY   It is much easier and safer to induce a multipara than a primigravida, and the success rate increases with parity.

FETAL MATURITY   In general the nearer the gestation is to 40 weeks the better the fetal results. When preterm termination of pregnancy is necessary, tests for fetal maturity should be performed to establish, as far as possible, that the fetus will be able to survive outside the uterus. These tests include clinical examination, ultrasonic measurement of the biparietal diameter of the head and circumference of the body, and determination of the L/S ratio, creatinine, bilirubin, and fat cells in the amniotic fluid.

DANGERS

1. Prolapse of the umbilical cord may occur if artificial rupture of the membranes is performed when the presenting part is not well engaged.
2. Fetal death, unexplained.
3. Prolonged labor.
4. Prematurity. Three major factors appear to be responsible for the morbidity and mortality in this situation:
   a. The erroneous assessment, on clinical grounds alone, of the infant's gestational age and the expected date of confinement.
   b. The decision to deliver the infants electively 2 to 3 weeks before term.

    c. The failure to use well-documented objective means for as-
sessing fetal size and pulmonary maturity, such as ultrasonography and the L/S ratio in the amniotic fluid.

5. Genital and fetal infection following a long period of ruptured
membranes.

6. Failure of induction may be defined as occurring (a) when the
uterus does not respond to stimulation at all or (b) when the
uterus contracts abnormally and the cervix does not dilate. As
long as the prerequisites are observed, the rate of successful labor inductions is over 90 percent. Some 10 percent of women are
delivered by cesarean section. It must be kept in mind that in
many cases the original indication for the induction and the cesarean are the same—e.g., diabetes or Rh immunization.

RIPENESS OF THE CERVIX

The changes in the uterine cervix that take place before the onset of
labor include physically detectable softening, shortening, and dilatation of the os. This process is known as ripening. The collagen fibrils
become disaggregated and no longer tightly bound by the glyco-
saminoglycans so that they will slide apart more readily and allow the
cervix to dilate.

    In most normal pregnancies the cervix is ripe at the onset of labor.
A ripe cervix is soft, less than 1.3 cm in length, admits a finger easily,
and is dilatable. The length of labor and the success of induction depend
on the degree of cervical ripeness. There are many situations, however,
where labor and vaginal delivery are indicated when the cervix is not
ripe. In such cases the cervix is unlikely to respond favorably to uterine
activity.

<table>
<tr><th rowspan="2"></th><th rowspan="2"></th><th colspan="4">POINTS</th></tr>
<tr><th>0</th><th>1</th><th>2</th><th>3</th></tr>
<tr><td rowspan="5">FACTOR</td><td>Dilatation of cervix (cm)</td><td>0</td><td>1–2</td><td>3–4</td><td>5–6</td></tr>
<tr><td>Effacement of cervix (%)</td><td>0–30</td><td>40–50</td><td>60–70</td><td>80</td></tr>
<tr><td>Consistency of cervix</td><td>Firm</td><td>Medium</td><td>Soft</td><td></td></tr>
<tr><td>Position of cervix in the vagina</td><td>Posterior</td><td>Mid</td><td>Anterior</td><td></td></tr>
<tr><td>Station</td><td>−3</td><td>−2</td><td>−1, 0</td><td>+1, +2</td></tr>
</table>

Figure 1. Bishop score.

Evaluation of the Cervix: Pelvic Score

Before inducing labor or using a modality to prime or ripen a cervix, one must differentiate between a cervix that is unprepared and one that is already ripe. The most readily used methods to make the assessment depend on the physical characteristics of the cervix.

Bishop was the first to attempt to quantify the physical examination of the cervix by the use of a numeric scoring system (Fig. 1). This is based on a number of criteria, including dilatation, effacement, consistency, and position of the cervix in the vagina. Each of the criteria is evaluated and assigned a number of points. Of all these parameters, dilatation is the most significant and position of the cervix the least important. The higher the score, the shorter will the length of labor be, and the more likely will induction be successful.

When a high score is present it can be assumed that cervical ripening has taken place and no further attempts to prime the cervix are needed. According to Bishop's system, the maximal total score is 13. When the score is 9 or more induction of labor is always successful. When the score is 4 or less, failure of induction is common, and preinduction cervical priming should be performed.

Lange and associates suggested that the factor of crucial significance to inducibility of labor is the condition of the cervix, and that cervical dilatation should be weighted by at least twice the value given it by Bishop. The results of their modified score are the same as those achieved by other methods, but theirs is simpler in that only three parameters are used: station of the presenting part, dilatation of the cervix, and length of the cervix. When the score is 5 to 7 the rate of successful induction is over 75 percent. When it is under 4, the rate of failure is considerable (Fig. 2).

Station	−3	−2	−1, 0	+1, +2
Points	0	1	2	3

Dilatation of cervix (cm)	0	1−2	3−4	>4
Points	0	2	4	6

Length of cervix (cm)	3	2	1	0
Points	0	1	2	3

Figure 2. Lange score.

Methods of Cervical Priming

Laminaria Tents

The use of laminaria tents to dilate the uterine cervix during pregnancy, given up many years ago because of the high rate of infection, has been revived as a consequence of the obviation of sepsis by modern methods of sterilization. *Laminaria digitata* is a species of seaweed. The dried stem is hygroscopic: when it comes in contact with moisture it swells to three to five times its original diameter. In so doing it brings about gradual softening and dilatation of the cervix. The most rapid swelling occurs in the first 4 to 6 hours and the maximal effect is achieved in 24 hours. The effect is entirely local. Uterine hyperactivity is rare. There is some evidence that the insertion of the tent leads to the production of endogenous prostaglandin, and this may play a part in the ripening process.

Indications

1. *First trimester abortions:* Precurettage or vacuum aspiration
2. *Midtrimester abortions:* In association with the intraamniotic injection of ecbolic solutions
3. *Term or preterm pregnancy:* To ripen the unfavorable cervix prior to induction of labor

Avantages

1. The cervix becomes soft and dilated; the Bishop score is improved.
2. The length of the first stage of labor is shortened.

Technique: Preinduction of Labor

1. In the evening before the day of induction two to five laminaria are placed in the cervix. The number depends on the capacity of the cervix. As many as possible are inserted.
2. Care is taken not to rupture the membranes.
3. A sterile gauze is placed against the cervix to hold the laminaria in place.
4. Next morning the laminaria tents are removed.
5. Amniotomy is performed.
6. An infusion of oxytocin may be started immediately. However, some obstetricians prefer to use oxytocin only if labor does not begin after 6 to 8 hours.

Complications

1. Mild pelvic cramps occur occasionally.
2. Cervical bleeding has been reported.
3. There is a small risk of infection, especially if the interval between the insertion of the tents and the emptying of the uterus is prolonged.

Prostaglandin (PG)

One of the main problems in inducing labor is the unripe cervix. Used intracervically or intravaginally, PGE_2 has been shown to be effective in ripening the cervix, and sometimes as an initiator of active labor. It is likely that the effect is twofold: (1) PG brings about biochemical changes in the collagenous matrix of the cervix that result in softening; (2) PG stimulates the uterus to contract gently and this leads to retraction and partial dilatation of the cervix.

The original preparations were suppositories of PG in a gel or in a wax base. In these vehicles, however, PG deteriorates rapidly and a fresh batch has to be made each day, an impractical situation. New types of gel are being investigated, however, and it is hoped that a stable product will be produced.

In the meantime oral tablets placed in the vagina have been shown to be effective in inducing ripening of the cervix. A dose of 2 to 4 mg of PGE_2 (depending on the ripeness of the cervix) appears to be adequate and safe. Large doses may cause excessive uterine contractions and fetal distress. A case of uterine rupture has been reported, and it is advised that once the patient is in labor, no more PG be given.

A good regimen is to put the PG tablets into the posterior fornix of the vagina the night before the induction is planned. Contractions of low amplitude begin within a couple of hours. These are similar to the contractions of early spontaneous labor. Not infrequently active labor begins during the period of cervical ripening, so that other procedures are unnecessary. The occasional occurrence of uterine hypertonus is controlled easily by an infusion of a tocolytic drug.

If labor has not started by the next morning and the cervix has become favorable, amniotomy is performed and, if necessary, an oxytocin infusion is set up. Successful ripening of the cervix and induction of labor is almost universal. In the rare cases where the cervix does not respond, the case must be reevaluated.

Oxytocin

Oxytocin does induce contractions of the pregnant myometrium, but it has not proved to be an efficient priming agent of the cervix. Given as an intravenous infusion oxytocin does improve the Bishop score, but to a much smaller extent than that achieved by intravaginal PGE$_2$, and prolonged treatment may be necessary. It appears that oxytocin is an inefficient ripening agent.

METHODS OF INDUCING LABOR

Medical Methods

Castor oil, 2 ounces, followed by soapsuds enema may succeed in inducing labor.

Oxytocin

Under the proper conditions oxytocin is an efficient inducer of labor. (See Chapter 40 for the details of the technique.)

Artificial Rupture of Membranes

Technique
1. The fetal heart is checked carefully.
2. Sterile vaginal examination is made to determine that the necessary conditions and prerequisites are present.
3. With a finger placed between the cervix and the bag of waters, the cervix is rimmed, stripping the membranes away from the lower uterine segment.
4. Pressure is maintained on the uterine fundus through the abdomen to keep the head well down.
5. Using a uterine dressing forceps, an Allis forceps, a Kelly clamp, or a membrane hook, the bag of waters is torn or punctured.
6. A gush of fluid from the vagina or the grasping of fetal hair in the clamp is proof of success.
7. The fetal heart is checked carefully.
8. Although the head may be pushed upward slightly to allow escape of the amniotic fluid, this must be done with caution for there is danger of umbilical cord prolapse.
9. Amnioscope. Artificial rupture of the membranes can be performed through a vaginal amnioscope. Advantages include:
    a. The procedure is carried out under direct vision, which adds to the safety.
    b. The color of the fluid and the presence of meconium can be ascertained before the membranes are ruptured.

    c. The presence of a low-lying umbilical cord or vasa previa can be ruled out.

    d. Amniotic fluid, uncontaminated by vaginal contents, can be collected for biochemical analysis.

    e. The amnioscope provides a sterile pathway to the cervix and reduces the danger of amnionitis.

Contraindications to Artificial Rupture of the Membranes

1. High presenting part
2. Presentation other than vertex
3. Unripe cervix
4. Abnormal fetal heart rate

Intraamniotic Injection of Ecbolic Solutions

The intraamniotic instillation of various solutions will induce labor. Some exert this effect by virtue of their hypertonicity. Others have a different mode of action. In most cases delivery of the products of conception takes place within 40 hours. Retained placenta, bleeding, and the need for curettage are common. This technique is feasible only after 16 weeks' gestation because of the difficulty of locating the amniotic sac before this time and the inadequate quantity of amniotic fluid.

Mechanism of Action

Hypotheses as to the mechanism of action include:

1. Normally progesterone blocks the onset of labor. The hypertonic solution disrupts the placenta and releases the local progesterone block; labor then follows.
2. Uterine volume is an important factor in controlling the onset of labor. The body attempts to equilibrate the hypertonic solution, the volume of intraamniotic fluid is increased, and uterine contractions begin.
3. The injected drug has a direct effect on the myometrium, stimulating it to contract.

Indications

This method is used for the induction of labor when the fetus is dead or when the termination of pregnancy is so essential to the interests of the mother that the fetus is being disregarded. This technique is useful in missed abortions. It works even when the cervix is unripe. This procedure is not employed to induce labor in a normal pregnancy or when the fetus is viable.

Technique

1. For maximum safety the placenta is localized and the diagnosis of fetal presentation confirmed by ultrasonic scan.
2. While premedication with an analgesic such as Demerol is helpful, general anesthesia must never be used as it would mask untoward reactions.
3. The patient is placed on an operating table in moderate Trendelenburg position.
4. An intravenous infusion of 5 percent glucose in water is instituted.
5. The bladder must be empty.
6. The procedure is performed under aseptic conditions. The abdomen is sterilized as well as possible.
7. Transabdominal amniotomy is performed under local anesthesia, using a 10-cm (4-inch) spinal needle with stylet. The needle is inserted halfway between the symphysis pubis and the umbilicus, 2.5 cm (1-inch) from the midline, toward the side where the fetal small parts are located.
8. The first bit of amniotic fluid removed may be tested to be certain it is not urine. If it is alkaline and positive for glucose and protein, it is probably amniotic fluid and not urine.
9. One of the dangers is that the needle may become displaced and injection made into the wrong area. To avoid this the needle must be fixed in position or, preferably, replaced by a catheter, which is easier to set and has less chance of moving out of the amniotic sac.
10. A three-way stopcock is helpful.
11. Amniotic fluid is removed and replaced with the drug being used. The amount of fluid withdrawn depends on the medication to be instilled. The injection is made slowly, with frequent aspirations to check the position of the needle or catheter and to make certain that it is not in a blood vessel.
12. After a small amount of drug has been injected the patient is observed for untoward effects. If these are absent the total dose is instilled. If abnormal reactions occur the procedure is discontinued.
13. The patient is returned to bed, the intravenous infusion maintained at a slow rate, and the patient kept under close supervision to await the onset of labor.

At the conclusion of the injection two laminaria tents may be inserted into the cervical canal to soften and dilate the cervix gradually so that the danger of cervical trauma may be reduced, including cervicovaginal fistula and cervical incompetence. Often the injection-to-delivery time is reduced. Care must be taken not to rupture the membranes. The laminaria tents are inserted after the injection is complete so that, if the intraamniotic injection is unsuccessful, the procedure can be reattempted the following week. Once the laminaria have been inserted the evacuation of the uterus cannot be postponed.

Postinjection Course

1. If labor does not begin by 24 hours an oxytocin infusion may be instituted.
2. Some physicians start an oxytocin drip routinely after the intraamniotic injection is made.
3. If induction of labor fails a second intraamniotic injection is made.
4. In rare cases hysterotomy may be necessary.
5. Retention of placenta or excessive bleeding requires immediate curettage.

Advantages

This method is an effective way of inducing labor and obviates the need for hysterotomy when the pregnancy must be terminated after the first trimester.

Dangers

1. Maternal death may result.
2. Infection may be introduced, especially when glucose is used.
3. Damage to placental vessels during amniotomy may allow fetal erythrocytes to enter the maternal circulation.
4. The bladder or bowel may be injured.
5. Intravascular injection may occur.
6. There may be water intoxication from overabsorption of saline into the maternal tissues.
7. Retained placenta or excessive bleeding occurs in 20 percent of cases.
8. Many patients show some changes in blood clotting, and a few develop a picture of consumption coagulopathy when hypertonic saline is used.

Ecbolic Agents

Hypertonic Glucose

Originally a solution of 50 percent glucose was employed with success. However, because of a high rate of infection, its use was discontinued.

Hypertonic Saline

A 20 percent solution is effective in inducing labor and is used widely. The amount of amniotic fluid removed ranges from 100 to 300 ml and is replaced with an equal quantity of saline. In the interests of safety no more than 200 ml of hypertonic saline should be injected.

The initial 10 ml of hypertonic saline is administered and the patient observed. Indications for discontinuance of the procedure include burning abdominal pain (myometrial or intraperitoneal injection) and sudden onset of headache, generalized flush, and thirst (suggesting intravascular injection). In the latter case 5 percent glucose in water is infused rapidly. In the absence of untoward symptoms the remainder of the saline is injected slowly.

The mechanism of action is not clear. Intraamniotic injection of saline leads to an increase in the production and release of prostaglandin, a substance known to stimulate the uterus to contract. The saline may also cause suppression of the synthesis of placental progesterone, thereby allowing myometrial activity to begin.

Complications

1. Hypernatremia is common, and, in most cases, it is insignificant. However, this complication accounts for most deaths. These fatalities are associated with rapid transfer of sodium chloride into the vascular system either by direct injection or through a tear in the uterine vessels. Death occurs from excessive dehydration of the brain.
2. Disseminated intravascular coagulation is rare. It may be related to a release of thromboplastin from the amniotic fluid into the maternal circulation. The removal of the products of conception results in rapid correction of the abnormality.
3. Hemorrhage and retained placenta require operative removal of tissue from the uterus.
4. The cervix may be lacerated. Occasionally, failure of the cervix to dilate leads to the fetus and placenta being extruded through the wall of the cervical canal, resulting in a cervicovaginal fistula.
5. If oxytocin is used, water intoxication may occur.
6. Hypertonic saline should not be used in women with cardiac disease, hypertension, severe renal abnormalities, or hemolytic processes.

Because of the rapid fetal death after injection of hypertonic saline, there are no live births with this method.

Urea

To avoid the dangers of hypertonic saline, urea may be employed. The mode of action is similar to saline in that decreases in circulating progesterone levels and increases in prostaglandin release have been reported. Fetal death and maceration occur in all cases.

Technique. Amniocentesis is performed in the usual way; 200 ml of amniotic fluid is removed and replaced with 200 ml of 5 percent dextrose in water containing 80 g of urea. The solution is injected slowly. The incidence of retained placenta and bleeding is higher than with saline. Operative evacuation of the uterus is necessary frequently.

Complications

1. Nausea and vomiting.
2. Urea is an osmotic diuretic and dehydration of clinical significance may occur, especially when there is vomiting.
3. If massive diuresis takes place, hyponatremia and hypokalemia may cause problems.
4. Coagulation defects are apparent but are not severe.
5. Infection and cervical laceration may occur.
6. Urea is contraindicated in patients with renal or hepatic impairment.

Advantages

1. There are no significant complications if inadvertent intravenous injection is made.
2. Intramural injection does not cause myometrial necrosis.

Prostaglandin F$_{2\alpha}$

Injected intraamniotically, this is an efficient agent in bringing about termination of pregnancy in the second trimester.

Technique. Amniocentesis is performed in the usual way. At least 1 ml of amniotic fluid is removed. One milliliter (5 mg) of prostaglandin F$_{2\alpha}$ is injected. The patient is observed for pain, vomiting, or bronchospasm. Then the rest of the 40 mg is injected. The patient may be ambulatory.

Advantages. Advantages of PG over saline include the following:

1. Injection-to-abortion time is shorter.
2. There is no significant change in heart rate, cardiac output, or intravascular volume.

3. There is no alteration in the clotting factors.
4. There is no risk of hypernatremia.
5. Myometrial necrosis does not occur even if the injection is made into the wall of the uterus.

Disadvantages

1. A number of patients will require a second injection.
2. The incidence of nausea, vomiting, diarrhea, dyspnea, flushing, and chest pain is higher than with saline.
3. Heavy bleeding, often necessitating blood transfusion, is more common than when saline is used.
4. Postabortal curettage, both for bleeding and retained secundines, is often necessary.
5. Prostaglandins do not cause fetal death in utero and the fetus may be born alive, leading to potential medical, psychological, and legal problems. This situation may be obviated by combining prostaglandin with urea.
6. Eight cases have been reported of sudden collapse and eventual death of women having intrauterine injections of $PGF_{2\alpha}$. The etiology is unknown.

Urea-Prostaglandin Combined

The induction to delivery time is shorter than with either agent alone. The risk of a live-born fetus is reduced.

BIBLIOGRAPHY

Binkin NJ, Schulz KF, Grimes DA, Cates W: Urea-prostaglandin versus hypertonic saline for instillation abortion. Am J Obstet Gynecol 146:947, 1983.

Gower RH, Toraya J, Miller JM: Laminaria for preinduction cervical ripening. Obstet Gynecol 60:617, 1982

Kazzi GM, Bottoms SF, Rosen MG: Efficacy and safety of *Laminaria digitata* for preinduction ripening of the cervix. Obstet Gynecol 60:440, 1982

Kennedy JH, Stewart P, Barlow DH, et al: Induction of labor: A comparison of a single prostaglandin E_2 vaginal tablet with amniotomy and intravenous oxytocin. Brit J Obstet Gynaecol 89:704, 1982

Lange AP, Secher NJ, Westergaard JG, et al: Prelabor evaluation of inducibility. Obstet Gynecol 60:137, 1982

Sawyer MM, Lipshitz J, Anderson GD, et al: Third-trimester uterine rupture associated with vaginal prostaglandin E_2. Am J Obstet Gynecol 140:710, 1981

Shepherd JH, Bennett MJ, Laurence D, et al: Prostaglandin vaginal suppositories: A simple and safe approach to the induction of labor. Obstet Gynecol
58:596, 1981
Shepherd JH, Knuppel RA: The role of prostaglandins in ripening the cervix
and inducing labor. Clin Perinatol 8:49, 1981
Steiner AL, Creasy RK: Methods of cervical priming. Clin Obstet Gynecol
26:37, 1983

42

Fetal Dysmaturity, Retarded Intrauterine Growth, Prolonged Pregnancy, Term Intrapartum Fetal Death

CLASSIFICATION OF FETAL STATUS

1. According to gestational age
   a. Preterm: less than 37 completed weeks (259 days) from the first day of the last menstrual period
   b. Term: from 37 to less than 42 completed weeks (259 to 293 days)
   c. Postterm: 42 completed weeks (294 days) or more
2. According to pattern of growth
   a. Appropriate for gestational age (AGA): between the 10th and 90th percentiles
   b. Large for gestational age (LGA): above the 90th percentile
   c. Small for gestational age (SGA): below the 10th percentile

FETAL DYSMATURITY

The term fetal dysmaturity refers to the syndrome in which either the infant's stage of development is less than expected for the period of gestation or it shows the regressive changes and signs of intrauterine hypoxia.

Children who demonstrate soft tissue wasting have the following appearance:

1. The weight is low in relation to body length.
2. The limbs are long and lean.
3. The baby looks undernourished and has only a small amount of subcutaneous fat.

4. The vernix is scanty or absent and when present is yellow or green.
5. The hair is abundant.
6. The nails are long.
7. The skin hangs in folds. There is a tendency to desquamation, especially on the palms and soles. The skin dries after birth and becomes parchment-like.
8. The skin, nails, umbilical cord, and amniotic fluid are stained with meconium.
9. In advanced cases the amniotic fluid becomes scanty and thick with meconium. There is a tendency to aspiration of this fluid with subsequent pulmonary complications.

INTRAUTERINE GROWTH RETARDATION

Infants whose intrauterine growth has been retarded have been described as being small for gestational age (SGA). The condition may be defined in two ways: (1) infants whose weight is below the 10th percentile for their gestational age, and (2) infants whose weight is two standard deviations below the mean weight for their gestational age. These babies do not have the same problems as premature infants, but have their own. These include asphyxia, hypoglycemia, hypocalcemia, polycythemia, hypothermia, and an increase in perinatal mortality.

Mechanisms of Growth Retardation

Slow growth of the fetus in utero may be a reflection of chronic uteroplacental insufficiency, a fetal anomaly beyond correction, or no more than a normal variation. The two mechanisms of intrauterine growth retardation are (1) a reduction in fetal growth potential (symmetrical), and (2) reduction of fetal growth support (asymmetrical).

Reduced Fetal Growth Potential: Early Onset Symmetrical Growth Retardation

One-third of clinically recognizable cases of fetal growth retardation are in this group. Most of these infants are small because of constitutional limitations. The insult occurs early in pregnancy, caused by a chromosomal aberration, a congenital anomaly, a viral infection, or severe maternal malnutrition. The basic defect is an interference with the hyperplastic phase of development. Beginning in the first trimester of pregnancy there is a persistently slow rate of growth and a reduction in absolute size. The total number of cells in the body, including those of the brain, is reduced. Because the brain and the body are affected equally, the ratio of the size of the head to that of the body is often normal. The head:abdomen ratio is within the mean for gestational age and shows the normal reversal, i.e., after 35 weeks the abdominal circumference is larger than that of the head. This type of growth retardation is symmetrical in that all organs are affected equally. It usually becomes evident before 32 weeks' gestation.

Reduced Fetal Growth Support: Late Onset Asymmetrical Fetal Growth Retardation

This form of reduction in or cessation of growth occurs in fetuses that start out with normal developmental potential. The basic defect implies impairment in the transplacental supply of nutrients. It is associated with hypertensive disorders and their associated reduction in uterine blood flow, chronic maternal malnutrition, and poor gain of weight during pregnancy. The decreased transplacental transfer of oxygen and nutrients leads to a decrease in soft tissue and muscle mass, and a decreased deposition of glycogen in the fetal liver.

Interference occurs with both hyperplasia and hypertrophy, and these infants appear wasted. There is a high association with fetal distress, meconium aspiration, asphyxia, and postpartum hypoglycemia. Hypoxia is probably the common denominator in this type of growth retardation. This group represents about 60 percent of cases of intrauterine growth retardation (IUGR).

Initially the growth of the body is reduced but, because the blood flow to the brain is maintained, the fetal head shows nearly normal growth, and its circumference remains greater than that of the body. This type of growth retardation has been described as being asymmetrical in that all organs are not affected to the same extent.

In most cases the disorder is not recognized until after 32 weeks of gestation.

Oligohydramnios

A reduced amount of amniotic fluid is found commonly in both varieties of fetal growth retardation; so often that the presence of a normal amount of amniotic fluid casts doubt on a diagnosis of IUGR. Oligohydramnios is significant in that it may be associated with an underlying congenital anomaly. In addition, the absence of the protective cushion of fluid may lead to compression of the umbilical cord, with eventual fetal hypoxia.

Etiology

The causes of intrauterine growth retardation are many and varied. Often it is difficult to implicate any single agent.

Fetal Factors

1. Congenital infection
2. Congenital malformation
3. Chromosomal abnormalities

Placental Factors

1. Decreased placental mass, absolute or relative
   a. Minor abruption
   b. Infarction
   c. Postterm pregnancy
   d. Multiple pregnancy
2. Intrinsic placental condition
   a. Poor implantation site
   b. Malformation
   c. Vascular disease
3. Decreased blood flow
   a. Maternal vascular disease
   b. Postural hypotension
   c. Hyperviscosity

Maternal Factors

1. Reduced availability of nutrients
   a. Poor diet
   b. Ileojejunal bypass
2. Decreased supply of oxygen
   a. High altitude
   b. Hemoglobinopathy
   c. Cyanotic cardiac disease
   d. Smoking
3. Ingestion of drugs
   a. Ethanol
   b. Hydantoin
   c. Coumarin

Diagnosis

Because of the high perinatal mortality, early diagnosis is important. However, it is difficult, being made in only one-third of cases. There is no reliable screening test. Often the growth-retarded infant is identified only after birth. On the other hand, overdiagnosis is a problem. Only one-third of infants suspected of being growth retarded turn out to be so. This leads to unnecessary investigation and interference.

The signs of intrauterine growth retardation or placental insufficiency are seldom elicited before 28 weeks of gestation. The clinical features are:

1. Failure of the uterus and fetus to grow at the normal rate over a 4-week period.
2. The uterine fundal height is at least 2 cm less than expected for the length of gestation.
3. Absence of maternal gain in weight.
4. Diminished fetal movements.
5. Often the uterus is irritable.
6. A reduced volume of amniotic fluid.

IUGR is more common:

1. In women with a previous SGA (small for gestational age) baby
2. When there has been a pregnancy loss in a former pregnancy
3. With poor maternal gain in weight
4. With maternal complications, especially those associated with reduced uterine and placental flow of blood
5. With maternal smoking of cigarettes

Antepartum Assessment

1. Menstrual history is important.
2. History of quickening and first auscultation of the fetal heart, around 18 weeks.
3. Clinical estimation of fetal size.
4. Serial ultrasonography is the most valuable tool in the detection of growth retardation. A scan is performed as soon as an abnormality is suspected. If a routine scan has been performed in early pregnancy, this is of great benefit. Ultrasonic examination is repeated every 2 to 3 weeks. Special attention is paid to the biparietal diameter of the fetal head, the ratio of the circumference of the head to that of the abdomen, the total intrauterine volume, the length of the femur, the presence of congenital fetal anomalies, and the amount of amniotic fluid.

    Because of the brain-sparing tendency in some cases, the cephalic measurements alone may be misleading. The head-to-body ratio is important. Up to 32 to 36 weeks in the normal pregnancy the abdominal circumference at the umbilicus is smaller than that of the head. By 36 weeks (sometimes earlier) the measurements are the same. After 36 weeks the circumference of the abdomen becomes larger than that of the head. In many cases of IUGR, the reversal of this ratio does not take place, and the head remains large in relationship to the body.

    Campbell described two ultrasonic patterns of biparietal

measurements seen with intrauterine growth retardation.

    a. *Low profile.* This pattern correlates with the group described as having reduced fetal growth potential. A persistently slow rate of growth is evident from early in the second trimester. Growth occurs steadily, but the absolute values are below the mean. These babies have symmetrical growth retardation.

    b. *Late flattening pattern.* This group correlates with that described under reduced fetal growth support. An abrupt slowing and eventual cessation of growth are seen following a period of normal development.

5. Amniotic fluid. On ultrasonography, a pocket of fluid over 1 cm, suggests that the amount of amniotic fluid is normal. If there is less than 1 cm. oligohydramnios is diagnosed. This is an indication of fetal jeopardy. It may be a sign of asphyxia, there is danger of compression of the umbilical cord, and the risk of aspiration of meconium is increased. Polyhydramnios may be associated with congenital anomalies.

6. A nonstress test is performed weekly. Some obstetricians prefer a weekly biophysical profile.

7. The mother carries out counts of fetal movement.

8. If these tests are normal, the pregnancy is allowed to continue.

9. Placental maturity: Sometimes it is difffcult to differentiate small for gestational age infants from small non-SGA infants. Recent studies have suggested that the combination of a small infant and an ultrasonic finding of a mature (grade III) placenta is evidence of intrauterine growth retardation. Placental maturity correlates with gestational age and not fetal size.

Antepartum Management

1. When IUGR is suspected, the pregnancy is monitored by clinical examination and ultrasonography is performed every 3 weeks (Fig. 1).

2. If fetal growth proves to be normal, the pregnancy is allowed to continue to term.

3. If growth is less than normal, ultrasonography is performed every 2 to 3 weeks and the nonstress test (NST) weekly or twice a week.

4. As long as growth continues and the NST test remains reactive (normal) spontaneous labor is awaited. There is no evidence that in mild cases of IUGR preterm delivery improves the results.

5. If there is arrest of growth or the nonstress test becomes nonreactive, a contraction stress test and/or a biophysical profile is performed.

6. If the CST and/or the biophysical profile are normal the NST is

carried out twice weekly. Should the NST become nonreactive, the CST and/or the biophysical profile are repeated.

7. If the CST and/or the biophysical profile are abnormal, amniocentesis is performed to determine fetal pulmonary maturity.

8. If the fetal lungs are mature, the baby should be delivered.

9. If the fetal lungs are immature and the baby is in jeopardy, there are two choices. Which route is selected depends on the infant's condition.

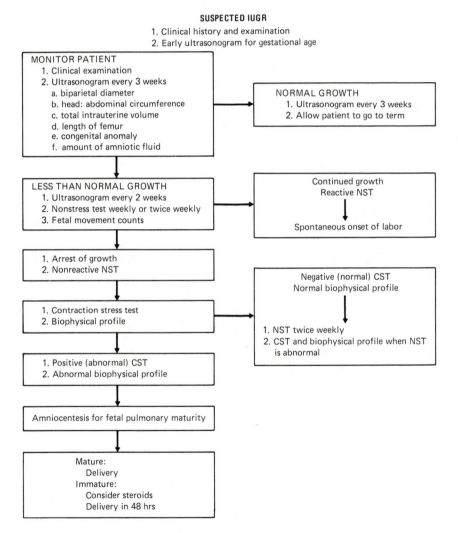

Figure 1. Management of intrauterine growth retardation.

    a. Deliver the baby immediately and take the risks of the respiratory distress syndrome.

    b. Give the mother glucocorticoids and deliver the infant in 48 hours.

Termination of Pregnancy

How this is done depends on the condition of the cervix.

1. Ripe cervix: Induction of labor by infusion of oxytocin and artificial rupture of membranes
2. Unripe cervix:
   a. Prostaglandin E_2 placed intravaginally in the evening to ripen the cervix, followed in the morning by infusion of oxytocin and artificial rupture of the membranes
   b. Cesarean section if immediate delivery is necessary
3. Liberal indications for cesarean section include:
   a. Fetal distress
   b. Malpresentation
   c. Failed induction
   d. Arrest of progress
   e. Previous cesarean section

Intrapartum Management

1. Delivery should take place in a hospital with specialized high-risk facilities, both obstetric and pediatric.
2. A neonatologist should be present at the birth.
3. The delivery should be atraumatic.
4. Continuous electronic fetal heart monitoring is essential.
5. Late decelerations are associated with a degree of asphyxia greater than in normally grown infants. Hence, earlier intervention may be necessary.

Postnatal Condition

1. Asphyxia neonatorum is common.
2. Meconium aspiration occurs more frequently than in normal infants. Gasping in utero in response to asphyxia appears to contribute to this problem. Aspiration of meconium before 34 weeks is seen rarely. The meconium acts as a foreign body and may obstruct the flow of air into the pulmonary alveoli. The nares, nasopharynx, and oropharynx should be suctioned as soon as the fetal head is born. Further clearing of the airway can be accomplished, when indicated, by laryngoscopy and

aspiration immediately after birth, especially when the meconium is thick.

3. Hypoglycemia is a frequent problem in SGA (small for gestational age) babies. This occurs both because the reserves of glycogen are inadequate secondary to intrauterine malnutrition, and because the gluconeogenic pathway is less responsive to hypoglycemia than that of the normally grown infant. The problem is compounded by an increased need for glucose and a limited oral intake. Levels of glucose in the blood of the neonate should be monitored every 2 to 3 hours and, where necessary, intravenous infusions of glucose given.

4. Hypocalcemia may occur. A serum level of calcium below 8 mg/dl in the mature SGA infant and below 7 mg/dl in the premature SGA infant is diagnostic. Oral or intravenous calcium gluconate will correct the problem.

5. Polycythemia is three times more common in growth-retarded newborns than in normal babies. It results from the increased production of red blood cells in response to hypoxia, and from the transfer of blood from the placental to the fetal circulation in the face of intrauterine hypoxia.

6. Hypothermia is caused by the decreased amount of stored body fat secondary to intrauterine malnutrition. These babies must be kept warm.

7. Congenital anomalies are seen in 10 percent of IUGR infants. Included in this group are Trisomy 18 and 21, neural tube defects, and Potter syndrome.

8. The respiratory distress syndrome is seen rarely. The stressed fetus seems to develop advanced pulmonary maturity.

9. In the neonatal period most babies who do not have congenital anomalies or severe asphyxia do well.

10. Nutritional management should support growth, but there must be no preoccupation with the rapid attainment of "normal" weight.

11. The neurologic behavior fits the age rather than the size of the newborn infant.

Long-term Effects

The perinatal morbidity and mortality is increased, but the long-term prognosis remains unclear. The evidence is conflicting.

1. Growth: It appears that these infants can be expected to have normal growth curves. Several studies have shown a pattern of catch-up to normal levels by 2 years of age.

2. Neurologic sequelae: This issue remains unresolved. A significant number of these children have long-term problems of
minimal cerebral dysfunction. Included are emotional malad-
justment, impaired hearing, decreased coordination and motor
skills, poor speech, reduced reading ability, and generally poor
performance at school. Major neurologic sequelae are less
common. The root of the problem is believed to be hypoxic
insults suffered during the intrapartum or the immediate neonatal period.

POSTTERM (POSTDATES, PROLONGED) PREGNANCY

In calculating the expected date of confinement, the Naegele rule is
that term is reached 40 weeks (280 days) after the first day of the last
normal menstrual period. This is based on the belief that conception
takes place on about the 14th day of the cycle. In many instances the
exact date of conception is not known.

By definition postterm pregnancy is one that has lasted 42 weeks
(294 days) or more. Included in this group are 12 percent of all pregnancies. The number of pregnancies that go to or past 43 weeks is 4 percent.
In many instances of suspected postterm pregnancy the gestation is not
as advanced as the patient believes.

Reasons for errors associated with the Naegele rule include these:

1. The menstrual history is unreliable. Many women do not remember when the last menstruation began.
2. Women whose cycle is longer than 28 days or whose ovulation is
late may deliver after the expected date.
3. Even under normal conditions the length of pregnancy varies.
4. Women have been known to falsify the menstrual history for social reasons.

Assuming that the expected date of confinement is known accurately, the following questions must be answered:

1. Does postterm pregnancy add any risk to mother and child?
2. At what stage do these dangers play a part?
3. How do they compare with the problems of artificial termination of the pregnancy?

Fetal Size and Condition

1. Most babies are of normal health and size.
2. A number of fetuses keep on growing, and the incidence of large

babies (over 4000 g) is higher than infants born at 40 weeks. This suggests that most fetuses remain well nourished. The large size may lead to disproportion and dystocia.

3. Fetal postmaturity: At birth about 5 percent of infants show signs of dysmaturity, being small, undernourished, and asphyxiated. This is a consequence of a reduction in the respiratory and nutritive functions of the aging placenta.

Fetal Mortality

Perinatal mortality and morbidity are increased in prolonged pregnancy. Quoted figures vary, but the probable rates of fetal death at 43 weeks are two, at 44 weeks three, and at 45 weeks five times that of babies born at term. The increased mortality is not confined to the malnourished postterm infant with the postmaturity syndrome, but occurs also in the infant whose growth appears to be normal. The highest perinatal mortality is found in elderly primigravidas. Fetal death may occur during pregnancy and in the neonatal period, but the highest incidence is during labor and delivery.

Recent studies have not confirmed the belief that the fetus has a special intolerance to labor in that there appears to be no greatly increased incidence of variable or late decelerations of the fetal heart rate (FHR). In most cases the postterm fetus tolerates labor well, and fetal death is an infrequent event. The majority of deaths do occur during labor, however, and can take place without warning. It may be that the placenta has sufficient reserve to support continued growth of the fetus in most women, but in some cases it is not enough to withstand the stress of labor.

The postterm woman must be monitored carefully and even minor signs of fetal distress must be taken seriously. There is no need for over-aggressiveness in anticipation of intrauterine hypoxia, however, and no justification for intervention during labor unless signs of fetal distress are documented.

Therapeutic Rationale

Some authorities advise that, because of the dangers of placental insufficiency, every pregnancy should be terminated at 42 weeks by whatever method is feasible.

Others disagree, pointing out that the diagnosis is often uncertain, that the dangers of prolonged pregnancy have been exaggerated, and that the hazards of induction under unfavorable conditions, such as an unripe cervix, are greater than those of delay. The latter is a real problem in that, in a number of cases of proven prolonged pregnancy, the cervix is unfavorable for induction. This is one of the reasons why routine induction of labor is unsuccessful so frequently.

While prolongation of pregnancy beyond 42 weeks may have an adverse effect on neonatal outcome in some cases, fetal death is rare. Induction of labor does not improve the results. What the latter practice does achieve is an increase in the rate of cesarean section because of failed induction. An uncomplicated postterm pregnancy is not an indication for the induction of labor. Early delivery is necessary only when tests of fetal health show that deterioration is taking place.

The situation is not ignored, however. Tests for fetal well-being are performed as soon as the diagnosis of postterm pregnancy is made, and repeated as often as necessary until the baby is born.

Investigation: Tests of Fetal Well-being

1. Clinical assessment to determine the true expected date of confinement.
    a. Menstrual history.
    b. Date of quickening and first auscultation of fetal heart.
    c. Size of uterus, height of fundus, abdominal girth.
    d. Ripeness of cervix
    e. Station of presenting part.
    f. Estimation of fetal size.
2. Fetal movement counts by the mother.
3. Nonstress test. A reactive result suggests that the fetus is in no danger for a week. The absence of a beat-to-beat variation in the fetal heart rate is an ominous sign.
4. Contraction stress test.
5. Biophysical profile.
6. Oligohydramnios, shown clearly by ultrasonogram, is more common in prolonged than in term pregnancy.
    a. It may be a sign of postmaturity.
    b. It carries with it the danger of compression of the umbilical cord.
    c. If meconium is passed, the reduced amount of amniotic fluid cannot dilute it effectively, and the danger of aspiration of thick meconium is increased.
7. Meconium in amniotic fluid: amnioscopy or amniocentesis. It is the opinion of some workers that meconium in the amniotic fluid is an ominous sign of fetal distress in the postterm pregnancy, that amniocentesis should be performed, and that, if meconium is present, the fetus should be delivered immediately.

While the passage of meconium is increased in postterm pregnancy, the significance is not known. It may well be that this is merely a sign of fetal maturity. Recent studies suggest that the search for meconium is of little value in the management of prolonged pregnancy, that the presence of meconium does not correlate well with a positive contraction stress test, and that there is no increase in perinatal death rates when meconium is present—as long as the other tests of fetal well-being are normal. The only real danger of the passage of meconium appears to be that of aspiration.

Management of Uncomplicated Postterm Pregnancy (Fig. 2)

Ripe Cervix
Induce labor.

Unripe Cervix

1. Monitor patient.
   a. Clinical examination: condition of the cervix twice weekly.
   b. Fetal movement count daily.
   c. Nonstress test twice weekly.
   d. Biophysical profile twice weekly.
2. If cervix ripens: induce labor.
3. Reactive (normal) NST: Allow pregnancy to go on until the cervix ripens or labor begins. Repeat NST twice weekly.
4. Nonreactive NST (abnormal).
   a. Repeat NST.
   b. Biophysical profile.
   c. Consider contraction stress test.
5. Tests are normal: Repeat NST and/or biophysical profile twice weekly.
6. Tests are abnormal: The pregnancy should be terminated.
   a. Induction of labor:
      i. Prostaglandin E_2 tablets (2 to 4 mg) in the posterior fornix of the vagina in the evening.
      ii. Oxytocin infusion and artificial rupture of membranes next morning.
   b. Cesarean section:
      i. Termination of pregnancy is urgent.
      ii. Abnormal presentation, e.g., breech.
      iii. Failure of induction.

Management of Complicated Postterm Pregnancy

In certain conditions the fetus is at high risk and the pregnancy should not go postterm. Included here are

1. Patients over 40 years of age
2. Patients with hypertension
3. Patients with diabetes
4. Previous unexplained stillbirth or neonatal death
5. Intrauterine growth retardation
6. Sensitized pregnancy in a woman who is Rh negative

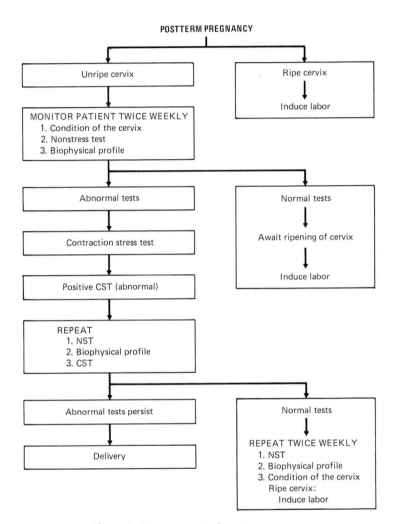

Figure 2. Management of postterm pregnancy.

Management of Labor

1. The fetus is at risk and careful monitoring of the fetal heart rate is essential.
2. An intravenous infusion should be in place.
3. The patient should lie on her side to obviate pressure on the large blood vessels, and so improve uterine perfusion.
4. Excessive sedation should be avoided.
5. Prolonged labor is dangerous; cesarean section should be considered after 12 hours if good progress is not being made.
6. Because there is an increased risk of fetal death during labor, any sign of fetal distress calls for the immediate delivery of the baby.

ANTEPARTUM FETAL DEATH

Fetal death after the 20th week of pregnancy accounts for half of the total perinatal mortality.

Etiology

1. Idiopathic. In half the cases no cause can be found, even after thorough investigation including autopsy.
2. Maternal complications.
   a. Preeclampsia.
   b. Bleeding disorders: abruptio placentae and placenta previa.
   c. Diabetes.
3. Fetal diseases.
   a. Congenital anomalies.
   b. Erythroblastosis.
   c. Infection following premature rupture of membranes.

Diagnosis

Symptoms

1. Cessation of fetal movement is often the first indication.
2. Disappearance of gestational symptoms.
3. Cessation of growth.
4. Decrease in size and tenderness of breasts.

Signs

1. Absence of fetal heart tones.
2. No palpable fetal movement.

3. Size of uterus is smaller than expected for length of gestation.
4. Ultrasonic techniques:
    a. Absence of fetal pulse.
    b. Loss of clarity of the outline of the body.
    c. An increase in the number of echos coming from within the fetal body.
    d. The fetal skull collapses between 5 and 10 days after death and the outline of the skull becomes irregular.
    e. Failure of fetal growth is demonstrable on serial films.
    f. Some weeks after death the fetal body becomes so disorganized that no internal structures can be recognized.
5. X-ray of the abdomen (see Chapter 38):
    a. Loss of fetal tone.
    b. Spalding sign: overlapping of the cranial bones.
    c. Gas in the fetus: heart, aorta, portal veins, umbilical arteries.
    d. Halo sign.
6. Failure of uterine growth noted on repeated examinations.
7. Decrease in the height of the fundus may result from collapse of the fetus and reduction in the volume of amniotic fluid.
8. Negative pregnancy test. The test may remain positive for variable times after fetal death. A week is not unusual.
9. Maternal excretion of estriol falls to undetectable levels 24 to 48 hours after fetal death.

Management

Expectant
Spontaneous labor and delivery will take place within 2 weeks of fetal death in 75 percent and by 3 weeks in 90 percent of patients. For this reason and because, in the past, attempts to induce labor by artificial rupture of membranes and infusion of oxytocin, in the presence of an unripe cervix, led to failure, hemorrhage, and intrauterine infection, many obstetricians preferred to wait until spontaneous labor began or until the cervix was favorable for induction.

Active
Because carrying a dead baby causes severe emotional stress for a woman, because of the risk of the development of hypofibrinogenemia, and because more effective methods of induction of labor are available today, most physicians prefer to terminate the pregnancy as soon as the diagnosis of fetal death is certain.

1. First trimester of pregnancy: Dilatation of the cervix and aspiration-curettage is the method of choice.

2. Second trimester: Abdominal amniocentesis and the injection of prostaglandin $F_{2\alpha}$, urea, or hypertonic saline into the amniotic sac will induce labor. Delivery occurs by between 20 and 40 hours. (See Chapter 41 for details of the technique.)
3. Third trimester:
   a. Ripe cervix. Whenever the cervix is favorable for induction, and there are no contraindications to its use, an infusion of oxytocin may be used to start labor. (See Chapter 41 for details of the technique.)
   b. Unripe cervix. Prostaglandin E_2 tablets (2 to 4 mg) are placed in the vagina in the evening to ripen the cervix. If labor has not begun by next morning, an oxytocin infusion is set up and amniotomy performed. (See Chapter 41 for technique.)

As long as good postpartum uterine contraction and retraction are maintained by an infusion of a solution of oxytocin of adequate strength, bleeding in the presence of reduced levels of fibrinogen is not a problem. The level of fibrinogen returns to normal within a few hours after delivery.

Complications

Disseminated Intravascular Coagulation
Prolonged retention of a dead fetus may lead to the development of a hemorrhagic diathesis. The sequence of events is believed to be as follows: Thromboplastin from degenerating fetal tissues is released into the maternal circulation. This causes maternal intravascular clotting and a reduction of the levels of fibrinogen in the maternal blood. It is unlikely that hypofibrinogenemia will develop before 4 to 6 weeks after fetal death has occurred. Even so, weekly measurements of the levels of fibrinogen should be made once fetal death has been diagnosed.

When the so-called dead fetus syndrome develops, active bleeding may occur at the time of delivery, and sometimes fibrinogen is needed. In such cases the need can be met better by administering cryoprecipitate rather than fibrinogen. If hemorrhage occurs whole blood should be given to restore the volume and to replace fibrinogen.

TERM INTRAPARTUM FETAL DEATH

Babies may die during labor. The definition of the term intrapartum fetal death includes the following: (1) documentation of fetal heart tones after the onset of labor, (2) birth weight over 2500 g, (3) gestation of 37 to 40 weeks, and (4) no sign of life after delivery of the child.

On an etiologic basis two large groups are noted. In half the cases there is a definite and acceptable explanation. In the rest there is no clearly defined cause of the fetal death, but associated conditions are present which may have played a part. The presence of these situations should prewarn the obstetrician to expect trouble.

1. Definite cause of death
   a. Difficult and traumatic delivery
   b. Prolapse of the cord
   c. Abruptio placentae
   d. Congenital anomalies incompatible with life
   e. Rh sensitization
   f. Ruptured uterus
2. Concomitant problems
   a. Highly significant conditions
      i. Prolonged gestation
      ii. Premature rupture of membranes
      iii. Tight cord around the neck
      iv. Paracervical block anesthesia
   b. Mildly significant conditions
      i. Intrapartum fever
      ii. Toxemia of pregnancy
      iii. Maternal hypotension
      iv. Breech (which easy labor and delivery)
      v. Abnormal sugar tolerance

BIBLIOGRAPHY

Gill DMF, Cardozo LD, Studd JWW, et al: Prolonged pregnancy: Is induction of labor indicated? A prospective study. Brit J Obstet Gynaecol 89:292, 1982

Harris BA, Huddleston JF, Sutliff G, Perlis HW: The unfavorable cervix in prolonged pregnancy. Obstet Gynecol 62:171, 1983

Kazzi GM, Gross TL, Sokol RJ, Kazzi NJ: Detection of intrauterine growth retardation: A new use for sonographic placental grading. Am J Obstet Gynecol 145:733, 1983

Miller FC, Read JA: Intrapartum assessment of the postdate fetus. Am J Obstet Gynecol 141:516, 1981

Perkins RP: Sudden fetal death in labor: The significance of antecedent monitoring characteristics and clinical circumstances. J Reprod Med 25: 309, 1980

Rayburn WF, Motley ME, Stempel LE, et al: Antepartum prediction of the postmature infant. Obstet Gynecol 60:148, 1982

43

Preterm Labor

Mary D'Alton

In 1948 the First World Health Assembly proposed that the definition of prematurity be based on a birthweight of less than 2500 grams. Since then the realization has come that birthweight may be quite discrepant from gestational age. In 1961 the Expert Committee of Maternal and Child Health of the World Health Organization recommended that the term "premature" be reserved for infants born before 37 weeks and that those infants born weighing less than 2500 g should be called "low birthweight." Many studies, however, continued to define prematurity as a birthweight of less than 2500 g. Because birthweight can be measured accurately, this practice is understandable, but it is important to remember that 15 percent of infants born after 37 weeks gestation will weigh less than 2500 g.

DEFINITION OF PRETERM LABOR

Labor is defined as the onset of regular uterine contractions accompanied by progressive dilatation and effacement of the cervix and descent of the fetal presenting part. Labor is preterm when it occurs in a patient whose period of gestation is less than 37 completed weeks (less than 259 days) from the first day of the last menstrual period. Preterm labor presents many challenges and the first one involves its diagnosis.

Among the problems that arise from a definition as simple as the one given above, is the need to make a clinical decision whether true preterm labor is in progress, whether pharmacologic agents should be given to inhibit labor, and/or whether steroid drugs should be prescribed to induce maturation of the fetal lungs. At the present time there is no certain objective way of identifying those contractions that will lead to changes in the cervix. If pharmacologic inhibition of preterm labor is to be effective, it must be instituted early. This poses a dilemma. On the one hand, if one elects to withhold therapy until the evidence in favor of labor is strong, such as progressive cervical dilatation, the process may advance to a degree where therapy is unlikely to be effective. On the other hand, unnecessary drug therapy with potentially harmful effects to mother and/or the fetus is unwarranted if there is only marginal evidence of preterm labor.

Diagnosis of Preterm Labor

In order to avoid unnecessary treatment, the following criteria are used in making a diagnosis of preterm labor in patients who have completed between 20 and 36 weeks of gestation:

1. Uterine contractions are occurring at a rate of four in 20 minutes or eight in 60 minutes.
2. The cervix is dilated to 2 cm or is effaced at least 80 percent.
3. Serial examinations, preferably by the same observer, reveal changes in the cervix.
4. The membranes are ruptured.

Significance of Preterm Labor

Preterm labor resulting in delivery before gestational age of 37 weeks accounts for 6 to 8 percent of all deliveries, but is associated with 75 percent of all perinatal deaths. The problem of preterm labor and delivery has grown as the incidence of other causes of perinatal morbidity and mortality has decreased. Over the past 20 years, with the advent of newborn special care units, there have been dramatic improvements in the neonatal survival rates of premature infants. To put this in historic perspective, the list that Hess compiled in 1922 of all known survivors of infants born weighing less than 1120 g comprised less than half a page. In 1973 Lubchenko and co-workers reported a 56 percent perinatal mortality for infants weighing 1001 to 1500 g, and only 10 percent of infants weighing less than 1000 g survived. Now the majority of infants born beyond 28 weeks' gestation do survive. Among the survivors of preterm birth, however, approximately 10 percent suffer from a permanent major handicap. The financial and emotional costs of newborn intensive care are staggering. Higher still are the costs of long-term care for the handicapped children, including institutionalization and special educational programs for those that are severely disabled.

Despite the progress in the field of perinatal medicine, the prematurity rate has not changed in North America over the last decade. Any intervention capable of preventing preterm labor or any therapy capable of postponing preterm delivery is potentially of great benefit in reducing perinatal mortality and morbidity and neurologic handicap of perinatal origin.

ETIOLOGY OF PRETERM LABOR

Idiopathic

In the majority of cases the cause of preterm labor remains unknown.

Fetal Factors

1. *Premature rupture of membranes (PROM):* Rupture of the membranes an hour before the onset of labor complicates 10 percent of pregnancies at term and 30 percent of preterm labors. In over 80 percent of patients with PROM the etiology cannot be ascertained.
2. *Multiple pregnancy:* McKeown and Record found the average duration of pregnancy to be 280.5 days for singleton pregnancies, 261.6 days for twins, 246.8 days for triplets, and 236.8 days for quadruplets.
3. *Polyhydramnios:* The incidence of polyhydramnios varies between 0.4 and 1.6 percent of all pregnancies. Approximately one-third of patients with polyhydramnios have a preterm delivery.
4. *Fetal anomalies:* Gross fetal anomalies, especially those associated with polyhydramnios (anencephaly), or with oligohydramnios (renal agenesis), are accompanied by an increased likelihood of preterm labor.

Maternal Factors

1. *Maternal disease*
   a. Pregnancy-induced hypertension: Although in itself, hypertension may not cause preterm labor, it may be of such severity to necessitate elective preterm delivery for maternal and/or fetal benefit.
   b. Renal disease: Acute pyelonephritis is associated with an increased incidence of preterm delivery, especially when associated with high fever.
   c. Appendicitis: This is an infrequent but serious complication

of pregnancy and is associated with preterm labor. Two theories are present to explain this relationship, namely, uterine irritation from the adjacent inflamed organ and, secondly, release of bacterial endotoxins with elevation of temperature.

2. *Structural defects of the uterus:* Some uterine anomalies are associated with preterm labor and delivery. Women whose mothers were given diethylstilbesterol while pregnant have a higher incidence of midtrimester preterm labor.

3. *Cervical incompetence:* The exact percentage of preterm labors and deliveries resulting from cervical incompetence is uncertain, but is probably small.

4. *History of preterm labor:* A strong correlation exists between past reproductive performance and preterm labor. A history of one previous preterm birth is associated with a recurrence risk varying from 25 to 50 percent and the risk increases with each succeeding preterm delivery.

5. *History of abortion:* The effect of prior induced abortion on subsequent pregnancy remains controversial. Studies from Hungary and Britain have reported significant increases in the prematurity rate following induced abortions. A North American study, however, has shown no deleterious effect. Whether different abortion techniques are responsible for these disparate results is unclear. Until this question is resolved it is prudent to consider the patient with previous abortions, especially with multiple abortions, at risk for preterm delivery.

6. *Socioeconomic status:* The number of preterm births rises with declining socioeconomic status. Important factors in this group include:
   a. Poor nutrition.
   b. Inadequate prenatal care.
   c. Low maternal age.
   d. Heavy work.

7. *Maternal smoking:* A number of reports describe a direct relationship between smoking and preterm births.

Placental Factors

1. *Antepartum hemorrhage:* Placenta previa and premature separation of the placenta have an incidence of preterm delivery four to five times the normal rate.

2. *Placental insufficiency:* Occasionally, when the supply of nutrients reaching the fetus is inadequate, preterm labor takes place.

PREVENTION OF PRETERM LABOR

Despite the introduction of pharmacologic agents to treat preterm labor, there is only minimal evidence that these interventions have actually decreased the number of births ending before 37 completed weeks of gestation. As with any medical problem, it is more desirable to have some method of preventing preterm labor rather than treating it once it is present.

Identification of the Patient at Risk

The first step in preventing preterm labor is to identify the patients at risk. These have been described above. High risk scoring systems are useful in helping to pick out those patients who require special observation and care.

General Measures

1. *Prenatal care:* An important feature of prenatal care is the ensuring that the diet is balanced and adequate. Epidemiologic data implicate poor nutrition as a causal factor in preterm delivery.
2. *Exercise:* While there is no evidence that mild exercise is harmful, overexertion should be avoided during pregnancy, especially in the high-risk patient.
3. *Smoking:* Patients should be encouraged to give up smoking. It is implicated in preterm delivery and is a cause of low birthweight.
4. *Coitus:* Semen is rich in prostaglandins and their presence in the vagina may cause uterine activity. Uterine contractions often follow orgasm. While coitus is not contraindicated in normal pregnancy, it may be worthwhile to curtail sexual activity in patients identified as being at risk for preterm labor.
5. *Patient education:* Instruction of the patient as to the subtle signs and symptoms of preterm labor, e.g., low backache, menstrual-like cramps, unusual vaginal discharge, and diarrhea may help to identify preterm labor at an earlier stage, and thus offer a better chance of successful therapy. Patients should be encouraged to communicate with their doctor if they experience any of these signs and symptoms.
6. *Vaginitis and cervicitis:* Local infection may play a role in the etiology of preterm labor and premature rupture of the mem-

branes. In these patients cultures should be performed and adequate therapy prescribed.

7. *Urinary tract infections:* Pyelonephritis is associated with an increased incidence of preterm labor. Asymptomatic bacteriuria is a forerunner of pyelonephritis and should be eradicated.

8. *Acute febrile illness:* Any sickness causing high fever may lead to preterm labor, and must be treated promptly and vigorously.

9. *Medical complications:* Conditions, such as pregnancy-induced hypertension and diabetes, require careful evaluation and control. This will obviate the need for elective preterm delivery in many cases.

Specific Measures

1. *Bed rest:* For most illnesses bed rest is a recommended part of therapy. There is no proof, however, that rest in bed can prevent the initiation of preterm labor. Most of the studies have been concerned with multiple pregnancy. Since it is a harmless intervention and may be of benefit, however, it is reasonable to advise bed rest for patients at high risk for preterm birth.

2. *Pharmacologic agents:*
   a. Tocolytic drugs: Beta-adrenergic agents have been employed with increasing frequency for the prevention of preterm labor in high-risk patients. They have not, however, been shown to be of value in preventing preterm delivery in multiple gestations.
   b. Hormones: A double-blind study using 17 beta-hydroxyprogesterone caproate in selected patients at high risk for preterm labor demonstrated encouraging results. Patients with a history of two abortions, two preterm births, or a combination of abortion and preterm birth were given either weekly injections of 17 beta-hydroxyprogesterone caproate or no treatment. Preterm delivery did not occur in the 18 patients receiving the progestational agent, whereas 9 of the 22 control patients had a preterm delivery. Larger trials are necessary to substantiate this. It should be remembered that progestin usage in the first trimester has been linked with anomalous fetal development. Although the use of progestin in the last half of pregnancy has not been implicated, the long-term safety has not been assessed fully.

3. *Special antenatal care:* A clinical evaluation of a program for preventing preterm birth was conducted at the University of California at San Francisco. The program included scoring and assigning patients according to their risk of having preterm de-

livery. Patients were educated about the subtle signs and symptoms of preterm labor. Those patients at high risk were followed weekly in a high-risk clinic. In-service education of the obstetric staff was also included in the program. The data indicated that during the year under review a significant decrease in the incidence of preterm delivery occurred when compared with previous experience in the same department. There was no control group in the study. Although the data are encouraging, historic comparisons when a new intervention is introduced are often inaccurate. Subsequent studies, hopefully, will prove more conclusively that this simple intervention of patient and provider education and frequent antenatal assessments will reduce the incidence of preterm labor.

4. *Cerclage of the incompetent cervix.*

INCOMPETENT INTERNAL CERVICAL OS

Clinical Picture

Some women with a history of repeated midtrimester abortions have an incompetent cervix. The internal os undergoes painless dilatation and is unable to maintain the pregnancy. The membranes bulge through the cervix, rupture, and a short, relatively painless labor ensues. The fetus is usually alive at birth, but is too premature to survive.

Etiology of Incompetent Cervix

1. Cervical trauma, previous pregnancy, or overdilatation of cervix at the time of curettage
2. Cervical surgery, e.g., cone biopsy
3. Congenital abnormalities
4. Idiopathic

Diagnosis of Incompetent Cervix

The diagnosis, difficult to establish with certainty, is based on history supported by examination of the cervix.

History
Previous midtrimester delivery following spontaneous rupture of the membranes, and associated with painless dilatation of the cervix is suggestive of cervical incompetence.

Examination of the Cervix

1. *Nonpregnant state*
   a. Hegar dilator: The ability to pass a No. 8 Hegar dilator through the internal os of the cervix in the nonpregnant patient is suggestive of, but does not prove, cervical incompetence.
   b. Hysterosalpingogram: This examination may show that the diameter of the os of the cervix is more than 8 mm.
2. *During pregnancy*
   a. Digital examination of the cervix: The finding of painless progressive dilatation in the second trimester where no other etiologic factors exist suggests the diagnosis of cervical incompetence.
   b. Ultrasonography: Two techniques of ultrasonic scanning have been used to detect cervical dilatation: Abdominal sector scanning may demonstrate dilatation of the cervix in some cases, but it fails to show the internal os and the cervical canal in others. It is thought that an internal os greater than 20 mm in diameter is abnormal. A new method is perineal scanning by the placement of the ultrasonic transducer on the perineum in a sterile glove. This method can demonstrate the internal os consistently, and can measure cervical dilatation. Although digital examination can provide information about dilatation and effacement, there is considerable interobserver variability. Perineal scanning is helpful occasionally to follow a patient who is thought to be at risk for an incompetent cervix.

Treatment of Incompetent Cervix

1. *Bed rest:* The rationale of this method of treatment is to help reduce the pressure of the uterine contents on the cervix. This form of therapy appears to be successful in some cases, but there is no proof that bed rest can prevent the onset of preterm labor. However, this is a harmless intervention, and, since it may do some good, it is reasonable to advise these patients to get as much rest as possible.
2. *Vaginal pessary:* This has had success on occasion. The idea is that, by changing the inclination of the cervical canal, the weight of the growing conceptus will be redistributed away from the internal os of the cervix.
3. *Cervical cerclage:* This is the predominant treatment at the present time. The aim of this procedure is to prevent the cervix

from dilating, to obviate the bulging and rupture of the membranes, and so to reduce the incidence of preterm labor and resultant prematurity. It must be emphasized that a prospective randomized trial has not yet been published to prove that cerclage is more effective than expectant management.

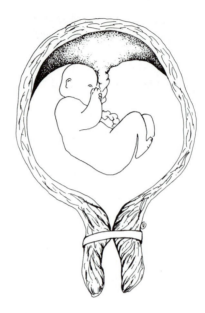

Figure 1. Cervical cerclage, McDonald method.

Cerclage Procedures

Two main types of cerclage are used. Both are effective, but the Mc-Donald technique is easier to perform.

1. *McDonald suture:* A purse-string suture is placed in the body of the cervix at the level of the internal os. The suture is tightened around the cervical canal and tied securely in front of the cervix. The suture materials that have been used include Mersilene, No. 2 proline, or No. 4 silk. The ends are left long enough to facilitate subsequent removal (Fig. 1).

2. *Shirodkar procedure:* This technique involves an incision in the anterior cervix, with advancement of the bladder, an incision in the posterior vaginal mucosa, and placement of a Mersilene suture submucosally between these two incisions. The suture is placed at the level of the internal os. The Mersilene is anchored with silk sutures. The mucosa is closed with chromic or vicryl sutures.

Timing of Cerclage

The classic time for cerclage has been at 14 to 16 weeks of gestation. The reason for this was that spontaneous abortion was unlikely to occur at this time, and the surgery could be done before the cervix dilated and

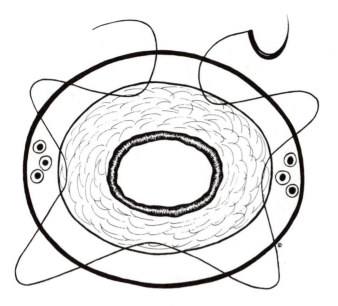

Figure 1. (cont.) Cervical cerclage, McDonald method.

effaced. Now, with ultrasound, a viable pregnancy can be demonstrated early in the first trimester and some obstetricians carry out the procedure at the 10th or 11th week. There is merit, however, in waiting until 14 to 16 weeks as ultrasound at this gestational age will not only confirm viability but will rule out some major congenital anomalies.

Although a cerclage may be placed in the nonpregnant state this offers no advantage.

Cerclage is not indicated after 28 weeks of pregnancy. Cervical manipulation at this time may cause preterm labor or premature rupture of the membranes, and bed rest is a more appropriate form of therapy at this gestational age.

Anesthesia for Cerclage

Conduction anesthesia is preferable. There is concern that general anesthesia may, at an early stage of pregnancy, cause fetal anomalies.

Postoperative Care

1. Bed rest for 24 hours is usual. The patient may have bathroom privileges.
2. There is no evidence that progestins, tocolytic drugs, or antibiotics are beneficial.

3. The patient is seen every 2 weeks for the remainder of her pregnancy and cervical examination is performed at each visit.
4. While there is no evidence that coitus is harmful after cerclage, many obstetricians advise against it.

Complications of Cerclage

1. *Intraoperative*
   a. Accidental rupture of membranes. This is more likely when, at the time of cerclage, the cervix is dilated and/or the membranes are bulging.
   b. Bleeding. Extensive bleeding may occur at the operative site. This is more common with the Shirodkar than with the Mc-Donald procedure.
2. *Early postoperative*
   a. Infection.
   b. Premature rupture of the membranes.
   c. Preterm labor.
      These complications are rare, but are potentially serious and call for the removal of the suture. Rupture of the uterus or laceration of the cervix may result if contractions are allowed to continue with cerclage in place.
3. *Late complication*
   a. Failure of the cervix to dilate during labor, caused by scarring at the site of the cerclage, is a rare complication. In most cases the cervix dilates rapidly.

Contraindications to Cerclage

1. Documented or suspected infection
2. Ruptured membranes
3. Vaginal bleeding
4. Uterine contractions
5. Fetal anomaly
6. Gestation of 28 weeks or more

Removal of Cerclage

Indicated

1. Labor
2. Rupture of membranes
3. Maternal or fetal infection
4. Vaginal bleeding

Elective. At 38 weeks' gestation the cerclage is removed and the onset of labor is awaited. The procedure is usually easy and no anesthesia is required.

TREATMENT OF PRETERM LABOR

General Measures

1. *Bed rest.* Lying down in the left lateral position is often successful in reducing the frequency and intensity of uterine contractions.
2. *Hydration.* An intravenous infusion of 500 ml Ringer lactate is given in 1 hour and then the intake is adjusted to 120 ml per hour.

Pharmacologic Control of Preterm Labor: Tocolysis

In considering pharmacologic treatment of preterm labor it is important to follow the old medical dictum *primum non nocere,* first do no harm. Before any attempt is made to arrest labor, it is mandatory to make certain that prolongation of the pregnancy is likely to be of benefit for the fetus and of no detriment to the mother. Only in the last 20 years have pharmacologic agents been used successfully to inhibit uterine contractions. The recognition of the tocolytic potential of the original agents used to inhibit premature labor, ethanol and isoxsuprine, occurred accidentally. Tocolytic agents developed in recent years have been synthesized specifically for this purpose.

To Treat or Not to Treat
The question as to whether pharmacologic agents should be used in the management of preterm labor has not been answered. These drugs are used widely, however, and those using them must be aware of the dangers to mother and fetus.

Reasons for Nontreatment
A number of authorities have advocated a hands-off policy for the following reasons:

1. Because of the inherent difficulties with the diagnosis of preterm labor, as many as 40 percent of patients will be treated unnecessarily.
2. In the few instances where randomized, controlled trials have

been carried out, tocolytic drugs have not been shown to be more effective than placebo.

3. All of the tocolytic drugs have adverse effects, some potentially serious, on the mother, fetus, and newborn.

General Contraindications to Tocolysis

1. *Maternal conditions requiring termination of the pregnancy*
   a. Severe hypertension, preeclampsia or eclampsia.
   b. Uncontrolled diabetes, especially with ketoacidosis.
   c. Chorioamnionitis.
   d. Severe vaginal bleeding, e.g., abruptio placentae.
2. *Fetal conditions*
   a. Fetal death.
   b. Fetal malformation incompatible with extrauterine survival.
   c. Fetal distress.
   d. Intrauterine growth retardation (IUGR).
3. *Gestational age.* When the pregnancy is over 34 weeks' duration, the fetal weight is over 2500 g, or pulmonary maturity is established, little is gained by prolonging the pregnancy. With special care in the nursery, the survival of premature infants in these groups is excellent.
4. *Imminent delivery.* Cervical dilatation greater than 4 to 5 cm renders attempts at tocolysis futile.

Available Agents

1. Betamimetic drugs
   a. Isoxsuprine (Vasodilan)
   b. Ritodrine (Yutopar)
   c. Terbutaline (Bricanyl)
2. Ethanol
3. Calcium antagonists
   a. Magnesium sulphate
   b. Nifedipine
4. Prostaglandin synthetase inhibitions
   a. Indomethacin
   b. Aspirin

Betamimetic Drugs

Mechanism of Action of Betamimetics
Adrenergic agents produce their effects by acting on two different receptors, the alpha adrenergic and the beta adrenergic. Myometrium

contains both alpha and beta receptors. Activation of the alpha-adrenergic receptors causes uterine contractions. In contrast, activation of the beta-adrenergic receptors inhibits uterine contractions. There is a subclassification of beta-adrenergic receptors into B_1 and B_2 receptors. B_1 receptors are dominant in the heart, adipose tissue, and intestine, while B_2 receptors are dominant in the blood vessels and uterus. Isoproterenol and epinephrine can decrease uterine activity but, because of their activation of both B_1 and B_2 receptors, their cardiovascular side effects limit their clinical use. B_2 agonists have a greater effect on the uterus than they have on the heart, and have made treatment of preterm labor a practical clinical consideration.

Eight beta agonists have been studied clinically in the treatment of preterm labor. Some general comments can be made which are true for all betamimetic agents.

The final step in contraction of the myometrium depends on the interaction between the contractile proteins, actin and myosin. This interaction is regulated by the intracellular calcium concentration. Serum ionized calcium is 10^{-3} M and is maintained within a narrow range. The intracellular calcium concentration is much lower than the serum calcium, and changes with contraction and relaxation of the uterus. In the relaxed myometrial cell the intracellular calcium concentration is 10^{-8}. The concentration must rise in excess of 10^{-7} M to initiate contractions. Thus the amount of free calcium available to the contractile apparatus determines whether the muscle contracts or relaxes. Calcium tends to enter the cell passively from sites of sequestration (mitochondria and sarcoplastic reticulum) and from the surrounding fluid. If the cell is to stay relaxed it must pump calcium back out again into the extracellular fluid or into the calcium storage areas. The calcium pump depends on cyclic AMP for energy which is formed from ATP in the presence of the enzyme adenylate cyclase.

Beta-adrenergic agents interact with surface receptors and activate adenylate cyclase. This increases the intracellular content of cyclic adenosine 3^1– 5^1 monophosphate (cyclic AMP). The increased level of cyclic AMP may initiate a series of cellular reactions providing energy for calcium extrusion from the cell and sequestration of calcium by intracellular storing mechanisms. The net result of this reaction is a reduction of free cytoplasmic calcium and inhibition of contractility. Cyclic AMP may also inhibit myosin light chain kinase thus diminishing the interaction between myosin and actin.

Contraindications to Betamimetic Drugs
In addition to the general contraindications listed previously, there are specific contraindications to the use of betamimetic agents.

Absolute Contraindications

    1. Maternal cardiac disease

Relative Contraindications. In the following conditions betamimetic drugs may be employed, but only with extreme caution and after thorough evaluation of the risk/benefit ratio:

    1. Uncontrolled diabetes mellitus
    2. Untreated hyperthyroidism
    3. Anemia

Preliminary Investigation

Before using betamimetic drugs the following tests should be performed:

    1. Urinalysis
    2. CBC and differential WBC
    3. Blood type
    4. Coagulation screen
    5. Blood glucose
    6. Electrolytes, BUN, creatinine
    7. Liver function tests
    8. Electrocardiogram

Management of Betamimetic Therapy

    1. *Pretreatment*
        a. Document uterine activity.
        b. Assess the cervix for effacement and dilatation.
        c. Determine whether the membranes are intact or ruptured.
        d. Maintain patient in bed with a lateral tilt to avoid supine hypotension.
        e. Infuse 500 ml of Ringer lactate in 1 hour.
        f. Then start the infusion of the betamimetic.
    2. *During treatment*
        a. The speed of the infusion is governed by the effect on uterine contractions and the side effects.
        b. The maternal pulse rate, blood pressure, and respirations are measured every 10 minutes while the speed of the infusion and the dosage are being regulated. Once a stable and effective dose is established, these measurements are repeated every 30 minutes until 1 hour after the infusion is discontinued.
        c. Nothing is given by mouth until 1 hour beyond the optimum

rate of infusion (rate at which the uterine contractions cease).

d. Intake and output of fluids is recorded accurately.

e. Blood glucose, potassium, and electrolytes are measured every 4 hours.

f. Continuous electronic fetal heart rate monitoring is carried on during therapy and for an hour afterwards.

g. If contractions are not controlled within 2 hours of starting therapy, or if they resume after having ceased, the cervix should be examined. If dilatation is taking place and delivery seems inevitable, the treatment must be discontinued to avoid harmful effects on the fetus.

Maternal Side Effects and Complications

1. *Cardiovascular*
   a. Tachycardia is common and is often accompanied by palpitations and nervousness.
   b. Hypotension, especially a decrease in the diastolic blood pressure.
   c. Elevation of pulse pressure.
   d. Increase in cardiac output by as much as 50 percent.
2. *Pulmonary edema.* This is a rare, but serious and even fatal problem. It is more likely to occur:
   a. When too much fluid is given and the cardiovascular system is overloaded. Total intake should be limited to between 1500 and 2000 ml of fluid and 4 to 6 g of sodium per day.
   b. When steroids are given concurrently to enhance fetal pulmonary maturity. These drugs can lead to the retention of sodium and water.
   c. When there is hypokalemia.
   d. In the presence of anemia.
   e. In patients with cardiac disease.
   f. In patients with multiple pregnancy.
3. *Metabolic*
   a. Increased levels of serum glucose. In diabetic patients betamimetic drugs may precipitate decompensation of the diabetic status and lead to ketoacidosis, requiring an increase in the dose of insulin. The problem is increased when glucocorticoids are administered concurrently.
   b. Increase in pyruvate.
   c. Increase in lactate.
   d. Decrease in serum potassium.
   e. Decrease in serum iron.

Fetal and Neonatal Effects

1. *Cardiovascular.* The fetal heart rate is increased.
2. *Pulmonary.* There is a suggestion that the incidence of the respiratory distress syndrome may be lower when the mother has been treated with a betamimetic drug.
3. *Metabolic*
   a. Neonatal hypoglycemia.
   b. Neonatal hypokalemia.
   These effects are more common when the infant is born sooner than 5 hours after the drug has been discontinued.

Discontinuation of Therapy: Indications

1. *Unacceptable side effects*
   a. Hypotension.
   b. Tachyarrhythmia.
   c. Chest pain.
   d. Pulmonary edema.
2. *Failure of therapy.* Persistance of labor when maximum dosage is being given.

Isoxsuprine (Vasodilan)

Isoxsuprine is a derivative of catecholamine. It is a potent inhibitor of all types of nonvascular smooth muscle.

Isoxsuprine was the first drug subjected to clinical study as a tocolytic agent. While no adequate randomized controlled trials have been carried out, several series report prolongation of gestation by more than 7 days.

Administration

1. Intravenous
   a. Isoxsuprine, 80 to 160 mg, is mixed in 500 ml of Ringer lactate.
   b. The initial dose is 0.1 mg per minute.
   c. The rate is increased by 0.1 mg per minute every 10 minutes until the contractions cease or the side effects become unacceptable.
   d. The usual effective dose is 0.25 to 0.5 mg per minute.
   e. The maximum dose is 0.9 mg per minute.
   f. The infusion is maintained for 12 hours after the contractions cease.
   g. Once labor has been controlled the rate of infusion is reduced

to two-thirds of the maintenance dose for 4 hours, one-third
for 4 hours, and then discontinued.
   h. Oral therapy is commenced 1 hour before the rate of the infu-
      sion is reduced.
2. Intramuscular or subcutaneous: Neither is recommended today.
3. Oral: After the intravenous infusion has been terminated isoxsuprine is given by mouth in a dose of 5 to 20 mg every 3 to 4
   hours until tocolysis is no longer necessary.

Complications

1. *Maternal:* Tachycardia occurs in 30 to 50 percent of women and
   severe hypotension in 10 percent. In the latter case the rate of
   the infusion must be reduced or discontinued. The incidence and
   degree of hypotension is greater with isoxsuprine than with
   other agents.
2. *Fetal and neonatal:* The problems are rare, but include tachycardia, hypotension, hypoglycemia, hypocalcemia, and necrotizing
   enterocolitis. These conditions are worse when the interval between discontinuance of the therapy and delivery is short.

Ritodrine (Yutopar)

Ritodrine hydrochloride was developed specifically for obstetric use. Its
predominant effects are on the beta-2 receptors and, hence, the cardiovascular side effects are less than those of isoxsuprine. A prospective
randomized trial in the United States of a comparison between ritodrine, ethanol, and placebo suggested that there was in the patients
treated with ritodrine:

1. A significant reduction in the incidence of neonatal death and
   respiratory distress syndrome (RDS)
2. A significantly higher proportion of infants achieving 36 weeks'
   gestation or a birthweight greater than 2500 g
3. A significant improvement in gestational age at delivery and in
   the number of days gained in utero

These results contributed to ritrodrine becoming the first drug ap-
proved by the FDA for the treatment of preterm labor in the United
States.

Administration

1. Intravenous
   a. Ritrodrine, 150 mg, is added to 500 ml of Ringer lactate.
   b. The initial dose is 0.1 mg per minute.

    c. The rate is increased by 0.05 mg per minute every 10 minutes until the contractions cease or the side effects are unacceptable.

    d. The effective dose lies between 0.15 and 0.35 mg per minute.

    e. The maximum recommended dose is 0.35 mg per minute.

    f. The infusion is continued for 12 hours after the uterine contractions cease.

2. Intramuscular or subcutaneous routes: These are not recommended at the present time.

3. Oral: This route is used for maintenance. Ten mg is given 30 minutes before the infusion is discontinued, 10 mg every 2 hours for 24 hours, followed by 10 to 20 mg every 4 hours until the need for tocolysis no longer exists.

Terbutaline (Bricanyl)

Terbutaline is a selective beta-2 stimulator, and appears to be effective in depressing uterine contractions. Maternal tachycardia is common, but other side effects seem to be minimal, and the drug is tolerated well.

Administration

1. Intravenous
    a. Terbutaline, 5 mg, is placed into a 100-ml container and 95 ml of normal saline is added. The concentration is 5 mg (50 µg) per 100 ml. This solution is added to 500 ml of Ringer lactate.

    b. The infusion is commenced at a rate of 10 µg per minute, and increased in increments of 5 µg per minute until the contractions cease or unacceptable side effects appear.

    c. The maximal rate of infusion is 50 µg per minute.

    d. If effective, the infusion is continued for 6 hours.

2. Subcutaneous
    a. The dose is 0.25 mg every 4 hours either a half hour before stopping the intravenous infusion or upon its completion.

    b. The subcutaneous administration is continued for 24 hours.

3. Oral
    a. The dose is 2.5 mg every 4 to 6 hours until tocolysis is no longer required.

Other Beta-sympathomimetic Agents

Included here are orciprenaline, nylidrine, fenetrol, salbutamol, and heroprenaline. These are in clinical use in various parts of the world.

The ideal beta agonist is one that is totally uteroselective, but this drug has not yet been found.

Ethanol

Mode of Action
Ethanol has an inhibiting effect on the release of oxytocin from the neurohypophysis, and this is the most probable explanation for its inhibitory action on the contractions of the pregnant uterus.

Efficacy
In controlled studies against placebo, ethanol has been shown to be more effective in approximately two-thirds of cases of preterm labor when the membranes are intact. When it was used as a control in clinical trials of betamimetic agents, however, ethanol was found to be less efficacious in all studies. Because of maternal and fetal side effects of ethanol and greater efficacy of other tocolytic agents, the use of ethanol in the treatment of preterm labor has decreased considerably.

Administration
The route is by intravenous infusion of a 10 percent solution of ethanol. The dose is 7.5 mg per kg of body weight per hour for 2 hours then 1.5 mg per kg of body weight for 10 hours. If contractions recur one or two additional courses can be employed.

Side Effects

1. *Maternal*
   a. Symptoms of intoxication: headache, restlessness, vomiting, and coma
   b. Aspiration pneumonia
   c. Lactic acidosis
2. *Fetal*
   a. An increased incidence of low Apgar scores
   b. A greater incidence of respiratory depression
   c. Muscular hypotonia

Ethanol crosses the placenta readily, reaching a fetal concentration equal to that of the mother rapidly. The level of activity of alcohol dehydrogenase in the newborn liver is low, and this results in slow elimination of the drug by the newborn infant. The effects are more marked if the drug has been given less than 12 hours prior to delivery.

Calcium Antagonists

Magnesium Sulphate

Mode of Action. The likely explanation is that magnesium sulphate acts by preventing the influx of calcium into the myometrial cell, thus keeping the intracellular concentration of calcium low and the uterus in a relaxed state.

Efficacy. Magnesium sulphate has been used with success in the management of preterm labor, but its effectiveness is no greater than other agents.

Administration. The route is intravenous.

1. A loading dose of 4 g of magnesium sulphate ($MgSO_4$) in 250 ml of Ringer lactate is infused over 20 minutes.
2. For maintenance 40 g of magnesium sulphate in a liter of Ringer lactate is infused at a rate of 50 ml per hour to achieve a dose of 2 g per hour.
3. Serum levels of 4 to 8 mg per ml are needed to achieve inhibition of uterine activity.
4. If effective, therapy is continued for 24 to 48 hours.

Side Effects

1. Maternal
   a. Patellar reflexes disappear at a level of 10 mEq/liter.
   b. Respiratory depression occurs at 12 to 15 mEq/liter.
   c. Cardiac arrest may take place when the level is over 15 mEq/liter.
2. Fetal: Magnesium crosses the placenta readily, and fetal and maternal levels are similar.
   a. Loss of beat-to-beat variability may be observed in the fetal heart rate tracing.
   b. Neonatal respiratory depression is seen if the level of magnesium in the blood is elevated.

Nifedipine

Nifedipine is one of a new class of drugs, i.e., slow channel calcium blockers. They are used to treat a variety of conditions, including angina associated with atherosclerotic coronary artery disease and spasm of the coronary arteries. Because calcium plays a pivotal role in myometrial contractions, and because calcium channel blockers have been shown to reduce myometrial activity, these drugs have been investigated in the management of preterm labor. Their mode of action is probably at the cell membrane, where they inhibit the influx of calcium through slow channels.

Nifedipine has been shown to arrest uterine contractions in isolated strips of myometrium and in healthy menstruating women, and to decrease the intensity of contractions induced by the administration of prostaglandin $F_{2\alpha}$ and prostaglandin E_2. It has been shown to inhibit myometrial activity induced by prostaglandin $F_{2\alpha}$ and oxytocin in the postpartum uterus.

The route of administration is oral. Nifedipine is absorbed rapidly and completely. The peak concentration occurs between 15 and 90 minutes following ingestion, and the half-life is 2 to 3 hours.

The experience with nifedipine in human pregnancy is limited. No untoward fetal affects have been noted to date, but at the present time nifedipine must be considered an experimental drug. It should not be used for the treatment of preterm labor until careful studies have proven its safety and efficacy.

Prostaglandin Synthetase Inhibitors
There is good evidence to show that prostaglandins mediate the uterine contractions of labor. Concentrations of prostaglandin F and prostaglandin E_2 in blood, urine, and amniotic fluid show significant elevations at the beginning of active labor.

Indomethacin

Indomethacin is the drug in this class that has been tested most extensively as a tocolytic agent.

Administration. Indomethacin is absorbed rapidly after oral or rectal administration and reaches a peak concentration in 1 to 2 hours.

1. Treatment is started by inserting a rectal suppository containing 100 mg of the drug.
2. Subsequent therapy is carried out by repeated rectal suppositories at 8- to 12-hour intervals, or 25 mg given orally every 6 hours.
3. The course of treatment should be as short as possible, preferably limited to 24 hours.

Efficacy. Indomethacin has been found to be effective in inhibiting labor.

Fetal Side Effects

1. Premature closure of the ductus arteriosus. There may be a danger to the fetus because of the ability of prostaglandin synthetase inhibitors to bring about closure of the ductus arteriosus. Clinical reports suggest that this event occurs rarely, and mainly when the fetus is near term.
2. Neuronal micronecrosis. In the brain of the rat fetus, indomethacin has been shown to increase the number of areas of neuronal micronecrosis.
3. Oligohydramnios. This has been observed in the Rhesus monkey, and is thought to result from renal vasoconstriction. The dose and duration of treatment, however, were much higher than those used in clinical human experience. Oligohydramnios following therapy with indomethacin has not been reported in humans.
4. Delay in pulmonary maturation. This has been reported in the rabbit. There is no evidence at present to show that the incidence of the respiratory distress syndrome has increased following treatment with indomethacin in humans.

Use of Indomethacin. Because of possible dangers to the fetus, the use of indomethacin and other antiprostaglandins to inhibit preterm labor is not advocated at the present time, and should be limited to investigational units. These drugs may be useful when treatment by betamimetic drugs fails to arrest preterm labor.

Aspirin

Acetylsalicylic acid has an antiprostaglandin effect and theoretically should be of benefit as a tocolytic agent. It is not recommended, however, to use aspirin at the present time for tocolysis.

MANAGEMENT OF PRETERM LABOR AND DELIVERY

In centers that are equipped to provide special care for the mother and infant at high risk, the survival rate of babies born preterm is such that no longer is it acceptable to ignore the tiny fetus (VLBW: very low birthweight) and to base management on maternal considerations alone. The delivery should take place in a hospital with special obstetric high-risk facilities and an intensive care nursery. Postnatal transfer of the baby to a tertiary care center is a less than satisfactory approach.

Gestational age rather than weight appears to be the more significant factor affecting survival. The use of 28 weeks' gestation as a cut-off point has been abandoned. As a number of babies born at 24 weeks gestation have survived, it is difficult to make any rule about a cut-off point. Optimal outcome depends on closely coordinated obstetric and neonatal care during labor, delivery, and early neonatal life.

Plan for Management of Preterm Labor

1. *Establish diagnosis.* Since the diagnosis of preterm labor has serious long-term implications, it is important to make the diagnosis as accurately as possible before therapy is instituted.
   a. Assess uterine activity
      i. The presence of four contractions in 20 minutes provides presumptive evidence for the diagnosis of preterm labor.
      ii. Uterine contractions should be assessed by an external electronic monitor. It is more accurate than palpation and provides a permanent record.
   b. Assess condition of the cervix. Points in favor of preterm labor include:
      i. Effacement of 80 percent.
      ii. Dilatation of at least 2 cm.
      iii. Evidence of cervical change as shown by serial examinations.
2. *Establish gestational age.* The cornerstone for establishing gestational age now lies with ultrasound and is performed by measuring the biparietal diameter and long bones such as femur and humerus. Several formulas are used to assess fetal weight, using the biparietal diameter, the abdominal circumference, and the femoral length. Fetal weight can be estimated within 10 percent of the actual weight. Ultrasonic examination will also diagnose multiple pregnancy, determine fetal presentation, and demonstrate the position of the placenta.

Two Possible Scenarios

1. *Diagnosis of preterm labor not confirmed:* In such situations no active treatment is indicated. The management consists of bed rest and observation, with discharge from the hospital if the contractions cease.
2. *Diagnosis of preterm labor is confirmed:* Active therapy is indicated to try and arrest the uterine contractions as long as there is no evidence of fetal compromise.
   a. Tocolytic treatment is instituted.

    b. In some cases amniocentesis is used to measure the L/S ratio to assess the degree of pulmonary maturity.

    c. Therapy with steroids is considered to induce fetal pulmonary maturity.

Steroids in the Prevention of Respiratory Distress Syndrome

Babies born with immature lungs are prone to develop RDS, a disease limited almost entirely to the premature infant and occurring rarely after 38 weeks of gestation. It is the most common cause of morbidity and mortality in these infants. The main etiologic factor is the deficiency of surfactant in the lungs. As a rule the lungs mature at approximately 35 weeks of gestation. At this time there is a large increase of pulmonary surfactant resulting in the lecithin/sphingomyelin (L/S) ratio in the amniotic fluid reaching 2 or more.

    Since Liggins and Howie first reported that antenatal administration of corticosteroids reduced the incidence of RDS, use of these agents to enhance fetal pulmonary maturity has become widespread.

Dose
The dosage of betamethasone is 12 mg to the mother by intramuscular injection, repeated in 12 hours; followed by 12 mg weekly until the fetal lungs achieve maturity. The drug reaches the fetus quickly, but the maximum effect does not occur until 48 hours.

Indications for Steroid Therapy
Precise indications remain controversial. Attempts at pharmacologic induction of pulmonary maturation should be reserved for certain situations:

1. Gestational age of less than 33 weeks.
2. The L/S ratio is unknown or less than 2:1.
3. The fetal membranes are intact. There is some evidence that, when the membranes have been ruptured for more than 24 hours, betamethasone does not reduce significantly the incidence of respiratory distress syndrome any further.
4. Delivery of the infant may be delayed without undue risk to the mother or fetus for 48 hours following the initiation of therapy to give the drug time to exert its full effect.

Contraindications to Steroid Therapy

1. Inability or inadvisability of delaying delivery for 48 hours
2. Gestational age of 34 weeks or greater
3. L/S ratio greater than 2

Side Effects of Steroids

At the present time there are no reports of serious side effects of this therapy on mothers or children. Infants of mothers who were treated in Liggins' original study have been followed prospectively for 7 years. These children have performed as well as controls in all the parameters evaluated which include growth and development, psychometric testing, general medical illnesses, neurologic abnormalities, ophthalmologic examinations, and pulmonary function.

There are not enough data at the present time, however, regarding long-term effects to warrant the indiscriminate use of these drugs. Analysis by the collaborative group on antenatal steroid therapy revealed that while its use reduced the incidence of RDS in the treated group to 12.6 from 18 percent in the placebo group, it did not affect the severity of the disease, nor was there any apparent effect in multiple pregnancy. No increase in postpartum complications was noted, including infection and hypertension. Conclusions were that the reduction of RDS occurred primarily in the 28- to 32-week gestational age group who delivered between 24 hours and 7 days from entry into the study.

Labor

Because infants who are premature are fragile they tolerate stress and hypoxia less well than term infants. Management of labor must take this into account. The labor and delivery of preterm infants must be attended by personnel skilled in obstetric management and neonatal resuscitation. Aims of management and the methods to achieve them include:

1. The ensuring of adequate fetal oxygenation throughout labor and delivery.
2. Prevention of traumatic delivery.
3. A skilled resuscitative team must be present at the birth.
4. Continuous electronic fetal monitoring (internal when the membranes have ruptured) is essential if hypoxia is to be detected in its early stage.
5. Scalp blood sampling is performed when indicated.
6. If fetal distress cannot be corrected by the administration of oxygen to the mother and a change in her position, cesarean section should be performed.

Analgesia and Anesthesia

During preterm labor, analgesics and sedatives must be used sparingly and with caution. The premature baby has limited abilities to metabolize these drugs and is more sensitive to their effects. A conduction technique, e.g., lumbar epidural block, is the analgesic of choice. It affords good relief of pain during labor, and makes possible a controlled delivery. If this is not available, narcotics are preferable to sedatives or tranquilizers because the depressing effects of the former can be reversed by narcon. Local anesthesia can be used for the delivery.

The Delivery

1. The birth should be gentle and slow to avoid rapid compression and decompression of the head.
2. Oxygen is given to the mother by mask during the delivery.
3. The membranes should not be ruptured artificially. The amniotic fluid acts as a cushion for the soft premature skull with its widely separated sutures.
4. An episiotomy may be indicated, as it reduces the pressure on the fetal head.
5. We prefer spontaneous delivery when possible. Low forceps, however, may be needed occasionally to guide the head over the perineum.
6. Breech presentation poses special problems. The preterm breech is at risk for prolapse of the umbilical cord and entrapment of the head. For these reasons cesarean section should be considered for any infant in a breech presentation whose weight is estimated at less than 2500 g.
7. Precipitous and unattended births are dangerous for the premature infant.
8. Every effort should be made to have an appropriate resuscitation team at the delivery.
9. If delivery is not imminent, transport of the mother to an appropriate center staffed and equipped for the high-risk infant offers the best prognosis for this infant.

Care of the Newborn Infant

See Chapters 11 and 51.

PREMATURE RUPTURE OF MEMBRANES

Spontaneous rupture of the membranes 1 hour or more prior to the onset of labor is defined as premature rupture of membranes.

Incidence and Etiology

Premature rupture of membranes (PROM) complicates approximately 10 percent of term and as high as 30 percent of preterm pregnancies.

Despite many theories about etiology, the cause of spontaneous rupture of fetal membranes prior to the onset of labor is unexplained in most cases. The most common known risk factors are:

1. Trauma
   a. Pelvic examination
   b. Coitus
2. Incompetent cervix
3. Chorioamnionitis
4. Polyhydramnios

Onset of Labor

Between 50 and 70 percent of patients with PROM will go into labor within 48 hours. The length of the latent period (between rupture of membranes and onset of labor) is influenced by the following:

1. Gestational age
   a. Near term labor begins within 24 hours in 80 to 90 percent.
   b. Before 36 weeks labor starts by 24 hours in 35 to 50 percent.
   c. A latent period of over 14 days occurs in only 10 percent of the preterm group.
2. The latent period is shorter when the fetus is large.
3. Primigravidas tend to have a longer latent period.
4. Intrauterine infection decreases the latent period.

The Diagnosis of Premature Rupture of the Membranes

Patients will often report a leak or gush of clear fluid from the vagina. Diagnosis should not be based on history alone, and further investigation is necessary before a definitive diagnosis of premature rupture of membranes is made.

1. *Sterile speculum examination:* Under sterile conditions a speculum is inserted into the vagina and the cervix is observed. Escape of fluid from the cervix may be seen spontaneously or following pressure on the abdomen. During the speculum examination for the diagnosis of premature rupture of membranes, a high vaginal swab is taken and sent for culture. *The cervix must not be examined digitally.* Digital examination increases the risk of ascending infection. This should be avoided unless a decision has been made to induce the patient.
2. *Nitrazine test:* Amniotic fluid is alkaline when compared to vaginal or cervical secretions. When the membranes rupture, the vagina is bathed with amniotic fluid which alters the pH. If the vaginal fluid is acid on the nitrazine test, the membranes are

definitely intact. If the fluid is alkaline on the nitrazine test, the membranes are probably ruptured. Nitrazine paper, however, will give an alkaline result if it is contaminated with blood, urine, or secretions caused by a vaginal infection. A positive nitrazine test should be confirmed by a fern test.

3. *Fern test:* A drop of vaginal fluid from the posterior fornix is placed on a slide, allowed to dry, and examined under the high power of a microscope. Sodium chloride from the amniotic fluid, when allowed to dry on a clean slide, will crystallize and will show a characteristic fern pattern. When this pattern is seen, it indicates that the membranes have ruptured. It is important not to obtain this sample from the internal cervical os because secretions in this area can appear to fern under the microscope even when the membranes are intact.

4. *Nile blue test:* A dried drop of vaginal fluid is stained with Nile blue. The presence of orange cells from fetal skin indicate that the membranes are ruptured.

5. *Ultrasound examination:* The finding of little or no amniotic fluid on ultrasonography is highly suggestive of ruptured membranes.

6. *Intraamniotic injection of dye:* Occasionally the diagnosis of premature rupture of the membranes is extremely difficult. In such situations, indigo carmine (0.5 cc mixed with 10 cc of sterile saline) can be injected into the amniotic cavity. Under ultrasonographic control a 22-gauge needle is inserted into a pocket of amniotic fluid and the dye is injected. The patient is then asked to wear a peripad and after a few hours the peripad and the vagina are inspected for the dye. Methylene blue dye should not be used as it has been associated with hemolytic anemia and hyperbilirubinemia in the infant.

Risks of Premature Rupture of Membranes

1. *Maternal risk:* The major complication following premature rupture of membranes is chorioamnionitis with or without generalized sepsis. In term pregnancies there is a direct correlation between the length of the latent period (rupture of membranes to delivery) and the development of maternal sepsis. This, however, does not appear to be the case for pregnancies less than 37 weeks' gestation, i.e., the risk of infection in the mother is not increased significantly by prolongation of the latent period. The danger of infection is related to the mode of delivery, being higher in women delivered by cesarean section.

2. *Fetal risk*

   a. Prematurity and respiratory distress syndrome. Approximately 20 percent of babies born after PROM weigh less than 2500 g. The major cause of perinatal death when the period of gestation is less than 34 weeks is RDS and not sepsis.

b. Infection. After 35 weeks, when the majority of fetuses have attained pulmonary maturity, sepsis takes over as the main cause of perinatal mortality and morbidity. Near term the incidence of fetal sepsis seems to correlate directly with the duration of ruptured membranes. In the preterm pregnancy, however, the rate of sepsis does not increase with the length of the latent period (rupture of membranes to delivery). It most be noted that the fetus can be infected even when there is no clinical evidence of chorioamnionitis. One of the most lethal types of infection in the newborn is that caused by group B beta hemolytic streptococcus. Every patient with premature rupture of membranes should have a vaginal culture on admission to hospital to identify the presence of group B beta-hemolytic streptococcus.

c. Prolapse of the umbilical cord. This is more common in premature infants with premature rupture of membranes.

d. Malpresentation. This is common, particularly breech.

e. Perinatal mortality. The overall figure is 5 percent. In premature infants it is 30 percent. Malpresentation increases the mortality and neonatal infection worsens the prognosis.

3. *Fetal Prognosis:* Fetal prognosis depends on:

a. Fetal maturity.

b. Intrauterine infection. Although neonatal infection following PROM is less than 5 percent, one of the most dangerous organisms is group B streptococcus. This bacterium has received much attention for its devastating effect on the infected premature neonate.

Management of Premature Rupture of Membranes

The two main approaches to management of patients with premature rupture of membranes are the conservative and the aggressive. The aggressive approach, based on fear of infection, consists of delivery within 24 to 48 hours of rupture of membranes. This may have merit when one is dealing with a population that is of extremely low socioeconomic class, but is not indicated for middle-class patients. The management of PROM depends on the gestational age.

Gestation Under 36 Weeks

1. Confirm the diagnosis.
2. Rule out chorioamnionitis. The signs and symptoms of cho-

rioamnionitis include fever, temperature over 38°C; persistent maternal tachycardia over 100 beats per minute; leukocytosis; purulent vaginal discharge; uterine tenderness. Persistent fetal tachycardia over 180 beats per minute suggests the presence of infection. Under these conditions the pregnancy must be terminated as soon as possible. Vaginal cultures are taken. Widespectrum antibiotics are prescribed during the induction of labor. Vaginal delivery is preferred. Cesarean section is performed only when induction fails or if there is a malpresentation. Unfortunately clinical criteria are neither sensitive nor specific. In some cases by the time the classic signs appear, the infection may be long standing and severe.

3. If there is no clinical evidence of chorioamnionitis and the gestational age is assessed to be less than 37 weeks we favor a conservative approach.

Conservative Management in Hospital

The purpose is to allow the fetus to reach a stage of maturity at which stage it can survive outside the uterus. The management is as follows:

1. Bed rest as long as there is leakage of fluid.
2. Temperature and pulse every 4 hours.
3. Daily white blood cell count.
4. Digital examination is not performed. This procedure increases the risk of infection.
5. Vaginal culture is carried out every week, or more frequently if there are symptoms.
6. Ultrasonography is performed weekly to assess the volume of amniotic fluid and the growth of the fetus.
7. No prophylactic antibiotics. The administration of antibiotics to the uninfected mother has not reduced fetal morbidity. The danger of using these drugs lies in the exposure of the infant to antibiotics and the masking of a neonatal infection.
8. The use of steroids to mature the fetal lungs. This is controversial in the face of premature rupture of membranes, as there is some evidence that suggests that premature rupture of membranes of itself may stimulate fetal pulmonary maturity. A prospective randomized study of the use of corticosteroids in the management of premature rupture of the membranes and premature gestation done by Garite did not find any significant difference in chorioamnionitis, respiratory distress syndrome, perinatal death rates, neonatal infections, cesarean section rates, birthweights, or gestational age when the steroid treatment group was compared with the placebo-treated group. Maternal postpartum endometritis among women delivered

vaginally was significantly higher for the steroid-treated group. The frequency of prolonged hospital stay was significantly higher for neonates in the steroid group. We do not advocate the use of corticosteroids to mature the fetal lungs in the presence of premature rupture of the membranes.

9. If infection occurs induction must be initiated.

Conservative Management at Home

Although we feel it is preferable that the patient remains in hospital where constant surveillance can be achieved, in occasional circumstances it may be permissible for the mother to go home. These include:

1. All parameters are stable including vital signs and fetal assessment.
2. There is no excessive loss of amniotic fluid.
3. No coitus, douches, or vaginal tampons are permitted.
4. Temperature is taken by the patient every 4 hours at home. If fever develops she returns to the hospital.

Induction of Labor

In the absence of complications labor is induced when the pregnancy reaches 37 weeks.

Gestation Over 36 Weeks

Classic obstetric teaching has been that the greater the duration of PROM the higher the risk of infectious morbidity and mortality for both the mother and the fetus. In the group close to term the incidence of serious respiratory distress syndrome is rare and the risk of infection becomes much more significant. Induction of labor is the management of choice in this gestational age group. An initial digital examination is done after confirmation of ruptured membranes.

Ripe Cervix

Labor should be induced. There is nothing to be gained by delay.

Unripe Cervix

There are two approaches:

1. Because 80 to 90 percent of patients will go into spontaneous labor within 24 hours, some obstetricians prefer expectant management during this period, and if labor does not begin at the end of 24 hours it is induced.
2. Ripening of the cervix is achieved by placing prostaglandin E_2 tablets in the posterior fornix of the vagina. Once the cervix becomes favorable, induction, using intravenous oxytocin, is carried out in the usual way.

Conclusion

Because of the inadequate and at times conflicting data, there is at the present time no generally accepted protocol for the management of premature rupture of the membranes. The outline that we have provided here gives our approach to the management of PROM in the term and preterm pregnancy. Possibly the most important management in the pregnancy with premature rupture of membranes prior to 37 weeks is transfer of the mother to a tertiary care institution that has an intensive care nursery.

BIBLIOGRAPHY

Barden TP, Peter JB, Merkatz IR: Ritrodrine hydrochloride: A betamimetic agent for use in preterm labor. Obstet Gynecol 56:1, 1980

Berkowitz RL, Hoder EL, Freedman RM, et al: Results of a management protocol for premature rupture of the membranes. Obstet Gynecol 60:271, 1982

Boylan P, O'Driscoll K: Improvement in perinatal mortality rate attributed to spontaneous preterm labor without use of tocolytic agents. Am J Obstet Gynec 145:781, 1983

Brazy JE, Little V, Grimm J, et al: Risk:benefit considerations for the use of isoxsuprine in the treatment of premature labor. Obstet Gynecol 58:297, 1981

Carson GD: Tocolytic therapy. Curr Prob Obstet Gynecol VI: 10, 1983

Collaborative Group on Antenatal Steroid Therapy: Effect of antenatal dexamethasone administration on the prevention of respiratory distress syndrome. Am Obstet Gynecol 141:276, 1981

Fuchs F: Prevention of premature birth. Clin Perinatol 7:3, 1980

Garite TJ, et al: Prospective randomized study of corticosteroids in the management of premature rupture of the membranes and the premature gestation. Am J Obstet Gynecol 141:508, 1981

Gibbs RS, Blanco JD: Premature rupture of the membranes. Obstet Gynecol 60:671, 1982

Harger JH: Cervical cerclage: Patient selection, morbidity, and success rates. Clin Perinatol 10:321, 1983

Lauersen NH, Merkatz IR, Tejani N, et al: Inhibition of premature labor: A multicenter comparison of ritodrine and ethanol. Am J Obstet Gynecol 127:837, 1977

Lipshitz J: Beta-adrenergic agents. Sem Perinatol 5:252, 1981

Mead PB: Management of the patient with premature rupture of the membranes. Clin Perinatol 7:243, 1980

Merkatz IR, Peter JB, Barden TP: Ritrodine hydrochloride: A betamimetic agent for use in preterm labor. II. Evidence of efficacy. Obstet Gynecol 56:7, 1980

Niebyl JR: Prostaglandin synthetase inhibitors. Sem Perinatol 5:274, 1981

Petrie RH: Tocolysis using magnesium sulfate. Sem Perinatol 5:266, 1981

Tejani NA, Verma UL: Effect of tocolysis on incidence of low birth weight. Obstet Gynecol 61:556, 1983

Ulmsten U, Anderson KE, Wingerup L: Treatment of premature labor with the calcium antagonist nifedipine. Arch Gynecol 229: 1–5, 1980

Wilson JC, Levy DL, Wilds PL: Premature rupture of membranes prior to term: Consequences of non-intervention. Obstet Gynecol 60:601, 1982

Prolonged Labor

44

GENERAL INFORMATION

By definition labor that lasts over 24 hours is classified as prolonged. As soon as signs are observed that indicate that adequate progress is not being made, however, the situation must be assessed immediately. Problems should be recognized and treated long before the 24-hour limit has been reached. Most prolonged labors represent extensions of the first stage. Whatever the reason, the cervix fails to dilate fully within a reasonable length of time.

Onset of Labor

Because it is difficult in many cases to be certain exactly when labor began, there is no unanimously accepted definition of the onset of labor. The definition based on the frequency, regularity, and duration of uterine contractions ignores the fact that patients with dysfunctional labor do have painful though irregular contractions.

The definition that insists on progressive effacement and dilatation of the cervix as an essential feature of real labor fails to recognize the important latent phase or preliminary stage of labor. During this period, despite regular uterine contractions, little recognizable change may take place in the cervix.

Perhaps, therefore, the best definition available may be the imprecise one that defines onset of labor as being the time at which the patient experiences uterine contractions that lead toward the birth of a baby.

Incidence and Etiology

The incidence of prolonged labor varies from 1 to 7 percent. Modern methods of diagnosis and treatment have reduced the frequency of this complication.

The principal causes of prolonged labor are:

1. Fetopelvic disproportion
2. Malpresentations and malpositions
3. Inefficient uterine action, including the rigid cervix

Accessory factors are:

1. Primigravidity
2. Premature rupture of the membranes when the cervix is uneffaced, closed, and hard
3. Excessive analgesia or anesthesia in the latent phase

These factors may act alone or in concert. A marked abnormality of one, or a minor deviation in several, can prevent successful termination of the labor. Whereas normal delivery is impossible in the presence of absolute cephalopelvic disproportion, a mild disparity between the size of the pelvis and that of the fetus can be overcome by strong and effective uterine contractions. The pelvis may be sufficiently large to accommodate an occipitoanterior presentation but too small for an occipitoposterior one. It is a matter of balance.

Rupture of the membranes in the presence of a ripe cervix and strong contractions never prolong labor. If, however, the bag of waters breaks when the cervix is long, hard, and closed, there is often a long latent period before progressive labor sets in.

Inefficient uterine action includes the inability of the cervix to dilate smoothly and rapidly, as well as ineffective uterine contractions.

GRAPHIC ANALYSIS OF LABOR

Friedman described a graphic analysis of labor (Fig. 1), correlating the duration of labor with the rate of cervical dilatation. On graph paper the cervical dilatation in centimeters is placed on the ordinate and the time on the abscissa. Joining the points of contact makes a sigmoid curve. The rate of cervical dilatation, as shown by the slope of the curve, is described in centimeters per hour.

The first stage of labor (from the onset of labor to full dilatation of the cervix) is divided into two periods, the latent phase and the active phase. By studying a large series, Friedman obtained figures for the lengths of the various phases. The upper normal limits represent the longest time that labor went on and still terminated normally. However, in slow or nonprogressing cases (as shown by a low rate of cervical dilatation) investigation must be instituted long before the maximum time limit has been reached.

Latent Period

This phase begins with the onset of labor and lasts until the beginning of the active phase of cervical dilatation, as shown by the upswing of the curve. The uterine contractions become orientated and the cervix softened and effaced. The slope of the curve is nearly flat, the cervical dilatation averaging only 0.35 cm per hour. At the end of the latent phase the cervix is around 3 cm dilated, well effaced, and soft.

In primigravidas the average length of the latent phase is 8.6 hours, with the upper limit of normal at 20 hours (Table 1). For multiparas the figures are 5.3 and 14 hours. Wide variations occur, and a prolonged latent period does not mean that the active phase will be abnormal.

Active Period

The active period lasts from the end of the latent phase to full dilatation of the cervix. The curve changes from the almost horizontal slope of the latent phase to a nearly vertical incline. As the second stage is being reached the curve flattens again. Effective labor begins with the active phase, the period of steady and rapid cervical dilatation.

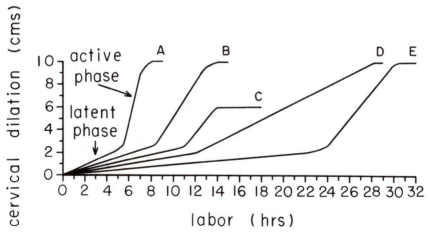

Figure 1. Normal and abnormal labor during the first stage. A, average multipara. B, average primigravida. C, secondary arrest of dilatation. D, primary dysfunctional labor. E, prolonged latent phase.

TABLE 1: LENGTHS OF THE PHASES OF LABOR

	Primigravidas		Multiparas	
	Average	Upper normal	Average	Upper normal
Latent phase	8.6 hrs	20 hrs	5.3 hrs	14 hrs
Active phase	5.8 hrs	12 hrs	2.5 hrs	6 hrs
First stage of labor	13.3 hrs	28.5 hrs	7.5 hrs	20 hrs
Second stage of labor	57 mins	2.5 hrs	18 mins	50 mins
Rate of cervical dilatation during active phase	Under 1.2 cm/hour is abnormal		Under 1.5 cm/hour is abnormal	

The vertical linearity of the curve makes possible the early recognition of deviations from the average. Premature flattening of the curve (indicating a reduction in the rate of cervical dilatation) calls for immediate investigation of the cause.

In the primigravidas of Friedman's series the average length of the active phase was 5.8 hours, and the upper limit of normal was 12 hours. The rate of cervical dilatation ranged from 1.2 to 6.8 cm per hour. A rate under 1.2 cm per hour is below normal and suggests dysfunctional labor.

In multiparas the average length of the active phase was 2.5 hours, with the upper normal limit at 6 hours. A rate of cervical dilatation less than 1.5 cm per hour is abnormal.

In the primigravidas the maximum duration of the normal first stage of labor (latent and active phases combined) was 28.5 hours (average 13.3), with the second stage maximum at 2.5 hours (average 57 minutes). In multiparas the figures were 20 hours (average 7.5) for the first stage, and 50 minutes (average 18 minutes) for the second stage.

CLASSIFICATION OF PROLONGED LABOR

Prolonged Latent Phase

A latent phase that exceeds 20 hours in the primigravida or 14 hours in the multipara is abnormal. Causes of a prolonged latent phase include (1) an unripe cervix at the onset of labor, (2) abnormal position of the fetus, (3) fetopelvic disproportion, (4) dysfunctional labor, and (5) the administration of excessive sedation.

The unripe cervix prolongs only the latent phase, and most cervices open normally once effacement is achieved. Even when the latent phase lasts over 20 hours, many patients advance to normal cervical dilatation when the active phase begins. While a long latent phase is worrisome, it does not endanger the mother or the child.

Prolonged Active Phase in the Primigravida

In the primigravida an active phase longer than 12 hours is abnormal. More important than the length of this phase is the speed of cervical dilatation. A rate less than 1.2 cm per hour is evidence of some abnormality and should alert the attendant.

Prolongation of the active phase is associated with (1) malpositions of the fetus, (2) fetopelvic disproportion, (3) injudicious use of sedation and analgesia, and (4) rupture of membranes before the onset of labor. It is followed by an increase in midforceps delivery, cesarean section, and fetal damage or death.

The prolonged active period can be divided into two main clinical groups: (1) those in whom there is a progressing albeit slow dilatation of the cervix, and (2) those in whom there is actual arrest of dilatation.

Primary Dysfunctional Labor

The rate of cervical dilatation is less than 1.2 cm per hour. Spontaneous increase in the rate of dilatation occurs rarely, and little can be done to speed up progress.

While, in the absence of other complications, the risk to mother and child is not great, the perinatal mortality is higher than in the general population. It is important that the diagnosis is made and that the patients are given special care. As long as progress is being made and there is no fetal distress, however, the phenomenon of slow cervical dilatation must be accepted.

Two-thirds of these patients deliver normally, 20 percent require midforceps, and 10 percent come to cesarean section. A few women go into secondary arrest of dilatation, for which the prognosis is more serious.

Secondary Arrest of Dilatation

During the active phase, previously advancing dilatation of the cervix stops. On the graph there is a flattening of the curve. Two hours of arrest is diagnostic.

There are two subgroups: (1) the uterine contractions become insufficient to maintain progressive dilatation of the cervix, and (2) cervical dilatation ceases in spite of strong and efficient uterine contractions.

While this is a different entity from the primary protracted active phase, both can occur in the same patient and the etiology can be related. Thus either a slowly dilating cervix or one that had been opening normally may stop advancing.

Accurate assessment of the situation and diagnosis of etiology is vital. Keeping in mind that inefficient uterine action is often associated with disproportion and abnormal position of the fetus, one must not blame the lack of progress on poor contractions until mechanical factors have been ruled out.

When ineffective labor (often myometrial fatigue) is the sole cause, half the patients resume progress after no more treatment than rest and an infusion of glucose in water. In this group amniotomy and oxytocin stimulation works well.

When there are complications such as disproportion or abnormal position, the treatment must be aimed in their direction.

Prolonged Active Phase in the Multipara

An active phase in the multipara lasting over 6 hours (average 2.5 hours) and a rate of cervical dilatation of less than 1.5 cm per hour are abnormal. While prolonged labor in a multipara is rare in comparison with the primigravida, it can, because of neglect and a false sense of security, lead to catastrophe. The fact that a normal birth occurred in the past does not mean it will be repeated. Careful observation, avoidance of traumatic vaginal deliveries, and consideration of cesarean section are important in the management of this problem.

The following are characteristics of prolonged labor in the multipara:

1. The incidence is less than 1 percent.
2. Perinatal mortality is higher than in primigravidas with prolonged labor.
3. The number of large babies is significant.
4. Malpresentations present a problem.
5. Prolapse of the umbilical cord is a complication.
6. Postpartum hemorrhage is dangerous.
7. Rupture of the uterus may occur in the grand multipara.
8. Most deliver spontaneously per vaginam.
9. Midforceps extractions are more frequent.
10. Cesarean section rate is high, around 25 percent.

Descent of the Presenting Part

Once active descent begins late in the first stage of labor, it should advance progressively throughout the course of the second stage. Interruption of descent is ominous and suggests that a serious problem exists. Diagnosis is based on the demonstration of there being no change in the station of the fetal presenting part over the period of at least 2 hours. Cephalopelvic disproportion and abnormalities of uterine action are seen often when descent arrests. Cesarean section, midforceps, forceps rotations, and failed forceps are noted frequently in association with this problem. With difficult vaginal operative deliveries maternal and fetal trauma are common.

INVESTIGATION OF PROLONGED LABOR

Graphic Analysis of Labor

By charting the progress of labor on a graph (Fig. 1) we can ascertain whether cervical dilatation is occurring at a normal rate, too slowly, or has ceased altogether. The type of abnormality can be diagnosed, and the point at which detailed investigation should be carried out is indicated.

Fetal Condition

The condition of the baby is evaluated by monitoring the fetal heart and by observing the passage of meconium.

Maternal Status

The patient's general physical and mental condition is assessed with respect to fatigue, morale, hydration, and nourishment.

Vaginal Examination

Vaginal examination is performed under sterile conditions, with the patient in the lithotomy position and the bladder and rectum empty. Rectal examinations have no place in problem cases when a decision must be made as to definite treatment. Errors are made too often as to the condition and dilatation of the cervix, a large caput is mistaken for the skull, and the position and station are diagnosed inaccurately. During the vaginal examination the following points are noted:

State of the Cervix

Is it open or closed, soft or hard, effaced or long, dilatable or resistant? Has any progress been made since the last examination? Is an anterior lip caught between the head and the symphysis? In the majority of cases the cervix ceases dilating when it is one-half to three-fourths open. In many of these instances it is erroneously considered to be fully dilated on rectal examination.

Station of Presenting Part

The station of the bony presenting part is determined. Is it at, above, or below the spines? Has engagement taken place? Is there a caput? Is molding excessive?

Position

The position must be diagnosed accurately. In all cases of prolonged labor, malpositions such as brow presentation and occiput posterior should be kept in mind.

Failure of Descent

What seems to be holding up the presenting part? Can it be pushed down? Is the cause of arrest in the bony pelvis or is it the cervix? Is the head too big for the pelvis? Or is the problem not the pelvis, the cervix, or the fetus, but in the uterine contractions, and will a few hours of really good labor achieve progress to successful delivery?

Uterine Contractions

The uterine contractions are assessed. Is the basic problem in the type of labor, or is the main problem elsewhere and the poor uterine action a secondary complication? If the contractions are judged to be efficient, then the reason for the failure of progress must be in another field. Since inefficient uterine action is almost entirely a disorder of primigravidas, multiparas with prolonged labors must be investigated for other factors carefully before a diagnosis of poor labor is made. A woman who has delivered a 7-pound baby with no trouble may not be able to do the same with a 9-pound baby.

The strength of the contractions may be assessed manually or by the use of an electronic monitoring system.

X-ray Examination

When diagnosis is difficult and imprecise because of considerable molding and a large caput succedaneum, x-ray may help in determining fetal station and position, as well as pelvic size and shape.

MANAGEMENT OF PROLONGED LABOR

Prevention

1. Good prenatal care and preparation for childbirth reduces the incidence of prolonged labor.
2. Labor should not be induced or forced when the cervix is not

ripe. A ripe cervix is less than 1.27 cm (0.5 inch) in length, effaced, patulous to admit at least a finger, and soft and dilatable.
3. False labor is treated by rest and sedation.

Supportive Measures

1. During labor the patient's morale should be bolstered. Encouragement is offered, and remarks that may worry the patient are avoided.
2. A fluid intake of at least 2500 ml is needed to prevent dehydration. In prolonged labor this is achieved by the intravenous infusion of crystalloid solutions (e.g, Ringer).
3. Food taken during labor is not digested well. It remains in the stomach with danger of vomiting and aspiration. Hence in long labors nourishment is given by intravenous feeding.
4. Elimination from bladder and bowel must be adequate. A full bladder and rectum not only cause discomfort and impede progress but are more liable to injury than empty ones.
5. While women in labor must be rested with sedation and relieved of pain by analgesia, this must be administered judiciously. An excessive amount of narcosis may interfere with contractions and can harm the baby.
6. The number of rectal or vaginal examinations should be kept to a minimum. It hurts the patient and increases the risk of infection. Each examination must be done for a definite purpose.
7. Should the findings at examination suggest that progress is being made and that delivery may be expected within a reasonable time, and if there is no fetal or maternal distress, supportive therapy is given and labor allowed to go on.

Prolonged Latent Phase

First the mechanical factors must be ruled out. Further treatment depends on the condition of the cervix.

Ripe Cervix
When the cervix is effaced, soft, and 2.5 to 3.0 cm dilated, augmentation of labor is indicated, and works well. This is accomplished by:

1. Oxytocin infusion
2. Amniotomy

Unripe Cervix
Treatment is supportive. The patient is provided with reassurance, nourishment by infusion of a solution of glucose, and medication to re-

lieve pain and induce sleep. Morphine, 15 mg, given subcutaneously, is an effective narcotic. Large patients may need 20 mg. In rare cases the dose may need to be repeated. This regimen will result in 4 to 8 hours of sleep. Following this, one of three courses follows:

1. About 10 percent will awaken having no uterine contractions and no pain. A retrospective diagnosis of false labor is made, and if the contractions do not recur the patient is discharged.
2. Some 85 percent of patients will go into efficient labor, dilate the cervix well, and proceed to delivery.
3. In some 5 percent the original type of ineffective labor resumes. The patient will, however, have had the benefit of rest, so she is in better condition. In these cases an oxytocin infusion is instituted. The patient will usually enter the active phase within 3 hours. Once the cervix dilates to 3 cm the membranes may be ruptured. Amniotomy alone is not good treatment for prolonged latent phase. Not only does it not work well, but it has the disadvantage of making an irreversible commitment to delivery within a limited period. This may lead to unnecessary operative intervention.

The prognosis is good. (1) Most patients proceed into the progressive labor of the active phase leading to vaginal delivery. (2) Some develop dysfunctional labor or secondary arrest of dilatation.

Cesarean section is almost never indicated in the latent stage of labor. Acute fetal distress, absolute cephalopelvic disproportion, and transverse lie are exceptions.

Primary Dysfunctional Labor

Mechanical factors must be ruled out. In some cases there is fetopelvic disproportion, and cesarean section is indicated. For the rest, medical management is carried out as long as the fetus and mother are in good condition. Nothing is done to complicate the situation further. Premature and traumatic vaginal operations are contraindicated. Slow progress is accepted. Support, reassurance, rest, fluids, and electrolytes are provided.

The results of amniotomy are not predictable, nor is there agreement as to whether it is a wise procedure in this situation. In some cases the progress of labor is improved; in others the arrest of labor seems to begin following artificial rupture of the membranes; and in many, amniotomy has no effect on the course of labor. In prolonged labor the incidence of ascending infection is increased once the membranes are ruptured; this danger must be kept in mind when amniotomy is being considered.

Reports concerning the value of an oxytocin infusion vary. Many workers feel it is ineffective in improving the progress of labor. However, we have had good results in some cases and feel it should be given a trial in managing this problem.

Results of medical treatment are as follows:

1. Two-thirds of the patients dilate the cervix slowly and proceed to vaginal delivery spontaneously or with the help of low forceps.
2. About 20 percent require midforceps.
3. Some 10 percent come to cesarean section because of arrest of progress or fetal distress.

Secondary Arrest of Dilatation

1. It is vital that mechanical factors be ruled out carefully. These include malpositions and malpresentations as well as disproportion.
2. In a large group there is disproportion, and cesarean section must be performed.
3. A few women are exhausted and are given support, rest, fluids, and electrolytes.
4. The majority of patients in whom there is no disproportion and no fetal distress are given an oxytocin infusion and the membranes are ruptured artificially. One of four courses follows:
   a. Rapid progress to full dilatation and vaginal delivery.
   b. Slow progress to full dilatation and vaginal delivery.
   c. Too slow progress so that after 4 to 6 hours cesarean section is done.
   d. No progress at all. At the end of 2 hours cesarean section is carried out.

Failure of Descent

1. Disproportion calls for cesarean section. With the decline of the use of difficult forceps deliveries the fetal results have improved.
2. No disproportion. The use of epidural anesthesia to relieve pain and promote relaxation often results in progress. If descent does not take place, stimulation by an oxytocin infusion, monitored by continuous recording of the FHR and the intrauterine pressure, will often bring about steady progress to vaginal delivery. If this treatment fails, cesarean section is performed.

Fetal and/or Maternal Distress

1. Fetal or maternal distress calls for early intervention.
2. If the cervix is fully dilated, the presenting part is low in the

pelvis, and there is no disproportion, the baby should be delivered by forceps if the presentation is cephalic and by cesarean section if it is a breech.

3. Preparations should be at hand for the treatment of postpartum hemorrhage and fetal distress.

Cervical Dystocia

The cervix may be holding up progress.

1. A thick anterior lip may be caught between the head and the symphysis pubis. This can be pushed over the head during a contraction.
2. There may be a thin, soft rim of cervix. This can also be pushed gently over the head.
3. In the past, when the cervix was well effaced and dilated to 7 cm, and the fetal head was well below the level of the ischial spines, Dührssen incisions of the cervix were performed and the head extracted with forceps. In modern times this procedure is carried out only in exceptional circumstances. Cesarean section is a better and safer means of delivery.
4. If the cervix is less than half open, vaginal delivery is impossible at that time. If immediate delivery is indicated, cesarean section must be performed.

DANGER OF PROLONGED LABOR

Maternal Dangers

Prolonged labor exerts a deleterious effect on both mother and child. The severity of the damage increases progressively with the duration of the labor, the risk rising sharply after 24 hours. There is a rise in the incidence of uterine atony, lacerations, hemorrhage, infections, maternal exhaustion, and shock. The high rate of operative deliveries aggravates the maternal dangers.

Fetal Dangers

The longer the labor, the higher the fetal mortality and morbidity, and the more frequently do the following conditions occur:

1. Asphyxia from the long labor itself.
2. Cerebral damage caused by pressure against the fetal head.

3. Injury as a result of difficult forceps rotations and extractions.
4. Rupture of the bag of waters long before delivery. This may result in the amniotic fluid's becoming infected and in turn may lead to pulmonary and general infection in the fetus.

Even when there is no obvious damage these babies require special care. While any type of prolonged labor is bad for the child, the danger is greater once there has been cessation of progress. This is especially true when the head has been arrested on the perineal floor for a long time, with continual pounding of the skull against the mother's pelvis.

Some workers feel that while prolonged labor increases the risk to the child during labor and the neonatal period, it has little effect on the infant's subsequent development. Others claim to have found that children born after extended labor were deficient intellectually as contrasted with babies born after normal delivery.

PROLONGED LABOR IN THE SECOND STAGE

Formerly it was a rule that the second stage of labor should not exceed 2 hours in a primigravida and 1 hour in a multipara. Experience has shown that after these periods the incidence of fetal and maternal morbidity rises. As a guide, this principle is still a good one, but under conditions of continous electronic monitoring the length of the second stage can be extended if there appears to be a good chance that progress will be made. Should fetal distress occur, however, immediate delivery must be carried out.

Etiology

1. Fetopelvic disproportion
   a. Small pelvis
   b. Large child
2. Malpresentation and malposition
3. Ineffective labor
   a. Primary inefficient uterine contractions
   b. Myometrial fatigue: secondary inertia
   c. Constriction ring
   d. Inability or refusal of the patient to bear down
   e. Excessive anesthesia
4. Soft tissue dystocia
   a. Narrow vaginal canal
   b. Rigid perineum

Management

Disproportion or Constriction Ring
Cesarean section is indicated.

No Disproportion
1. An oxytocin drip improves the uterine contractions.
2. Artificial rupture of the membranes is indicated if the bag of waters is intact.
3. The patient should be placed on the delivery table and urged to bear down with each contraction.
4. Forceps are used to further descent and rotation of the head.
5. An episiotomy overcomes the unyielding perineum.

When these methods of treatment fail or when operative vaginal delivery is considered to be too traumatic for safe delivery, cesarean section is indicated. The detailed descriptions of these procedures are found in the chapters concerned with each problem.

BIBLIOGRAPHY

Drouin P, Nasah BT, Nkounawa F: The value of the partogramme in the management of labor. Obstet Gynecol 53:741, 1979

Friedman EA: Disordered labor. Objective evaluation and management. J Family Pract 2:167, 1975

Friedman EA, Sachtleben MR: Station of the fetal presenting part. Arrest in nulliparas. Obstet Gynecol 47:129, 1976

Maltau JM, Anderson HT: Epidural anesthesia as an alternative to cesarean section in the treatment of prolonged, exhaustive labor. Acta Anesthesiol Scand 19:349, 1975

45

Fetopelvic Disproportion

Fetopelvic disproportion refers to the inability of the fetus to pass through the pelvis. Disproportion may be absolute or relative. It is absolute when under no circumstances can the baby pass safely through the birth canal. Relative disproportion is present when other factors contribute to the problem. Minor degrees of pelvic contraction can be overcome by efficient uterine contractions, dilatability of the soft tissues, favorable attitude, presentation, and position of the fetus, and moldability of the fetal head. On the other hand, poor contractions, rigid soft parts, abnormal positions, and inability of the head to mold properly can make vaginal delivery impossible.

THE PASSAGE

Pelvic Size

While the important question is the relationship between a given pelvis and a particular fetus, in some cases the contraction of the pelvis is such that no normal fetus can pass through. The reduced size may be at any level: the inlet, midpelvis, or outlet. Sometimes the pelvis may be small in all planes— the generally contracted pelvis.

Inlet Contraction
Inlet contraction is present when the anteroposterior diameter (obstetric conjugate) is less than 10 cm or the transverse diameter is less than 12 cm. Inlet contraction may result from rickets or from generally poor development.

Effects on the fetus are:

1. Failure of engagement.

2. Increase in malpositions.
3. Deflexion attitudes.
4. Exaggerated asynclitism.
5. Extreme molding.
6. Formation of a large caput succedaneum.
7. Prolapse of the umbilical cord. This becomes a complication since the presenting part does not fit the inlet well.

Effects on labor include:

1. Dilatation of the cervix is slow and often incomplete.
2. Premature rupture of the membranes is common.
3. Inefficient uterine action is a frequent accompaniment.

Midpelvic Contraction

Midpelvic contraction is basically a reduction in the plane of least dimensions, the one that passes from the apex of the pubic arch, through the ischial spines, to meet the sacrum usually at the junction of the fourth and fifth segments.

When the distance between the ischial spines is less than 9.0 cm, or when the sum of the interspinous (normal is 10.5 cm) and the posterior sagittal (normal is 4.5 to 5.0 cm) distances is less than 13.5 cm (normal is 15.0 to 15.5 cm), contraction of the midpelvis is probably present. To obtain accurate measurement of these diameters x-ray pelvimetry is essential. Clinical suspicion of a small midpelvis is aroused by the finding on manual examination of a small pelvis, the palpation of large spines that jut into the cavity, and the observation that the distance between the ischial tuberosities is less than 8.0 cm.

Midpelvic contraction is a common cause of dystocia and operative delivery. It is more difficult to manage than inlet contraction, for if the fetal head cannot even enter the inlet there is no doubt that abdominal delivery is necessary. However, once the head has descended into the pelvis, one is loath to perform cesarean section, hoping that the head will come down to a point where it can be extracted with forceps. A danger here is that with molding and caput formation the head may appear lower than it actually is. Instead of the projected midforceps delivery, one is engaged in a high forceps operation, often with disastrous results for both mother and infant.

Midpelvic contractions may prevent anterior rotation of the occiput and may direct it into the hollow of the sacrum. Failure of rotation and deflexion attitudes are associated frequently with a small pelvic cavity.

Outlet Contraction

Outlet contraction is present when the distance between the ischial tuberosities is less than 8 cm. Dystocia may be expected when the sum of the intertuberous diameter and the posterior sagittal diameter is much less than 15 cm. Diminution of the intertuberous diameter and the subpubic angle forces the head backward, and so the prognosis depends on the capacity of the posterior segment, the mobility at the sacrococcygeal joint, and the ability of the soft tissues to accommodate the passenger. The sides of the posterior triangle are not bony. While outlet contraction causes an increase in perineal lacerations and a greater need for forceps deliveries, only rarely is it an indication for cesarean section. Because the bituberous diameter can be measured manually, however, and since it may warn us that there is contraction higher in the pelvis, it should always be assessed as part of the routine examination.

Delay at the outlet may be caused by a rigid perineum. The tissues do not stretch well; and when they tear, a large uncontrolled laceration results. Treatment is by mediolateral episiotomy as soon as the problem is recognized.

Dwarfism

Dwarfism is defined as a height of less than 4 feet 10 inches at maturity. Vaginal delivery is possible in women with proportionate dwarfism. Respiratory embarrassment in the latter half of pregnancy, however, may make it impossible to await the onset of labor. Most patients are delivered by cesarean section between 35 and 37 weeks of gestation. The babies are often of adequate size and do well postnatally.

Influence of Pelvic Shape

The obstetric capacity of the female pelvis is governed by its size and shape or configuration. By radiologic techniques accurate classification by shape is more reliable than precise measurement of diameters. Hence, with the exception of cases of extreme contraction, we feel that in attempting prognosis the type of pelvis is more important than the size. These factors complement each other. A poor class of pelvis may be compensated for by being large, or a relatively small pelvis may function well because of a favorable shape.

Gynecoid. The gynecoid or normal female pelvis offers the best diameters in all three planes for the uncomplicated passage of the fetus.

Android. The android or male pelvis has a bad obstetric reputation. With reduced posterior segments in all pelvic planes, the occiput has a tendency to enter the inlet posteriorly, is impeded in rotation in the midpelvis, and is forced posteriorly at the outlet. The results are arrest of descent, failure of rotation, and lacerations of the perineum and rectum.

Anthropoid. In the anthropoid pelvis the reduced transverse measurements in the various planes are only relative and are compensated for by large anteroposterior diameters. The head descends often in the occipitoposterior position with surprising ease and is born frequently face to pubis. In general the prognosis is better than that of the android or platypelloid types.

Platypelloid. In the platypelloid pelvis there is interference with entry of the presenting part into the inlet, and there may be difficulty at the lower levels as well. In this group is found the highest incidence of cesarean section.

Mixed. There are also mixed types of pelves. A gynecoid or anthropoid pelvis may have an android-like narrowing at the midpelvis or the outlet. Thus the head enters the pelvis but becomes arrested lower down. Minor forms of funneling are common and are frequent causes of forceps extractions. In these situations the size of the fetal head, the degree of flexion, and the capacity for molding are critical factors. Even a slight variation in the presenting dimensions makes a great difference in the ease or difficulty of the delivery.

Abnormal Pelves

There are numerous varieties of grossly abnormal pelves associated with deformity and contraction. Fortunately these are not common and do not play a prominent part in the problem of fetopelvic disproportion.

Kyphoscoliosis. The incidence of kyphoscoliosis complicating pregnancy is low, occurring in but 1:6000 labors in America. In South Africa the rate was reported as 1:2400 pregnancies. The etiology includes tuberculosis (most frequent), osteomalacia, rickets, poliomyelitis, trauma, and congenital abnormality. When the lesion is in the thoracic area there is little or no reduction of pelvic capacity, but the enlarging uterus may decrease cardiopulmonary function. These patients tolerate pregnancy and labor fairly well as long as there are no significant problems prior to the pregnancy, and a number deliver vaginally. Dorsolumbar and lumbosacral kyphoses, on the other hand, are accompanied by marked pelvic deformity. Cesarean section is required in most of these cases because of pelvic contraction and cephalopelvic disproportion. Women with impaired cardiopulmonary reserve should not become pregnant. If they do, abortion is considered.

Bony Disease of the Femurs and Acetabula. By causing abnormal pressures on the pelvis during development, such disease may result in asymmetry and reduction of pelvic capacity.

Fractured Pelvis. This may also cause difficulties. Automobile accidents are the main cause. The effect on the pregnancy is twofold: (1) In women who were pregnant at the time of the mishap, fetal loss is the more frequent complication. (2) In pregnancies subsequent to the fracture, cesarean section is more common because the contracted and grossly misshapen pelvis causes disproportion. Cesarean section is a better method of long-term management than orthopedic surgery to try to correct the pelvic deformity.

Rare Abnormalities

Naegele Pelvis. The absence or imperfect development of one wing of the sacrum leads to an obliquely contracted pelvis. It was described by Naegele in 1803. He discussed six features of the deformity: (1) complete fusion of one sacroiliac joint; (2) absent or imperfect development of one-half of the sacrum with narrowing of the anterior sacral foramina on the side corresponding to the ankylosis; (3) ipsilateral narrowing of the hip bone and its sciatic notch; (4) apparent displacement of the sacrum to the ankylosed side with rotation of its anterior surface to the same side, plus contralateral displacement of the pubic symphysis; (5) ipsilateral flattening of the lateral wall of the pelvis; and (6) the other side of the pelvis not being more spacious than a normal pelvis. The condition is extremely rare. In most cases the deformity is of congenital origin. The diagnosis is made by x-ray examination. Vaginal delivery by means of a difficult forceps operation is hazardous. Cesarean section is the procedure of choice.

Robert Pelvis. Robert described the symmetrically transversely contracted pelvis caused by the absence of both sacral alae in 1842. It is extremely rare, fewer than 20 being reported. It is believed to be a congenital anomaly. The sacral alae are absent, and the innominate bone is positioned medially so that there is transverse contraction at the inlet, midpelvis, and outlet. Diagnosis is by radiologic examination. The method of delivery is cesarean section. Vaginal birth is impossible.

Split Pelvis. There is failure of union between the pubic bones. This is often associated with nonunion of the walls of the bladder and the anterior abdomen.

Assimilation Pelvis. This is an elongated pelvis in which the last lumbar or first coccygeal vertebra resembles a sacral vertebra and seems to be part of the sacrum rather than the lumbar spine or the coccyx.

Osteomalacic Pelvis. There is softening of the bones that bend into the cavity of the pelvis. This reduces all the diameters greatly.

Spondylolisthetic Pelvis. The last lumbar vertebra is displaced forward and downward over the sacral promontory. Symptoms such as pain in and weakness of the back begin in the second and third trimester and become worse in succeeding pregnancies. The sheering force applied to the lower lumbar vertebrae is increased by the protuberant pregnant uterus and, in association with the relaxation of the pelvic ligaments, is responsible for precipitating the symptoms.

Management of Spondylolisthesis

1. During pregnancy corsets and braces help.
2. Prolonged labor and abnormal fetal positions are seen frequently, and an assessment of progress must be made carefully after 8 to 12 hours.
3. Midforceps and cesarean section are necessary often.
4. The lithotomy position is harmful; the legs should be held in the horizontal position.

Soft Tissues

While poor dilatability of the muscles and fascia of the pelvis rarely causes severe disproportion in itself, in cases of borderline bony disproportion or poor uterine action it may make the difference between vaginal delivery or cesarean section. The rare case has been reported of a septum in the vagina causing obstruction. It must be excised before the baby can be born.

Neoplasms

Myoma of the Uterus

Most patients who have myomas of the uterus experience few problems during pregnancy apart from vague abdominal discomfort or tenderness. In the majority of cases the myoma is in the corpus of the uterus, rises out of the pelvis as pregnancy progresses, and causes no obstruction. Occasionally the myoma is in the lower segment of the uterus or in the cervix and obstructs the birth canal. If the myoma remains impacted in the pelvis and prevents descent of the fetus, cesarean section must be performed. While a pedunculated myoma can be removed safely following cesarean section, myomas located in the myometrium should be left in situ; the danger of hemorrhage is too great.

During pregnancy myomas may undergo red or carneous degeneration causing severe pain; treatment is symptomatic and expectant. The neoplasm may interfere with the efficiency of the uterine contractions and lead to prolonged and disordered labor. Postpartum hemorrhage may take place as a result of a faulty mechanism of the third stage and retention of the placenta. In the puerperium the myoma may undergo necrosis, infection, and suppurative degeneration. This can lead to general sepsis and is a serious complication.

Ovarian Tumor

The most common ovarian neoplasms complicating pregnancy are the benign cysts, especially dermoids and serous or pseudomucinous cystadenomas. When an ovarian neoplasm is discovered in early pregnancy, it should be removed at around 18 weeks of gestation, unless there are pressing reasons for earlier action. Oophorocystectomy in the first trimester increases the chance of abortion.

In most cases ovarian neoplasms are outside of the true pelvis and do not obstruct the birth canal. Occasionally incarceration in the pelvis occurs. In such cases labor becomes obstructed, and cesarean section should be performed. The cyst is removed at the same time. If vaginal delivery does take place the ovarian neoplasm must be removed during the puerperium. During active labor there is danger of torsion, necrosis, hemorrhage into the cyst, or rupture.

Cancer of the Cervix

For patients with carcinoma-in-situ, vaginal delivery is permitted. Treatment of invasive cancer depends on the extent of the disease and the length of gestation. In early pregnancy the disease is treated and the fetus disregarded. When the pregnancy has reached a stage where the fetus can survive outside the uterus, cesarean section is performed, because labor and vaginal delivery may lead to cervical tears, hemorrhage, and spread of the disease. Treatment of the malignancy follows the termination of the pregnancy.

THE PASSENGER

Fetal Size

Fetal size is important. Rarely is a baby too large for any pelvis. The essential problem is the relationship of the child to the pelvis. The question that must be answered is: Can this baby pass through this pelvis?

Fetal Macrosomia: The Oversized Fetus

The classic definition of the excessively large fetus is one weighing 4500 g. By this definition about 1 percent of all deliveries involve macrosomic infants. In almost 10 percent of births the baby weighs more than 4000 g. The incidence of fetal morbidity is higher than for infants of normal size.

Predisposing Factors

1. Multiparity
2. Maternal age over 35 years

3. Tall women: over 170 cm
4. Prepregnant weight over 70 kg
5. Gain of over 20 kg during pregnancy
6. Maternal diabetes
7. Macrosomia in a previous pregnancy
8. Delivery 7 days or more postterm
9. Two-thirds of oversized infants are male

Diagnosis
Prediction of fetal macrosomia is based upon:

1. General predisposing factors.
2. The weight of previous infants.
3. Maternal diabetes.
4. Abdominal palpation is accurate in only 50 percent of cases.
5. Ultrasonic measurements of the fetal head, thorax, and abdomen are the most useful parameters.

Labor

1. In most cases the presentation is cephalic.
2. The total length of labor is not prolonged, but the second stage is.
3. Shoulder dystocia occurs frequently.
4. There does not appear to be any special risk to the fetus during the first stage of labor. The incidence of abnormalities of the fetal heart rate is not increased.

Delivery

1. Many babies are born spontaneously or by low forceps.
2. There is a higher incidence of midforceps, cesarean section, and operations to relieve shoulder dystocia.
3. The risks that the macrosomic infant encounters are associated with the mode of delivery, which may result in trauma.

Maternal Complications

1. Lacerations of the genital tract
2. Postpartum hemorrhage
3. Separation of the pubic symphysis

Fetal Complications

1. Infant mortality is increased.
2. Severe asphyxia or postasphyxia encephalopathy occurs more frequently in macrosomic infants delivered by midforceps or by cesarean section than those born spontaneously or by low forceps. The

overall incidence of these conditions does not seem to be higher in macrosomic infants than controls.

3. Meconium aspiration is more common in infants undergoing difficult births.
4. Brachial and facial palsies are more common in macrosomic infants, especially when there is shoulder dystocia.
5. Compression of the brain, fracture of the skull, and intracranial hemorrhage are seen more often in macrosomic infants following complicated births.
6. Fractures of the clavicle and humerus.

Management

1. A trial of labor is indicated because most large infants will be delivered spontaneously or by low forceps.
2. Easy midforceps procedures, when the head is at a station of plus 2 are permissible.
3. Difficult midforceps operations that involve excessive force in rotation and traction should be avoided in favor of cesarean section.

Attitude and Position

In borderline pelves a well-flexed head in a good occipitoanterior position may deliver normally, while face presentation or an occipitoposterior becomes arrested.

Moldability

Moldability of the fetal head may be critical. The ability of the head to change its shape to fit the pelvis may enable it to negotiate the birth canal safely. Excessive molding can damage the brain, and this must be considered in deciding whether vaginal delivery is to be awaited. A reduction of more than 0.5 cm in the biparietal diameter is considered dangerous.

Fetal Abdominal Enlargement

This rare condition may cause dystocia. The diagnosis is made after the head is born and the trunk cannot be delivered. The fetal mortality is high because (1) intrauterine death may take place, (2) the causal condition is incompatible with extrauterine life, and (3) the trauma of a difficult birth may be lethal.

There are several varieties:

1. Generalized edema of all organs and cavities. This is associated with diabetic mothers, erythroblastosis, and toxemia of pregnancy.

2. Ascites (3 to 4 liters) is often associated with abnormalities of the urinary tract and is more common in males. Perforation of the abdomen or thorax is usually necessary before birth can be effected.
3. There may be distention of the urinary tract caused by vesical neck obstruction.
4. Polycystic kidneys may cause dystocia.
5. Fluid collection in and distention of the female genital tract may result from vaginal atresia.
6. Cystic or tumorous liver may be present.

UTERINE CONTRACTIONS

Strong uterine contractions should not be allowed or relied upon to push a baby through a pelvis when there is absolute disproportion. In borderline cases, however, when there are minor degrees of disproportion, uterine efficiency may be the essential difference between success and failure.

INVESTIGATION OF DISPROPORTION

In attempting to determine whether a given baby can be born per vaginam without serious injury to itself or to the mother, the following investigative procedures are carried out: history, abdominal palpation, vaginal examination, radiologic studies, and trial labor.

History

To an extent the information sought varies with the parity of the patient. If there have been previous pregnancies and labors the details of these are of great help in determining the prognosis. In primigravidas other information is elicited to aid in making the decisions.

Multiparas

1. The number of children and the number of pregnancies.
2. The size of the babies at birth, especially the largest. Many women tend to have progressively larger babies, and the knowledge that a 6-pound child was delivered with no difficulty does not guarantee the same success with an 8-pound baby.
3. The condition of the children at birth, including any damaged children or intrapartum deaths.
4. Length of labor.

5. Method of delivery.
6. Maternal lacerations.

Most labors and deliveries subsequent to the first are easier. The pelvic joints and soft tissues, once stretched, offer less resistance.

Primigravidas

1. The age of the patient: For the purpose of childbearing a woman is said to be as old as her cervix. While some clinics consider that a woman is not an elderly primigravida until she reaches 40, in many institutions 35 years of age is taken as the dividing line. Many elderly primigravidas ripen the cervix well, push the presenting part into the pelvis even before labor has started, and have an easy, spontaneous delivery. An equal number, however, have difficulties. Hence all older women who are pregnant for the first time merit careful investigation.
2. Type of menstrual cycle: This is important. Women whose menses were late in starting, irregular, and attended with severe dysmenorrhea have a tendency toward difficult labor.
3. Sterility: Women with a history of involuntary sterility for 7 or 8 years often have worrisome labors with uterine dysfunction, soft tissue dystocia, and operative deliveries.
4. Familial history: Information about the patient's mother and sisters is important. A history of dystocia with injured or dead babies calls for an especially careful investigation.

Failure of Engagement

While any doubt as to pelvic adequacy must be resolved by thorough examination, one of the most common problems is the unengaged head in the primigravida near term. In the majority of primigravidas with normal pelves the head engages about 3 weeks before term. Breeches, on the other hand, often do not engage until good labor has set it.

In about 5 percent of primigravidas the head is unengaged at term. Since most of these deliver per vaginam there is no need to panic, but the persistence of nonengagement is an indication for study to determine the cause for the failure of descent. In many cases the high station is related to the cervix and uterus being unprepared. The head cannot enter the pelvis until the lower uterine segment is formed.

Abdominal Palpation

The patient lies on her back on the examining table in as relaxed a condition as possible. First the position is ascertained. Then with one hand the examiner presses the head gently but firmly into the pelvic brim. The fingers of the other hand are applied to the area of the abdomen above the pubic symphysis. As pressure is being applied the examiner determines whether the head will enter the inlet of the pelvis or whether it overrides the pubis and fails to enter the superior strait. If the head can be pushed into the pelvis it suggests that there is no disproportion at the inlet. If it does not go in, further investigation must be carried out.

Causes of failure to descend or overriding include:

1. Disproportion
2. Malpresentation or malposition
3. Underdeveloped lower uterine segment
4. Polyhydramnios
5. Placenta previa
6. Soft tissue tumor blocking the pelvis
7. Full bladder or rectum
8. Patient not close enough to term, a situation often associated with an underdeveloped lower segment

Vaginal and Combined Abdominopelvic Examination

This is the most important procedure in the assessment of fetopelvic disproportion. The patient should be positioned on a table in the lithotomy position to ensure adequate examination.

The inner walls of the inlet, cavity, and outlet of the pelvis are palpated to estimate their capacities and to search for abnormalities. The length, dilatation, and consistency of the cervix are determined. The elasticity of the soft tissues (muscles, fascia, and ligaments) are checked to see whether they are likely to stretch and allow the head to pass through, or whether they will remain taut and prevent descent.

The position of the presenting part is noted, as well as its ability to flex. Extreme asynclitism is a bad sign. Pressure is applied to the presenting part over the pubis and to the fundus of the uterus to see whether it can be forced down to the level of the ischial spines, or further. If this can be accomplished by manual pressure, then it can be assumed that strong uterine contractions will have no difficulty in doing the same.

These examinations should allow the patient to be placed into one of three categories:

1. No disproportion is present. This infant should go through this pelvis.
2. There is absolute fetopelvic disproportion.
3. The fetopelvic relationship is borderline. A trial of labor is indicated.

Radiographic Examination

Occasionally x-ray pelvimetry adds additional information and helps in making a decision.

Trial Labor

This is a clinical attempt to evaluate the extent of cephalopelvic disproportion. The patient is allowed to labor under close supervision to see if the natural forces of labor can overcome real or suspected disproportion. It is also an excellent measure of the labor mechanism, which often determines the success or failure of the trial.

First a careful study is made of the pelvic adequacy in the light of the size and presentation of the baby. If gross disproportion is encountered cesarean section should be elected.

It is preferable that the patient go into labor spontaneously. Induction is carried out only in special cases, but augmentation of labor by artificial rupture of membranes or an infusion of oxytocin is permissible once labor is well under way.

During the labor the following factors are evaluated:

1. Mental and physical condition of the mother
2. Fetal heart rate as well as other signs of fetal distress, such as the passage of meconium
3. Force and coordination of the uterine contractions
4. Dilatation of the cervix
5. Descent of the presenting part
6. Degree of molding and the formation and size of the caput succedaneum

The exact length of a trial of labor varies with each case, is a matter of judgment, and can be determined only by the attending obstetrician and his consultant. Sufficient time is allowed for the physician to decide whether there is fetopelvic disproportion and, if so, to what extent, and to evaluate the effectiveness of the uterine contractions. Good labor often overcomes minor degrees of disproportion.

Needless rectal or vaginal examinations should be avoided. They are painful and predispose to infection. At the end of a reasonable period of labor a careful vaginal examination is made under aseptic conditions to evaluate the state of the cervix, the fetal position and presentation, and the station of the presenting part. On the basis of these findings the decision is made as to the success or failure of the trial.

Favorable progress of cervical effacement and dilatation, descent of the head into the pelvis, and the demonstration that the lower part of the pelvis is adequate are the criteria for continuing the trial. A poor labor mechanism with irregular, desultory, and ineffective contractions, the lack of effacement and progressive dilatation of the cervix, and failure of the head to enter the inlet and descend to the ischial spines serve as evidence that the trial of labor has failed and that other means of delivery should be sought.

Augmentation of Labor

The hypothesis is that many patients who do not make good progress in labor fail to do so because of unrecognized inefficient uterine action. On this basis, before a diagnosis of disproportion is made, and before operative measures to effect delivery are employed, a trial of augmentation of labor by an infusion of oxytocin should be carried out. During the trial the fetal heart rate and the uterine contractions are monitored. This procedure is a test of the functional capacity of the pelvis and the ability of the cervix to dilate. There is no intention of forcing the head through a pelvis that is too small for it.

If the head does not descend well, if the rate of cervical dilatation is less than 1 cm per hour, and if delivery does not take place within the allotted time, cesarean section is considered. The achievement of an easy vaginal delivery excludes disproportion and avoids cesarean section.

Contraindications to Augmentation of Labor

1. Fetal distress.
2. Malpresentations.
3. Disproportion.
4. Existence of effective uterine contractions.
5. Previous cervical scarring.
6. Previous myomectomy, hysterotomy, or cesarean section.
7. Parity over 5 is not an absolute contraindication, but augmentation carries a greater risk of uterine rupture than in the less parous woman.
8. Bicornuate uterus.
9. Lack of adequate monitoring.

TREATMENT OF FETOPELVIC DISPROPORTION

Cesarean Section

Cesarean section is the method of choice when a marked degree of disproportion is present. The low transverse incision in the uterus is preferred by most.

Forceps Delivery

When the degree of disproportion is small, when the arrest is related to failure of flexion or rotation, and when the presenting part is well below the ischial spines, forceps may be used to effect delivery. If, however, the presenting part is at the level of the spines or higher, and if extraction by forceps would entail a difficult and traumatic procedure, cesarean section should be performed.

Induction of Premature Labor

Induction of premature labor, to try to deliver the baby while it is smaller, was once a popular procedure to overcome disproportion. The drawbacks are:

1. Prematurity with its attendant complications
2. Poorly formed lower uterine segment with its resistant tissues
3. Unripe cervix
4. Inefficient function of the uterus, which is stimulated into labor before its polarity and coordinate action have been established
5. Prolonged labor

For these reasons we feel that it is preferable to allow the patient to have a trial of labor at term and to perform cesarean section if necessary rather than induce labor prematurely.

Craniotomy

Craniotomy has no place in the planned treatment of disproportion. It is permissible only for dead babies in situations in which the fetus is not deliverable intact. Its aim is to spare the mother an operative abdominal delivery.

Symphysiotomy

Performed first in 1777 by Signault, symphysiotomy was abandoned because of the frequency of complications and the growing safety of cesarean section. In 1920 Zarate resurrected the procedure in Argentina, and Seedat and Crichton, working in Africa, published their modified technique in 1962. Symphysiotomy widens the space between the pubic bones, enlarges the pelvic capacity permanently, and is, in certain situations, an alternative to cesarean section. In some areas of the world, cesarean section, especially when the indication is cephalopelvic disproportion, is associated with a high incidence of uterine rupture because the patient does not return to hospital for consideration of repeat cesarean section with subsequent pregnancies.

Advantages

1. It takes only 5 minutes to perform.
2. It can be done anywhere.
3. Local anesthesia is adequate.

4. The uterus is unscarred.
5. The pelvis is enlarged permanently; the next delivery will be easier.

Indications

1. Moderate cephalopelvic disproportion. Symphysiotomy is an alternative to cesarean section or a difficult forceps delivery.
2. Difficulty with the aftercoming head in a breech presentation.
3. Patients who are poor surgical risks.

Prerequisites

1. Effective uterine action, spontaneous or induced by oxytocin
2. Less than 80 percent of the fetal head above the pelvic brim
3. Cervical dilatation of at least 8 cm

Contraindications

1. Inefficient uterine contractions.
2. Cervical dilatation less than 8 cm.
3. Previous cesarean section.
4. Fetal head more than 80 percent above the pelvic brim, especially if the membranes are ruptured.
5. True conjugate less than 8 cm.
6. Severe disproportion.
7. Malpresentation such as transverse lie or brow.
8. Suspected uterine rupture.
9. Deformity of the pelvis, back, or hips.
10. Marked obesity. The excessive weight puts too great a strain on the pelvis.
11. Baby estimated to weigh over 8 pounds.

Technique

With the patient in the lithotomy position and a Foley catheter in the bladder, the skin and subcutaneous tissue over the symphysis are infiltrated with a local anesthetic (Fig. 1). A 2-cm incision is made in an anteroposterior direction. The left hand is placed in the vagina to displace the urethra and catheter to one side and to prevent the knife from penetrating too deeply. The scalpel is positioned vertically with the cutting edge pointing inferiorly. The pubic joint is entered at the junction of the upper and middle thirds, and the lower two-thirds of the joint is incised. The knife is then turned 180° and the upper one-third of the joint is cut. The separation of the symphysis should be less than 2.5 cm.

During delivery the patient's legs must be controlled to prevent excessive separation of the symphyseal joint. The fetal head is pressed posteriorly, away from the anterior vaginal wall. The vacuum extractor may be used, but forceps should be avoided. Episiotomy increases the room posteriorly. After delivery the skin is closed with a single stitch.

Delay in Delivery
This may be caused by:

1. Inadequate uterine contractions
2. Insufficient separation of the joint
3. Inadequate episiotomy
4. Excessive residual disproportion
5. Fetal abnormality

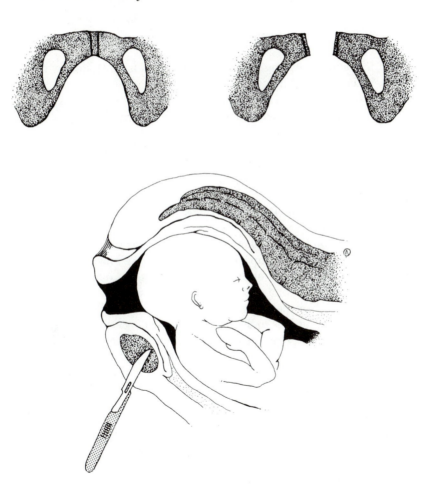

Figure 1. Symphisiotomy.

Postoperative Care

1. The Foley catheter is left in the bladder for 5 days.
2. A belt around the trochanters makes the woman more comfortable.
3. The patient remains in bed, preferably on her side, for 3 to 4 days.
4. She sits up out of bed on the 5th day, walks with the help of a cane on the 6th, and by the 10th day no longer needs the belt.
5. Undue muscular effort is avoided for 6 weeks.

Complications

1. Urinary tract.
   a. Infection is the most common.
   b. Vesicovaginal and urethrovaginal fistula.
   c. Stress incontinence is rare.
2. Hemorrhage.
   a. Venous bleeding in the incisional area is controlled by pressure.
   b. Postpartum hemorrhage.
3. Tears of the anterior vaginal wall.
4. Instability of the symphyseal joint occurs occasionally when the separation was excessive.
5. There may be temporary difficulty in walking, but most women are able to resume previous physical activity.

PREGNANCY IN PATIENTS UNDER 15 YEARS OF AGE

A study of pregnant girls under 15 years of age was made and the findings compared with a paired group between the ages of 19 and 25. Only two complications occurred more often in the youngsters, namely, pregnancy-induced hypertension and pelvic contraction, especially at the inlet. It is probable that the bony pelvis had not reached its potential size at the time of delivery. A trial of labor is indicated, but the incidence of cesarean section is higher than average. There is no expected increase in maternal or infant mortality and morbidity.

GRAND MULTIPARITY

The definition varies, but parity of 6 seems to be an acceptable figure. During pregnancy the grand multipara has an increased incidence of:

1. Anemia
2. Toxemia of pregnancy
3. Placenta previa
4. Abruptio placentae

Complications of Labor and Delivery

1. Malpresentations, such as transverse lie and breech
2. Postpartum hemorrhage
3. Disproportion caused by a large baby
4. Rupture of the uterus
5. High incidence of midforceps

Management

1. Delivery should take place in a hospital.
2. Careful monitoring of labor and fetal heart is needed.
3. Oxytocin should be used rarely and with great care.
4. Cesarean section is performed when there is failure of progress or suspicion of disproportion.
5. Postpartum oxytocin drip is given to prevent hemorrhage from uterine atony.

Despite her problems the grand multipara can go through pregnancy, labor, and delivery safely. However, there must be no false sense of security.

BIBLIOGRAPHY

Boyd ME, Usher RH, McLean FH: Fetal macrosomia: Prediction, risks, proposed management. Obstet Gynecol 61:715, 1983

Duenhoelter JH, Jimenez JM, Baumann G: Pregnancy performance of patients under fifteen years of age. Obstet Gynecol 46:49, 1975

Golditch IM, Kirkman K: The large fetus. Obstet Gynecol 52:26, 1978

Hartfield VJ: A comparison of the early and late effects of subcutaneous symphysiotomy and of lower segment cesarean section. J Obstet Gynaecol Brit Commonw 80:508, 1973

Kopenhager T: A review of 50 pregnant patients with kyphoscoliosis. Brit J Obstet Gynaecol 84:585, 1977

Modanlou HD, Dorchester WL, Thorasian A, Freeman RK: Macrosomia—maternal, fetal, and neonatal implications. Obstet Gynecol 55:420, 1980

O'Driscoll K, Foley M, MacDonald D: Active management of labor as an alternative to cesarean section for dystocia. Obstet Gynecol 63:485, 1984

46

Cesarean Section

Cesarean section is an operation by which the child is delivered through an incision in the abdominal wall and the uterus. The first professional cesarean was performed in the United States in 1827. Before 1800 cesarean section was performed rarely and was usually fatal. In London and Edinburgh in 1877, of 35 cesareans performed 33 resulted in the death of the mother. By 1877 there had been 71 cesarean operations in the United States. The mortality rate was 52 percent, mainly because of infection and hemorrhage.

INDICATIONS FOR CESAREAN SECTION

Indications for cesarean section are absolute or relative. Any condition that makes delivery via the birth canal impossible is an absolute indication for abdominal section. Among these are extreme degrees of pelvic contraction and neoplasms blocking the passage. With a relative indication, vaginal birth is possible but the conditions are such that cesarean section is safer for the mother, the child, or both.

Pelvic Contraction and Dystocia

1. Fetopelvic disproportion
2. Malpresentation and malposition
3. Uterine dysfunction
4. Soft tissue dystocia
5. Neoplasms
6. Failure to progress

Previous Uterine Surgery

1. Cesarean section
2. Hysterotomy
3. Myomectomy
4. Cervical suture

Hemorrhage

1. Placenta previa
2. Abruptio placentae

Toxemia of Pregnancy

1. Preeclampsia and eclampsia
2. Hypertension
3. Renal disease

Fetal Indications

1. Fetal distress
2. Previous fetal death or damage
3. Prolapse of the umbilical cord
4. Placental insufficiency (IUGR)
5. Maternal diabetes
6. Rhesus incompatibility
7. Postmaternal death
8. Maternal genital herpes

Miscellaneous

1. Elderly primigravida
2. Previous vaginal repair
3. Congenital uterine anomaly
4. Poor obstetric history
5. Failed forceps

Frequency of Cesarean Section

The rate of cesarean section has risen steadily from an incidence of 3 to 4 percent of 25 years ago to the present 10 to 20 percent. A figure of 15 percent seems to be acceptable. Not only has the operation become safer for the mother, but the number of infants damaged by prolonged labor and traumatic vaginal operations has been reduced. In addition, concern for the quality of life and the intellectual development of the child has widened the indications for cesarean section.

The largest increase in the use of cesarean section is in those cases described as having "dystocia." While conditions such as disproportion, malpresentation, and incoordinate uterine action are included in this group, in many instances the exact diagnosis is not made, and the diagnosis of "dystocia" represents slow progress in labor from whatever cause. The use of cesarean section for these patients is part of a more aggressive management of poor progress in labor and the abandonment of difficult midforceps operations.

While it appears clear that the replacement of high forceps and difficult midforceps operations by cesarean section has reduced the perinatal morbidity and mortality in this area, the available evidence does not support the contention that the great expansion in the rates of cesarean section for other indications has contributed significantly to the reduction in the rates of perinatal mortality in recent years. Certainly, the more frequent use of cesarean section has led to an increase in the rate of maternal morbidity.

Pelvic Contractions and Mechanical Dystocia

Fetopelvic Disproportion. Fetopelvic disproportion includes the contracted pelvis, the overgrown fetus, or a relative disparity between the size of the baby and that of the pelvis. Contributing to the problem of disproportion are the shape of the pelvis, the presentation of the fetus and its ability to mold and engage, the dilatability of the cervix, and the effectiveness of the uterine contractions.

Malposition and Malpresentation. These abnormalities may make cesarean section necessary when a baby in normal position could be born per vaginam. A great part of the increased incidence of cesarean section in this group is associated with breech presentation. Today over half of babies in breech presentation are born by cesarean section.

Uterine Dysfunction. Uterine dysfunction includes incoordinate uterine action, inertia, constriction ring, and inability of the cervix to dilate. Labor is prolonged and progress may cease altogether. These conditions are often associated with disproportion and malpresentations.

Soft Tissue Dystocia. Soft tissue dystocia may prevent or make normal birth difficult. This includes such conditions as scars in the genital tract, cervical rigidity from injury or surgery, and atresia or stenosis of the vagina. Forceful vaginal delivery results in large lacerations and hemorrhage.

Neoplasms. Neoplasms that block the pelvis make normal delivery impossible. Invasive cancer of the cervix diagnosed during the third trimester of pregnancy is treated by cesarean section followed by radiation therapy, radical surgery, or both.

Failure to Progress. In this group are included such conditions as cephalopelvic disproportion, ineffective uterine contractions, poor pelvis, large baby, and deflexion of the fetal head. Often an exact diagnosis cannot be made and is academic in any case. The decision in favor of cesarean section is made on the failure of the labor to achieve cervical dilatation and/or fetal descent regardless of the etiology.

Previous Uterine Surgery

Cesarean Section. In 1916, E.B. Cragin expressed the opinion that, in women who had had a previous cesarean section, the risk of uterine rupture was so high and the consequences of such an accident so costly that a repeat cesarean section should be performed prior to the onset of labor. His dictum, "Once a cesarean, always a cesarean," has been observed for many years, but the concept is being reevaluated because of the increasing incidence of cesarean section, the high rate of maternal morbidity with abdominal delivery, and the lower risk of rupture when the original incision was transverse and confined to the lower segment of the uterus. Under certain conditions a trial of labor is permissible for women who have had a cesarean section. When successful, maternal morbidity, length of stay in hospital, and period of convalescence are reduced. The faster recovery enables the woman to participate earlier in the care of the infant, herself, and her family. Recent data suggest that about half the women who have been delivered by cesarean section can have a trial of labor in future pregnancies.

Hysterotomy. Pregnancy in a uterus in which a previous gestation was terminated by hysterotomy is attended by danger of uterine rupture. The risk is similar to that of classical cesarean section. Hysterotomy should be avoided whenever possible, keeping in mind that the next pregnancy might necessitate cesarean section.

Extensive Myomectomy. Myomectomy in the past is an indication for cesarean section only if the operation was extensive, the myometrium disorganized, and the incision extended into the endometrial cavity. The previous removal of pedunculated or subserous fibromyomas does not call for cesarean section.

Cervical Cerclage. In some cases where there has been a cervical suture or repair of an incompetent os, cesarean section may be necessary because of fibrosis of the cervix.

Trial of Labor After Previous Cesarean Section

Prerequisites

1. A previous lower segment transverse incision with no extension, as documented by the hospital record and the operative note.
2. The previous indication for cesarean section no longer exists.
3. Cephalic presentation.
4. No disproportion.
5. No previous uterine rupture.
6. Expectation of a normal labor and delivery.
7. No medical or obstetric complications.
8. Readily available blood, operating facilities, and in-house anesthesia.
9. Patient understands and accepts the risks.

Contraindictions

1. More than one previous cesarean section
2. Previous fundal or lower segment vertical incision, or T-shaped extension
3. Unknown incision
4. Advice by the surgeon who did the first operation against a trial of labor
5. Abnormal presentation, such as brow, breech, or transverse lie
6. Contracted pelvis or disproportion
7. Recurring indication
8. Urgent medical or obstetric indication for delivery
9. Unavailability of blood, or refusal of patient to accept blood transfusion
10. Operating room away from the delivery suite; inability to perform immediate cesarean section
11. Patient's refusal to undergo a trial of labor

Guidelines for Management of the Trial

1. Ideally, the onset of labor is spontaneous.
2. The patient should come to hospital immediately if:
   a. She thinks that labor has begun.

      b. The membranes have ruptured.

      c. There is vaginal bleeding.

3. On admission to hospital:
   a. The maternal-fetal status is evaluated.
   b. An intravenous infusion is set up.
   c. Blood is cross-matched and available.
   d. Cardiotachometry is established.
4. During labor:
   a. The fetal heart is monitored.
   b. The uterine contractions are assessed by an electronic system or by a hand on the abdomen almost continually.
   c. Maternal vital signs are checked every 15 minutes.
   d. The patient is never left unattended.
   e. The physician must be on the labor floor at all times.
   f. Labor should progress normally.
5. While the use of oxytocin to stimulate labor is not contra-indicated, it must be used with great care and only in selected cases.
6. There has been concern that epidural block might mask the symptoms and signs of impending or actual rupture of the uterus. This does not appear to be justified, however, and epidural block has been used with success.
7. Delivery should be spontaneous or by low forceps. Difficult vaginal operations are contraindicated.
8. Following the delivery the cavity of the uterus is explored for evidence of rupture.
9. The trial continues until vaginal delivery occurs or cesarean section is performed. Most patients should be delivered by 8 hours.
10. The main indications for discontinuing the trial and performing cesarean section are:
    a. Arrest of progress.
    b. Fetal distress.
    c. Suspicion that the scar is giving way.

Results and Safety

A recent review of the English literature from 1950 to 1980 indicated that properly conducted vaginal delivery following cesarean section in a previous pregnancy is relatively safe.

1. The incidence of uterine rupture ranged from 0 to 2.8 percent, with an average of 0.7 percent.
2. No maternal deaths were the result of uterine rupture.

3. Perinatal mortality associated with rupture of the uterus was 0.93 per 1000 births.
4. Approximately 70 to 80 percent of patients whose indication for the first cesarean section is nonrecurrent can be expected to deliver safely per vaginam. This rate is reduced in patients whose prior cesarean section was performed for cephalopelvic disproportion.
5. Patients with a previous vaginal delivery seem to have a better prognosis for successful vaginal birth than those without a previous vaginal delivery.
6. A classic cesarean section scar increases the probability of uterine rupture in a subsequent pregnancy, the rupture is more likely to be complete, and the incidence of fetal death is higher.
7. A trial of labor is highly acceptable to most patients.

Hemorrhage

Placenta Previa.   Cesarean section in all cases of central and many cases of partial placenta previa has reduced both fetal and maternal mortality.

Abruptio Placentae. Abruptio placentae occurring before or during early labor may be treated by rupture of the membranes and oxytocin drip. When the hemorrhage is severe, the cervix hard and closed, or uteroplacental apoplexy suspected, cesarean section may be necessary to save the baby, to control hemorrhage, to prevent afibrinogenemia, and to observe the condition of the uterus and its ability to contract and control the bleeding. In some cases hysterectomy is necessary.

Toxemia of Pregnancy

These states must be considered:

1. Preeclampsia and eclampsia
2. Essential hypertension
3. Chronic nephritis

Toxemia of pregnancy may require termination of the pregnancy before term. In most cases induction of labor is the method of choice. When the cervix is not ripe and induction would be difficult, cesarean section is preferable.

Fetal Indications

DISTRESS Fetal distress, severe bradycardia, irregularity of the fetal heart rate, or late patterns of deceleration, sometimes necessitates emergency cesarean section. The rate of cesarean section is high in monitored patients. This is not surprising since the main indications for monitoring are those which predispose to fetal hypoxia. However, fetal distress is not the prime reason for increasing the rate of cesarean section. Problems associated with dystocia are the main indications for abdominal delivery. A new indication for cesarean section is described as fetal intolerance of labor. This is seen in patients who have desultory labors. Stimulation by oxytocin may result in abnormalities of the FHR. Often an emergency cesarean section is performed, but a normal baby with no evidence of asphyxia is delivered.

PREVIOUS FETAL DEATH OR DAMAGE Especially in older women who have given birth to more than one dead or damaged baby, cesarean section may be elected.

PROLAPSE OF THE UMBILICAL CORD Prolapse of the umbilical cord in the presence of an undilated cervix is managed best by cesarean section, provided the baby is in good condition.

PLACENTAL INSUFFICIENCY In cases of intrauterine growth retardation or postterm pregnancy, when clinical examinations and various tests suggest that the baby is in jeopardy, delivery may be necessary. If induction is not feasible or fails, cesarean section is indicated. There is an increased ability of pediatricians to salvage small babies and, when the need exists, cesarean section may offer these infants the best chance for survival and a good chance for normal development.

MATERNAL DIABETES The fetus of the diabetic mother is inclined to be larger than normal, and this can lead to difficult labor and delivery. Although these infants are large they behave like prematures and do not withstand well the rigors of a long labor. Death during labor and the postnatal period is common. In addition, a number of babies die in utero before term is reached. Because of these dangers to the fetus and because a high proportion of pregnant diabetics develop toxemia, the pregnancy may require termination before term. When conditions are favorable and a rapid and easy labor is anticipated, induction of labor can be carried out. However, if there are urgent reasons for immediate delivery, if induction fails, or if good progress in labor is not made, cesarean section should be performed.

RHESUS INCOMPATIBILITY When a fetus is becoming progressively damaged by the antibodies of a sensitized Rh-negative mother and when induction and delivery per vaginam would be difficult, the pregnancy may be terminated by caesarean section in selected cases for fetal salvage.

POSTMORTEM CESAREAN Post mortem cesarean sections were performed in Rome as early as 715 BC, when Numa Pompilius decreed that if a pregnant woman died, the fetus was to be cut out of her abdomen. The intent of the decree was not to save the life of the infant, but to obviate its being buried with the mother. In 237 BC the first reported infant who survived postmortem cesarean section was Scipio Africanus. He grew up to become the Roman General who defeated Hannibal. Some 15 percent of infants born in these circumstances are in good condition. Their survival depends on how soon they are extracted, their maturity, the nature and duration of the maternal illness, the performance of cardiopulmonary resuscitation on the mother, and the availability of neonatal intensive care.

HERPES VIRUS HOMINIS INFECTION OF THE GENITAL TRACT This is a cause of serious, often fatal, infection of the newborn infant. When genital herpes infection is present at term the risk of clinically apparent infection in the infant delivered per vaginam has been estimated at being between 40 and 60 percent. In about half of these the infection will be severe or fatal. Herpes infection in the newborn is almost always acquired from the mother's infected birth canal, either as an ascending infection after the membranes have ruptured, or during passage through the vagina. In the latter situation there is contamination of the child's eyes, scalp, skin, umbilical cord, and upper respiratory tract. The possibility of transplacental transmission is small, certainly far less important than direct contact during labor and delivery. The greatest hazard to the baby exists when the primary genital infection occurred 2 to 4 weeks prior to delivery. The risk of fetal infection at term is greater during primary genital herpes infection than during recurrent genital herpes. Often it is difficult to distinguish between these two. Fetuses at risk receive some maternal antibodies transplacentally, and this may play some part in limiting infection.

The danger of the occurrence of asymptomatic genital infection and reactivation at term makes weekly culturing of the cervix and other sites of previous infection, beginning at 36 weeks, an integral part of the management of all women with culture-verified herpes infection during pregnancy. The choice of route of delivery is predicated upon the results of the most recent genital culture, provided it has been performed 3 or more days before the onset of labor.

Vaginal delivery is permitted if the cultures are negative, indicating that the infection has not been reactivated, if there are no visible vulvar lesions, and there is no vulvar pruritus or paresthesia. In most pregnancies vaginal delivery is safe and cesarean section can be avoided.

Cesarean section is indicated for women with documented or clinically suspicious cases of genital herpes infection at the time of labor. Although the risk of fetal infection is higher when the membranes have been ruptured for 4 to 6 hours, cesarean section should be performed in all cases of proven or strongly suspicious cases of herpes infection regardless of the duration of labor or the length of time that the membranes have been ruptured.

Breast feeding by infected mothers is permissible, provided that direct contact between the infant and infected areas in the mother is avoided. Nursing is prohibited when herpetic lesions are present on the breast.

Miscellaneous

ELDERLY PRIMIGRAVIDITY   Elderly primigravidity is difficult to define. While the age varies from 35 to 40 years, other factors are equally important. These include the presence or absence of a good lower uterine segment, elasticity or rigidity of the cervix and the soft tissues of the birth canal, ease of becoming pregnant, number of abortions, fetal presentation, and coordination of the uterine powers. When all these points are favorable vaginal delivery should be considered. When the adverse factors are present cesarean section may be the wiser and safer procedure.

PREVIOUS VAGINAL REPAIR   Fear that vaginal delivery will cause a recurrence of cystocele, rectocele, and uterine prolapse may lead to an elective cesarean section.

CONGENITAL UTERINE ANOMALY   Not only does an abnormal uterus often function badly, but in the case of anomalies such as a bicornuate uterus one horn may block the passage of the baby from the other. In such cases cesarean section must be performed.

POOR OBSTETRIC HISTORY   When a previous delivery has been difficult and traumatic with extensive injury to the cervix, vagina, and perineum, or when the baby has been injured, cesarean section may be selected for subsequent births.

FAILED FORCEPS   Failed forceps is an indication for cesarean section. It is wiser to turn to abdominal delivery than to drag a baby through the pelvis by force.

TYPES OF CESAREAN SECTION

Position of the Patient on the Operating Table

The practice of placing a wedge under the patient's right hip to tilt her to her left side at the time of cesarean section is well established. This permits the uterus and its contents to fall away from the inferior vena cava and the aorta. The return circulation from the patient's lower extremities to the right heart is improved, supine hypotension is prevented, and good placental perfusion is maintained.

Skin Incisions

Vertical Incision
The incision employed most often for cesarean section has been the midline, vertical, hypogastric incision, extending from the symphysis pubis to the umbilicus, and above the umbilicus when necessary. The advantages of this approach are that it provides excellent exposure, and entry into the abdominal cavity can be made rapidly. In cases of acute fetal distress, when time is of paramount importance, the vertical incision is the one of choice.

Transverse Incision
The Pfannenstiel transverse suprasymphyseal incision has been gaining steadily in popularity. The incision in the skin is semilunar just above the pubic hairline, the angles inclined slightly upward towards the anteriorsuperior iliac crests. This incision has several advantages. The cosmetic result is far better than the vertical incision; the scar is narrow and often is partly hidden by the hair on the mons pubis. Many women are demanding the "Bikini cut." The abdominal wall, postoperatively, is stronger because of the perpendicular relationship between the incisions in the fascia, the muscles, and the peritoneum, and because there is less side-to-side tension on the scar. Postoperative pain is reduced and the patient can be active much sooner. Dehiscence is rare. The disadvantages of the Pfaanenstiel incision are that the exposure may not be as good as with the vertical incision, and the fact that the procedure is time consuming and should not be used when an acute emergency exists.

Lower Segment of Uterus: Transverse Incision

Because it permits safe abdominal delivery even when performed late in labor and even when the uterine cavity is infected, the lower segment transverse incision (Fig. 1A) has revolutionized obstetric practice in the following respects:

1. It allows the obstetrician to change his mind.
2. It has resulted in the concepts of trial of labor, trial of oxytocin stimulation, and trial forceps.
3. The need for traumatic forceps delivery has been virtually eliminated.
4. The indications for cesarean section have been widened.
5. Maternal morbidity and mortality are lower than with upper segment procedures.
6. The uterus is left with a stronger scar.

In our opinion this is the procedure of choice. The abdomen is opened and the uterus exposed. The vesicouterine fold of peritoneum (bladder flap), which lies near the junction of the upper and lower uterine segments is identified and incised transversely; it is dissected off the lower segment and, with the bladder, is pushed downward and retracted out of the way. A small transverse incision is made in the lower segment of the uterus and is extended laterally with the fingers, stopping short of the area of the uterine vessels. To avoid injury to the fetus by the sharp blade of the scalpel, this incision can be made easily by the scalpel handle. The fetal head, which in most cases lies under the incision, is extracted or expressed, followed by the body, and then the placenta and membranes. The transverse incision is closed with a single or double layer of continuous catgut. The bladder flap of peritoneum is sewn back to the wall of the uterus above the incision so that this area is covered completely and isolated from the general peritoneal cavity. The abdomen is closed in layers.

Advantages

1. The incision is in the lower segment of the uterus. However, one must be certain it is in the thin lower segment and not in the inferior part of the muscular upper segment.
2. The muscle is split laterally instead of being cut; this leads to less bleeding.
3. Incision into the placenta is rare.
4. The head is usually under the incision and is extracted easily.
5. The thin muscle layer of the lower segment is easier to reapproximate than the thick upper segment.

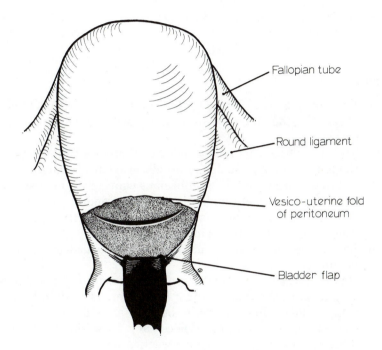

A. Lower segment transverse incision.

Figure 1. Cesarean section incisions.

6. The entire incision is covered by the bladder flap, thus reducing spill into the general peritoneal cavity.
7. Rupture of the transverse scar in a subsequent pregnancy poses only a small threat to the mother and fetus.
   a. The incidence of rupture is lower.
   b. This accident occurs rarely before term. Hence the patient is in the hospital under close observation.
   c. The loss of blood from the less vascular lower segment is less than from the corpus.
   d. Rupture of the low transverse incision is followed only rarely by expulsion of the fetus or by a separation of the placenta, so that there is a chance to save the baby.

Disadvantages

1. If the incision extends too far laterally, as may occur if the baby is very big, the uterine vessels can be torn, causing profuse hemorrhage.
2. The procedure is not advisable when there is an abnormality in the lower segment, such as fibroids or extensive varicosities.
3. Previous surgery or dense adhesions which prevent easy access to the lower segment make the operation onerous.
4. When the lower segment is not well formed, the transverse operation is difficult to perform.
5. Sometimes the bladder is adherent to a previous scar, and it may be injured.
6. On rare occasions, because of a narrow lower uterine segment or a large baby, the infant cannot be delivered through the transverse incision. To make more room a J-shaped (Fig. 1B) or a T-shaped (Fig. 1C) extension is necessary. These should be avoided if possible because they have a weakening effect on the uterus. Future deliveries should be by repeat cesarean section.

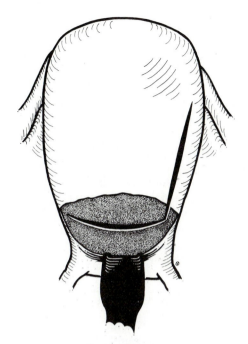

B. J incision.

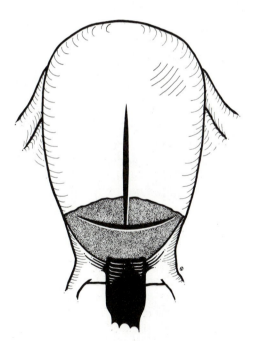

C. T incision.

Figure 1. (cont.) Cesarean section incisions.

Lower Segment of Uterus: Vertical Incision

The exposure is the same as with the transverse incision. The vertical incision (Fig. 1D) is made with the scalpel and is enlarged with blunt scissors to avoid injury to the baby.

The vertical incision has an advantage in that it can be carried upward when necessary. This may be needed when the baby is large, when the lower segment is poorly formed, when there is a fetal malposition such as transverse lie, or when there is fetal anomaly such as conjoined twins. Some obstetricians prefer this incision for placenta previa.

One of the main disadvantages is that since the muscle is cut there is more bleeding from the incised edges; often, too, the incision extends inadvertently into the upper segment, and the value of a completely retroperitoneal closure is lost.

Classical Cesarean Section: Upper Segment of Uterus

A longitudinal midline incision (Fig. 1E) is made with the scalpel into the anterior wall of the uterus and is enlarged upward and downward with blunt-nosed scissors. A large opening is needed since the baby is often delivered as a breech. The fetus and placenta are removed and the uterus is closed in three layers. In modern times there is almost no justification for classical cesarean section. Technical difficulty in exposing the lower segment is the only indication for the upper segment procedure.

Indications

1. Difficulty in exposing the lower uterine segment
   a. Large blood vessels on the anterior wall
   b. High and adherent bladder
   c. Myoma in the lower segment
2. Impacted tranverse lie
3. Some cases of anterior placenta previa
4. Certain uterine malformations

Disadvantages

1. Thick myometrium is cut, large sinuses are opened, and bleeding is profuse.
2. The baby is often extracted as a breech with greater aspiration of amniotic fluid
3. Should the placenta be attached to the anterior wall of the uterus the incision cuts into it and may lead to dangerous loss of blood from the fetal circulation.

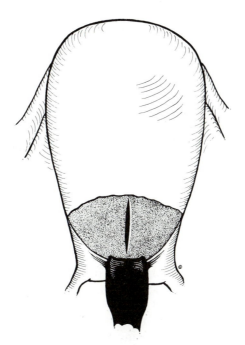

D. Lower segment vertical incision.

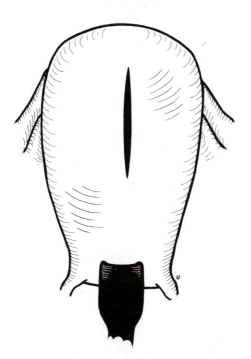

E. Upper segment classical vertical incision.

Figure 1. (cont.) Cesarean section incisions.

4. The incision lies uncovered in the general peritoneal cavity, and there is greater chance of seepage of infected uterine contents with resultant peritonitis.
5. There is a higher incidence of adhesion of abdominal contents to the line of closure in the uterus.
6. There is a higher incidence of uterine rupture in subsequent pregnancies.

Extraperitoneal Cesarean Section

The extraperitoneal operation was devised in the preantibiotic era to obviate the use of hysterectomy in grossly infected cases to prevent general and often fatal infection. The purpose of the procedure was to avoid the spillage of infected amniotic fluid into the peritoneal cavity and subsequent peritonitis and abscess. Among the methods are those described by Latzko, Norton, and Waters.

The technique of extraperitoneal cesarean section is relatively difficult unless one has special training; accidental entry into the peritoneal cavity occurs, negating the purpose of the procedure, and there is an increase in injury to the bladder. Better prenatal care, reduction in the incidence of prolonged labor and the neglected patient, the availability of blood, and the use of effective antibiotics to combat infection, have almost eliminated the need for the extraperitoneal procedure. It is employed rarely today.

Delivery of the Placenta

There is a tendency to rush the delivery of the placenta at cesarean section. This may lead to profuse bleeding. It is our experience that, in the absence of any reasons to do otherwise, it is better to wait a few minutes for the placenta to separate from the wall of the uterus. Its delivery becomes easy and bleeding is minimal.

MORTALITY AND MORBIDITY FOLLOWING CESAREAN SECTION

Maternal Mortality

The gross uncorrected mortality rate in the United States and Canada is approximately 30:10,000 cesarean sections. In many clinics the rate is much lower, well under 10:10,000. However, Evrard and Gold found the risk of maternal death associated with cesarean section to be 26 times greater than with vaginal delivery. They noted a tenfold increase in the risk of maternal death inherent in the operation itself. The increasing use of cesarean section to protect the baby may lead to a higher danger for the mother.

Factors That Add to the Risk

1. Age over 30
2. Grand multiparity
3. Obesity, over 200 pounds
4. Prolonged labor
5. Prolonged period of ruptured membranes
6. Numerous vaginal examinations
7. Low socioeconomic status

Causes of Maternal Death

1. Hemorrhage
2. Infection
3. Anesthesia
4. Pulmonary embolism
5. Renal failure following prolonged hypotension
6. Intestinal obstruction and paralytic ileus
7. Heart failure
8. Toxemia of pregnancy
9. Rupture of uterine scar
10. Miscellaneous causes not related to the operation, e.g., cancer

Reasons for a Decline in Mortality Rate

1. Adequate blood transfusion
2. Use of antimicrobial drugs
3. Improved surgical methods
4. Better anesthetic techniques and specially trained anesthesiologists
5. The realization that patients with heart disease do better with vaginal delivery than with cesarean section
6. Basic treatment of toxemia of pregnancy by medical rather than by surgical methods

Maternal Morbidity

Maternal morbidity is defined as a temperature of 100.4° F (38°C) or over occurring on any 2 of the first 10 days postpartum, exclusive of the first 24 hours. It is more common after cesarean section than after normal delivery, the incidence being between 15 and 20 percent. Antimicrobials, blood transfusions, better surgical technique, use of the lower segment operation, and improved anesthesia have all contributed to the decrease in postcesarean maternal morbidity.

Almost half of the patients undergoing cesarean section develop operative or postoperative complications, some of which are serious and potentially lethal. It must be accepted that cesarean section is a major operation with the attendant risks. Standard morbidity for cesarean section is around 20 percent.

Serious Complications

1. *Hemorrhage*
   a. Uterine atony.
   b. Extension of uterine incision.
   c. Difficulty removing the placenta.
   d. Hematoma of the broad ligament
2. *Infection*
   a. Genital tract.
   b. Incision.
   c. Urinary tract.
   d. Lungs and upper respiratory tract.
3. *Thrombophlebitis*
4. *Damage to the urinary tract,* with or without the formation of a fistula, occurs in less than 1 percent of cesarean sections. Most important is the recognition of the injury at the time it happens. Those that are discovered during the operation can be repaired immediately, and the return of normal function is likely. Late diagnosis necessitates a second operation and considerable discomfort in the interim. Postoperative pain in the flank after a difficult cesarean section with much bleeding calls for an intravenous pyelogram.
   a. Bladder injury is caused mainly during the development of the bladder flap over the lower uterine segment and the displacement of the bladder caudad. In repeat cesarean section, adhesions and scar tissue from the previous operation may make the dissection difficult. Defects in the bladder caused by accidental entry are repaired with a double layer of 3-0 chromic catgut. Drainage of the bladder is continued for 10 days. In most of these cases, when the injury is recognized and repaired, healing takes place. Occasionally a fistula develops between the bladder and the vagina.

   A rare complication of cesarean section is a vesico-uterine fistula. This condition occurs during the performance of a low cesarean section when unrecognized injury to the bladder takes place or the bladder is included in the closure of the uterine incision. The fistula is between the bladder and the uterus at the site of the incision for the cesarean section. These patients have incontinence, the urine passing from the bladder into the uterus and thence through the cervix into the vagina. Urinary infection may develop. Investigation: (1) Methylene blue dye instilled in the bladder enters the vagina. (2) Cystoscopy reveals the site of the fistula and determines the relationship of the fistula to the ureteral orifices. (3) An intravenous or a retrograde pyelogram will evaluate the upper urinary tract.

Because a number of these conditions will undergo spontaneous closure, a trial of conservative management is reasonable. This consists of continuous drainage of the bladder by urethral catheter and antibiotics to prevent infection. If this management fails, surgical closure of the fistula is performed. An abdominal approach is preferred. Early repair has been carried out successfully. It is probably advisable to wait, however, until uterine involution has taken place.

   b. Ureteral injury is caused by extension of the transverse incision in the lower uterine segment or the vagina, and during attempts to control profuse bleeding in the broad ligament. The ureter may be cut, crushed, tied, or devitalized. If there is suspicion that a ureter has been injured, the bladder may be opened and the ureteral orifices inspected. One way of diagnosis is to inject 10 ml of indigo carmine intravenously and observe the efflux of blue urine from the ureters, indicating that they are intact. Or the dye may be seen in the surrounding tissue, suggesting that the ureter has been cut. If recognized, repair should be carried out immediately.

5. *Intestinal complications:*
   a. Lacerations should be repaired immediately by a double-layer of 3-0 chromic catgut.
   b. Obstruction may be paralytic or mechanical. Volvulus accounts for some 25 percent of intestinal obstruction associated with pregnancy. The sigmoid is the most common site. Volvulus of the transverse colon, the small bowel, or the cecum occurs less frequently. The diagnosis of intestinal obstruction in the postcesarean patient is difficult and is often delayed. The treatment is surgical.

6. *Inadvertent vaginal incision* during cesarean section. The patient at risk is a parturient whose cervix is fully dilated, and who has been pushing in the second stage of labor for some time.

The operator, thinking he is making the incision in the thinned-out lower uterine segment, makes the incision into the vagina. Possible complications include injury to the bladder or ureter, vesical fistula, laceration of adjacent ligamentous structures, and hemorrhage. Management requires meticulous hemostasis, careful search for tears in the bladder, and anatomic closure of the vagina. The problem can be avoided by making the incision in the lower uterine segment above the reflection of the vesi-couterine peritoneum.

Prevention of Infection

Along with the rise in the rates of cesarean section there has been an increase in the incidence of maternal febrile morbidity, infections of the endometrium and wound, and prolonged hospitalization. There is evidence that the incidence of infection can be reduced by the perioperative administration of an antibiotic before the local defense mechanisms are overwhelmed.

High-Risk Factors. Because the benefits of prophylactic antibiotic therapy to low-risk patients appears to be minimal, and because there are adverse effects from the administration of antibiotics, it may be best to restrict this regimen to patients who are at high risk for postoperative infection. The factors involved include:.

1. Low socioeconomic status
2. Gestational age less than 38 weeks
3. Obesity
4. Hematocrit under 30 percent
5. Rupture of membranes over 8 hours before delivery
6. Labor lasting over 12 hours before the cesarean section is performed
7. More than three vaginal examinations during labor
8. Use of both an intrauterine pressure catheter and a scalp electrode for FHR monitoring, especially if they were in place for more than 9 hours

When none of these factors is present, the use of prophylactic antibiotics does not decrease the rate of infection. When one or more is present the patient is at increased risk for infection, and prophylactic antibiotics should be used.

Clamping of the Umbilical Cord. Although a high level of antibiotic in the tissues before surgery is desirable, it has been shown that the administration of the drug immediately after the clamping of the cord is as effective in preventing maternal infection as when it is given preoperatively. This technique eliminates the risk of antibiotic exposure to the unborn infant as well as the masking of a neonatal infection. Hence, antibacterial agents given to women at high risk should be withheld until the umbilical cord has been clamped.

Adverse Effects. Toxic effects on the mother from prophylactic antibiotic therapy are rare. These include (1) Primary hypersensitivity, including rash, fever, and pruritus. In most cases discontinuance of the antibiotic and observation are adequate treatment. If there is a history of allergy to an antibiotic, it should not be employed. (2) Anaphylactic shock is a possibility. (3) Most other side effects occur with long-term therapy and are not seen in association with prophylactic treatment.

Antibiotic of Choice. When used prophylactically, a single antibiotic with broad-spectrum coverage against most pelvic pathogens appears to be as effective as a combination of two or more drugs, and would be associated with fewer side effects. No one drug has been shown to be more effective than others. The cost of drugs has to be considered. Popular antibiotics include a combination of penicillin and gentamycin, cephalothin, and cephoxitin.

Dosage and Duration of Treatment. The current trend is to administer the drug for a short period; continuation after 12 hours does not seem to be of any benefit. One regimen is to give cephalothin or cephoxitin 2 grams intravenously as soon as the umbilical cord has been clamped, and to repeat it in 6 and 12 hours. Some investigators have reported that a single dose given when the cord is clamped is just as effective as the multiple dose method.

Fetal Mortality

Fetal mortality associated with cesarean section is higher than that of vaginal delivery. Some of the reasons follow.

1. Conditions such as toxemia of pregnancy, erythroblastosis, and placenta previa that require treatment by cesarean section result in premature, small infants.
2. Iatrogenic prematurity. On occasion the performance of an elective cesarean on a date determined entirely by the menstrual history has led to the birth of a premature infant. In some cases respiratory distress syndrome developed, and occasionally the baby died. It is important, therefore, that an accurate assess-

ment of fetal gestational age be made before the pregnancy is terminated. Methods of achieving this include:

a. Clinical parameters, including the date of the onset of the last menstrual period, uterine size at the first prenatal visit, date of quickening, date when the fetal heart tones were first heard using an ordinary fetal stethoscope, and date of an early positive pregnancy test, taken in combination, correlate well with the gestational age of the fetus.

b. Ultrasonography. Measurement of the crown-rump length between the 8th and 14th week of gestation permits dating to within ± 5 days, and by measurement of the biparietal diameter between 15 and 25 weeks dating is possible to ± 10 days. Serial ultrasonic scans will narrow the spread.

c. Amniocentesis with measurement of the L/S ratio in the amniotic fluid is an accurate way of determining fetal pulmonary maturity. It is, however, an invasive technique and carries a small risk. For this reason many physicians restricted its use to situations where other methods of determining the maturity of the fetus leave serious doubt.

d. Some obstetricians delay the cesarean section until the onset of spontaneous labor. This is an effective way of obviating the delivery of a premature infant. The major drawbacks to this approach are the risks of operating on a woman with a full stomach, and the small danger (reported to be less than 1 percent) of uterine rupture. The patient must come to hospital at the first sign of labor.

3. While respiratory complications such as atelectasis and hyaline membrane disease and the respiratory distress syndrome are more common in premature infants, the incidence is higher when the premature baby is born by cesarean section.

4. Conditions such as placenta previa, abruptio placentae, diabetes, preeclampsia, eclampsia, essential hypertension, chronic nephritis, and prolapse of the umbilical cord result in babies whose general condition and powers of resistance and recuperation are low. When these conditions need treatment by cesarean section fetal mortality is increased.

There has been a decline in the mortality rate of infants born both by cesarean section and by vaginal delivery. The great majority of fetal deaths are associated with prematurity. On the one hand cesarean section has reduced the number of babies damaged by traumatic vaginal procedures. On the other hand a number of babies are born alive who have congenital defects incompatible with continuing or reasonable existence.

Cesarean Hysterectomy

This is the performance of a cesarean section followed by removal of the uterus. Whenever possible total hysterectomy should be performed. However, since the subtotal operation is easier and can be done more quickly, it is the procedure of choice when there has been profuse hemorrhage and the patient is in shock, or when she is in poor condition for other reasons. In such cases the aim is to finish the operation as rapidly as possible

Indications

1. Hemorrhage from uterine atony after failure of conservative therapy.
2. Uncontrollable hemorrhage in certain cases of placenta previa and abruptio placentae.
3. Placenta accreta.
4. Gross multiple fibromyomas.
5. In certain cases of cancer of the cervix or ovary.
6. Rupture of the uterus, not repairable.
7. As a method of sterilization when continuation of menstruation is undesirable for medical reasons.
8. Severe chorioamnionitis. There is danger of the peritoneal cavity becoming infected both when the uterus is incised and from the seepage through the incision after it has been repaired. In such cases, and especially if future childbearing is not an issue, it may be safer to remove the infected uterus.
9. Defective uterine scar.
10. Extension of incision into the uterine vessels resulting in bleeding that cannot be stopped by ligature.

Complications

1. Morbidity rate of 20 percent.
2. Increased loss of blood.
3. The incidence of damage to the urinary tract and the intestines is higher than with cesarean section or hysterectomy alone.
4. Psychological trauma due to loss of the uterus.
5. Maternal mortality. If the conditions that create the need for cesarean hysterectomy are eliminated, the mortality is not higher than that from cesarean section or hysterectomy alone.
6. Postoperative hemorrhage. There is a significant danger of this complication occurring. About 1 percent of patients require reoperation in the immediate postoperative period for the control of intraperitoneal bleeding.

As a Method of Sterilizion

When used for sterilization this procedure has certain advantages over tubal ligation, including a lower rate of failure and the removal of an organ that may cause trouble later on. However, the complications are such that cesarean hysterectomy is not recommended as a routine procedure for sterilization.

THE OBESE PREGNANT PATIENT

Definition of Obesity

There is no clear and universally acceptable definition of obesity; the incidence is not established. A maternal weight of 90 kg (200 pounds) has been used frequently to designate the upper limit of normal. This does not take into consideration the woman's height, however.

Abnormalities of Labor

Obese mothers are usually older, more parous, and have an increased incidence of medical complications, such as hypertension and diabetes mellitus. If women with these problems are eliminated, there is no evidence that obesity per se is associated with a higher incidence of abnormalities of labor (uterine dysfunction, fetal malpositions). There is no increase in the use of oxytocin to augment labor.

Fetopelvic Disproportion

The incidence of primary cesarean section is no higher in obese women than in others. From this finding it can be inferred that obesity is not a cause of disproportion.

Fetal Growth and Neonatal Outcome

1. The mean birthweight of infants born to obese mothers is greater.
2. The incidence of macrosomia (over 4000 g) in obese women is twice that of nonobese women.
3. The incidence of low birthweight babies (under 2500 g) in obese women is reduced by half.
4. Preterm labor is less common.
5. Postterm pregnancy is more common.
6. Neonatal outcome is as good as in nonobese patients.

Cesarean Section in the Obese Woman

Major surgery of any type in the obese patient is associated with an increase of intra- and postoperative complications. In pregnancy there are special problems. There are no contraindications to cesarean section, however, and the procedure should be performed without delay if obstetric indications are present.

Care of the Skin
Preoperative care of the skin including cleansing and local therapy of intertrigo is important.

Prophylactic Antibiotics
The incidence of wound infection is high. Obesity increases the risk of serious maternal sepsis following cesarean section. Hence, prophylactic antibiotics should be prescribed for these patients.

Mini-dose Heparin
The incidence of thrombosis and embolism is higher in obese patients. Reasons for this include prolonged operative time and the postoperative period of immobilization. Low-dose heparin may reduce the danger of embolization, and is probably worth using in massively obese women who undergo cesarean section. Subcutaneous injection of 5000 units of heparin is given every 8 to 12 hours, beginning before the operation and is continued until the patient is fully ambulatory. This dose does not cause maternal bleeding and does not cross the placenta. Some anesthetists believe that epidural anesthesia is contraindicated when heparin is being administered.

Anesthesia
Because of the increased incidence of medical problems including chronic hypertension, preeclampsia, coronary artery disease, diabetes mellitus, and pulmonary insufficiency, anesthesia in the obese may be difficult. Consultation with the anesthetist should, when possible, be obtained well before the operation.

Respiratory Function
In obese women total respiratory compliance is reduced because of a heavy chest wall and increased abdominal pressure on the diaphragm. The amount of work needed to breathe is increased. The residual volume and functional residual capacity are lower.

Choice of Anesthesia

Emergency Cesarean Section. In this situation general anesthesia is best.

Nonemergency Cesarean Section.   Because of the reduction in respiratory function continuous epidural anesthesia does offer certain advantages, and is chosen by some anesthetists, even though placing the catheter may be difficult in obese women. Other anesthetists prefer general anesthesia.

Abdominal Wall Incisions

Pfannenstiel (Transverse) Incision

The transverse incision is demanded by patients because of the cosmetic result. It is performed after the panniculus has been retracted cephalad.

Advantages

1. Once the panniculus has been retracted, the amount of subcutaneous adipose tissue is less than in the nonobese
2. The closure is more secure because the abdominal muscles tend to pull the sides of the incision together.
3. Postoperative pain is less than with the vertical incision, and this facilitates early mobility and deep breathing.
4. As a rule, transverse incisions heal well.

Disadvantages

1. The area of the transverse incision is warm and moist, is difficult to clean, there is a high growth of bacteria, and intertrigo is common.
2. Delivery of a large baby may be difficult
3. The vertical incision can be enlarged to make more room; the transverse incision cannot.
4. Retraction of the panniculus may have an adverse effect on maternal cardiovasculatory functions. However, there is no clear evidence of this.
5. The transverse incision takes longer.

Vertical Incision

1. Low
2. High, periumbilical

These carry the same advantages and disadvantages, except that in the upper abdomen the layer of subcutaneous tissue that has to be cut is much less. The lower uterine segment can be reached with either incision.

Advantages. Speed: it takes less time to enter the abdominal cavity.

Disadvantages

1. There is an increased risk of dehiscence compared with the transverse incision.
2. There is more pain.
3. The patient is less mobile.

Closure of the Incision

Special attention is needed in the obese patient.

Transverse Incision. The standard layered closure is adequate.

Midline Vertical Incision. Some surgeons advocate a layered closure with the addition of through-and-through retention sutures.

Others prefer the use of internal retention sutures of the Smead-Jones variety (Fig. 2).

Drains. The placing of surgical drains at the time of closure is important in obese patients. This can be accomplished by a Hemovac drain placed through a small puncture wound lateral to the incision, and extending the suction catheter the entire length of the incision above the fascia. Another method is to lay a small Penrose drain in the subcutaneous layer, making it exit through one end of the incision, and removing it in 24 hours. This ensures that serum and liquified adipose tissue, good culture media, are removed from the wound.

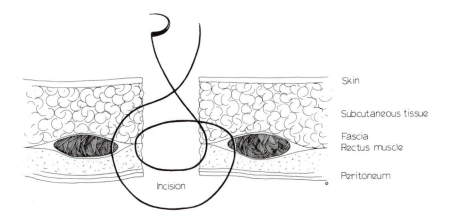

Figure 2. Smead-Jones closure.

Postoperative Complications

1. Longer postoperative recovery period.
2. Wound infection.
3. Wound dehiscence.
4. Atelectasis.
5. Pulmonary embolism.
6. Maternal morbidity and mortality are increased.

BIBLIOGRAPHY

Alinovi V, Herzberg FP, Yannopoulos D, et al: Cecal volvulus following cesarean section. Obstet Gynecol 55:131, 1980

Bryan B, Strickler RC: Inadvertent primary vaginal incision during cesarean section. Canad J Surg. 23:581, 1980

Buckspan MB, Simha S, Klotz PG: Vesicouterine fistula: A rare complication of cesarean section. 62:645, 1983

Chervenak FA, Shamsi HH: Is amniocentesis necessary before elective repeat cesarean section? Obstet Gynecol 60:305, 1982

Cunningham FG Leveno KJ De Palma RT, et al: Perioperative antimicrobials for cesarean delivery: Before or after cord clamping? Obstet Gynecol 62:151, 1983

DePace NL, Betesh JS, Kotler MN: 'Postmortem' cesarean section with recovery of both mother and offspring. J Am Med Assoc 248:971, 1982

Eisenkop SM, Richman R, Platt LD, et al: Urinary tract injury during cesarean section. Obstet Gynecol 60:591, 1982

Gross TL: Operative considerations in the obese pregnant patient. Clin Perinatol 10:411, 1983

Lavin JP, Stephens RJ, Miodovnik M: Vaginal delivery in patients with a prior cesarean section. Obstet Gynecol 59:135, 1982

Ledger WJ: Management of postpartum cesarean section morbidity. Clin Obstet Gynecol 23:621 1980

O'Driscoll K, Foley M: Correlation of decrease in perinatal mortality and increase in cesarean section rates. Obstet Gynecol 61:1, 1983

Park RC, Duff WP: Roll of cesarean hysterectomy in modern obstetric practice. Clin Obstet Gynecol 23:601, 1980

Perkins RP: Role of extraperitoneal cesarean section. Clin Obstet Gynecol 23:583, 1980

Rayburn, WF: Prophylactic antibiotics during cesarean section: An overview of prior clinical investigations. Clin Perinatol 10:461, 1983

Wallace RL, Eglinton GS, Yonekura ML, Wallace TM: Extraperitoneal cesarean section: A surgical form of infection prevention? Am J. Obstet Gynecol 148:172, 1984

47

Dystocia: Uterine Abnormalities

PROLAPSE OF THE UTERUS

Prolapse of the uterus during pregnancy is rare but troublesome. As a rule the uterus rises out of the pelvis by the end of the fourth month. Occasionally it fails to do so. In most cases it is only the cervix, with or without an associated hypertrophic elongation, that protrudes through the vagina. Occasionally the whole uterus is involved. No pregnancy has carried to term with the uterus completely out of the vagina.

Complications

Antepartum

1. Abortion and premature labor
2. Cervical edema, ulceration, and sepsis
3. Urinary retention and infection
4. Need for prolonged bed rest

Intrapartum

1. Cervical dilatation may begin outside the vagina, offering resistance to progress.
2. The edema and fibrosis may cause cervical dystocia.
3. Lacerations of the cervix are common.
4. Obstructive labor may lead to uterine rupture.
5. Fetal mortality is higher.

Postpartum
Puerperal infection is increased.

Treatment

Antepartum

1. Bed rest in Trendelenberg position to reduce edema and permit repositioning of the uterus
2. Local antiseptics to the cervix
3. Pessary to maintain the position of the uterus

During Labor

1. Most patients have a normal vaginal delivery, but arrest of progress may ensue.
2. If cervical dystocia develops, several procedures may be considered:
   a. Dührssen incisions of the cervix.
   b. Pitocin augmentation of labor.
   c. Cesarean section.

Postpartum

A pessary should be inserted to elevate the uterus and support the ligaments.

ANOMALIES OF THE UTERUS

Abnormal fusion of the Müllerian ducts or failure of absorption of the septum lead to a variety of congenital malformations of the uterus. The reported incidence is between 1:1200 and 1:600 fertile women. Most Müllerian anomalies are never detected because of the absence of clinical symptoms. Only about 25 percent of women with uterine anomalies have serious reproductive problems. Concurring renal abnormalities are common.

Fetal wastage occurs in all trimesters, including abortion, early or late, and preterm labor and delivery. Malpresentation, especially breech, is common. Women with uterine anomalies are in a high-risk group and have to be controlled carefully during pregnancy, labor, and delivery.

The theoretical reasons for reproductive failure include:

1. Poor vascularization of the endometrium
2. Distortion of the uterine cavity
3. Incompetent cervix
4. Luteal phase deficiency

5. Absence of binding sites for estrogen and progesterone in some areas of the malformed uterus

Diagnosis

During pregnancy a uterine anomaly may be suspected when the following conditions are present:

1. Notching and broadening of the uterine fundus
2. Abnormal lie
3. Recurring breech
4. Trapped or retained placenta
5. Prolonged third stage of labor
6. Habitual abortion
7. Axial deviation of the uterus
8. Flanking of the fetal limbs
9. Cervix located in the lateral fornix of the vagina
10. Presence of a vaginal septum

In any suspicious case hysterography should be performed postpartum.

Complications

1. Breech presentation.
2. Transverse lie; the fetus often assumes the hammock position with the head in one horn and the feet in the other.
3. Incoordinate uterine action is common and failure of progress is treated best by cesarean section.
4. Premature rupture of membranes.
5. Placenta previa.
6. Obstruction of descent of the fetus by the nonpregnant horn.
7. Obstruction by a thick vaginal septum.

Labor and Delivery

In many cases labor will progress without incident and terminate in a normal delivery. Therefore, a trial of labor is indicated. Failure of progress is treated by cesarean section. The incidence of the latter is higher than in normal patients.

Postpartum Complications

1. Retained placenta
2. Subinvolution of the placental site
3. Postpartum hemorrhage

Arcuate Uterus

The uterine fundus has a midline curved indentation that projects into the cavity of the uterus (Fig. 1). The external contours of the uterus are not affected and, seen through a laparoscope, the uterus appears normal. Hysteroscopy and hysterosalpingography help in establishing the diagnosis. It is rare for this abnormality to lead to fetal loss from either abortion or preterm delivery. Most pregnancies are normal and the diagnosis is not made.

Septate Uterus

The longitudinal septum may be complete (Fig. 3), extending down to the internal or external os of the cervix, or incomplete or partial (Fig. 2), when it extends part way from the uterine fundus. Fetal loss in the first half of pregnancy is common. In such cases the septum should be excised.

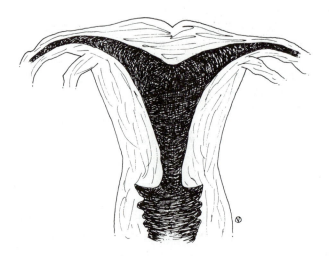

Figure 1. Arcuate uterus.

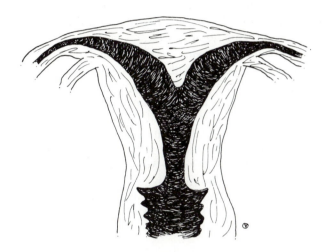

Figure 2. Septate uterus, partial.

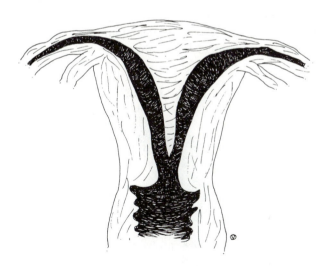

Figure 3. Septate uterus, complete.

Unicornuate Uterus

This is a uterus with a single horn (Fig. 4). A normal vagina and a single normal tube are present in most cases. The other half of the uterus is absent or rudimentary. In many patients the kidney is absent on the same side as the uterine abnormality.

In this condition there is an increased incidence of difficulty or inability to conceive, spontaneous abortion, preterm labor, abnormal presentation of the fetus, and intrauterine growth retardation. A possible explanation of the latter is that, with one uterine artery being absent, there is inadequate perfusion of the uterus and reduced fetal nutrition. On the other hand, there may be insufficient room in the uterus for normal growth. An incompetent cervix is often present.

If there is a rudimentary horn, transmigration of sperm or ova can occur with a resultant pregnancy. In such cases the rudimentary horn should be excised. If the patient is unable to conceive, removal of the contralateral ovary and rudimentary horn may be followed by a successful pregnancy.

Bicornuate Uterus

The division down the middle of the uterus is complete to the internal os (Figs. 5, 6). Diagnosis is made by palpation, postpartum exploration of the uterine cavity, during curettage, by hysteroscopy, hysterosalpingography, and laparoscopy. Abortion, incompetent cervix, premature rupture of membranes, preterm labor, abnormal presentation (especially

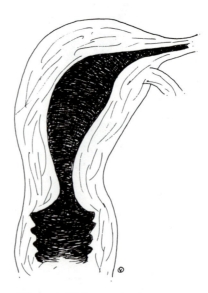

Figure 4. Unicornuate uterus.

breech and transverse lie), and cesarean section are all more common than when the uterus is normal. Fetal salvage is good in many cases. When fetal loss recurs, a unification operation should be performed.

Labor proceeds to vaginal delivery in many cases. Cesarean section is indicated only for obstetric reasons and not because of the anomaly per se. Dystocia may be caused by uterine inertia, obstruction by the nongravid horn, and hypertrophy of a septum. Occasionally the non-pregnant horn may rupture during labor.

Retained placenta occurs in some 20 percent of cases and may lead to postpartum hemorrhage.

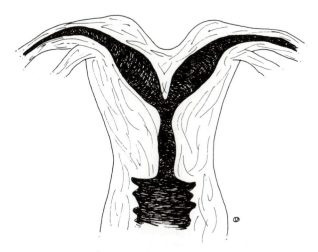

Figure 5. Bicornuate uterus.

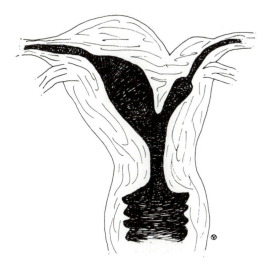

Figure 6. Bicornuate uterus with a rudimentary horn.

Double Uterus: Uterus Didelphys

The reported incidence of complete duplication of the female reproductive tract is between 1:1500 and 1:15,000 pregnant women (Fig. 7). The cervices are externally united and the uterine fundi are externally separate. In most cases there are two vaginas. The halves of the uterus are often of different sizes.

Ineffectual contractions, desultory labors, and slowly dilating cervices are common during the first stages of labor. Postpartum atony leading to hemorrhage is observed often. Sloughing of a decidual cast from the nonpregnant uterus can cause excessive bleeding. The cervix of the nongravid uterus may interfere with the descent and rotation of the fetal presenting part, and may so obstruct progress that cesarean section is necessary. Many women have normal vaginal deliveries, however. Preterm labor is common, but fetal survival is over 50 percent. Surgical unification is indicated only when fetal wastage occurs repeatedly.

TORSION OF PREGNANT UTERUS

Uterine torsion is defined as rotation of the uterus on its long axis of more than 45°. Torsion of the pregnant uterus is rare; only 129 cases have been described up to 1969. The condition was first reported in animals in 1662 and in the human 200 years later. The exact cause is not known, but some uterine malformation or tumor is present in many instances.

Most pregnant uteri show a slight degree of rotation, to the right in 80 percent and toward the left in 20 percent. In most abnormal situations the rotation has been 180°, although a case was reported of a 540° torsion associated with uterine necrosis.

In 20 percent of cases no causative factor is apparent. Predisposing conditions include:

1. Malpresentation, especially transverse lie
2. Uterine myomas
3. Anomalies of the uterus
4. Pelvic adhesions
5. Ovarian cyst
6. Uterine suspension
7. Abnormal pelvis
8. Placenta previa

Preoperative diagnosis is rare. The picture is one of an acute abdominal crisis, including pain, shock, bleeding, obstructed labor, and

symptoms referable to the intestinal and urinary tracts. The most serious complication is uterine rupture.

Acute torsion results in compromise of the uterine circulation. The
overall maternal mortality rate, around 13 percent, increases as term
is approached and is directly proportional to the degree of torsion. The
perinatal mortality rate of 30 percent also varies with the degree of rotation of the uterus.

Treatment at or near term is by cesarean section. Before viability
of the fetus has been reached laparotomy is performed, the uterus is
rotated to its normal position, and the pregnancy is allowed to continue
to term.

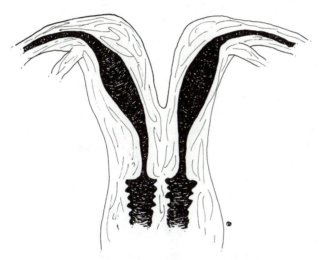

Figure 7. Double uterus: uterus didelphys.

SACCULATION OF THE UTERUS

Sacculation of the uterus (Fig. 8), a rare entity, defined as a diffuse ballooning of a portion of the wall, may be primary or secondary to incarceration of the retroverted uterus. In the primary variety, if the sac involves the lower part of the uterus, it will present as a pelvic mass. In sacculation of the retroverted uterus the saccule represents the stretched anterior wall, while the pelvic mass represents the uterine fundus. The saccule is a functional, transitory pouch, contains all layers of myometrium, and is present only during pregnancy. In half of the reported cases the placenta was located in the sacculation; in one-fourth, part of the fetus was in the pouch; and in the remainder the sacculation was empty. The sacculation may be in the anterior or the posterior wall of the uterus.

Etiology

The causation of sacculation is obscure. Hypothetical explanations include:

1. An embryologic abnormality of the uterus, the Müllerian ducts having failed to fuse completely.
2. A myometrial defect leading to attenuation of the muscle during gestation. The increased intrauterine pressure makes the thin area bulge out. Once the fetus is expelled the pouch collapses and disappears.

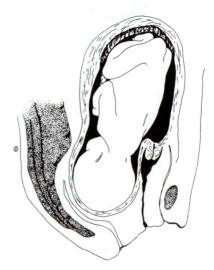

Figure 8. Sacculation of the uterus.

3. Faulty innervation of a segment of the uterus, resulting in a functional disturbance and a ballooning of the affected area.
4. Weakening of part of the uterine wall by trophoblastic digestion, placenta accreta, adenomyosis, curettage, or myomectomy.

Symptoms and Signs

1. There is abdominal pain.
2. The patient experiences a sensation of heaviness.
3. In anterior sacculation the presenting part is felt in front of and above the pubic symphysis.
4. The vagina is elongated and the cervix is high.
5. Dysuria, caused by an elongation of the urethra and compression of the neck of the bladder, is present.

Diagnosis

Diagnosis is difficult, having been achieved preoperatively in only 2 of 38 reported cases. In most situations the diagnosis is made at laparotomy performed during the first trimester for suspected ectopic pregnancy, and at cesarean section in treating dysfunctional labor. An x-ray of the abdomen may help. Amniography has been useful in establishing the true state of affairs. Postpartum hysterosalpingography may show a defect, but in most cases a normal picture is seen.

Retroverted Uterus

In most cases a pregnant retroverted uterus will correct its position and grow out of the pelvis; the pregnancy will proceed normally. If this does not happen one of three events may occur: (1) The uterus will contract and expel its contents. (2) The uterus continues to grow until, at 14 to 16 weeks' gestation, the retroverted gravid uterus becomes incarcerated in the pelvis. (3) In the rare case of incarceration a part of the uterine corpus remains imprisoned in the pelvis, while the anterior wall expands into the abdomen to accommodate the growing fetus. This sacculation was described by Oldham in 1860.

Examination will reveal a large, cystic, tender mass (the body of the uterus) which fills the posterior cul de sac and often bulges into the vagina. The cervix is displaced upward above the symphysis pubis and is hard to see or reach (Fig. 9).

The urethra is compressed and elongated. Frequency of urination is common. Occasionally there is retention of urine, causing overflow and infection. If retention is complete, catheterization must be performed or the bladder may rupture.

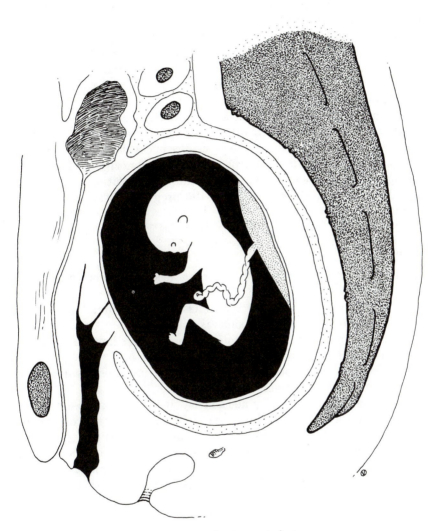

Figure 9. Incarcerated retroverted uterus.

Course of Labor

In primary sacculation the uterine fundus is in the correct position, polarity is maintained, and there is a chance for vaginal delivery. Rupture of the uterus is rare in progressing cases. In some situations, especially when the presenting part is in the sacculation, the cervix does not dilate but is displaced more and more upward as the sac is pushed down. In neglected cases prolonged labor may lead to fetal and even maternal death as a result of infection, necrosis of the sac, and rupture of the uterus. Retained placenta is common.

In sacculation secondary to retroversion the uterine forces are misdirected and the cervix fails to dilate even in the presence of strong contractions. Cesarean section is the procedure of choice. Once the baby is delivered the uterus corrects its position and no abnormality is evident. If diagnosed in the early part of pregnancy, the position of the retroverted uterus can be corrected and the pregnancy can proceed normally.

Management

1. During the first trimester nothing need be done since the pregnancy will go to term.
2. At term a trial of labor is permissible, as vaginal delivery may occur, especially if the pouch is empty.
3. At term, when labor is prolonged or progress has ceased, cesarean section is the treatment of choice.
4. Sacculation secondary to retroversion requires cesarean section. Vaginal delivery is impossible.
5. Cesarean section may not be easy. It is essential to determine the level reached by the cervix and to ascertain the exact height of the elongated vagina. The vagina may be so thin that it resembles peritoneum, and there is danger of making the incision into the vagina instead of the lower uterine segment. It may be wise to deliver the uterus from the abdomen before the incision into it is made.

BIBLIOGRAPHY

Andrews MC, Jones HW Jr: Impaired reproductive performance of the unicornuate uterus: Intrauterine growth retardation, infertility, and recurrent abortion in five cases. Am J Obstet Gynecol 144:173, 1982

Ansbacher R: Uterine anomalies and future pregnancies. Clin Perinatol 10:295, 1983

Heinonen PK, Saarikoski S, Pystynen P: Reproductive performance of women with uterine anomalies. Acta Obstet Gynecol Scand 61:157, 1982

Nielsen TF: Torsion of the pregnant uterus without symptoms. Am J Obstet Gynecol 141:838, 1981

Spearing GJ: Uterine sacculation. Obstet Gynecol 51:115, 1978

Visser AA, Giesteira MUK, Heyns A, Marais C: Torsion of the pregnant uterus. Case reports. Brit J Obstet Gynaecol 90:87, 1983

48

Embryotomy: Destructive Operations on the Fetus

INDICATIONS

The purpose of destructive operations on the unborn child is to reduce its size (head, shoulder girdle, or body) and so enable the vaginal delivery of a baby which is too large to pass intact through the birth canal. This procedure is tolerable only on a fetus that is dead or so deformed that survival is impossible. The risk of abdominal delivery to the mother has decreased to the point where embryotomy on the living normal child is never justified. Indeed the operation is so unpleasant and the dangers to the mother are such that destructive procedures are rarely performed today. After delivery the birth canal must be examined thoroughly to be certain that no injury has been caused by the instruments or the sharp edges of the skull bones.

CONTRAINDICATIONS

1. Living normal fetus
2. Markedly contracted pelvis
3. Cervix less than three-fourths dilated (full dilatation preferable)
4. Neoplasms obstructing the pelvis

DANGERS

1. Lacerations of the vagina, cervix, and uterus, as well as fistulas in the bladder or rectum
2. Uterine rupture, especially through the thinned-out lower segment, when labor has been obstructed

3. Hemorrhage from lacerations and uterine atony
4. Infection
5. Risks attendant on prolonged deep anesthesia

CLASSIFICATION OF DESTRUCTIVE OPERATIONS

Living Fetus

1. Needle drainage in hydrocephaly
2. Fracture of the clavicle or arm
   a. Shoulder dystocia
   b. Breech with nuchal arms

Dead Fetus

1. Craniotomy
   a. When delivery of the intact head is impossible
   b. Hydrocephaly
2. Decapitation
   a. Neglected transverse lie
   b. Interlocked twins
3. Cleidotomy
   a. Shoulder dystocia
   b. Breech with nuchal arms
4. Spondylectomy
   a. Breech with hydrocephaly
5. Evisceration or morcellation
   a. Hydrops fetalis with marked ascites
   b. Monsters

TYPES OF EMBRYOTOMY

CRANIOTOMY   Craniotomy is the opening of the skull. This can be done by perforating the head with Smellie scissors, evacuating the brain, and delivering the head by applying scalp traction with a tenaculum. Sometimes following craniotomy the head is crushed and extracted by special instruments (cranioclast, basiotribe).

The purpose of the operation is to reduce the bulk of the head. The only indication acceptable today is hydrocephalus. The excess cerebrospinal fluid can be removed, even in a live infant, by inserting a large-bore needle (16 to 18 gauge) through the scalp. The size of the head is reduced and its delivery made possible.

The most direct approach to encephalocentesis is vaginal. The needle is inserted through the cervical os and into the cranial cavity through a fontanelle or suture. The sagittal sinus should be avoided. If necessary, the needle can be pushed through one of the cranial bones. When the presentation is breech, drainage of the cerebrospinal fluid can be achieved by spondylectomy or, if the head is reachable, by direct entry into the ventricles beneath the occipital plate or behind the ear.

When the head cannot be reached through the vagina, an alternative route is the transabdominal one. The needle is passed through the abdominal and uterine walls, and through the fetal cranial bones into the interior of the skull.

SPONDYLECTOMY   Spondylectomy is the transection of the spine of the delivered thorax. In a breech presentation this may allow drainage of cerebrospinal fluid. It is done when the back is anterior and the head and neck are out of reach. In cases of hydrocephalus when there is communication between the ventricles and the spinal cord, the fluid may be drained from the brain in this way, thus obviating the need for craniotomy.

DECAPITATION   Severing the head from the body may be done for neglected transverse presentations when the child is dead and version and extraction or cesarean section are contraindicated. It may be done also when twins have become interlocked, chin to chin. A blunt hook is placed over the neck to steady the fetus, and decapitation is performed with scissors. The fingers of the other hand are used to protect the mother's soft tissues. After decapitation the body is extracted by pulling on an arm or a lower limb. The head is delivered either by forceps or by inserting a finger in the mouth and exerting traction on the jaw. This must be done slowly.

CLEIDOTOMY   Cleidotomy is indicated when there is shoulder dystocia and a dead fetus. One or both clavicles are cut with scissors. The shoulder girdle then collapses, and delivery is accomplished.

EVISCERATION   Evisceration is the removal of organs from the abdomen and thorax to reduce the body size of the fetus.

MORCELLATION   Cutting the fetus into pieces is necessary on rare occasions before vaginal delivery can be accomplished.

BIBLIOGRAPHY

Smale LE: Destructive operations on the fetus. Am J Obstet Gynecol 119:369, 1974

49

Medical Complications of Pregnancy: Intrapartum Management

Peter Garner

CARDIAC DISEASE

Intrapartum and Postpartum Circulatory Changes

Cardiac output increases by 40 percent during pregnancy, and the elevation continues to term. Contractions of the uterus during labor lead to a further increase in venous return to the heart and an associated rise in central venous pressure and arterial blood pressure. The cardiac output is lower in patients who are supine between contractions because obstruction of the inferior vena cava by the weight of the pregnant uterus diminishes venous return.

After delivery of the fetus and placenta, the tonic contraction of the uterus reduces its size and forces the blood from the myometrium into the maternal circulation, leading to a rise in the blood volume. This is increased further by reabsorption of fluid from the tissues. The rise in circulatory volume is associated with an increased cardiac output.

The acute and significant hemodynamic changes that occur during labor, delivery, and the immediately postpartum period may strain the heart to an extent that failure is precipitated in women with structural cardiac disease.

Timing of Delivery

Heart disease is not an indication for induction of labor, and timing of delivery is based solely on obstetric considerations. Vaginal delivery at term provides the optimal conditions for successful outcome in the pregnant cardiac patient. Induction of labor may be considered occasionally when precise timing is required to facilitate changing or discontinuation of drug therapy. A mother on long-term anticoagulant therapy is such an example.

Supervision During Labor

Intrapartum care of the patient who has a cardiac disorder of any degree must be meticulous. Pulse, respiratory rate, blood pressure, and systemic venous pressure should be assessed every 20 minutes during the first stage of labor, and every 10 minutes during the second stage.

Warning Signs

1. *Pulse:* Irregularity of the pulse or a steadily rising rate, especially if it is over 100 beats per minute.
2. *Blood pressure:* Diminution in pulse pressure reflecting a reduction in stroke volume, or an elevation in diastolic pressure as a consequence of generalized vasoconstriction.
3. *Lungs:* An increase in the rate of respiration and the presence of severe dyspnea are significant indications of trouble. The lungs should be auscultated frequently; the finding of basal pulmonary rales is an indication that cardiac failure may be developing.
4. *Systemic venous pressure:* This is elevated in heart failure and is recognized by observing the extent of the distention of the jugular vessels.

Seriously Ill Patients

In addition to the above, seriously ill women require continuous monitoring by electrocardiography and central venous pressure measurement.

1. *Electrocardiogram:* A continuous ECG provides an accurate and analyzable recording of the heart rate. Changes in the ECG may be difficult to interpret because circulatory alterations occurring during labor and delivery can result in the appearance of clinical and electrocardiographic changes that simulate organic cardiac disease. A midsystolic ejection murmur and S_3 heart sound are heard frequently during normal delivery. The electrocardiogram may demonstrate left axis deviation, a Q wave in lead 3, and transient changes in ST segment and T waves.
2. *Central venous pressure:* In normal term pregnancy the central venous pressure (CVP) ranges from 2.0 to 4.5 cm of water. This is

50 percent lower than in the nonpregnant state. During the first stage of labor the CVP increases slightly at the onset of each contraction. During the second stage the uterine contractions and the bearing down efforts of the patient lead to a marked increase of the CVP, peaking at delivery. An increase in the CVP usually indicates an elevated right ventricular diastolic pressure, suggesting the onset of right-sided congestive heart failure.

Ominous Signs in the Cardiac Patient During Labor

1. Right- or left-sided heart failure
2. Sudden onset of atrial fibrillation
3. Systemic embolism

All of these situations are associated with increased maternal mortality and fetal loss.

Medical Management During Labor

Maternal Position

Maternal position during labor is important. When the woman lies supine, the pressure of the pregnant uterus on the inferior vena cava leads to a reduction in the venous return to the heart. This may cause hypotension and reduced perfusion of the uterus. Pressure of the uterus on the inferior vena cava and fluctuations in maternal hemodynamics can be avoided by having the laboring patient lie on her side in a semirecumbent position.

Analgesia During Labor

Pain and anxiety increase the cardiac load, and must be controlled to avoid stressing an already taxed cardiovascular system. Systemic analgesics, such as Demerol, often combined with sedatives or tranquilizers, should be administered early to allay stress and apprehension.

Continuous lumbar epidural block is effective in relieving pain during labor and delivery. Maternal hemodynamic response to uterine contractions is not changed by epidural block, but maternal supine hypotension may occur as a consequence of vasodilatation of the lower limbs. Epidural block is contraindicated in patients receiving anticoagulants.

In patients with mild mitral stenosis and left-to-right shunts (acyanotic) epidural block is a safe method of controlling pain. Patients with moderate or severe mitral stenosis or right-to-left shunts (cyanotic) have difficulty increasing their cardiac output, and are at risk of developing severe hypotension during epidural block. This may lower placental blood flow and reduce fetal oxygenation. In this situation an analgesic, such as Demerol, with or without supplementation by a sedative or tranquilizer, is preferred.

Treatment of Cardiac Failure During Labor

Management of cardiac failure during labor is similar to that of the nonpregnant patient.

1. *Morphine:* Morphine is administered by the subcutaneous or intramuscular route in doses from 15 to 20 mg. This allays anxiety and reduces adrenergic vasoconstrictor stimuli to the arteriolar and venous beds.
2. *Diuretic:* Intravenous fursemide or ethacrynic acid (40 to 100 mg) will cause rapid diuresis and reduction of the blood volume.
3. *Digitalis:* A rapidly acting glycoside such as digoxin (0.5 to 0.75 mg) is given intravenously. Following this digitalizing dose, the usual daily oral maintenance dose is 0.25 to 0.5 mg. Digitalis glycosides improve myocardial contractility, slow the heart rate and atrioventricular conduction.
4. *Aminophylline:* Aminophylline (6 mg/kg of body weight) given intravenously reduces bronchoconstriction and augments myocardial contractility. If necessary, a further 3 mg/kg by intravenous injection may be repeated 30 minutes after the first dose.
5. *Vasodilators:* Vasodilator therapy using hydralazine (intravenously) or nitroglycerin (intravenous, sublingual, or as an ointment) may be considered. Vasodilator therapy is particularly useful in the treatment of acute pulmonary edema or refractory congestive heart failure because it reduces left ventricular afterload.
6. *Oxygen:* This is administered by face mask or by nasal prongs.
7. *Rotating tourniquets:* These are placed on the extremities to reduce the venous return to the heart.

Delivery

Most cardiac patients are at greatest risk at the time of delivery and in the immediate postpartum period. Increases in venous return, loss of blood, and pain occur simultaneously.

Route of Delivery

Unless there are serious obstetric reasons for performing cesarean section, vaginal delivery is best. Nonobstetric maternal factors should not change this approach. Hemodynamic changes associated with labor and vaginal delivery are less than with cesarean section, and morbidity and mortality rates are lower.

Method of Delivery
It is desirable to shorten the second stage of labor, as maternal bearing down markedly increases venous pressure. The ideal delivery is by simple low forceps under local or regional anesthesia. Shortening the length of the second stage should be elected only if it can be accomplished easily and safely. A difficult midforceps extraction may lead to trauma, hemorrhage, and shock, conditions which are tolerated poorly by pregnant patients with cardiac disease.

Third Stage of Labor
Following delivery, prompt removal of the placenta and bimanual compression of the uterus will minimize blood loss. Oxytocic drugs should be used with caution. Oxytocin may be given slowly by the controlled intravenous administration of a dilute solution. A 5 to 10 unit bolus of oxytocin may cause hypotension, tachycardia, and an increase in cardiac output, and should not be used. Patients at special risk for developing acute pulmonary edema may receive furosemide at the same time as the oxytocin. In general the risk of mild pulmonary edema, which can be treated, is less than the danger of uncontrolled postpartum hemorrhage. Ergonovine or methylergonovine produce elevation of central venous pressure and transient hypertension, and should be avoided.

Delivery of the Patient in Cardiac Failure
If cardiac failure occurs when the cervix is fully dilated and the fetal head is deep in the pelvis, prompt delivery with forceps should be carried out unless spontaneous birth will occur in a few minutes. A difficult delivery or cesarean section may precipitate cardiac failure rather than prevent it, and it is safer to obtain cardiac stability medically and then wait for labor to progress.

Anesthesia

Vaginal Delivery
In suitable patients lumbar epidural block is an excellent technique (described above in section on relief of pain during labor). In others delivery can be accomplished under pudendal block or local infiltration.

Cesarean Section
In patients with rheumatic or congenital heart disease, cesarean section is performed best under general anesthesia. Following thorough

preoxygenation, anesthesia is induced with a small dose of thiopentone or methohexital. Succinylcholine is used to facilitate endotracheal intubation. Nitrous oxide with 50 percent oxygen is then administered. It is a popular agent because it causes few changes in maternal hemodynamics. Transient rises in cardiac output, arterial blood pressure, and pulse rate are noted during intubation and extubation.

Special Considerations

Prevention of Endocarditis
Patients with heart disease risk developing bacterial endocarditis during labor and delivery. The pathogens most often involved have been commensals of the genital tract such as gram-negative organisms and anaerobic streptococci. Many antibiotics have been used alone or together to prevent the development of endocarditis. The combination of ampicillin 8 mg per kg of body weight and gentamycin 1 mg per kg given intravenously every 8 hours for three doses, starting with the onset of labor, provides a broad, effective, and safe bactericidal prophylaxis during parturition.

Cardiac Arrhythmias
Arrhythmias are encountered during labor. Many disturbances are minor and self-limiting. In patients with heart disease, however, they may result in pulmonary edema. Standard drug therapy can be used during labor for acute treatment of arrhythmias, including digoxin, quinidine, beta-adrenergic blocking agents, procainamide, lidocaine, and verapamil.

Thromboembolism
In view of the high incidence of thromboembolism in pregnant cardiac patients, the need for anticoagulation should be assessed. Anticoagulation is required in all individuals with mechanical valve prostheses, and those with valvular disease who have a history of systemic emboli. Warfarin derivatives cross the placenta and increase the dangers of abnormal fetal development and intracranial hemorrhage at delivery. Women on oral anticoagulants should be converted to heparin at 36 weeks' gestation in preparation for delivery. Bleeding should not be a problem at delivery when heparin is used, if meticulous hemostasis is effected during repair of lacerations and episiotomy. Hemorrhage does not occur from the placental site because this is controlled by contraction of the uterus rather than by blood clotting. Where possible heparin should be stopped a few hours prior to delivery (half-life 60 to 90 minutes) and restarted postpartum. Epidural anesthesia is contraindicated.

Elastic Stockings

Elastic support stockings for the legs are valuable during labor, delivery, and the puerperium, as venous pooling in the large dilated leg veins can reduce venous return significantly.

The Puerperium

In the immediate postpartum period, a large amount of extravascular fluid is returned to the circulation and cardiac output rises transiently. Careful monitoring of maternal vital signs should continue in the early puerperium, as pulmonary hypertension and edema may still occur. Hemodynamic changes accompanying parturition return to the normal nonpregnant level by 2 weeks postpartum. Postpartum hemorrhage, infection, and thrombophlebitis are all serious complications in the woman with cardiac disease. Because of this she should be observed carefully in hospital for a week following delivery.

Lactation

Breast feeding usually poses no problems to the cardiac patient. Most cardiac drugs, antibiotics, and anticoagulants appear in only trace amounts in breast milk. One exception is the anticoagulant phenindione which enters breast milk, but patients taking other anticoagulants such as warfarin and heparin may breast feed safely.

Effect of Cardiac Disease on Fetus and Newborn Infant

Fetal loss is higher in pregnancies complicated by cardiovascular disease than in normal pregnancies, but there has been a gradual decrease in perinatal mortality. Retarded fetal growth and preterm labor are found when cardiac disease is associated with maternal hypoxemia. Neonates born to women with congenital heart disease have a 2 to 4 percent risk of having a congenital cardiac abnormality.

HYPERTENSION IN PREGNANCY

Hypertension complicates approximately 10 percent of pregnancies and is, therefore, the most common medical problem requiring special attention in the intrapartum period. Although there is marked regional variation, approximately three-quarters of these patients have pregnancy-induced hypertension (preeclampsia) and the remaining one-quarter have chronic hypertension of various types. A classification of hypertension in pregnancy is useful in defining risks, and in planning for potential complications that may arise in the intrapartum period.

Classification

1. Pregnancy-induced hypertension
   a. Preeclampsia, mild or severe
   b. Eclampsia
2. Chronic hypertension (preceding pregnancy) of any etiology
3. Chronic hypertension with superimposed preeclampsia or eclampsia
4. Late or transient hypertension

Whatever the cause of the hypertension, the potential complicating factors include placental insufficiency, abruptio placentae, renal changes, and maternal convulsions. Intrapartum management is aimed at preventing these complications by optimal timing and control of delivery.

Diagnosis of Preeclampsia

The diagnosis of preeclampsia is based upon the development of hypertension after the 20th week of gestation. Only rarely will it occur at an earlier date. Proteinuria is a late event and the degree varies widely. Edema is often included in the "triad" of preeclampsia, but since it also occurs in many normal pregnancies it should be deemphasized.

Mild Preeclampsia: Intrapartum Management

Many patients who have mild preeclampsia can be treated on an outpatient basis. Admission to hospital for observation, assessment, and treatment is necessary when the following findings have been noted on at least two occasions 6 or more hours apart:

1. The diastolic blood pressure is above 90 mm Hg.
2. The diastolic blood pressure is 20 mm Hg above the reading in early pregnancy.
3. The mean arterial pressure (MAP) exceeds 105 mm Hg.

In most cases the rise in blood pressure signalling onset of preeclampsia will occur only after 37 weeks of gestation, so prolonged hospitalization is necessary rarely. Careful monitoring of both maternal and fetal progress is essential, as preeclampsia has a variable course. The hypertension of mild preeclampsia will often settle down on bed rest alone, without the need for antihypertensive or sedative therapy.

Monitoring of Maternal Condition

1. Frequent measurement of blood pressure.
2. Serial testing of renal function:

a. Serum uric acid. A level rising above 400 mmol/L (6.5 mg/100 ml) is a bad sign.
b. Creatinine.
c. Blood urea nitrogen.
d. Total urinary protein excretion, measured on a 24-hour specimen.

Termination of the Pregnancy

Preterm induction of labor is not necessary in a patient with resolving hypertension and an unfavorable cervix as long as the tests for fetal well-being are normal. It is preferable, however, that the pregnancy does not go past term.

Active Labor

When active labor commences frequent observation should be made of:

1. Blood pressure
2. Urinary output
3. Signs of central nervous system irritability such as headache, visual signs, and hyperreflexia

If the blood pressure rises during labor or signs of central nervous system irritability begin, then antihypertensive or sedative/anticonvulsive therapy is instituted (see severe preeclampsia).

Analgesia and Anesthesia

Lumbar epidural block provides:

1. Relief of pain and anxiety
2. A modest, but valuable, reduction in blood pressure

Severe Preeclampsia: Intrapartum Management

The goals of medical management of severe preeclampsia are to maintain the health of the mother and fetus until the definitive or final treatment, namely the delivery of the baby, can be carried out. The following are sought:

1. Prevention of convulsions
2. Stabilization of blood pressure
3. Maintenance of an adequate urinary output
4. Prevention of other sequelae, such as disseminated intravascular coagulation

Continuation Versus Termination of Pregnancy

When moderately severe preeclampsia occurs before the 30th week of pregnancy, it is occasionally possible, in selected cases, to carry the pregnancy from, for example, 28 weeks to delivery at 32 weeks. At this time there is a 95 percent chance of neonatal survival in a modern special care neonatal unit. Any deterioration in maternal status, however, signals the need for immediate delivery whatever the fetal maturity. Most patients with severe preeclampsia require initial stabilization and delivery within 24 hours.

Fetal Pulmonary Maturity

When a decision is made to terminate the pregnancy before the 34th week, the question arises as to the advisability of the administration of corticosteroids to accelerate fetal lung maturation. There is considerable controversy as to their use in severe preeclampsia. A delay in delivery of 48 hours in this situation increases the risk of intrauterine fetal death. It has been suggested that the stress of severe preeclampsia is sufficient to increase fetal corticosteroid secretion. The consensus of opinion is that corticosteroid administration is probably not indicated in severe preeclampsia.

General Measures During Labor

1. The patient is nursed in a quiet, darkened room.
2. The vital signs are evaluated and recorded on a flow sheet every 15 minutes.
3. The intake and output of fluid is measured every hour.
4. Continuous electronic fetal monitoring is instituted.
5. Initial laboratory investigations include:
   a. Complete blood count.
   b. Serum electrolytes.
   c. Serum creatinine.
   d. Serum uric acid.
   e. Blood urea nitrogen.
   f. Urine for protein and glucose.
6. In the most severe cases the following additional tests are carried out:
   a. Platelet count.
   b. Serum fibrinogen.
   c. Prothrombin and thrombin times.
   d. Liver function tests.
   e. Blood gases.
7. Intravenous fluid (0.9 normal saline or Ringer lactate) is administered, beginning at a rate of 75 ml per hour. The rate may be altered when the biochemical parameters are known.

Stabilization of Blood Pressure

Very high blood pressure must be controlled because it damages small arteries and arterioles, and can lead to retinal changes, renal impairment, disseminated intravascular coagulation, left ventricular failure, and even fatal cerebral hemorrhage. Blood pressure levels of 170/110 correspond to mean arterial pressure of 130 mm Hg and require urgent treatment. Preeclamptic hypertension is caused by arteriolar constriction. Hypotensive agents which act on arterial smooth muscle are the drugs of first choice. The aim of treatment is to achieve a diastolic blood pressure of 95 to 100 mg Hg.

1. *Hydralazine* may be given intramuscularly (10 to 20 mg) repeated as necessary, or intravenously by continuous infusion (40 mg in 500 cc normal saline titrated to keep the blood pressure at or below 150/100). The major side effects are headache, nausea, and reflex tachycardia. The latter symptom can be prevented by concurrent use of methyldopa or propranolol. Marked hypotension may result in some sensitive patients, and this can be avoided by using an initial testing dose of 5 mg. There is no evidence that the gradual lowering of the blood pressure is dangerous to the fetus because of reduction of placental perfusion, providing the fall is not extreme.

2. *Diazoxide* has been used effectively in the treatment of severe preeclampsia. The usual bolus dose of 300 mg IV may cause dangerous hypotension and fetal death. A titrated dose of a small 30 mg bolus every 60 seconds has been suggested. Intrapartum use of diazoxide should be reserved for patients who do not respond to hydralazine, and where dangers of severe hypertension pose a threat to maternal well-being. Side effects include hypotension, uterine relaxation, antidiuresis, and hyperglycemia.

3. *Methyldopa* is the most popular drug used in the treatment of essential hypertension in pregnancy. However, its use in the intrapartum treatment of preeclampsia is limited. In mild cases it can be given orally; a loading dose of 500 mg is followed by 250 to 500 mg every 6 hours. In severe preeclampsia the administration is by intravenous injection of 250 to 500 mg every 6 hours. The maximum antihypertensive effect takes place in 4 to 6 hours. Side effects include bradycardia, hypotension, and mental depression.

4. *Alpha- and beta-adrenergic blocking agents* have been introduced for the treatment of preeclampsia. Beta-blocking agents such as propranolol have been used mainly for the treatment of essential hypertension in pregnancy. Intrauterine growth retardation and neonatal hypoglycemia and bradycardia have been noted with their use. Maternal and fetal outcome is generally good if careful monitoring is carried out. A combination of hydralazine and propranolol has been used in the intrapartum management of preeclampsia. The combined alpha- and beta-

blocking agent labetalol reduces blood pressure without significantly altering heart rate or cardiac output. Initial studies indicate this is an effective drug suitable for management of preeclampsia. The dose is 200 to 400 mg b.i.d.

Anticonvulsant Treatment

The main aim of medical therapy is to prevent the progression of preeclampsia to eclampsia. Signs suggestive of central nervous system irritability such as hyperreflexia, headache, and visual changes should be treated vigorously by sedative or anticonvulsant therapy.

1. *Magnesium sulfate:* The agent of choice varies regionally, but most North American centers use magnesium sulphate. Magnesium depresses neuromuscular transmission by presynaptic inhibition. It has little effect on blood pressure and no sedative action. It should be given as a loading bolus of 4 g (IM or slowly IV) followed by intravenous infusion of 2 to 3 g per hour. The therapeutic range of magnesium is 2.0 to 2.8 mmol/L (5 to 7 mg/100 ml), and serial magnesium levels should be performed every 4 hours during infusion. Toxic side effects may be seen at 4 to 6 mmol/L (10 to 15 mg/100 ml), presenting as hyporeflexia, respiratory, and cardiac depression. Since magnesium sulphate is excreted entirely by the kidneys, it should be given cautiously if renal function is impaired. Calcium gluconate (5 to 10 ml of a 10 percent solution by slow IV injection) will rapidly reverse toxic side effects.

2. *Diazepam* is used widely as a sedative/anticonvulsant. It depresses the reticular-activating center and basal ganglion without depressing medullary centers. Large doses can adversely affect the neonate by causing respiratory depression, hypotonia, and impaired suckling reflex after birth. An initial bolus of 10 mg diazepam is given intravenously followed by an intravenous infusion of 40 mg diazepam in 500 ml of 5 percent dextrose solution. When other measures are not effective or in an emergency diazepam is a valuable drug in controlling convulsions.

3. *Diphenylhydantoin:* Dilantin may be used when seizures cannot be controlled by other measures. It is administered slowly in an intravenous dose of 150 to 250 mg.

Maintenance of Fluid and Acid-base Balance

The fluid balance in severely preeclamptic or eclamptic patients is maintained by replacing intravenously the urinary volume plus insensible loss. This requires urinary catheterization and accurate input-output charting. The fluid should be a crystalloid solution such as

Ringer lactate, normal saline, or normal saline in 5 percent dextrose in water (so-called 2/3 – 1/3). A moderate degree of oliguria is a frequent manifestation of severe preeclampsia, but reverses in the 24 hours following delivery. In the presence of severe oliguria (less than 25 ml per hour) central venous pressure monitoring (CVP) may assist in accurate correction of hypovolemia. Measurement of urinary electrolytes, creatinine, and osmolality will help in diagnosis of the type of oliguria. If the central venous pressure indicates that hypovolemia and prerenal oliguria exist, a fluid challenge with normal saline (500 cc over 15 to 30 minutes) should be considered. Furosemide (40 to 120 mg IV bolus) or mannitol (25 g IV over 10 to 15 minutes) are alternative measures. Acidemia may occur after eclamptic seizures as a result of impaired renal function or lactic acid accumulation.

Essential Hypertension: Intrapartum Management

Women with essential hypertension are at increased risk for the development of obstetric complications such as abruptio placentae and preeclampsia. Antihypertensive treatment has proven efficacy in preventing maternal complications of hypertension, and should be continued throughout pregnancy and delivery. Antihypertensive therapy, however, has not decreased the incidence of abruptio placentae and preeclampsia.

Continuation of Pregnancy
In women who have essential hypertension the pregnancy can be carried to term providing that:

1. Maternal hypertension is well controlled.
2. There is no superimposed preeclampsia.
3. The tests of fetal health in utero are normal.

Therapy
Methyldopa, hydralazine, and clonidine are all safe antihypertensives for use in pregnancy. Beta-adrenergic blockers such as propranolol and oxyprenolol are being used more widely in pregnancy, and are safe as long as careful fetal monitoring is used. Transient fetal bradycardia and hypoglycemia have been noted when beta-adrenergic blockers are used, and a neonatologist should attend the delivery. Antihypertensive drugs should be continued during labor, and the blood pressure and pulse rate should be monitored carefully. Oxytocin has little pressor activity and may be used during labor. Ergot preparations should be avoided.

DIABETES MELLITUS

Diabetes mellitus occurring in the pregnant patient may be associated with many fetal and maternal complications, but the main obstetric concern is the prevention of intrauterine death during the last month of pregnancy. The goal of management of the pregnant diabetic is to time the day of delivery so that fetal maturity is achieved while avoiding death in utero. With improved antenatal diabetic control and close obstetric monitoring, intrauterine death in the final weeks of pregnancy is now rare, but may still occur. The risk of the respiratory distress syndrome in the newborn after 38 weeks' gestation in the diabetic mother is extremely low. Carrying the pregnancy beyond the 38th week, therefore, adds few benefits, but still carries the risk of sudden fetal demise even in a "well-controlled" diabetic.

Timing of Delivery

The old dictum that insulin-dependent diabetes (type I) should be delivered at an arbitrarily selected point in gestation, has given way to individualized care. Special systems of classification of diabetes in pregnancy (White, Peterson) were introduced to help predict outcome of pregnancy. Although these classifications underline risk factors associated with diabetic pregnancy, tight diabetic control and meticulous maternal fetal monitoring now allow individual care and timing of delivery. The value of such classifications is, therefore, diminished.

Termination of Pregnancy at 38 Weeks or Later
This is considered when:

1. Good control of the diabetes mellitus has been maintained. The fasting blood sugar is less than 5.0 mmol/L (90 mg/100 ml), and the p.c. blood sugar is less than 7.5 mmol/L (140 mg/100 ml) measured by daily home capillary blood glucose monitoring. Hemoglobin A_{1c} measurement is a useful check for reliability of glucose control in pregnancy.
2. Antepartum testing of the fetus has been normal. Testing includes a nonstress test, the contraction stress test where indicated, and ultrasonic biophysical profile. Some centers continue to use daily measurement of maternal estriol as an adjunct to monitoring of the fetoplacental unit, but estriol levels should not be relied upon as a single determinant of fetal well-being.
3. Amniotic fluid. The lecithin:sphingomyelin ratio is 2:1 or more, and phosphatidylglycerol is present.

Termination of Pregnancy Before 38 Weeks
Indications for preterm delivery include:

1. Poorly controlled diabetes mellitus as indicated by home capillary blood glucose monitoring above the levels indicated above, HbA_{1c} levels above normal, fetal macrosomia, polyhydramnios, or diabetic ketoacidosis.
2. Abnormal antepartum testing of the fetus.
3. Associated risk factors such as diabetic nephropathy with hypertension, preeclampsia, pyelonephritis, advanced maternal age (greater than 35 years), intrauterine death in a previous pregnancy, and diabetic disease of the large blood vessels including calcification.
4. Deteriorating vision due to proliferative diabetic retinopathy in spite of laser treatment.

Mode of Delivery

Spontaneous Labor
Spontaneous labor and vaginal delivery take place occasionally.

Induction of Labor
Induction of labor is considered when the diabetes is well controlled and fetal testing is normal in the following situation:

1. The pelvis is adequate.
2. The fetus is not macrosomic. Fetal hyperinsulinemia, resulting from poorly controlled diabetes mellitus, leads to a tendency for such infants to be large. This causes difficulty during delivery, including problems of cephalopelvic disproportion, shoulder dystocia, and injury to the brachial plexus. The existence of obvious fetal macrosomia (weight estimated at greater than 4000 g) may necessitate cesarean section without trial of labor in order to avoid these complications.
3. The presentation is cephalic and the head is well engaged in the pelvis.
4. The cervix is ripe, soft, well effaced, admits a finger easily, and is dilatable. The use of intravaginal prostaglandin E_2 to induce ripening of the cervix has been successful in diabetic pregnancies. Repeated attempts at induction of labor in the presence of an unfavorable cervix are stressful for the fetus and should not be attempted.
5. Babies of diabetic mothers may be large but they often behave like premature infants, and do not tolerate long labor. If there is

lack of progress in labor after 8 hours of stimulation by oxytocin, cesarean section should be performed.

6. Continuous electronic fetal monitoring is essential during labor.

Cesarean Section

Elective. Maternal diabetes mellitus is not an indication for cesarean section per se, but 50 percent of insulin-dependent (type I) diabetics are delivered by this route. Cesarean section is preferred by many obstetricians for the following reasons:

1. Exact timing of delivery is arranged allowing the perinatal/ neonatal team to give optimal care.
2. Better control of blood glucose levels are possible over a shorter period of time.
3. A relatively atraumatic birth can be achieved.

Indicated. Indications for cesarean section include:

1. Arrest of progress with suspicion of disproportion due to a large fetus
2. Fetal distress before or during labor
3. Previous stillbirth
4. Poor diabetic control

Analgesia and Anesthesia

1. *Labor:* Continuous lumbar epidural block provides excellent relief of pain and is the method of choice. When this is unavailable small doses of narcotics may be used.
2. *Vaginal delivery:* Epidural anesthesia or pudendal block are effective.
3. *Cesarean section:* General anesthesia has the advantage that normal fetal acid-base balance can be achieved more easily. Regional anesthesia, however, has a low incidence of vomiting and an earlier return to oral food intake which is beneficial in the diabetic patient. Anesthetics that may increase endogenous catecholamine release, hyperglycemia or metabolic acidosis (chloroform, cyclopropane, methoxyflurane) should not be used.

Care of the Newborn Infant

Whatever the method of delivery:

1. A neonatologist must be present.
2. There must be a special care nursery to look after the newborn baby.

Management of Diabetes During Labor and Delivery

The assessment of pregnant diabetic patients in a Maternal/Fetal Day Care Unit provides optimal metabolic control and fetal assessment, and has allowed most diabetics to remain home until the day prior to delivery.

Induction of Labor

On the morning of planned induction of labor, food and subcutaneous insulin are withheld. Intravenous 5 percent dextrose in water is started at 100 to 150 ml/hr (5 to 7.5 g dextrose per hour) by infusion pump. Well-controlled gestational diabetics seldom require insulin supplementation during labor in spite of the additional stress during this period. Bedside capillary blood glucose estimations are performed every 2 to 3 hours, with optimal control of blood glucose being 4.5 to 5.5 mmol/L (80 to 100 mg %). Insulin-dependent diabetics (type I) usually require insulin supplementation during labor. This is preferably given by a continuous insulin infusion pump at a rate of 1 to 3 units of regular insulin per hour. The maintenance of euglycemia during labor helps prevent neonatal hypoglycemia.

Cesarean Section

The patient undergoing planned cesarean section has food withheld from midnight the preceding day, and arrangements are made for the cesarean section to be performed early in the morning. Blood glucose is estimated prior to the operation, and intravenous 5 percent dextrose in water started at 100 cc/hr. As insulin requirements fall immediately after delivery, care is taken not to cause postpartum hypoglycemia by administering too much insulin preoperatively. The dosage and type of insulin used preoperatively should be individualized but an approximate estimate is one-third of the term morning insulin dosage.

Postpartum Management of Diabetes

Vaginal Delivery

Following vaginal delivery the majority of gestational diabetics will require no further dietary or insulin control. Less than 5 percent of gestational diabetics continue to have carbohydrate intolerance after delivery. Insulin-dependent diabetics should be placed on their prepregnancy diet and insulin dosage unless breast feeding is planned. A fully established breast feeding infant obtains 600 calories per day from breast milk, and the maternal diet and insulin should be adjusted accordingly. Diabetes mellitus is not a contraindication to nursing but greater vigilance is required in terms of diabetic control.

Cesarean Section

The postcesarean section patient poses the greatest difficulty in diabetes control. She is not eating, is not active, and may be considering breast feeding. Intravenous 5 percent dextrose in water at 100 cc/hr should be continued until the patient is taking oral feeding. Bedside capillary blood glucose estimations should be performed every 6 hours and insulin given according to a blood glucose sliding scale.

Perinatal Morbidity

1. Congenital malformations are more common than in the general population, especially if euglycemia has not been maintained in the first trimester.
2. Hypoglycemia in the neonate results from hyperplasia of the fetal pancreatic beta cells which leads to hyperinsulinemia. Once again the incidence and degree of neonatal hypoglycemia is related to maternal blood glucose control during pregnancy and labor.
3. Hypocalcemia is a common finding.
4. Hyperbilirubinemia may occur.
5. Respiratory distress syndrome (RDS) is a major contributor to neonatal death in infants of diabetic mothers. Fetal hyperinsulinemia may retard lung surfactant synthesis. Even when gestational age and method of delivery are taken into consideration, infants of diabetic mothers are five times more likely to develop RDS.

DISSEMINATED INTRAVASCULAR COAGULOPATHY (DIC)

Intrapartum Etiologic Conditions

1. Intrauterine death with retained fetus
2. Severe preeclampsia
3. Premature separation of the placenta
4. Retained placenta
5. Amniotic fluid embolism
6. Hemorrhagic shock
7. Transfusion reaction

Clinical Features

1. Purpura and ecchymoses

2. Bleeding from venipuncture sites and skin sutures
3. Gastrointestinal and genitourinary bleeding

Laboratory Investigation

1. Delayed clotting of blood or lysis (whole blood clot in a plain glass tube).
2. Examination of peripheral blood smear for erythrocyte fragmentation and reduced numbers of platelets.
3. Progressive thrombocytopenia.
4. Decreasing plasma concentration of fibrinogen.
5. Presence of fibrinogen-fibrin degradation products (FDP-fdp). Occasionally low titers of FDP-fdp may be found during normal delivery.
6. Thrombin time, prothrombin time, and partial thromboplastin time may be abnormal in DIC, but in many cases these parameters are normal.

Intrapartum Management of DIC

1. Evacuation of uterine contents. The primary treatment of DIC in the intrapartum period is correction of the underlying disorder. Emptying of the uterus following premature separation of the placenta, intrauterine death, and retained placenta immediately reverses the coagulopathy. Immediate delivery in severe preeclampsia is usually sufficient to arrest DIC. Vaginal delivery is possible in the majority of instances, without the need for heparin or fibrinogen administration. In most cases the abnormalities of coagulation return to normal within 24 hours.
2. Blood transfusion. Hemorrhage and shock are treated vigorously with fluid and red blood cell replacement and appropriate supportive measures.
3. Fibrinogen. Rarely, it may be necessary to correct fibrinogen levels in women who require cesarean section. Fibrinogen levels of 1.0 to 1.5 g/L (100 to 150 mg/100 ml) will provide good hemostasis. Cryoprecipitate is the richest source of fibrinogen, but fresh frozen plasma can be used.
4. Heparin. The value of heparin in reversing intrapartum DIC is controversial. Its use in abruptio placentae, amniotic fluid embolus, and severe preeclampsia is not proven, and it should not be given in the presence of active bleeding.
5. Epsilon aminocaproic acid. This substance, a fibrinolysis inhibitor, should not be used in the intrapartum management of DIC as it may precipitate thrombotic episodes.

IMMUNE THROMBOCYTOPENIC PURPURA (ITP)

ITP is an autoimmune disease of unknown etiology in which the patient produces IgG antibodies against her own platelets. The immunoglobulin damages the platelets which are then sequestered and destroyed by the reticuloendothelial system, including the spleen. Clinically, however, there is usually no splenomegaly. Petechiae, particularly involving the mucous membranes, may appear and purpura is seen over the upper chest, neck, and limbs. More seriously, severe visceral or intracranial bleeding may occur. The platelet count is less than 100,000 per mm^3, but bleeding diatheses are not usually seen unless the count is less than 20,000 per mm^3. There is an increased percentage of large platelets. Bleeding time is prolonged and clot retraction is poor. Increased levels of platelet-associated IgG are usually found.

Effects on Pregnancy and the Fetus

The course of ITP is not affected by pregnancy, and the maternal risk is small. The disease, however, may affect the fetus adversely because maternal IgG antibodies cross the placenta and cause fetal thrombocytopenia. This is transient in the neonate lasting 1 to 12 weeks, but 35 to 70 percent of infants born to mothers with ITP are affected. If the infant survives delivery and the early neonatal period, the chance of full recovery is excellent.

The factors determining the development of fetal thrombocytopenia are not known, but there is little relationship between maternal and fetal platelet count. An association between neonatal platelet count and level of maternal platelet-associated IgG antibody has been suggested, but has not been proven.

Administration of corticosteroids to the mother antepartum does not reduce the incidence of thrombocytopenia in the fetus. This may reflect the low concentration of prednisolone in the cord blood of prednisone-treated mothers. Betamethasone or dexamethasone may be more effective. Supplementary intravenous corticosteroids should be given during delivery if the patient has received them during gestation.

Route of Delivery

The major danger to the fetus occurs during labor and delivery. Perinatal mortality is associated with intrauterine death from maternal hemorrhage, fetal intracerebral hemorrhage, and prematurity. In order to reduce the risk of intracranial hemorrhage at vaginal delivery, routine cesarean section has been proposed if the fetus is affected. Identification of the affected fetus, however, poses the greatest diagnostic dilemma. Fetal morbidity is high when maternal platelet counts are less than 100,000 per mm^3, but affected fetuses can be found in women with normal platelet counts, particularly when splenectomy has been performed. Fetal scalp sampling has been proposed to aid diagnosis of thrombocytopenia and to indicate the need for cesarean section. Scalp sampling is not possible in all cases as the cervix has to be partly open, which presupposes that some labor has taken place. If the fetal scalp sample platelet count is over 50,000 per mm^3, vaginal delivery is safe. Bleeding from the fetal scalp incision is minimal and is controlled by firm pressure. Because the identification of the unaffected fetus is so difficult and uncertain, many authorities feel that cesarean section is the method of delivery of choice.

Maternal Bleeding

Maternal hemorrhage can occur during the second stage from the episiotomy or lacerations, or from the incisions of cesarean section. Maternal bleeding is uncommon unless the platelet count is less than 20,000 per mm^3. The use of platelet transfusions is not recommended except in life-threatening situations, since the platelets are rapidly destroyed by the antiplatelet antibodies. Postpartum hemorrhage from the uterus is not a problem because bleeding is controlled by myometrial contractions and retraction. Splenectomy can be considered during cesarean section in selected patients.

VENOUS THROMBOEMBOLIC DISORDERS

Incidence

Pregnancy, delivery, and the puerperium are high-risk periods for the development of deep venous thrombosis and thromboembolic disorders. Study by fibrinogen leg scanning has shown that 3 percent of patients develop venous thrombi after normal delivery. Although the incidence of clinically diagnosed deep venous thrombosis is similar to the nonpregnant state in the weeks prior to delivery, there is a marked increase in the incidence postpartum (10 per 1000 deliveries). Predisposing factors include traumatic, complicated, or cesarean section deliveries. The incidence of nonfatal pulmonary embolization in the peripartum period ranges from 1 to 12 per 1000 deliveries.

Diagnosis

Diagnosis of deep venous thrombosis prior to delivery is achieved best by the use of impedance plethysmography and limited venography. The latter can be performed with minimal risk to the fetus if shielding by an abdominal lead apron is used. Doppler ultrasound examination is useful for proximal vein thrombosis, but is less reliable for calf vein thrombosis. ^{125}I-fibrinogen leg scanning should be avoided during pregnancy. Diagnosis of venous thromboembolism in the puerperium is assessed best by ascending venography. Doppler ultrasound, impedance plethysmography, and ^{125}I-fibrinogen leg scanning are useful adjuncts in selected patients. Fibrinogen leg scanning should not be used in nursing mothers.

Management

Patients who develop acute venous thromboembolism in the third trimester should be treated by continuous intravenous heparin for 10 to 14 days. The average pregnant patient requires a bolus dose of 70 units of heparin per kilogram body weight, with infusion of 300 to 400 units of heparin per kilogram body weight every 24 hours. Optimal anticoagulation corresponds to an activated partial thromboplastin time (APTT) of two-and-one-half times the pretreatment level, or a plasma heparin level of 0.2 to 0.4 units per ml. Following the course of full heparinization, subcutaneous heparin (10,000 units b.i.d.) is given. Heparin should be discontinued with the onset of labor, but restarted several hours after delivery. If the episode of venous thromboembolism started in the first or second trimester, heparin should be continued for 1 week following delivery or until full mobilization is achieved. If the episode occurred in the third trimester, subcutaneous heparin should be continued for a total of 3 months. Venous thromboembolism occurring in the postpartum period should be treated by full heparinization for 7 to 10 days followed by oral anticoagulants for a further period of 6 to 12 weeks.

ASTHMA

Asthma occurs in 1 percent of pregnant women. Pregnancy has no consistent effect on the course of asthma, but asthma may have a deleterious effect on both pregnancy and labor. Asthmatic mothers tend to have a higher incidence of hyperemesis, preeclampsia, antepartum hemorrhage, and induced labor than normal women. There is an increase in prematurity, low birthweight, perinatal mortality, and neonatal mortality. Outcome is worse in women with severe asthma.

Most medications used for treatment of asthma in the nonpregnant state can be used safely during pregnancy and labor.

Labor

Mild asthmatics should continue their oral medication or aerosol therapy during labor, and most can be controlled adequately in this way. Ventilation, however, rises sharply in the first stage of labor and peaks at delivery. Oxygen consumption increases more than twofold, and acute exacerbation of asthma may occur during this time.

Management of Acute Attack of Asthma

1. Oxygen. This is given by nasal prongs or 0.24 Venturi mask.
2. Bronchodilatation. This can be achieved by giving aminophylline orally or by infusion (0.9 mg/kg/hr after a loading dose of 5.6 mg/kg). Aminophylline toxicity has been noted in newborns whose mothers received intravenous aminophylline during labor, but the side effects were transient and this factor should be weighed against the severity of the asthmatic attack. Epinephrine (0.3 to 0.5 ml of a 1:1000 solution) is equally effective. Bronchodilators such as salbutamol, metaproterenol, and terbutaline inhibit uterine contractility when given intravenously and the use of these drugs is best avoided during labor. However, terbutaline (0.25 to 0.5 mg) can be given at the time of the initial exacerbation of the asthma without deleterious effect.
3. Corticosteroids. Intravenous or oral corticosteroids may be needed to control severe asthma not responsive to bronchodilator therapy. Beclomethasone aerosol is preferable in pregnancy to oral steroids. Asthmatic women who come to delivery while taking systemic steroids should be covered with parenteral steroids during labor. A good regimen for preparing the steroid-dependent asthmatic patient for labor and delivery is hydrocortisone 100 mg IM at the onset of labor, followed by hydrocortisone 100 mg IM every 8 hours for 24 hours.

Induction of Labor

1. Prostaglandins. The use of prostaglandins in induction of labor in the asthmatic patient is controversial. Significant airway constriction has occurred after $PGF_{2\alpha}$ (intraamniotic) and PGE_2 (intramuscular) administration. Bronchospasm following intravaginal administration has not been reported, but these agents should be used with caution in the asthmatic patient.
2. Oxytocin. This drug has no effect on bronchial smooth muscles, and may be used.

Analgesia

Care must be taken in the use of narcotic analgesics during labor in the asthmatic patient as they may depress respiration, dry secretions, and provoke bronchospasm.

Lactation

Breast feeding is safe in asthmatic patients as the drugs used in the treatment of asthma do not appear in significant concentrations in the breast milk.

BIBLIOGRAPHY

Carloss HW, McMillan R, Crosby WH: Management of pregnancy in women with immune thrombocytopenic purpura. J Am Med Ass 244:2756, 1980

Chesley LC: The control of hypertension in pregnancy. Obstet Gynecol Annual 10:69, 1981

Cines DB, Dusak B, Tomaski A, et al: Immune thrombocytopenic purpura and pregnancy. N Engl J Med 306:826, 1982

Cohen AW, Gabbe SG: Intrapartum management of the diabetic patient. Clin Perinatol 8:165, 1981

Gabbe SG, Quilligan EJ: General obstetric management of the diabetic pregnancy. Clin Obstet Gynecol 24:91, 1981

Hall JG, Paul RM, Wilson KM: Maternal and fetal sequelae of anticoagulation in pregnancy. Am J Med 68:122, 1980

Kelton JG: Management of the pregnant patient with idiopathic thrombocytopenic purpura. Ann Int Med 99:796, 1983

Moseley P, Kerstein MD: Pregnancy and thrombophlebitis. Surg Gynecol Obstet 150:593, 1980

Pritchard JA, Cuningham FG, Pritchard SA: The Parkland Memorial Hospital protocol for treatment of eclampsia. Am J Obstet Gynecol 148:951, 1984

Redman CWG: The use of antihypertensive drugs in hypertension in pregnancy. Clin Ob Gyn 4: 3, 1977

Rotmensch HH, Elkayam U, Frishman W: Antiarrhythmic drug therapy during pregnancy. Ann Int Med 98:487, 1983

Soler NG, Malins JM: Diabetic pregnancy: Management of diabetes on the day of delivery. Diabetologia 15:441, 1978

Turner ES, Greenberger PA, Patterson R: Management of the pregnant asthmatic patient. Am Int Med 6:905, 1980

Ueland K: Intrapartum management of the cardiac patient. Clin Perinatol 8:155, 1981

West TET, Lowy C: Control of blood glucose during labor in diabetic women with combined glucose and low-dose insulin infusion. Brit Med J 1:1252, 1977

50

The Puerperium

NORMAL CHANGES

The puerperium begins after the delivery of the placenta and lasts until the reproductive organs have returned to approximately their prepregnant condition. The length of the puerperium is about 6 to 8 weeks.

Uterus

Involution. After the delivery of the placenta and membranes, uterine contractions reduce the size of the uterus so that it can be felt as a hard globular mass lying just below the umbilicus. Myometrial contraction and retraction compress the blood vessels of the uterus, and so control bleeding until the vessels are thrombosed. Uterine involution is rapid, and the size of the uterus, 1000 to 1200 g immediately postpartum, falls to 500 g at the end of a week. By 2 weeks the uterus cannot be palpated by abdominal examination, and by 6 weeks the uterus lies within the pelvis, and is back to its nonpregnant weight of 50 to 70 g. This reduction is the result mainly of a decrease in the size of the myometrial cells rather than of their number.

Afterpains. Uterine contractions go on throughout the early puerperium, causing the so-called "afterpains." The pain may be sufficiently distressing to require analgesia. Afterpains are less severe or absent in primiparas. The puerperal uterine contractions are more intense during nursing, and involution of the uterus occurs more rapidly and more completely in the mother who breast feeds her baby.

Placental Site.   Involution of the placental site takes up to 6 weeks. Immediately after delivery the placental site is elevated, irregular, friable, and is composed of thrombosed vascular sinusoids. These undergo gradual hyalinization. Most of the decidua basalis is shed over a period of weeks and is replaced by regenerating endometrium. Failure of normal involution of the placental site may lead to late postpartum hemorrhage.

Lochia.   The superficial layer of decidua surrounding the placental site becomes necrotic, and is sloughed off during the first 5 to 6 days. This postpartum vaginal discharge, made up of a mixture of blood and necrotic decidua is called "lochia." It is red for 2 to 3 days (lochia rubra), becomes paler as the bleeding is reduced (lochia serosa), and by 7 days it is yellowish white (lochia alba). The flow of lochia lasts from 3 to 6 weeks.

Regeneration of Endometrium.   The deeper part of the decidua, that contains some endometrial glands, remains intact and is a source of a new lining of the uterine cavity. Restoration of the endometrium is rapid; by the seventh day it resembles the nonpregnant state, and is complete by 16 to 21 days.

Cervix

Immediately following delivery the cervix is floppy and ragged, with several small tears and bleeding points that are insignificant. The cervical os closes gradually. It admits two to three fingers for the first 4 to 6 days, and by the end of 10 to 14 days is dilated to barely more than 1 cm.

The glandular hypertrophy and hyperplasia of pregnancy regress gradually and this process is complete by about 6 weeks. The squamous epithelium that was lacerated during delivery heals and undergoes rapid reepithelialization, but not all cervices regain their prepregnant appearance. Persistence of glandular epithelium on the exocervix is described as a cervical erosion.

Vagina

Following delivery the vagina is a spacious, smooth-walled cavity with poor tone. Gradually the vascularity and edema decrease, and by 4 weeks the rugae reappear, but the latter are less prominent than in the nullipara. The vaginal epithelium appears atrophic for some time (longer in lactating women), but looks normal by 6 to 10 weeks.

Lacerations of the lower vagina and perineum heal gradually. Perineal care is a matter of hygiene. Showers and washing with soap and water are sufficient for most patients. Hot sitz baths reduce perineal tenderness and promote healing of episiotomy and lacerations. The suggestion has been put forward that ice baths, by causing vasocontraction, by reducing edema, inflammation, and bleeding, by decreasing the excitability of nerve endings, and by relieving muscular irritability and spasm relieve pain more effectively and for a longer period than hot baths. The drawback to this treatment is that the patient has to endure the sensation of cold, burning, and aching until the numbness and analgesia supervene.

Fallopian Tubes

The cells decrease in size and number. Two weeks after delivery the tubal epithelium is similar to that seen in the menopause, with atrophy and deciliation. After 6 to 8 weeks, the normal structure has been regained.

Ovary and Ovulation

The puerperal period is one of relative infertility, especially for the woman who is lactating. In nonlactating mothers the initial postpartum ovulation occurs on an average of 10 weeks, but it may take place earlier. In women who breast feed, ovulation is delayed, as long as 28 weeks in those who lactate for 6 months. Lactation reduces the incidence of pregnancy, but is unreliable as a method of contraception.

The occurrence of the first menstruation varies, but 70 percent of nonlactating women have menstruated by 12 weeks following delivery. The return of menstruation is more gradual in lactating women. By 36 weeks nearly 70 percent do menstruate. Menses within the first 6 weeks are rarely ovulatory.

Mammary Glands

In the early puerperium the breasts undergo marked changes. Between the second and fourth days the breasts become engorged, the vascularity is increased, and areolar pigmentation increases. There is enlargement of the lobules resulting from an increase in the number and size of the alveoli.

At this time lactation begins, controlled by various hormones, including estrogen, progesterone, prolactin, human placental lactogen, and insulin. The production of milk occurs spontaneously, but is enhanced by suckling. Once lactation is established, the most important stimulus for the continuation of the production of milk is suckling. A message is sent via the nervous system to the hypothalamus and there is an increase in the production and release of oxytocin. Oxytocin stimulates the myoepithelial cells of the alveoli of the breast to contract, causing milk to be transported to, and sometimes through, the nipple. This is the "let-down" reflex.

Some mothers are unable to breast feed their infants for a variety of reasons, including: (1) insufficient milk, (2) inverted nipples, (3) diseases of the breast, (4) the need to take drugs that are excreted in the milk and are harmful to the baby.

Mothers who decide to stop breast feeding have to do no more than discontinue suckling, wear a good support, and avoid stimulation of the nipples in any way. The release of oxytocin is inhibited, milk remains in and accumulates in the alveoli, and the back pressure causes production to be arrested. Drugs do not seem to be effective once lactation has been established.

In women who do not wish to breast feed, lactation can be suppressed in 60 to 70 percent by the use of a tight brassiere and the avoidance of stimulation of the nipple. The use of estrogen, or a combination of estrogen and androgen, can increase the rate of successful suppression by 10 to 20 percent, but they must be given immediately after the birth has taken place. The exact mode of action is not known. Unfortunately these hormones have some undesirable effects: (1) In a number of patients there is a rebound phenomenon. The patient feels fine in hospital, but after she goes home and the effect of the drug wears off, the breasts become engorged and painful. (2) In some women who take estrogen there is excessive bleeding. (3) There is some risk that estrogen may increase the incidence of thrombophlebitis. Bromocriptine, an inhibitor of prolactin, appears to be effective and may turn out to be the drug of choice for the suppression of lactation.

Cardiovascular System

The cardiac output increases during the first and second stages of labor, and rises even higher right after the birth. The reduction in the size of the uterus squeezes an additional amount of fluid into the circulation. After a short interval the cardiac output decreases to about 40 percent above the prelabor levels, and returns to normal by 2 to 3 weeks. The decrease of the heart rate is partly responsible for the reduced cardiac output. Alterations in the blood volume result from loss of blood at delivery, and from the mobilization and excretion of extravascular fluid.

Urinary Tract

The dilatation that takes place during pregnancy in the urinary collecting system does not return to normal for over 6 weeks. The combination of loss of tone, trauma to the bladder during delivery, and anesthesia, especially of the conduction variety, may lead to retention of urine, necessitating catheterization.

Gastrointestinal Tract

Return to normal of the mobility of the intestines, which is decreased during pregnancy, takes place gradually. The use of excessive analgesia may delay this process. Laxatives or an enema may be required to promote elimination.

PUERPERAL MORBIDITY

Puerperal infection is still a threat to the mother. The incidence in North America is around 5 percent. In the 1930s puerperal morbidity was defined as "a temperature of 38°C (100.4°F) or higher, the temperature to occur on any 2 of the first 10 days postpartum exclusive of the first 24 hours, and to be taken by mouth by a standard technique at least four times daily." This definition has lost some of its validity because women do not stay in hospital for 10 days any longer, and the use of antibiotics results often in a rapid fall in the temperature before the criteria can be fulfilled.

Factors that Increase the Risk for Puerperal Infection

1. During pregnancy
   a. Low socioeconomic status
   b. Inadequate nutrition
   c. Anemia
   d. Obesity
   e. Lack of prenatal care
   f. Coitus during late pregnancy
2. During labor
   a. Frequent vaginal examinations: over three
   b. Prolonged rupture of membranes
   c. Prolonged labor
   d. Chorioamnionitis
   e. Prolonged intrauterine fetal monitoring may be a factor
3. During delivery
   a. Cesarean section
   b. Operative vaginal delivery
   c. Devitalization of tissue from episiotomy and lacerations
   d. Hemorrhage

Cesarean Section
The rate of infection in women who undergo cesarean section is much higher than in those who deliver vaginally, and the infections are more severe. Infections are worse when the incision was classic, in the upper segment of the uterus. The rate of infection is higher in women who were in labor before the cesarean section than in those whose surgery was elective.

Prolonged Labor
It seems certain that prolonged labor is an etiologic factor in puerperal infection. It is not clear, however, whether prolonged rupture of membranes, frequent vaginal examinations, and internal fetal monitoring are etiologic factors per se, or play a role only in being part of prolonged labor.

Bacterial Flora

In women without signs of infection it is probable that the postpartum uterus is sterile. The vagina and cervix do contain large numbers of potentially pathogenic bacteria, and these organisms enter the uterine cavity. The longer the labor, the greater is the chance of infection. Numerous bacteria are involved in puerperal infection. The common ones include:

Aerobic Bacteria

Gram-positive Cocci

1. *Group B streptococcus*. This organism plays a significant part in puerperal infection. The onset of clinical symptoms occurs soon after delivery. The patient is ill, with a high fever, and a thin acrid discharge. This bacterium causes dangerous infection in the newborn. The response to penicillin is good.
2. *Group D streptococcus*. Included here are the enterococci. These infections respond to treatment with a combination of penicillin and an aminoglycoside, such as gentamycin.

Gram-negative Bacilli

1. *Escherichia coli*. This organism is a common cause of genital and urinary infection. About 80 percent of *E. coli* are sensitive to ampicillin. Most of the rest respond to aminoglycosides.
2. *Gardnerella vaginalis*. This bacterium is being recovered from an increasing number of cultures. It is sensitive to most antibiotics.

Anaerobic Bacteria

These are present in a large number of endometrial samples.

Gram-positive Cocci

1. *Peptostreptococci* and *peptococci* are prone to infect necrotic debris, and cause a foul-smelling discharge. They are sensitive to penicillin.

Gram-negative Bacilli

1. *Bacteroides* are implicated frequently in puerperal infection. These bacteria are associated with the following clinical situations:
   a. The infection is adjacent to a mucous membrane that contains anaerobes.
   b. There is devitalized tissue present.
   c. There is a foul-smelling odor.
   d. An abdominal abscess has developed.
   e. Thrombophlebitis or embolism complicate the picture.
   f. Gas has formed in the tissues.
   g. Conventional antibiotics have not cured the condition.
   The two more virulent organisms are *B. fragilis* and *B. bivus*. They are sensitive to clindamycin and metronidazole, and many to cefoxitin and doxycycline.

Gram-positive Bacilli

1. *Clostridium perfringens* is an occasional, but serious offender. Early cases respond to medical treatment. Signs of spread beyond the uterus (formation of gas, hemolysis, renal failure) call for surgical exploration and possible hysterectomy.

Perineal-vaginal Infections

These local disturbances are common, especially when small hematomas are present. The latter may result from incomplete hemostasis when an episiotomy or lacerations are repaired. The perineum is swollen, painful, red, and tender to touch. Frequently there is an indurated area that is especially tender.

The mainstay of treatment is the hot sitz bath, two or three times a day for 20 minutes. In almost all cases the sutures give way, drainage occurs, pain is relieved, and no further treatment is necessary. As long as there is no injury to the bowel, healing is universal and the patient may go home. It is in only the rare case that the sutures have to be removed and the area opened surgically (see Chapter 34).

Uterine Infections

Infections of the uterus run the gamut from the mildest and most superficial varieties of endometritis through myometritis, parametritis, pelvic abscess, and general peritonitis.

Superficial Endometritis, Deciduitis, Sapremia

These patients do not have a fever and are not ill. The only symptom is a
foul-smelling lochia. The old term for this condition is "sapremia." The
bits of necrotic tissue in the uterus are invaded by saprophytes, organisms that attack dead tissue, and putrefaction takes place, giving rise
to the bad smell. One of the worst odors is caused by the inadvertent
leaving of a sponge in the vagina, preventing adequate drainage. Treatment consists of promoting drainage by keeping the patient ambulant.
Occasionally an ergot preparation is used to increase uterine contractions and expel the retained dead tissue.

Endometritis

In this condition the infection has affected the true endometrium and
often has spread into the myometrium. The patient has a fever, complains of malaise, anorexia, and abdominal pain. In most cases the
uterus is tender to palpation. The fever ranges from 38°C (100.4°F) in
mild cases to 40°C (104°F) in severe infections, when chills may occur.

Cultures should be performed of swabs from the vagina, cervix,
and, if possible, the cavity of the uterus. The latter is difficult because of
contamination from the cervix. A specimen of urine must be cultured as
well to rule out infection of the urinary tract.

Treatment consists of bed rest, hydration, and antibiotics, chosen
on the basis of the culture. While waiting for the report of the culture, a
drug such as ampicillin is prescribed. Curettage is performed only if
retention of placenta is suspected.

Endoparametritis, Pelvic Cellulitis, Pelvic Peritonitis

The infection has progressed and spread into the broad ligaments.
There is inflammation and induration. Under treatment the condition
may resolve or it may progress to the formation of an abscess.

Treatment is by bed rest, hydration, and antibiotics. Abscesses
have to be drained by posterior colpotomy if there is a fluctuant mass
pressing against the vault of the vagina, or by laparotomy if the abscess
is out of reach by the vaginal route. In the most severe cases the uterus,
tubes, and ovaries have to be removed.

Generalized Peritonitis

The condition has spread to the general peritoneal cavity, either by
gradual progression or by the rupture of a pelvic abscess. These patients

are seriously ill, and the problem is complicated often by ileus, paralytic or mechanical, causing distention of the abdomen and vomiting.

Treatment is by bed rest, hydration by the intravenous route, appropriate antibodies, and nasogastric suction. If ileus does not resolve, surgery may be required to relieve the obstruction and effect drainage of the pus.

Diagnosis of Uterine Infection
This may be difficult in the early stages because so many postpartum patients have low-grade abdominal pain, and a 1-day fever. On the other hand a number of infected patients do not have a fever.

The presence of a low grade fever of 38 to 38.6°C (100.4 to 101.5°F) calls for physical examination of the patient, but antibiotic therapy should not be prescribed unless there are other signs of infection. Most of these will settle down within 24 hours.

In patients with high, persistent, or swinging temperatures a thorough general and pelvic examination is mandatory. The main sites of infection include the genital tract, the urinary tract, the lungs, the veins, and the breasts.

Laboratory tests include cultures of vagina, cervix, endometrial cavity, aerobic and anaerobic, and urine, complete blood count, and a chest x-ray. Blood cultures may be helpful.

Antibiotic Therapy
This is the mainstay of modern treatment. The results from the culture will indicate the bacteria that are present and the antibiotics to which they are sensitive. Because of the persistence of the high volume of intravascular fluid in the postpartum patient, high doses of antibiotics are needed to maintain adequate levels of the drug in the tissues.

While waiting for the culture to be completed empiric antibiotic therapy should be initiated. The regimen chosen is that which will be effective against most of the common aerobic and some, at least, of the anaerobic bacteria. Combinations include ampicillin, penicillin plus an aminoglycoside (gentamycin, tobramycin, or kanamycin), or penicillin and tetracycline, or a cephalosporin. If these prove to be ineffective within 48 hours the patient should be reexamined to look for other causes of infection, and the therapy reassessed on the basis of the cultures.

For patients who are seriously ill, and in whom an anaerobic infection appears to be present, drugs that are especially effective against anaerobes (clindamycin, chloramphenicol, or metronidazole) are administered plus an antibiotic that inhibits aerobic organisms; an aminoglycoside is preferred. Combinations used frequently are an aminoglycoside plus clindamycin or metronidazole.

Single antibiotic regimes that are effective against both aerobic and anaerobic bacteria include doxycycline, cefoxitin, and the newer penicillins (carbenicillin, ticarcillin, and piperacillin). The efficacy in comparison with the older combinations is not yet known, and their expense is still a consideration.

THROMBOEMBOLIC DISEASE

The etiologic factors associated with thrombophlebitis occurring in pregnancy include:

1. The sluggish flow in the dilated veins of the pelvis.
2. The trauma to the pelvic blood vessels by the fetal head.
3. The hypercoagulability that exists in pregnancy and the puerperium.
4. The effects of hormones, such as estrogen, given to suppress lactation may increase the levels of the clotting factors.
5. Uterine infection that has spread to the broad ligamants may affect the pelvic blood vessels.

The sites of the disease include the deep veins of the pelvis and lower limbs, and the superficial vessels of the leg and thigh.

The incidence of thrombophlebitis is less than 1 percent. The marked reduction of recent times has been ascribed to better health of pregnant women, early ambulation postpartum, and elimination of traumatic deliveries.

Superficial Thrombophlebitis

In most cases the saphenous vein is affected. The main symptom is pain. Examination reveals tenderness along the vein and, in most instances, hard segments of palpable thrombosis. It is unusual to find marked increases in fever and pulse rate. Once thrombosis of the deep veins has been ruled out, limited superficial thrombosis is treated by analgesia, hot packs, and support by elastic bandage or stocking. Embolism occurs rarely, if ever.

Deep Thrombophlebitis

When the veins of the leg are involved, symptoms include pain, worse on walking, fever, and, sometimes, malaise. The diagnosis is made by finding tenderness of the deep veins, increased heat of the affected leg, and evidence of venous obstruction as shown by the increased circumference of the leg. Confirmation can be attained by Doppler ultrasonography and, if necessary, by venography.

When the deep veins of the pelvis are affected, fever may be the only presenting symptom. Sometimes the first sign may be the occurrence of pulmonary embolism.

Treatment is by anticoagulation, preferably with heparin given subcutaneously or intravenously. The aim is to increase the clotting time of the blood by a factor of 2 or 3. The acute symptoms subside in 7 to 14 days, and the treatment can be changed to low-dose subcutaneous heparin or coumadin. The period of therapy is 6 weeks. During the acute phase bed rest, a cradle to protect the leg, and hot packs are important adjuncts to the treatment.

Pulmonary Embolism

Pulmonary embolism is often difficult to diagnose. The sudden onset of pain in the chest, cough, fever, tachycardia, and tachypnea, with or without hemoptysis are strongly suggestive signs. Scan of the lungs or pulmonary angiography help in making the diagnosis, but are not conclusive in all cases. This is a potentially lethal condition and anticoagulative therapy should be instituted immediately, even if the diagnosis is uncertain. Relief of symptoms is often rapid and dramatic.

Septic Thrombophlebitis

Septic thrombophlebitis is defined as clotting that occurs in the veins as a result of infection. Occasionally puerperal infection spreads into the walls of the engorged pelvic blood vessels causing inflammation and thrombosis. The most commonly involved bacteria are anaerobes, such as bacteroides, peptostreptococci, and peptococci.

The pathologic process is as follows:

1. The intimal lining of the affected veins is damaged by bacterial invasion.
2. The process extends along the intima itself or through the perivenous lymphatics.
3. The clotting process is initiated by the damaged intima.
4. The clot formed subsequently is invaded by microorganisms.
5. The suppurative process of liquification takes place, fragmentation of the clot occurs, and, finally, septic embolization follows.

The clinical diagnosis may not be evident immediately, and delays have occurred in patients who received inappropriate treatment for fever of unknown origin. In some cases there is an acute onset of severe lower abdominal pain, fever, and signs of an acute abdominal situation.

One must be certain that no acute surgical disorder exists, such as appendicitis, torsion of an adnexa, or abscess, in which case a delay in surgical therapy could be serious.

The diagnosis in the preembolic phase is difficult to make, and is often a matter of excluding other causes of fever. Fever, chills, tachycardia, and tachypnea are noted in many cases. Blood cultures drawn at the time of the spikes of fever are positive in half the cases. Often the exact diagnosis is made only when the abdomen is opened because a different condition is suspected, and the thrombosed pelvic veins are discovered. In this situation the veins (often the ovarian is involved) should be ligated to prevent embolism, anticoagulation instituted to arrest the thrombotic process, and antibiotics given to combat the infection.

In many instances septic thrombophlebitis is suspected only when treatment of a uterine or pelvic infection with appropriate antibiotics fails. These patients have fever, pelvic pain, and tachycardia, but local signs, such as evidence of an abscess, are absent. The administration of therapeutic doses of heparin results in a dramatic fall of the fever within 24 to 48 hours. Antibiotics should, of course, be continued. If the expected response takes place, heparin should be given for 10 days. If lysis of the fever does not take place in 48 to 72 hours, it is unlikely that thrombophlebitis is the cause of the symptoms, and search for other conditions, such as abscess, should be made. In rare occasions, when septic emboli occur, surgical exploration of the pelvis is necessary.

URINARY TRACT INFECTION

Infection of the urinary tract occurs against the background of the hypotonicity that develops during pregnancy, the trauma exerted on the bladder as the fetus passes through the pelvis, and the catheterization that is often necessary both during labor and in the postpartum period.

The offending organism is *E. coli* in close to 90 percent of cases. In women with persistent or repeated infections, bacteria such as Proteus, Pseudomonas, Enterobacter, and Klebsiella are often grown in culture of the urine. These latter are more resistent to therapy.

Cystitis

The most frequent variety of urinary tract infection is limited to the bladder. The presenting symptoms are frequency and dysuria. Rarely is there fever or malaise. The causative bacteria are, in most cases, sensitive to simple and relatively safe antibiotics such as oral sulfonamides, nitrofurantoin, trimethoprin-sulfamethoxazole, and ampicillin.

Treatment consists of culture of the urine, the forcing of fluids to flush out the urinary tract, and antibiotics. The length of the period of treatment has been set at 7 to 14 days, but recent evidence suggests that shorter courses of between 2 to 4 days are sufficient in many cases.

Pyelonephritis

In contrast to the women with cystitis, those who have pyelonephritis are sick. They have fever (40°C or 104°F), shaking chills with spikes of fever, pain in the back and flank, and tenderness in the costovertebral angle.

Although most of these infections respond to treatment with ampicillin—*E. Coli* is the most frequent organism—it is important to culture the urine to see what other bacteria might be present.

Treatment includes bed rest in the flat position to avoid kinking of the ureters, the administration of large amounts of fluid (intravenous infusion may be necessary as some patients cannot take much by mouth), and antibiotics–ampicillin is usually effective. In severe cases the antibiotic is given intravenously. Patients with pyelonephritis respond to therapy more slowly than those with only cystitis, and a longer course of treatment—often 6 weeks—may be necessary. Intravenous pyelography is considered 2 months postpartum to look for any residual structural damage.

INFECTION OF THE BREAST

Mastitis occurs almost entirely among women who are breast feeding at the time of the infection, or who did breast feed for a short interval. The common route of infection is via a fissure in the nipple. The source of the pathogen is usually from the infant. The occasional infection appears to be blood borne. In 95 percent of cases *Staphylococcus aureus* is involved.

Clinical Picture

Most infections are clinically evident during the second and third weeks postpartum, but they may occur earlier or later.

The symptoms include fever—as high as 39 (102) to 40.6°C (105°F), pain, chills, anorexia, headache, and malaise. The affected breast is erythematous, tender, and an indurated area may be palpated. Fissures in the nipple may be observed.

The further course of the disease is in one of two directions. The mastitis may resolve or it may progress to the formation of an abscess.

Treatment

Some cases of mastitis respond to therapy with ampicillin. However, because most strains of *S. aureus* produce penicillinase, which makes them resistant to penicillin, antibiotics such as cloxicillin, dicloxacillin and the cephalosporins, which are resistant to penicillinase, are preferred. Erythromycin and the aminoglycosides are also effective. If treated early, many cases of mastitis resolve.

If an abscess develops it must be incised and drained. It is important not to incise an area of mastitis prematurely, before the abscess has formed and fluctuation is evident.

Before an abscess has formed breast feeding can be continued from both breasts unless extensive fissures are present. Once an abscess has formed, breast feeding from the affected brest should cease, but the milk pumped from the breast to prevent stasis. After the abscess has been drained and has cleared up, breast feeding may be resumed.

LATE POSTPARTUM HEMORRHAGE

See Chapter 32.

BIBLIOGRAPHY

Cohen MB, Pernoll ML, Gevirtz CM, Kerstein MD: Septic thombophlebitis: An update. Obstet Gynecol 62:83, 1983

Droegemueller W: Cold sitz baths for relief of postpartum perineal pain. Clin Obstet Gynecol 23:1039, 1980

Eschenbach DA, Wager GP: Puerperal infections. Clin Obstet Gynecol 23:1003, 1980

Kochenour NK: Lactation suppression. Clin Obstet Gynecol 23:1045, 1980

Monheit AG, Cousins L, Resnik R: The puerperium: Anatomic and physiologic readjustments. Clin Obstet Gynecol 23:973, 1980

51

The Newborn Infant

Michael J. Hardie

ADAPTATION TO EXTRAUTERINE LIFE

Following delivery the newly born child must undergo those major physiologic changes by means of which he adapts to his new environment and his new way of life. The most vital of these are:

1. The establishment of regular breathing and exchange of gases
2. Alterations in the circulation

Respiration

In utero the fetal lung produces fluid which passes through the tracheobronchial tree until it reaches the oropharynx. There it is swallowed or mixes with the pool in the amniotic cavity. In animals, catecholamines secreted by the fetus during labor decrease lung fluid production. During vaginal delivery the thorax is compressed as it traverses the birth canal. This expresses some fluid from the upper airways. Most of what remains is absorbed by the pulmonary capillaries and lymphatics.

The mechanical expansion of the lungs at first breath and the rise in alveolar PO_2 lead to a rapid decrease in pulmonary vascular resistance and an increase in pulmonary blood flow. A number of factors are involved in the initial stimulus to respiration. Perhaps the most important is the fall in PO_2 and the rise in PCO_2 which follow the cessation of umbilical circulation. Tactile, thermal, and proprioceptive inputs also play significant roles.

Circulation

The changes in the circulation include:

1. Absolute and relative pressure changes
2. Closure of fetal channels

Changes in Pressure

Fetal circulation is characterized by relatively high right ventricular and pulmonary artery pressures. These are maintained by elevated pulmonary arteriolar resistance and by the presence of a large ductus arteriosus. The ductus equalizes pressures between the pulmonary artery and aorta and directs most of the right ventricular output into the systemic circulation. Systemic pressures are decreased by the presence of the umbilical circulation, which acts as a low pressure shunt.

As outlined above, with the first breath, there is a drop in pulmonary vascular resistance and consequently in right ventricular pressure. Clamping of the umbilical cord leads to a sudden rise in systemic vascular resistance. Left ventricular pressure is elevated above that of the right ventricle.

Closure of Fetal Vascular Channels

1. *Foramen ovale.* The increase in pulmonary venous return leads to a rise in left atrial pressure. This compresses the valve of the foramen ovale and produces functional closure of the interatrial septum. Anatomic closure takes place over a period of months or years.
2. *Ductus arteriosus.* The ductus arteriosus closes functionally over the first 24 to 72 hours of life. This process is related to the rise in arterial oxygen saturation, and is mediated by prostaglandins.

CARE OF THE INFANT IN THE DELIVERY ROOM

See Chapter 11.

PERINATAL ASPHYXIA

Asphyxia results from impairment of fetal blood supply and/or impairment of fetal gas exchange prior to or during delivery. In mild asphyxia apnea is the principal clinical manifestation. In severe cases the neonate is flaccid and pale with hypotension and bradycardia.

When fetal blood supply and oxygenation are adequate, energy requirements during labor and delivery are met by aerobic glycolysis. Uterine contractions reduce placental blood flow and compress the umbilical cord. There is a transient decrease in oxygen supply and build-up of carbon dioxide, for which the normal fetus can readily compensate.

If, however, the supply of blood or oxygen falls below a critical level, the production of energy changes to less efficient anaerobic glycolysis. During this process lactic and pyruvic acids accumulate with the development of increasingly severe metabolic acidosis. The causes of asphyxia may be divided into two large groups:

1. Central causes, which originate before or during delivery
    a. Perinatal anoxia
    b. Intracranial trauma or hemorrhage
    c. Narcosis due to maternal drugs or anesthetics
    d. Congenital anomalies of the central nervous system
2. Peripheral causes, mainly respiratory, where problems begin after delivery
    a. Respiratory distress syndrome
    b. Congenital pneumonia
    c. Aspiration of meconium or amniotic fluid
    d. Congenital anomalies, such as respiratory obstruction or pulmonary hypoplasia.

In the first group the infants are either born with apnea or breathing ceases after a few ineffectual gasps. In the second category, breathing begins fairly promptly but is, or soon becomes, labored or inadequate.

Prevention

The optimal management of asphyxia of the newborn is prevention. This demands recognition of factors during pregnancy, labor, and delivery which increase the risks to the fetus. These include:

During Pregnancy

1. Maternal causes
    a. Anemia
    b. Hemorrhage
    c. Cardiorespiratory disease
    d. Toxemia of pregnancy
    e. Advanced maternal age
    f. Grand multiparity
2. Placental causes

    a. Placental disease such as infection or infarction

    b. Hemorrhage caused by placenta previa, vasa previa, or abruptio placentae

3. Umbilical cord causes

    a. Prolapse

    b. Knots and entanglements

    c. Compression

4. Fetal causes

    a. Prematurity

    b. Intrauterine growth retardation

    c. Congenital anomalies

    d. Prolonged rupture of the membranes leading to amnionitis

    e. Anemia, as in Rhesus incompatibility

During Labor and Delivery

1. Interference with placental circulation by abnormally intense or lengthy uterine contractions
2. Maternal hypotension from compression of the inferior vena cava, or from spinal anesthesia
3. Prolonged labor
4. Difficult delivery, with or without forceps

Preventive Management

1. Trauma must be kept to the minimum. Prolonged labor and difficult vaginal operations should be avoided whenever possible.
2. Oxygen is given to the mother for at least 5 minutes before and during difficult deliveries.
3. Excessive narcosis and deep prolonged inhalation anesthesia should not be used. Local or conduction anesthesia is preferable. If inhalation anesthesia must be used, one is chosen that gives the mother and infant the highest oxygen saturation with the least physiologic alterations. Conduction anesthesia sometimes causes hypotension in the mother. Posturing the mother on her left side corrects this problem in most cases.
4. Careful monitoring is necessary so that fetal distress, discussed in Chapter 37, can be diagnosed and prompt treatment carried out both during the labor and after birth.

Apgar Score

Apgar elaborated a method of grading newborns: 0, 1, or 2 points are awarded for each of five signs, depending on their presence or absence (Table 1): The grading is done at 1 minute after birth and may be re-

TABLE 1. APGAR SCORING OF NEWBORNS

Sign	0 Points	1 Point	2 Points
Heart rate	Absent	Under 100	Over 100
Respiratory effort	Absent	Slow, irregular	Good, crying
Muscle tone	Limp	Flexion of extremities	Active motion
Reflex irritability: response to catheter in nostril	No response	Grimace	Cough or sneeze
Color	Blue-white	Body pink, extremities blue	Completely pink

peated at 5 minutes. Most children are normal and fall in the 7 to 10 point range. A score of 3 to 6 indicates mild to moderate depression. When the Apgar score is 0 to 2 the infant is severely depressed.

The Apgar scoring system has become established as the method by which the condition of babies is assessed immediately after birth. Recent investigations have shown that the Apgar score by itself is not a totally accurate index of the health of the neonate, and that the predictive value of the system is limited. Analyses of blood from the umbilical cords of infants from mothers in the high-risk category revealed that many acidotic babies were born in a vigorous condition, with high Apgar scores, and that numerous infants with low Apgar scores did not have acidosis at birth. The conclusion is that, while the scoring of the infant's condition by the Apgar criteria is important, other tests and examinations are necessary to obtain a complete picture.

Treatment of Asphyxia

The management of the depressed infant may be based conveniently on the Apgar score.

Mild to Moderate Depression: Apgar Score 3–6
These infants have normal heart rates, some muscular tone, and frequently make respiratory efforts.

1. The infant is placed so that head is dependent, dried, and warmed under a radiant heater.
2. Oropharyngeal suction is performed.
3. If meconium is present or there is concern regarding obstruction of the airway, laryngoscopy is carried out so that the larynx and trachea can be suctioned under direct vision.

4. Oxygen is given by mask.
5. Cutaneous stimulation is applied to the extremities.
6. If the mother has received a narcotic recently, an appropriate antagonist is given. Naloxone, available as Narcan Neonatal, is administered intravenously or intramuscularly in a dose of 0.01 mg per kilogram.
7. In the absence of improvement, the neck is extended moderately. A small airway may be inserted. The face mask is applied tightly around the mouth and nose. Bag and mask ventilation is instituted at a rate of 30 to 40 breaths per minute. Care must be taken to make certain that adequate expansion of the chest takes place.

Severe Depression: Apgar Score 0–2
Such an infant is bradycardic atonic, and pale. There is no respiratory activity other than an occasional gasp.

1. Laryngoscopy. No time should be wasted. Laryngoscopy is performed immediately, the airway cleared, and the trachea intubated.
2. Ventilation is begun with oxygen at a rate of 30 to 40 breaths per minute. The lungs should be auscultated to ensure that the endotracheal tube is properly positioned and that oxygen is reaching the lungs. Ventilation should produce a rise in arterial Po_2 and a drop in Pco_2, with a consequent rise in pH. In the presence of severe asphyxia, however, there may be persistence of the fetal circulatory pattern, with pulmonary vasoconstriction and shunting of pulmonary blood flow through the ductus arteriosus.
3. If the baby's respiratory center has been depressed by narcotics administered to the mother during labor, the drug of choice to reverse this effect is Narcan in the dose of 0.01 mg per kilogram preferably intravenously.
4. When there is inadequate response to ventilatory treatment, correction of the metabolic acidosis should be undertaken using sodium bicarbonate. The best route of administration is via the umbilical vein, which can be catheterized easily in most cases. An appropriate initial dose of sodium bicarbonate is 2 mEq per kilogram given over a period of several minutes. The solution should be diluted with equal parts of sterile water to lower the osmolality.
5. If the heart beat has been present at or just before birth but then the rate falls or ceases, external cardiac massage should be

started. The fingers of both hands support the back and pressure is applied with both thumbs on the sternum. The sternum is depressed 1 to 2 cm at a rate of 100 to 120 per minute. Epinephrine may be given as a 1 in 10,000 solution in the dose of 0.1 ml per kilogram. It is administered best through an umbilical venous catheter, or may be given directly into the endotracheal tube.

6. When the condition of the baby or the response to resuscitation seems inappropriate, he should be examined thoroughly to rule out a congenital abnormality such as diaphragmatic hernia or Potter syndrome. One should exclude also a complication such as obstruction of the endotracheal tube or pneumothorax.

Consequences of Perinatal Asphyxia

Severe perinatal asphyxia has profound effects on almost every organ system. Some of the more important of these are:

1. *Central nervous system:* Anoxic-ischemic encephalopathy may result in extensive neural damage or destruction. The neonatal period may be complicated by seizures, disturbances of tone and activity, and signs of damage to the brain stem, such as apnea and instability of temperature. The rate of mortality is significant, and morbidity occurs in the form of mental retardation and cerebral palsy.

2. *Respiratory system:* Asphyxia increases the incidence of respiratory distress syndrome probably because of damage to the surfactant producing type 2 alveolar cells. Pulmonary hemorrhage is another serious complication which may occur in the asphyxiated infant.

3. *Cardiovascular system:* Profound hypoxia can cause acute cardiac failure. In such cases the electrocardiogram will show changes consistent with myocardial ischemia.

4. *Urinary system:* The kidney is sensitive to ischemia. Anuria or oliguria result from acute tubular necrosis. Cortical necrosis may occur. In most cases the changes are reversible but occasionally chronic renal disease results.

BIRTH INJURY

Birth injuries are usually the result of traumatic vaginal deliveries. The frequency of birth injury has decreased significantly with the declining use of high and midforceps and vaginal breech deliveries.

Fracture of the Skull

Most skull fractures are the result of difficult forceps deliveries. The two common varieties are linear fractures, which usually require only observation, and depressed (ping-pong) fractures. Here the periosteum is intact but the bone is pushed inward. Some of these resolve without treatment. Negative pressure, applied with a vacuum extractor, may be used to elevate the depressed area. Occasionally neurosurgical intervention is needed.

The underlying brain may be damaged, and the presence of a fracture should alert the physician to the possibility of cerebral contusion or hemorrhage.

Intracranial Hemorrhage

Anatomy

The brain is enclosed in a tough membrane, the dura mater. The falx cerebri and the tentorium cerebelli are extensions of the dura inside the skull and act as scaffolding to support the brain. The falx occupies a vertical plane between the two cerebral hemispheres. The tentorium lies in a horizontal plane separating the cerebral hemispheres above from the cerebellum below. Venous sinuses are enclosed in the margins of the falx and tentorium.

Etiology

1. Prolonged labor, especially when obstructed
2. Cephalopelvic disproportion
3. Difficult forceps deliveries
4. Breech extraction
5. Delivery of preterm infants
6. Unattended deliveries
7. Precipitous births

Symptoms and Signs

Symptoms and signs may not appear for 24 to 48 hours or longer. They include:

1. A high pitched cry
2. Signs of increased intracranial pressure, i.e., bulging fontanelles, split sutures, increased circumference of the head
3. Irritability and convulsions
4. Focal cerebral signs, such as hemiparesis or deviation of the eyes.

5. Pressure on vital centers leads to apnea, bradycardia, disturbances of tone, and possibly death
6. Anemia
7. Otherwise unexplained findings, such as heart failure, hypoglycemia, or thrombocytopenia

Sites of Bleeding

1. *Subdural hematoma:* This type of hemorrhage is the result of difficult labor and delivery. Venous sinuses are torn and blood collects between the dura mater and pia-arachnoid. Prognosis depends on the site and size of the hematoma.
2. *Subarachnoid hemorrhage:* Primary subarachnoid hemorrhage may follow trauma or asphyxia. A typical clinical presentation is the development of seizures between the second and tenth days in a previously well infant. The prognosis is generally good.
3. *Intracerebellar hemorrhage:* This is a lesion seen mainly in the small preterm infant. Trauma is involved in some cases. It is associated frequently with intraventricular hemorrhage.
4. *Intraventricular hemorrhage:* Intraventricular hemorrhage is seen almost exclusively in preterm infants of less than 32 weeks' gestation. Routine ultrasonic screening has revealed frequencies of 30 to 50 percent in very low birthweight infants. Most frequently the bleeding originates in one of the vascular areas of the subependymal germinal matrix. Trauma is not a factor in intraventricular hemorrhage. Etiologic factors include asphyxia and sudden changes in cerebral blood pressure and blood flow.

   If the hemorrhage is massive, the infant will present with shock and collapse. Death may ensue within a few hours. A smaller or more gradual hemorrhage can be asymptomatic. A drop in hemoglobin may be noted. Blood drains from the lateral ventricles through the cerebrospinal fluid pathways into the subarachnoid space in the posterior fossa. Obstruction of cerebrospinal fluid flow at any level gives rise to secondary hydrocephalus.

Diagnosis of Intracranial Hemorrhage
Where the history and clinical findings raise the possibility of intracranial hemorrhage further investigations must be undertaken.

1. Lumbar puncture will produce blood-stained cerebrospinal fluid if there is a subarachnoid or intraventricular hemorrhage. In the cerebrospinal fluid the protein will be increased and the glucose reduced.

2. In the presence of subdural hemorrhage over the convexity of the hemispheres, a subdural tap is both diagnostic and therapeutic.
3. The diagnosis of intracranial hemorrhage was improved dramatically with the introduction of CT scanning, which allows accurate location of a hematoma and assessment of its extent.
4. Diagnostic ultrasonography has added a further dimension. Not only can a diagnosis be made with confidence, but it can be made in the nursery without moving the baby from his incubator.

Treatment of Intracranial Hemorrhage

1. The most important aspect of management is prevention, particularly the avoidance of traumatic delivery and perinatal asphyxia.
2. The infant's condition should be stabilized. A blood transfusion may be required. Adequate ventilation and oxygenation must be ensured. If seizures occur they are treated with anticonvulsants.
3. The baby should be transferred without delay to a center which has the necessary diagnostic facilities and a neurosurgical service.

Extracranial Hemorrhage

Two types of extracranial hemorrhage occur.

Subgaleal Hemorrhage

The galea aponeurotica is a tendinous layer which extends from the frontal to the occipital areas of the skull. Bleeding can occur into the loose connective tissue which separates this layer from the periosteum. Rarely the hemorrhage is massive, resulting in anemia or shock.

Cephalhematoma

This is the name given to a collection of blood between the periosteum of the skull and the bone it covers. Most commonly it is found in the parietal region and presents as a fluctuant swelling limited by the sutures. It is a common lesion, occurring in 1 to 2 percent of live births, and, while seen more often following traumatic and instrumental deliveries, it also occurs following uneventful spontaneous births.

It is reported that 10 percent of cephalhematomas are accompanied by underlying skull fractures. The blood loss is rarely large enough to cause any significant drop in hemoglobin but the resorption of the hematoma may contribute to a rise in bilirubin.

No treatment is indicated. The blood resorbs gradually in 6 to 12 weeks. Calcification may occur, especially around the edges of the hematoma.

Injury to the Spinal Cord

Injuries to the spinal cord are unusual. The most common sites of damage are the lower cervical and upper thoracic regions. Rarely is there an associated fracture or dislocation of the vertebral bodies, because the spinal column is much more elastic than the spinal cord.

Excessive longitudinal traction, especially when accompanied by flexion or torsion, is the most important etiologic factor. Vaginal breech delivery is involved in 75 percent of cases, especially when the head is hyperextended.

Clinical Outcome

Clinical outcome may be divided into 4 groups:.

1. Stillbirth or early neonatal death because of lower brain stem injury.
2. Respiratory failure leading to death or permanent ventilator dependence.
3. Long-term survival with paralysis or weakness of the limbs.
4. Survival with minimal neurologic damage. Most of these later develop spasticity and may be diagnosed erroneously as having cerebral palsy.

Management

There is no specific therapy. It is important to rule out other possible conditions which might lead to a similar picture, e.g., an occult dysrhaphic lesion or a neuromuscular disorder. There is little evidence that there is a place for neurosurgical intervention in spinal cord injury. Supportive care, including mechanical ventilation and physiotherapy, will minimize disability in less severely affected cases.

Injury to Peripheral Nerves

Brachial Plexus

Paralysis of the arm from injury during birth was described by Smellie in 1764 but it was Erb who, in 1872, localized the most common lesion to the fifth and sixth cervical roots which supply the upper trunk of the brachial plexus. The reported incidence of this injury is around 1:1000 births.

The neural lesion results from lateral traction on the shoulder or neck. It occurs during breech delivery when there is difficulty with the arms and in cephalic presentations with shoulder dystocia.
Two basic types are described:

1. *Erb palsy,* involving C-5 and C-6. The arm hangs limply by the side and is rotated internally. The elbow is extended but flexion

of the wrist and fingers is preserved, giving rise to the so-called "waiter's tip" position. The possibility of phrenic nerve injury (C-3, 4, and 5) should be considered and diaphragmatic paralysis excluded.

2. *Klumpke paralysis* involving C-8 and T-l. There is weakness of the wrist and finger flexors and of the small muscles of the hand. A true isolated Klumpke palsy is extremely rare. The term is sometimes loosely applied when there is a total brachial plexus palsy.

Management

There is no specific treatment. Early immobilization is followed by passive movements with a view to preventing contractures. The prognosis will depend on the severity of the lesion. Around 90 percent of those affected can be expected to have normal function by the age of 1 year. If the nerve roots are avulsed the damage will be permanent.

Facial Nerve

Injury to the seventh cranial (facial) nerve occurs, generally, distal to its emergence from the stylomastoid foramen of the skull. The result is weakness of the muscles on the affected side of the face. The characteristic signs are the failure of one side of the mouth to move and the eyelid to close. It has been believed that injury to the nerve takes place most commonly during forceps deliveries, the result of direct damage by the tips of the blades. One study, however, failed to show any increase in the incidence of facial nerve palsy following forceps delivery as compared with spontaneous birth. The site of injury appeared to be related rather to the fetal position in utero, leading to the suggestion that the lesion might result from pressure on the face from the sacral promontory.

Management

Treatment is limited to the protection of the eye when it is involved. Methylcellulose eye drops are applied, or the eye may be taped shut to avoid corneal injury.

The prognosis for affected infants is good. In most cases there is some return of function in 2 to 3 weeks and complete recovery by 2 to 3 months.

Other Injuries

Bony Injuries

1. *Fracture of the clavicle.* This is the most common bony injury and usually occurs in association with shoulder dystocia. Most fractures are of the greenstick type but complete fractures also oc-

cur. The diagnosis may be suspected by noting decreased or absent movements of the arm on the affected side. Tenderness, deformity, and crepitus may be elicited at the site of the injury. Usually no treatment is required other than care in handling the infant.

2. *Fractures of the humerus or femur.* These occur rarely, and result from traumatic delivery.

Sternomastoid Muscle

A firm painless swelling may be palpated in the midportion of the sternomastoid muscle at birth or within the first 1 to 2 weeks. It was postulated that this was fibrosis related to a hemorrhage into the muscle following birth trauma. Pathologic examination of such a tumor may show mature fibrous tissue, suggesting that the lesion originated earlier, that is during intrauterine life.

In the absence of treatment, shortening of the muscle can occur with the production of torticollis (wry neck) and eventual deformation of the skull. A regular program of passive stretching of the involved muscle should avoid this outcome and obviate the need for surgical intervention.

Abdominal Injury

Abdominal trauma is uncommon, but can have serious consequences. In infants presenting with shock, pallor, and abdominal distention, intraperitoneal bleeding must be considered. There may be bluish discoloration of the overlying skin. Paracentesis is diagnostic.

1. *Hepatic rupture.* The liver is the organ most often injured or lacerated. A subcapsular hematoma may develop, increasing in size until it ruptures into the peritoneal cavity. Infants are at increased risk if:
   a. They have hepatomegaly or coagulation disorder.
   b. They are asphyxiated at birth.
   c. They are preterm or postterm.
   d. They are delivered as breeches.
2. *Splenic Rupture.* This accident is less common than injury to the liver. Splenomegaly increases the danger of its occurrence, but in most cases the damaged organ is of normal size.

RESPIRATORY DISTRESS SYNDROME

Respiratory distress syndrome (RDS, hyaline membrane disease) is a disorder which is a consequence of an infant being born before the lungs are functionally mature. As such it affects mainly preterm infants.

In the mature lung, surface active phospholipids (collectively referred to as surfactant) are produced by alveolar type 2 cells. Surfactant molecules form a layer over the interior of the alveoli effectively reducing surface tension during expiration and preventing collapse.

The infant's first breath requires the production of negative pressure much greater than that needed for subsequent inspirations. The first expiration is accompanied by positive intrathoracic pressure, but some air remains trapped in the alveoli and so a functional residual capacity is built up over the first few breaths.

In the immature lung, where surfactant is deficient, progressive alveolar collapse will tend to occur with each expiration. It is almost as if the first inspiration is repeated with each breath. Worsening lung compliance increases the work of breathing. Areas of atelectatic alveoli cause intrapulmonary shunting. The result of these changes is increasing respiratory failure and hypoxia.

Recovery may occur in time as surfactant production increases or the baby may die of exhaustion or hypoxia. At autopsy the lungs are collapsed and airless. Histologically the bronchioles and alveoli are lined with hyaline membranes, composed of fibrin and cellular debris.

Clinical and Laboratory Findings

The baby, who is almost always preterm and who may require resuscitation at birth, shows evidence of respiratory difficulty immediately or within the first few hours of life. There is indrawing of the sternum and lower ribs on inspiration, flaring of the alae nasi, and an audible expiratory grunt. The baby is cyanotic in room air but his color improves with the administration of oxygen.

The condition may stabilize. More typically, however, there is deterioration over the first 24 to 48 hours. The baby's oxygen requirements increase. As he tires, he becomes increasingly hypercarbic and begins to have apneic spells. Hypoxia and acidosis may cause a reversion to the fetal circulatory pattern with pulmonary vasoconstriction, a rise in pulmonary artery pressure, and right-to-left shunting through the still patent ductus arteriosus.

Since the signs of respiratory distress are nonspecific, a chest x-ray is most important for diagnosis. This will show small, poorly aerated lungs with a granular appearance, the result of areas of microatelectasis. The airways stand out against the opaque lung fields as air bronchograms.

Treatment

Therapy is essentially supportive. Oxygen is given as necessary. A neutral thermal environment is provided to minimize oxygen consumption.

Hypotension or hypovolemia are treated by blood volume expansion with plasma or albumen. Anemia is corrected by transfusion with packed red blood cells. Blood gases, glucose, calcium, and electrolytes are monitored carefully.

In the presence of ongoing deterioration, continuous positive airway pressure may decrease atelectasis and improve oxygenation. If the response to this treatment is inadequate, mechanical ventilation is instituted.

Prevention

The maturity of the lung can be assessed in utero by the measurement of the lecithin/sphingomyelin (L/S) ratio in the amniotic fluid. Lecithin is the main surface active phospholipid present in the fetal lung. For most laboratories an L/S ratio of greater than 2:1 indicates the presence of functional maturity. Some centers have found the measurement of other components of surfactant, especially phosphatidylglycerol (PG), to be equally or more helpful than the L/S ratio itself.

When the maturity of the fetus is less than 32 weeks, the administration of betamethasone to the mother may accelerate lung maturation. Several centers are experimenting with the use of "surfactant replacement" by administering intratracheally to the newborn infant a variety of synthetic phospholipid preparations derived from animal pulmonary or human amniotic fluid.

MECONIUM ASPIRATION SYNDROME

Unlike the respiratory distress syndrome, which is a disease of the preterm infant, this condition is usually seen in term or postterm babies. Meconium staining of the amniotic fluid can probably be regarded as a physiologic finding which does not, in itself, indicate the presence of asphyxia. The great majority of infants who are born with meconium staining are well at birth and have no respiratory problems.

If asphyxia occurs prior to delivery, the fetus may be stimulated to make respiratory movements and thereby draw meconium into the upper airways. Following delivery further gasping will draw this material deep into the respiratory tract. Meconium causes chemical irritation and physical partial or complete obstruction of small airways.

Clinical and Laboratory Findings

The infant shows signs of respiratory distress, with grunting, indrawing, and cyanosis in room air. Severe hypoxia may result from the persistence of a fetal circulatory pattern. Chest x-ray shows the presence of areas of pulmonary collapse and hyperinflation. "Air-leak" with pneumothorax or pneumomediastinum is a common complication. The picture is frequently complicated by other signs of perinatal asphyxia such as seizures and anuria.

Prevention

The most important form of management is prevention. In the presence of meconium staining, the fetus should be carefully monitored to detect early evidence of distress. If fetal distress develops, delivery should be accomplished promptly, by cesarean section if necessary.

At the time of birth the upper airways must be suctioned carefully by the obstetrician, prior to delivery of the shoulders in a case of cephalic presentation. When delivery is complete, laryngoscopy should be carried out, and if there is evidence of meconium, thorough tracheo-bronchial aspiration should be undertaken.

Treatment
The treatment of established meconium aspiration syndrome is mainly supportive and follows the general principles described above for respiratory distress syndrome. If mechanical ventilation is required, minimal pressures should be used to reduce the risk of pneumothorax. Persistent fetal circulation may have to be treated with hyperventilation or drugs. Antibiotics should be started because of the risk of bacterial contamination of the aspirated material. There is also evidence that the presence of meconium facilitates bacterial growth.

CONGENITAL MALFORMATIONS

Of the many congenital malformations which occur, only a few examples which may complicate labor and delivery are described.

Neural Tube Defects

Failure of normal closure of the neural tube in early embryonic life gives rise to a spectrum of abnormalities of the central nervous system of which the most important are anencephaly and spina bifida.

Anencephaly
Anencephaly is the absence of the vault of the skull with complete or partial absence of the brain. What brain tissue there is is uncovered and unprotected. The diagnosis is frequently made incidentally by ultrasonography in early pregnancy. Anencephaly is the most common cause

of polyhydramnios and should be suspected in all cases of unexplained excess amniotic fluid. In later pregnancy the diagnosis may be suspected by inability to feel the fetal head and by hyperactive movements of the fetus following rectal or vaginal examination, due to stimulation of the exposed brain by the examining finger.

Most anencephalics deliver without difficulty. Since the head is small, it does not dilate the cervix well and traction may be necessary to pull the shoulders through. These infants do not survive.

Spina Bifida

Spina bifida cystica is a defect most commonly of the lumbar or lumbosacral spine in which there is an external saccular protrusion. When the sac is composed of meninges and spinal fluid but no neural elements, it is referred to as a meningocele. If spinal cord and nerves are included, it is called a myelomeningocele. The great majority of the latter are accompanied by hydrocephalus.

Diagnosis

Anencephaly is not a difficult diagnosis to make in utero by ultrasonography or x-ray.

Spina bifida may also be diagnosed in utero by ultrasonography. When there is a family history of spina bifida or hydrocephalus, the patient should be examined carefully to rule out a congenital anomaly.

Screening for an open lesion is possible by measurement of alphafetoprotein in the maternal blood or in amniotic fluid. About 5 percent of neural tube defects are closed and will go undetected by this test.

There is some preliminary evidence that recurrence rates of neural tube lesions may be reduced by supplementing the maternal diet with vitamins in early pregnancy.

Management of Neural Tube Defects

Anencephaly

Anencephaly is invariably lethal, and nothing can be done for the baby. If possible, the pregnancy should be terminated when the diagnosis is established.

Spina Bifida

The treatment of spina bifida involves surgical closure of the back lesion followed, where necessary, by relief of the hydrocephalus by a shunt inserted between a lateral ventricle and the peritoneal cavity. There is almost always some degree of neurologic impairment below the level of the lesion, involving the lower limbs and control of bowel and bladder.

Hydrocephalus

Hydrocephalus is the accumulation of cerebrospinal fluid in the ventricles of the brain. These become dilated. The amount of fluid varies between 500 and 1500 ml, although much larger quantities have been reported. The obstetric problem is one of gross disproportion between the head and the pelvis. Breech presentation occurs in some 30 percent of cases.

Diagnosis

Abdominal Examination. When the head is very large the abnormality is recognizable by palpation.

Vaginal Examination. During labor, when the head is presenting, the enlarged fontanelles, the widely separated sutures, and the cystic consistency of the head are noted. In breech presentation associated anomalies, such as spina bifida and talipes, may be clues.

Radiography. X-ray will confirm the diagnosis in most cases, but sometimes the divergence of the x-rays leads to misinterpretation.

Ultrasonography. A biparietal diameter over 11.0 cm is suggestive of hydrocephalus. Hydrocephalus may be present, however, when the biparietal diameter is smaller than the stated figure. More sensitive diagnostic findings are the size of the ventricles and the thickness of the cortical mantle of the brain. In addition, these parameters help in estimating the degree of damage to the brain and in deciding the type of therapy.

Management

Intrauterine Shunt
Ultrasound examination has enabled the diagnosis of hydrocephalus to be made in early pregnancy and also for the assessment of ventricular size in the fetus. This has led to attempts to treat the condition in utero by inserting a shunt between a lateral ventricle and the amniotic fluid. The results of these efforts have been disappointing to date.

Vaginal Delivery
Where the hydrocephalus is severe, the risk to the mother is of uterine rupture during obstructed labor. Because of the disproportion, the lower segment of the uterus becomes distended and thin, and rupture may take place spontaneously, or as the result of obstetric manipula-

tions. After labor is in progress and the cervix is dilated, fluid is evacuated through a large bore needle. This makes the head smaller and delivery ensues. In breech presentations, where the aftercoming head cannot be extracted, the obstetrician must resist the temptation to pull the head through by force, since this ruptures the lower uterine segment. The fluid should again be drained by perforating the skull.

Cesarean Section

Preterm. In selected cases of mild to moderate hydrocephalus, especially if the presence of other abnormalities can be excluded, there may be a place for early delivery by cesarean section, with a view to reducing brain damage.

Term. Occasionally cesarean section must be performed at term for the following reasons:

1. A maternal indication
2. A persistent transverse lie
3. Constriction ring dystocia
4. Failure of decompression
5. Nondescent of the fetal head
6. Uncertainty as to the diagnosis in the presence of a live child when labor does not progress

Potter Syndrome

The original description of Potter syndrome related renal agenesis to oligohydramnios, intrauterine growth retardation, pulmonary hypoplasia, abnormalities of the limbs, and a characteristic facial appearance. The renal abnormality appears to be primary and the lack of urine production results in oligohydramnios which causes compression of the fetus. The other features are thought to be results of this external pressure. The syndrome is lethal, with severe pulmonary hypoplasia leading to neonatal asphyxia and respiratory failure. Pneumothorax is a frequent complication of resuscitatory efforts in these infants.

A similar picture has been described in other urinary tract abnormalities that give rise to anuria or oliguria, such as lower urinary tract obstruction. Pulmonary hypoplasia can also result from other causes of oligohydramnios. Of particular concern is premature rupture of the membranes in midtrimester with continuation of the pregnancy.

The diagnosis can often be made or suspected by ultrasonic examination if there is poor fetal growth and severe oligohydramnios. A search for the kidneys and the bladder will usually confirm or exclude the diagnosis.

Amniotic Band Syndrome

The amniotic band syndrome represents the occurrence of a collection of fetal malformations, sometimes severe, associated with fibrous bands that entangle or entrap various fetal parts in utero, leading to deformation, malformation, or disruption. Oligohydramnios is seen.

The band may encircle or compress the umbilical cord, cutting off the flow of blood, and resulting in fetal death. Ring constrictions of fingers and toes are common, and in rare cases a limb may be amputated.

The reported incidence ranges from 1:10,000 to 1:5000 live births. There is no known rate of recurrence, no familial pattern, and no association with teratogenic agents.

The etiology is unclear.

PERINATAL MORTALITY

Perinatal mortality is the index most frequently used to assess the quality of reproductive care. It is defined as the sum of intrauterine deaths plus deaths in the first 7 days of life of infants weighing more than 500 g at birth, expressed per 1000 total births.

Etiology

Stillbirth

Deaths prior to or during delivery (stillbirths) are most commonly caused by anoxia. These may be associated with:

1. Placental insufficiency where the placenta is small or its function impaired by infarcts or disease. There is usually evidence of decreased fetal growth and these deaths may be avoidable by careful monitoring and early delivery when indicated.
2. Antepartum hemorrhage, especially abruptio placentae. This accident can occur as an unexpected emergency 1 to 2 months before term and may result in immediate fetal death caused by extensive placental separation.
3. Umbilical cord problems. Prolapse of the cord carries a high risk of fetal death. Knots or loops in the cord are considered causes of fetal death only when they are very tight and no other cause can be found.
4. Abnormalities of labor and delivery such as breech presentation and prolonged labor.
5. Maternal disease, especially diabetes. The risk of sudden unexpected fetal death has been much reduced by improved medical care of the pregnant diabetic.

Neonatal Death

Early neonatal deaths are most commonly related to:

1. Preterm delivery with its attendant complications, especially respiratory distress syndrome and intraventricular hemorrhage. Some infants, born at 25 weeks' gestation or less, though weighing over 500 g, show inadequate lung development to allow for gas exchange.
2. Congenital malformations. Abnormalities causing early death include extensive lesions of the central nervous system and severe forms of congenital heart disease, especially the hypoplastic left heart syndrome. Pulmonary hypoplasia, incompatible with life, accompanies Potter syndrome and many cases of diaphragmatic hernia.
3. Infection. Bacterial infections remain a serious problem in the neonatal period. The organism most frequently associated with overwhelming infection is the Lancefield group B, beta-hemolytic streptococcus. This organism is a common commensal of the female genital tract and the infant can become colonized at or prior to delivery. Pneumonia or generalized sepsis may result which, especially in the preterm infant, have a very high mortality rate.
4. Intrapartum asphyxia or trauma. Deaths from these causes have been reduced due to better fetal monitoring and the more judicious use of cesarean section. However, ill-advised forcep deliveries or unexpected complications continue to cause occasional neonatal deaths.

BIBLIOGRAPHY

Brans YW, Cassady G: Neonatal spinal cord injuries. Am J Obstet Gynecol 123:918,1975

Brown BJ, Gabert HA, Stenchever M: Respiratory distress syndrome, surfactant biochemistry, and acceleration of lung maturity: A review. Obstet Gynecol Surv 30:71, 1975

Faix RG, Donn SM: Immediate management of the traumatized infant. Clin Perinatol 10:487, 1983

Fiedler JM, Phelan JP: The amniotic band syndrome in monozygotic twins. Am J Obstet Gynecol 146:864, 1983

Frigoletto FD, Birnholz JG, Greene MF: Antenatal treatment of hydrocephalus by ventriculoamniotic shunting. JAMA 248:2496, 1982

Hardy AE: Birth injuries of the brachial plexus: Incidence and prognosis. J Bone Joint Surg 63:98, 1981

Illingworth RS: Why blame the obstetrician? A review. Brit Med J 24 Mar 1979:797

Johnson ML, Pretorius D, Clewell WH, et al: Fetal hydrocephalus: Diagnosis and management. Sem Perinatol 7:83, 1983

Koh KS, Paul RH: Preventing fetal distress. Contemp OB/GYN 15:27, 1980

Mayer PS, Wingate MB: Obstetric factors in cerebral palsy. Obstet Gynecol 51:399, 1978

Moessinger AC, Blanc WA, Byrne J, et al: Amniotic band syndrome associated with amniocentesis. Am J Obstet Gynecol 141:588, 1981

Ostheimer GW: Resuscitation of the newborn infant. Clin Perinatal 9:177, 1982

Seeds JW, Cephalo RC, Herbert WNP: Amniotic band syndrome. Am J Obstet Gynecol 144:243 1982

Sykes GS, Johnson P, Ashworth F, et al: Do Apgar scores indicate asphyxia? Lancet 1:494, 1982

Towbin A, Turner GL: Obstetric factors in fetal-neonatal visceral injury. Obstet Gynecol 52:113, 1978

Index